Gracey's Meat Hygiene

This book is dedicated to the memory of two great veterinarians

Dr Joseph Forde Gracey (1918–2001)
and
Dr James Andrew Storrar (1947–2006)

Gracey's Meat Hygiene

Eleventh Edition

Edited by

David S. Collins
MVB, DVPH(MH), MRCVS

Robert J. Huey
TD, MVB, DVPH(MH), MRCVS

WILEY Blackwell

Library of Congress Cataloging-in-Publication Data

Gracey's meat hygiene / edited by D.S. Collins, R.J. Huey. – Eleventh edition.

    p. ; cm.

    Meat hygiene

    Preceded by Meat hygiene / J.F. Gracey, D.S. Collins, R.J. Huey. 10th ed. c1999.

    Includes bibliographical references and index.

    ISBN 978-1-118-65002-8 (cloth)

I. Collins, D.S. (David S.), editor.   II. Huey, R.J. (Robert J.), editor.   III. Gracey, J.F. Meat hygiene.

Preceded by (work):   IV. Title: Meat hygiene.

    [DNLM: 1. Meat.   2. Food Inspection.   3. Food Safety.   4. Meat-Packing Industry.

5. Quality Control.   WA 707]

    RA602.M4

    363.19′29–dc23

2014016565

A catalogue record for this book is available from the British Library.

Contents

Contributors

David S Collins, MRCVS
Veterinarian, Belfast, UK

Robert J Huey
Chief Veterinary Officer
Department of Agriculture and Rural Development
Veterinary Service
Belfast, Northern Ireland, UK

Glenn Kennedy
Veterinary Sciences Division
Agi-Food and Biosciences Institute
Belfast, UK

Rosemary Lee
Department of Agriculture and Rural Development
Northern Ireland, UK

Chris Loughney
Country Manager UK-IE
Ecolab Food and Beverage Division
Northwich, Cheshire, UK

Malcolm J Taylor, BSc(Hons), MSc
Senior Scientific Officer
Food Science Branch
Agri-Food and Biosciences Institute
Belfast, UK

Preface

The aim of the book's authors is to maintain the standard of the previous edition and to produce a textbook which is of practical use to the veterinarian working in the slaughter and meat processing industry.

The world of meat hygiene has undergone a lot of changes since the publication of tenth edition in 1999. While we have introduced the concepts of 'system control' and integrated food safety management, we have kept this to a high level and attempted to keep clear of the legislation which is subject to frequent change.

We have chosen to remove much of the text in the previous edition on animal disease, which is covered more comprehensively in other texts. In chapters on microbiology and pathology, we have also provided details that the front-line veterinarian should know and again concentrated on principles rather than specific detail.

While building on the work of those who have contributed to the previous editions, we have introduced new authors and new chapters to the book to reflect current trends. Chris Loughney builds on the work of Stan Brown in updating the sanitation chapter, Malcolm Taylor assisted with the editing of the work of Bill Reilly and others on microbiology and Glenn Kennedy produced a completely new chapter, with a new approach on the complex area of residues of veterinary medicines and contaminants.

Reflecting the increasing importance and changes in the priorities of society, Rosemary Lee has produced a comprehensive chapter on health and safety for all staff working in the potentially hazardous environment of the meat slaughter establishment. Her practical and authoritative text is a must read for all with a responsibility for management of staff in this workplace.

D.S. Collins & R.J. Huey

Acknowledgements

This edition is dedicated to two public health veterinarians, Dr J.R. (Joe) Gracey and Dr J. Andrew Storrar.

Both these men were passionate about Veterinary Public Health and Animal Welfare.

Joe qualified in 1942 from the Royal (Dick) Veterinary College and after a period in John Boyd Dunlop's private practice, he of tyre fame, in Belfast, served in the Royal Army Corps in Burma during the Second World War reaching the rank of Major.

He obtained his PhD from Queen's University in 1959, having taken the subject of his thesis a survey of livestock diseases in over 600 farms and 18 abattoirs. The abattoir records which he produced were the precursor of the centralised meat inspection recording system which now prevails throughout Northern Ireland. The results were used at that time to identify means of increasing production and furthering animal welfare on farms long before the concept of integrated meat inspection systems had even been considered by other regions.

In 1961, he became Belfast City Veterinarian and was internationally known as an authority on meat hygiene, veterinary public health, animal husbandry, humane slaughter and for his involvement with Belfast Zoo.

He was appointed a fellow of the Royal Society of Health and a fellow of the Royal College of Veterinary Surgeons.

He was also responsible, with others, for the design of the Belfast Meat Plant at the Duncrue Complex which replaced the old victorian abattoir at Stewart Street, Belfast.

Joe was a team player and understood the necessity of bacteriologists, engineers, meat plant operators, farmers, transport and personnel administrators working together to achieve satisfactory outcomes in the running of a food processing business.

It is often said of Joe Gracey that he was a man ahead of his time, and even in semi-retirement, he was pursuing the possibility of better identification and recording of animal disease and production data with the use of the latest developments in computerised information technology.

Throughout his career, he had demonstrated unflagging zeal and infectious enthusiasm for the great benefit of those who had been privileged to work with him and of the veterinary profession as a whole.

Andrew qualified in 1978 from the University of British Columbia at Saskatchewan, Canada. He returned to the United Kingdom where he joined his father's practice in Chester. In doing so, he became the fifth generation to be a veterinarian, one of his sons continuing as the sixth-generation veterinarian.

Andrew became especially involved in meat hygiene when he was the Official Veterinarian for several meat slaughter and processing establishments, one of which carried out slaughter on many casualty animals. This provoked Andrew to explain the welfare applications of handling animals between farm and slaughter with particular interest in farm emergency slaughter. Andrew was the first president of Veterinary Public Health Association to serve for four terms and was for several years the Association's representative of the British Veterinary Association's Animal Welfare Foundation.

Like Dr Gracey, Dr Storrar was also a Major in the Royal Army Veterinary Corps. He served with the corps as a veterinary officer not only in support of the regulars but also in support of humanitarian and emergency relief operations with the UK Civil Affairs Group and within Medical Intelligence.

It had been Dr Storrar's intention to assist the book's authors with the text for the eleventh edition. He commenced this work during his illness which took him from us much too soon.

The authors also wish to thank the many colleagues throughout the 'meat hygiene' community who have assisted with the production of this eleventh edition.

In particular, the authors wish to acknowledge the help and cooperation they received from the many associations, firms and individuals of the previous editions of 'Meat Hygiene' who continued with their support in preparing this eleventh edition.

Members of the Agri-Food and Biosciences Institute, Northern Ireland, were very generous with their time in advising on pathology, bacteriology and animal production. The authors thank Tony Patterson, Helen Hartley, Ronald Annett, Alistair Carson, Francis Lively and Elizabeth Ball. Glenn Kennedy and Malcolm Taylor kindly contributed to sections on residue detection and microbiology respectively.

The staff of the Department of Agriculture and Rural Development for Northern Ireland (DARDNI) have assisted with the production of a number of chapters. Jean Wales, John O'Neill, Pat Treanor and David Cassells assisted with their knowledge of legislation and operational practice. Anne Lacey helped with the chapter on exotic meat production. The Department's senior Health and Safety advisor Rosemary Lee lent her significant expertise to the new 'Health and Safety' chapter.

Joe Lawson and Mark Elder of Moy Park Ltd., UK, shared their knowledge of poultry matters as did Roy Driessen, Marel Stork Poultry Processing and Margaret Hardy, St David's Poultry Team, Dungannon, UK.

Conor King, Managing Director of Enisca Ltd., an engineering company specialising in effluent and water treatment, lent his significant expertise to the chapter dealing with meat plant infrastructure.

Jim Ross, previously with Food Standards Agency, Northern Ireland, and now with the Food and Veterinary Office of the EU Commission, gave statistical advice.

As longstanding members, past presidents and long-term supporters of the UK Veterinary Public Health Association, the authors have profited from the accumulated knowledge of members and the excellent scientific meetings they organise. In particular, the authors would wish to mention Jason Aldiss, Jane Downes, Kenneth Clarke and Milorad Radakovic. In addition, advice on practical meat hygiene was offered by members of the Association of Meat Inspectors, particularly Peter Watson and Ian Robinson.

The development of digital photography has permitted additional illustration of this edition with again a significant contribution being made by staff from the DARDNI, namely Graham Fallows, John Hood, Harold Moore, Sarah Jackson, David Armstrong and Stephen Coogan. The authors are also grateful to all those who provided useful photographs which have not been included either due to space constraints or due to difficulty in making the illustrations relevant to the text.

Illustrations and advice have also been received from Karen von Hollenberg, Hal Thompson and Ron Siddle.

Finally, authors David and Robert both wish to thank their long-suffering families who had to withstand years of evenings, weekends and holidays in the company of 'the book'. In particular, Peter Huey, Robert's son, is acknowledged, who with his knowledge of IT helped to get this work over the line.

1

The food animals

HEALTH is a state of complete physical, mental and social well-being and not merely the absence of disease or infirmity.

World Health Organisation chronicle (1978)

Meat is normally regarded as the edible parts (muscle and offal) of the food animals which consume mainly grass and other arable crops, namely, cattle, sheep, goats, pigs, horses, deer, reindeer, buffalo, musk oxen, moose, caribou, yak, camel, alpaca, llama, guanaco, vicuna, etc. In addition, poultry have become a major meat-producing species, while rabbits, guinea pigs, capybara and various game animals and birds provide a substantial amount of protein, particularly in localised areas. Fish and other seafood have also been an important part of man's diet since earliest times.

Although, theoretically, hundreds of animals could supply meat for human consumption, in practice, only a relatively small number of species are used today. This is all the more remarkable since it represents in general the instruction of the Levitical law of the Old Testament, most of which is in accord with modern sanitary science. The animals suitable for the food of man had to part the hoof and chew the cud. Only those fish with fins and scales were wholesome. It is true that today we eat pig, rabbit and hare, but it is recognised that they are subject to parasitic infestation. There appears to be little doubt that the dangers of trichinosis and of Cysticercus cellulosae were recognised 1400 years before the birth of Christ. In many parts of the world, horseflesh forms an important article of human diet. The Danes reintroduced the consumption of horseflesh into Europe during the siege of Copenhagen in 1807; slaughter of horses for human consumption is now well established in Denmark, Belgium, Holland and Germany.

All the above animals, including fish, are converters, that is, they utilise green vegetable material with varying efficiency to produce protein. Even micro-organisms can be classified as converters in that they use carbohydrates from plants to make protein from simple nitrogenous compounds. Especially when an animal eats something which is inedible for man or could not easily be made into food for man, it is considered valuable as a source of food; so when pigs and poultry, and even other animal species, are used as scavengers to eat scraps, by-products, etc., they are very useful indeed. However, when food which could be utilised by human beings is fed to livestock, the question of efficiency becomes more problematic. Nevertheless, other factors, such as the production of manure for fertiliser usage, variety in the human diet, etc., have to be borne in mind.

Not only did the Creator command the earth to 'bring forth grass, the herb yielding seed and the fruit tree yielding fruit after his kind' (Genesis 1:11). He also 'made the beast of the earth after his kind, and cattle after their kind, and everything that creepeth upon the earth after his kind' (Genesis 1:25). For both plant and beast, 'God saw that it was good' (Genesis 1:12 & 25). They were both to be used as food for man.

In more recent times, efforts have been made to domesticate certain *wild animals*, although many of these have been used as food since ancient times. In Africa and Russia, elands are being domesticated, as well as antelope in the latter country. Kangaroos are being kept for meat in Australia, and in South America, the large rodent capybara, which is a semi-aquatic vegetarian, is being used as a source of meat, although it is not especially palatable. There are probably many other wild species which could be utilised in meat production and would have some advantages over the domesticated

Gracey's Meat Hygiene, Eleventh Edition. Edited by David S. Collins and Robert J. Huey.
© 2015 John Wiley & Sons, Ltd. Published 2015 by John Wiley & Sons, Ltd.

animals since they exist on less valuable land, need only rough grazing, are more disease resistant and act as a tourist attraction. Some problems, however, arise in connection with feeding, protection from predators, slaughter and meat inspection.

Recent innovations have included the breeding of wild boar in England and buffalo in Germany, France and Poland. Wild boars introduced from Germany and Denmark into England are used to produce purebreds as well as crosses with established breeds of pigs. Differences in quality and flavour are said to exist between the wild variety and the various crosses. Litter sizes average six piglets and only one litter is produced yearly. Slaughtered at 12–14 months, wild boar has a live weight of about 59 kg and a dead weight of around 45 kg. The meat is very lean with an acceptable flavour, but stress is sometimes associated with abattoir slaughter, which may necessitate on-farm handling. In Great Britain, the keeping of wild boar is subject to the Dangerous Wild Animals Act.

Buffalo meat is said to be more tender, leaner and gamier than beef, with lower levels of cholesterol. Although expensive in France, it is cheaper than beef in Canada. The name buffalo is often applied to the bison (*Bison bison*) of North America, a different species of the order Bovidae. There are several species; the Indian buffalo (*Bubalus bubalis*), sometimes called the water buffalo or arna, is the only one to be domesticated. It is found in many parts of the Old World, with significant numbers in Hungary, Italy and France.

The future for meat and meat products will depend mainly on consumer demand and the prices at which they can be profitably produced. As living standards rise, so also does the consumption of meat. Factors such as the cost of production, feed conversion efficiency, land use and availability, consumer taste, price to consumers, diet, attitudes of people to meat production methods, use of protein from non-animal sources, etc. will all play a part in determining future demands.

Procedures such as genetic engineering, embryo transfer, sexed semen, cross-breeding and twinning will continue to be utilised in attempts to produce more productive livestock with improved milk and meat quality. But if close attention is not paid to the vital importance of disease resistance, we may well see the development of stock susceptible to existing and novel conditions, some of which may have serious public health implications. Consumer attitudes must always be borne in mind by research workers and those engaged in the agriculture and food industries, which will only prosper in a climate of real consumer confidence in the quality and safety of food.

In order to address this point, much food from animals is produced under 'Farm Quality Assured Schemes'. These provide customers with some assurance that the animals have been reared in a manner which involves animal welfare and environmental issues and are fit to produce wholesome, safe food products. This complements the 'farm-to-fork' approach to meat production with control over all the nutritional, welfare, housing and other management factors, as well as ensuring the traceability of the food product. Veterinarians have a pivotal role in this discipline, both on the farm and at the meat plant.

Dietary factors

Concern about the amount of fat, especially saturated fat, in the diet, has been given prominence in the Western world due to the adverse effects on human health. According to the Living Costs and Food Survey (2011), the amount of dietary energy derived from fat was 38.1% for UK adults, with 14.2% of this energy being from saturated fats. While these values are lower than 20–30 years ago, the amount of fat in British diets is still higher than current recommendations. The Scientific Advisory Committee on Nutrition (SACN) states that the amount of dietary energy derived from saturated fat should not exceed 11%.

Steps have been taken to have legislation which require total fat and saturated fatty acid content labelling on a wide variety of foodstuffs. While much of the intake of fat is derived from milk and dairy products, meat and meat products, margarine, cooking fat and salad oils, some comes from vegetable sources, where it is either produced in a saturated form, for example, coconut oil, or converted into such during manufacture. An increase in dietary unsaturated fatty acids has been shown to reduce the risk of cardiovascular disease (CVD) and possibly some cancers, asthma and diabetes. It is possible to modify animal diets to increase the amount of unsaturated fatty acids in meat, milk and eggs and to decrease the n-6:n-3 fatty acid ratio (Woods and Fearon, 2009).

The sources of fat in the average British diet are given in Table 1.1.

If people respond to the SACN recommendations and there are indications that this is already the case, there will be major changes in food consumption which will inevitably have an impact on production methods in agriculture, especially in milk and livestock production, despite the fact that not all is known about the aetiology of the most common cause of death in most industrialised countries. In the United Kingdom, in 2006, 30% of all deaths in men and 22% of all deaths in women under 75 were ascribed to CVD. Factors such as heredity, blood pressure, obesity, blood haemostasis, physical inactivity, water hardness, smoking and alcohol consumption are also involved in the causation of this serious condition.

Table 1.1 Average British diet fat consumption (g/person/day) (FAOSTAT) 2009

Food group	Consumption (g/person/day)
Milk and dairy products (excluding butter)	21
Meat	36.5
Fish	1.5
Eggs	2.8
Total fats (including butter and vegetable oils)	60.3
Fruit	0.7
Vegetables	0.5
Cereals	4

Source: Reproduced with permission from FAO (2011). © FAO.

Consumer demand is now for leaner meat in smaller, waste-free cuts, which is easy and quick to prepare. On the livestock breeding and rearing side, changes have taken place with emphasis on animals which produce leaner carcases. Appropriate grading and certification standards are applied in meat plants. Quite apart from the health aspect, overfat stock are too costly to produce, and farmers will have to realise that energetic competition will have to be faced from vegetarians (sincere and insincere), 'animal welfarists' and a wide range of branded convenience and 'health foods', many not based on a meat content.

In the United Kingdom, the annual consumption of meat and meat products, which represent about 26% of the total household expenditure on food, amounted to approximately £16 037 million in 2011.

It is estimated that only 60% of the world's population eats 18 kg or more of meat per year, which is regarded as the nutritional minimum. The remaining 40% represents some 1500 million people who consume less than this amount. This stark fact is exemplified by countries in equatorial Africa and OPEC where the average annual consumption is only 10 kg per head and in the underdeveloped countries of Asia where it is as low as 3 kg. Table 1.2 shows the average annual meat consumption per person in the European Union (EU) (FAOSTAT).

World livestock production

In general, those countries with the highest meat consumption rates are also the major producers. Some parts of the world such as Argentina, Australia, New Zealand and Denmark are large exporters of meat and meat products, while the United States, Britain and Germany import large quantities, although the former also have a considerable export trade as have many other countries.

Table 1.2 Annual consumption of meat in the EU (kg/person/year) (FAOSTAT) 2009

	Bovine	Sheep and goat	Pig meat	Poultry
Austria	16.4	1.1	65.6	17.9
Belgium	18.0	1.6	33.6	21.5
Bulgaria	4.9	1.7	23.4	21.4
Cyprus	5.8	6.0	37.6	26.9
Czech Republic	8.0	0.2	44.7	25.1
Denmark	26.0	1.1	48.3	18.9
Estonia	12.5	0.6	26.8	19.4
Finland	18.2	0.5	35.5	18.8
France	25.5	3.3	31.0	22.3
Germany	12.8	0.8	54.6	17.3
Greece	18.1	13.1	27.7	13.7
Hungary	4.6	0.1	43.8	26.4
Ireland	22.1	4.2	33.6	26.0
Italy	23.6	1.3	42.8	17.3
Latvia	6.5	0.3	34.8	19.5
Lithuania	4.6	0.2	50.6	22.6
Malta	20.7	1.5	30.5	26.0
The Netherlands	18.1	0.9	34.0	22.7
Poland	4.9	0.1	50.4	21.4
Portugal	18.3	2.4	42.9	28.7
Romania	7.8	3.2	31.9	21.0
Slovakia	5.0	0.2	36.2	17.4
Slovenia	20.8	1.0	39.5	26.5
Spain	14.3	2.8	48.9	27.5
Sweden	24.9	1.4	36.0	15.4
United Kingdom	19.8	5.29	26.2	32.2

Source: Reproduced with permission from FAO (2011). © FAO.

Many factors operate to determine levels of food animal populations, economics playing the principal role, but disease outbreaks, weather conditions, overproduction, consumer preference, feed availability, etc. are also important reasons, along with trade barriers imposed by individual states, often on ill-defined, even unjustified, grounds.

Beef production globally, in the next 20 years, is expected to rise by only by 6%: 61 million tonnes carcase weight in 2010 and 64.5 tonnes in 2025.

Sheep meat production on a global basis is rising slowly, primarily as a result of rising production in China. Expected improved world prospects for the wool trade had encouraged extra production in Australia. In eastern Europe and countries of the former Soviet Union, production continues to contract. World pork consumption has increased by 27% from 1997 to 2005 with China being the largest producer (Orr and Shen, 2006).

Poultry production continues to expand throughout the world, but growth rate has slowed somewhat in the past year. Annual poultry meat production was reported to be 79.4 million tonnes in 2008 (FAOSTAT).

UK meat plants and throughputs

In 2008, 28.8 million animals (cattle, sheep and pigs) were slaughtered in the United Kingdom (Department of Food and Rural Affairs (DEFRA), 2008). Latest estimates indicate that there are approximately 360 abattoirs in the United Kingdom which is a significant reduction from the level of 2062 abattoirs, reported in Great Britain alone in 1968 (see Table 1.3, Table 1.4 and Table 1.5).

Cattle

In 2011, the world cattle population was 1399.9 million with 195 million buffaloes (Food and Agriculture Organisation of the United Nations (FAO), 2011). The numbers in the main countries are as follows (in millions): Brazil, 212.8; India, 210.8; United States, 92.7; China, 83; and Ethiopia, 53.4.

In the United Kingdom, beef and milk account for about one-third of the total agricultural output. Britain now pro-

duces almost 80% of its beef requirement, compared with about 50% just before the Second World War. The remaining 20% is imported mainly from Ireland and Argentina. About 52% of the home-produced beef is derived from the dairy herd, that is, from calves reared for beef. Specialised beef cattle and their crosses provide 48% of the home kill.

Breeds

In Britain's dairy herd, the Holstein/British Friesian is the dominant breed. About one-third of mature dairy cows and almost half of the dairy heifers are mated with beef bulls, mostly Limousin and Angus and a smaller proportion with Belgian Blue due to concerns regarding incidence of calving difficulties with the latter breed, in order to increase the beef potential of calves not required as dairy herd replacements.

Exotic breeds have been introduced into the United Kingdom in an attempt to improve beef production. The first of these (in 1961) was the French Charolais, which is typical of the large cattle breeds of western Europe with their mature body size, rapid growth rate and lean carcases. Charolais and Belgian Blue, are, however, liable to some difficulty in calving, often necessitating caesarean section, but this is apparently regarded as an acceptable risk by many farmers. British Charolais, through selective breeding, have easier calvings.

Other breeds which have been imported include Blonde d'Aquitaine, Brown Swiss, Limousin, Murray Grey (which was developed in Australia but has been in the United Kingdom for decades and is now widely considered to be British), Piedmontese, Romagnola, French Salers and Simmental. The Luing was evolved from Beef Shorthorn and Highland cattle on the island off the west coast of Scotland.

British breeds have been exported to many other countries to improve local strains, as live animals, frozen embryos or semen.

Throughout the world, there are numerous breeds of domestic cattle used for meat and milk production and also in some cases as draught animals (see Fig. 1.1, Fig. 1.2, Fig. 1.3, Fig. 1.4, Fig. 1.5, Fig. 1.6 and Fig. 1.7 for cattle bred for beef). Most are humped Zebu cattle or cross-breeds of these with cattle of European origin. In addition, the domestic buffalo, the water buffalo of Asia,

Table 1.3 Total throughputs (2008) in the United Kingdom

Animal group	Number slaughtered ('000)
Cattle	
Prime cattle (steers, young bulls and heifers)	2 028.4
Adult cattle (cows and adult bulls)	559.2
Steers	999.2
Heifers	758.9
Young bulls	270.3
Cows	541.4
Adult bulls	17.8
Calves	44.2
Sheep	
Ewes and rams	2 344.5
Other sheep and lambs	14 352.4
Pigs	
Sows and adult boars	235.0
Clean pigs	9 191.8

Source: Reproduced with permission from DEFRA (2008). © DEFRA.

Table 1.4 Throughputs in the United Kingdom by species in 2009

Species	England	Scotland	Wales	Northern Ireland	Total
Cattle	1 467 185	499 811	144 856	453 726	2 565 578
Sheep	9 509 298	1 527 533	3 933 577	582 299	15 552 707
Pigs	7 025 834	592 898	30 198	1 354 767	9 003 697
Poultry	694 773 788	50 654 143	47 734 287	102 076 083	894 238 301

Table 1.5 Numbers of approved red meat slaughterhouses (RSL) and poultry meat slaughterhouses (PSL) in the United Kingdom in 2009

Country / Type	England	Scotland	Wales	Northern Ireland	Total
RSL	207	37	25	13	282
PSL	74	5	4	7	90
Number of establishments	281	42	29	20	372

Source: Reproduced with permission from United Kingdom Food Standards Agency. © DEFRA.

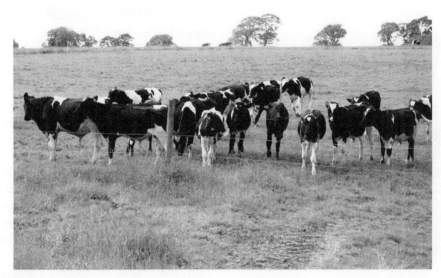

Figure 1.1 Friesian bulls.

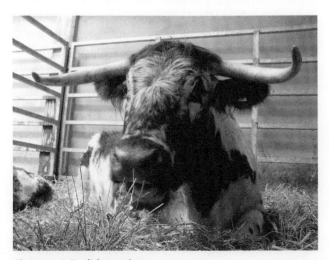

Figure 1.2 English Longhorn.

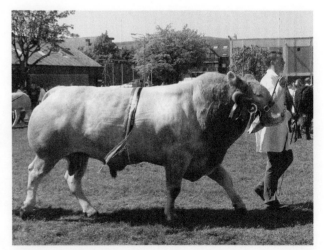

Figure 1.3 Blonde D'Aquitaine.

is an animal of great importance mainly in the Far East (India and China) but is also found in the Caribbean, Middle East and the former USSR (it has to be distinguished from the buffalo of North America, which is not a buffalo at all but a bison, and from the African wild buffalo, which has never been domesticated). Many consider that the full potential of the water buffalo as a meat and milk producer has not yet been realised. A breed of Droughtmaster cattle (*Bos taurindicus*) has been developed by cross-breeding the Zebu or Brahman

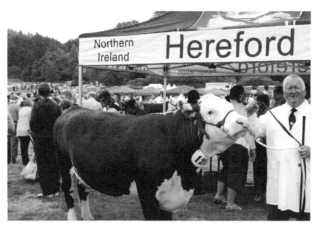

Figure 1.4 Hereford.

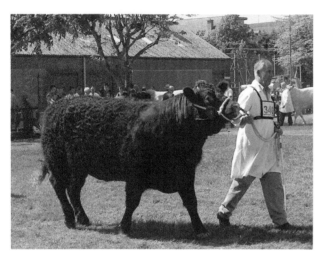

Figure 1.5 Salers.

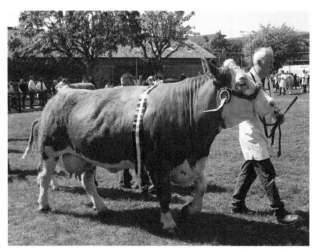

Figure 1.6 Simmental.

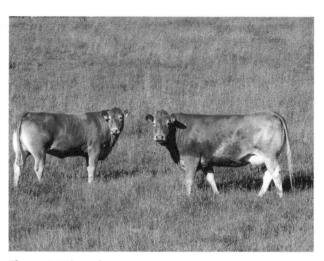

Figure 1.7 Limousin.

(*Bos indicus*) of the tropics with British beef breeds, notably Shorthorn and Hereford (*Bos taurus*). The Droughtmaster is said to combine the hardiness and disease resistance of the Zebu with the productivity and early maturity of the British breeds. Since 1974, Droughtmasters have been exported from Australia to many tropical countries including Nigeria, Ghana, Pakistan, New Guinea, Solomon Islands and Taiwan.

Systems of beef production

Beef production systems vary from almost range conditions to semi-intensive and intensive units. The efficiency of animal production is the ratio of output to input: the main outputs are meat, milk, hides, fur and by-products, and the principal inputs are feed, land, labour, capital, energy and water.

In the United Kingdom, consumer demand has dictated that meat be lean with a minimum of fat cover, tender, nutritious, palatable and, not least, relatively inexpensive. Accordingly, it is now the custom to slaughter not only cattle but all animals and poultry at much earlier ages. The economically important beef production systems in Britain usually involve slaughter of cattle at between 15 and 24 months of age. Even lower slaughter ages are adopted for certain specialist beef systems; for example, in the so-called barley beef system, calves are weaned early and fed concentrates ad lib to slaughter at 11 months of age and 400 kg, with an overall feed conversion ratio of 5.5:1. At the other extreme, there may be a high utilisation of grass with a lower overall live weight gain, with animals slaughtered at 2 or more years of age at carcase weights of 499 kg and over. A popular intermediate system is 18-month beef in which autumn-born calves are fed through the winter, kept on grass from 6 to 12 months of age and then finished during their second winter on hay, silage and feed grains.

In Britain, the term 'fatstock' used to mean exactly what it said. The meat industry was traditionally based on well-finished animals with substantial fat depots. However, the term fatstock is no longer appropriate;

'leanstock' or 'meatstock' is more suitable. Changes in the grades of fatness of livestock will probably be promoted by the production of intact males; use of bulls for larger, leaner, late-maturing breeds on the dairy herd; and genetic selection of types with efficient feed conversion rates, rapid growth rates and less fat.

Most male cattle in Britain today are reared as castrates (steers or bullocks) (80% of male cattle are reared as castrates), with the remaining 20% finished as young bulls, and these percentages have remained constant over the period 1998–2008 (DEFRA, 2008). The practice of castration was adopted to prevent indiscriminate breeding, to make animals more docile and less dangerous to man and to facilitate fattening. Only the latter factor can be regarded as significant today, since modern husbandry methods for the most part eliminate the breeding problem and present consumer demand is for lean meat. While bulls are more dangerous to handle than steers, experience has shown that the problem has been over-emphasised. It has also been well demonstrated under experimental and practical farm conditions that bulls grow faster (by 12%), convert food more efficiently (by 8%) and produce heavier (by 10%) and leaner carcases than steers. Bull beef production is much more important in Europe, especially in Italy, Germany and eastern Europe, than it is currently in Britain.

In Europe, bulls are reared in intensive feedlot systems largely based on maize silage and also in grass-finishing systems with slaughter ages of 24–30 months. The main breeds are Simmentals and Friesians. In New Zealand, grass-finishing systems have been used over the last 25 years.

In the period from 1985 to 2005, the production of bull beef in the United Kingdom increased by 66%. However, between 2005 and 2008, production has decreased by almost 40% (DEFRA, 2008). Some sections of the meat trade have considered bull beef to be of inferior conformation and tenderness as well as being subject to dark, firm and dry (DFD) meat. However, trials have shown most of these objections to be ill judged. In fact, young bull carcases are heavier and leaner than steers of the same age. Careful handling of young bulls will obviate the DFD problem (which is not confined to bulls), and chilling efficiency will offset any tendency to meat toughness, bull beef being inclined to cool more rapidly than steer beef.

Young bull beef must be distinguished from the inferior product supplied by old cull bulls, which is much darker in colour. Investigations by the UK Meat and Livestock Commission on groups of young bulls and steers transported and slaughtered under comparable commercial conditions have shown that bull flesh is only marginally darker than that of the steers, and there are only a few dark cutters among the bulls. The solution is to avoid pre-slaughter stress by gentle, efficient handling, keeping social groups intact and providing for immediate slaughter. Some of the other meat trade criticisms can be ascribed to pure conservatism. In the United Kingdom, full use is made of grassland and grass products in cattle-rearing systems, unlike in certain EU countries, for example, Germany, where bulls are housed for beef production. In the United Kingdom, prime stock is 49.3% steers, 13.3% young bulls and 37.4% heifers. In Europe, over 50% of prime stock is young bulls.

Growth promoters

Probiotics are benign bacteria which are administered by mouth to animals (calves, lambs and piglets) sometimes at birth and/or after disease. The introduction of a probiotic into the digestive tract is claimed to ensure more efficient feed conversion, earlier slaughter and a healthier animal. Unlike antibiotics, which often kill useful intestinal micro-organisms and create undesirable residues, probiotics are said to be natural products without any side effects.

Prebiotics are ingredients that stimulate the growth and/or function of beneficial intestinal micro-organisms.

Definitions

Bull

An uncastrated bovine.

Heifer

A female up to its first calf.

Cow

A female which has had one or more calves.

Steer or bullock

A castrated male (usually castrated at 6–12 weeks old).

Stag

A male bovine castrated late in life, therefore presenting a more masculine conformation than the bullock.

Sheep

Figures produced by FAO (2011) indicate that there are 1.04 billion sheep on a global scale. The principal sheep-producing countries in the world are the following (in millions): China, 138.8; India, 74.5; Australia, 73; Sudan, 52; Iran, 49; the United Kingdom, 31.6; New Zealand, 31.1; Pakistan, 28; Ethiopia, 25.5; South Africa, 24.3; Turkey, 23; and Spain, 17.

Sheep were probably among the first animals to be domesticated by man. They can be found under a wide range of environments throughout the world, and, just like goats, their system of husbandry has changed very little over the centuries in most countries. In the main, this can be classed as an extensive grazing system, the most natural for the three main species of meat animals: cattle, sheep and pigs. This system probably explains why sheep have the fewest lesions and condemnations at post-mortem compared with cattle and pigs, at least under UK conditions.

Various breeds are adapted to living in areas of high altitude where wind, rainfall, low temperatures and snow are common. The hill ewe lives a very hazardous life exposed to these adverse elements, and with low food intake, especially during pregnancy, it is little wonder that up to one-third of body weight can be lost and that neonatal mortality is high. Indeed, of all the farm animals, the relative mortality rate is highest in sheep. Other breeds can be found in desert or semi-desert regions where high temperatures or fluctuating high and low temperatures predominate, with arid conditions and sparse vegetation. With some breeds, such as those kept under lowland conditions in Britain, stocking rates can be as high as 20 ewes and their lambs per hectare; under hill and other extensive systems, the rate may be as low as one sheep to 20 hectares.

The quality of forage consumed by sheep varies from good grass under semi-intensive husbandry to low-quality (high-cellulose) plants, such as thorn scrub, rushes and heather, where the stock are relatively few in number. The ability of sheep to eat plants of little use to man and to survive in places which cannot easily be cultivated is very much in their favour. On the other hand, except for specialised breeds like the Finnish Landrace and Russian Romanov, which can produce over three lambs per ewe a year, low reproductive rates, difficulties with husbandry (e.g. fencing and labour) and the disposition towards carcases of fairly high fat content are definite drawbacks. It has been shown that with housing of ewes and subjecting them to artificial photoperiods and hormone treatment, they can produce a lamb crop every 8 months and an average of 2.2 lambs per ewe yearly. Unless fecundity can be improved by suitable breeding methods and leaner carcases ensured, it is possible that in many hill areas sheep may be replaced by goats or deer.

In addition to meat, sheep produce wool and, in some countries, milk, which is used in the making of cheese.

In the United Kingdom, there are some 50 breeds of sheep classified by habitat and type of wool. They are kept mainly for meat production, with wool as an important secondary product. Two major systems of sheep farming exist: hill sheep farming, by far the larger of the two, where the sheep are hardy and thrifty, small in size, long of wool, late in maturity and low in fecundity; and lowland sheep farming, in which short-woolled breeds predominate, possessing characteristics of early maturing, higher carcase weights and superior lambing percentages.

True hill breeds include the North Country Cheviot, South Country Cheviot, Scottish Blackface, Swaledale, Welsh Mountain, Exmoor Horn, Herdwick, Rough Fell, Derbyshire Gritstone and Lonk. Hill flocks provide store stock for fattening on lowland farms along with cast ewes which are retained for a year or two for further breeding. The famous Halfbred, which is the product of the Border Leicester ram and the Cheviot ewe, is one of the foremost utility sheep in Britain. Although the flesh of the Border Leicester carries an excessive amount of fat, its prolificacy and milk yield potential when blended with the hardiness of the Cheviot make the resulting cross an excellent animal, the dams bred to Down rams being very popular for fat lamb production in lowland areas. Another example of this close association between hill and lowland breeds is the use of the Border Leicester ram on Scottish Blackface ewes, the cross being known as the Greyface. Another Halfbred, the Welsh Halfbred, results from the crossing of the Border Leicester with Welsh Mountain ewes. The Mule is a cross-bred ewe which has grown in popularity in the United Kingdom; it now makes up 20% of the UK ewe flock. The term Mule covers a number of Blue-faced × hill breed ewe crosses. The most common of these are the Blue-faced Leicester × Scottish Blackface cross and the Blue-faced Leicester × (Welsh) Hardy Speckled Face. Reported prolificacy levels are higher in Mules than Greyfaces. Where certain hill sheep, for example, Scottish Blackface ewes, are grazed on lowland pastures, the good feeding can result in up to 200% lamb crops.

Lowland breeds are represented by the short-woolled downland types (the Suffolk, Dorset Horn and Dorset Down, Southdown, Oxford Down, Ryeland and Shropshire) and the long-woolled breeds of Leicester (Lincoln Longwool, Kent or Romney Marsh, Wensleydale and the Blue-faced or Hexham Leicester). The three most common terminal sires used in the industry at present are Suffolk, Texel and Charolais.

The Dorset Horn, a white-faced short-woolled sheep, has a much-extended mating season and can produce three crops of lambs in 2 years. In this way, it resembles the Merino. Breeds like these along with Finnish Landrace (high prolificacy), East Friesland (good milking potential) and the Île-de-France (excellent carcase quality) could feature in cross-breeding programmes. It is possible that many of the present British breeds may disappear with the development of new hybrids: it is certain that some 50 breeds are unnecessary for successful sheep production. Indeed, this has already taken place with the appearance of the Colbred sheep, named after Oscar Colborn, a Cotswold farmer who crossed Cluns, Dorset Horns, Suffolks and East Frieslands in order to increase fecundity, mothering ability and carcase quality. More recently, French Texels, Beltex, Berrichon du Cher, Rouge de l'Ouest and Charolais have been imported for crossing purposes. The Cambridge breed of sheep is another recently developed breed which is very prolific.

British breeds of sheep are not found extensively in Europe, although Cheviots and some lowland types occur in Scandinavia, but many have found their way to other parts of the world. In Australia, about 75% of the 126 million sheep are Merinos, the remainder being crosses with certain British breeds. In New Zealand, the Romney Marsh predominates, followed by Corriedales, Merinos and Southdowns and their crosses. In the United States, the Rambouillet is the main representative of the Merino, and a lot of cross-breeding occurs, with larger sheep units under confined systems of management becoming more important. However, it is doubtful whether sheep grazing in the United States will expand very much. In South Africa and the USSR, the most important breed is the Merino. Fat-tailed and fat-rumped sheep are found in the Middle and Far East; the Awassi breed is an important coarse wool type in the eastern Mediterranean and Iraq, where the wool is used mainly for making carpets.

In some parts of Europe, milk or dairy sheep are of significance: the common breeds are East Friesland (Holland), Cochurro, Lancha and Mancha (Portugal and Spain).

In recent years, more attention is being given to the production of fine wools, cashmere and mohair which the textile industry needs and presently has to import. In addition to sheep, Angora goats and rabbits, alpacas and llamas also produce quality fibres. Judicious crossing of British sheep with Merinos, for example, Merino de l'Ouest from France, produces sheep capable of high lambing percentages, good growth rates and carcase quality as well as fine fleeces.

In addition to better feeding methods, improvements in sheep production are currently centred on the use of hormones to increase the number of lambs born and out-of-season lambing, hybridisation to produce a superior stock of leaner types, oestrous synchronisation, early weaning and artificial rearing of lambs. Intensification on grass and fodder is possible as long as farmers are aware of the problems involved.

In the United Kingdom, the demand for young and small carcases means that lamb is the more important product. Lambs are usually slaughtered at between 36 and 50 kg live weight giving a dressed carcase of 17–23 kg. 'Mutton' is derived from lambs not attaining a finished condition before weaning and from ewes, wethers, hoggets and rams.

As in the case of cattle and pigs, use has been made of entire ram lambs to produce leaner carcases. Work carried out at the Meat Research Institute, Bristol, and in New Zealand has shown that carcases from entire ram lambs grade about one fat class lower than those from ewes at the same weight without deterioration in eating quality. The entire ram lambs had lower values of subcutaneous and intramuscular fat, and a higher proportion of the total fat in the rams was deposited subcutaneously where it can be removed by trimming – an important commercial consideration. Some 30% of the New Zealand kill is now composed of entire ram lambs, non-castration being encouraged.

Research work on carcase and meat composition and tenderness of meat from ram, wether and ewe Dorset Down-cross and Suffolk-cross lambs slaughtered at 20 weeks of age showed that differences in meat quality were very small, tenderness of ram meat being ensured by efficient refrigeration control. The fact that the rams, especially the Suffolk crosses, grew faster, yielded larger joints and had good carcase conformation in addition to meat tenderness would indicate potential for ram lamb production in the United Kingdom (Dransfield *et al.*, 1990). When the adverse aspects of castration – namely, sepsis, which often leads to pyaemia and sometimes death – the improvement in welfare and labour and equipment costs are considered, the lead given by New Zealand would seem a good one to follow.

The desirable features required by the butcher in both lamb and mutton carcases of any breed are short stocky plump legs, thick full loin, broad full back, thick fleshy ribs with a wide breast and shoulder, a good depth of chest cavity, a short plump neck and overall lean content (Fig. 1.8, Fig. 1.9 and Fig. 1.10).

Definitions

Lamb

A sheep from birth to weaning time (generally at 3½–4½ months old). Butchers apply a more generous interpretation to the term 'lamb' and use it to denote a sheep from birth until shearing time the following year; by this interpretation, a sheep 13 months old is still classed as lamb.

Hogget

A 'lamb' in its second year, often with two permanent incisors replacing the lamb teeth.

Tup or ram

The uncastrated male.

Wether

The castrated male sheep (usually castrated before 1 week of age with a rubber ring or at 3 weeks to 3 months old by other methods).

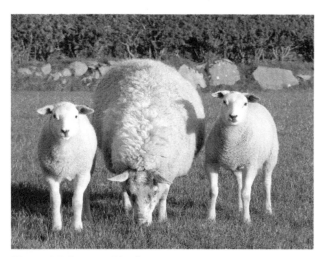

Figure 1.8 A ewe and lambs.

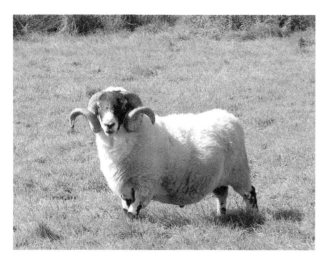

Figure 1.9 A Blackface ram.

Gimmer

A female which has not yet borne a lamb.

Ewe

A female which has borne lambs.

Cast ewe

One which has been removed from the breeding flock.

Pigs

According to the most recent world census data, 2011, there were 963 million pigs worldwide. The leading 12 pig-producing countries in order of numbers slaughtered are the following (in millions): Republic of China, 672.3; United States, 111; Germany, 59.7; Vietnam, 44.2; Spain, 41.7; Brazil, 34.9; Russian Federation, 29; France, 24.8; Philippines, 24.3; Poland, 22; Denmark, 20.9; and Japan, 16.4. The number of pigs slaughtered worldwide was 1382.6 m (FAOSTAT). Over the past decade, pig production in China, the United States and Vietnam has grown significantly. In 1997, in the Netherlands, a severe outbreak of classical swine fever led to a major culling programme which removed 40% of the Dutch annual production (6% EU total annual output) during that year. Since then, the Dutch government has decided to introduce stringent new legislation which limits the size of the national herd to 80% of the 1996 herd size.

Pig breeds

A breed is defined as 'A group of animals that has been selected by man to possess a uniform appearance that is inheritable and distinguishes it from other groups of

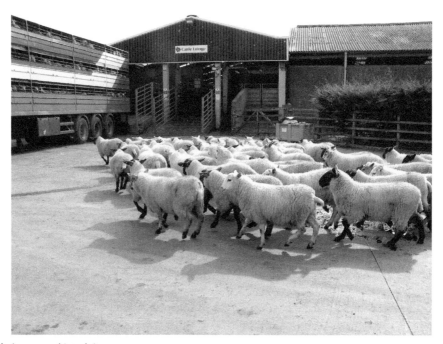

Figure 1.10 Sheep being moved into lairage.

animals within the same species'. In essence, a breed relies on being recognisable because it possesses a number or combination of features, for example, coat colour, body conformation, head shape, etc.

As the pig was domesticated, it was selected for a variety of different characteristics such as fertility, mothering ability, muscle and fat deposition, durability and amenability to handling under a variety of husbandry systems. This process continues today on two distinct levels. There are those who breed *pedigree* pigs with the aim of preserving the 'purity' of their breed and the *commercial* pig-producing companies and pig farmers who use cross-bred varieties to utilise hybrid pigs to optimise production traits. Through selection, there are now estimated to be some 300 different breeds of pigs.

Unlike some species, the pig has suffered little from man's selection to maximise production and appearance. The most noted exception was the introduction of the halothane gene following the introduction of the Piétrain breed. This breed was chosen with the aim of increasing muscle production via the double muscle gene carried naturally by the Piétrain breed. However, pigs which carry the double recessive halothane gene tend to drop dead if stressed, and those that do survive and are slaughtered express a high frequency of pale, soft and exudative (PSE) muscle tissue such that the meat appears pale and suffers from high drip loss, making it less suitable for processing and sale. For many years after this gene was introduced, the commercial breeding companies tested breeding stock by exposing all potential breeding pigs to the anaesthetic gas halothane because it was found that if 10-week-old pigs which were double recessive for this gene were exposed to this gas, they would become rigid; pigs not carrying the gene retained a relaxed posture. Recently, a gene probe has been developed which is cheaper and more welfare acceptable. This new test has also made it possible for the breeding companies to retain some of the benefits of this gene in terms of muscle production without the risk of pigs being stress susceptible and producing PSE meat.

More recently, breeding companies in the United Kingdom and France have imported and experimented with genes introduced by crossing European breeds with the Meishan breed which originates in China. The Meishan is a highly prolific breed with the potential of producing up to 30 piglets per litter. The aim is to introduce the genes for prolificacy while retaining the leaner carcase characteristics of the European breeds.

Pig breeds in the United Kingdom

In the United Kingdom, pedigree pig breeding is carefully recorded by the British Pig Association (BPA), which began keeping breeding records in 1884 when the association was known as the National Pig Breeders Association (NPBA). The aim of the NPBA was to

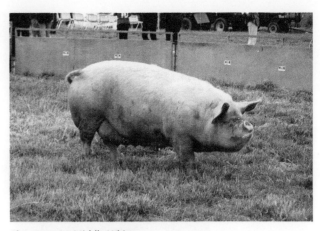
Figure 1.11 Middle White.

'maintain the purity and improve the breeds of swine in the United Kingdom of Great Britain and Ireland by the means of livestock inspection and herdbook recording all pedigree pure-bred pigs'.

Today, the BPA recognises 14 pedigree pig breeds: Large White, Landrace, Welsh, Berkshire, British Hampshire, British Saddleback, Duroc, Gloucester Old Spot, Large Black, Middle White, Tamworth, Mangalitza, Oxford Sandy and Black and Piétrain (Fig. 1.11, Fig. 1.12, Fig. 1.13 and Fig. 1.14). The main breeds used commercially are Large White, Landrace, Duroc, Hampshire and Piétrain.

Commercial breeding companies in the United Kingdom supply approximately three-quarters of all the replacement gilts bought by commercial pig farmers. These companies use pedigree pigs at the top of their breeding pyramids to produce cross-bred grandparent and parent pigs.

Increasingly, the force which has been driving the selection made by the breeding companies is coming from the retail sector where the demand is for a leaner, 'healthier' carcase which produces a tender, succulent meat not showing signs of PSE or excessive drip loss and which has sufficient intramuscular fat to provide flavour. Added to this is a new demand which places emphasis on the production system used, with the requirement being for what are termed 'high-welfare' production systems but which equate to loose housing systems. These demands influenced the choice of breed used by the breeding companies in their breeding programmes. For example, although the traditional crosses of the White breeds still account for 84% of all commercial indoor production, sales of Duroc crosses to produce hardier pigs, more suited to the more demanding outdoor environment, are on the increase.

Pig production

The United Kingdom, with some 25% of its pigs outdoors, has the highest percentage of *outdoor production* in Europe. The availability of suitable outdoor sites will

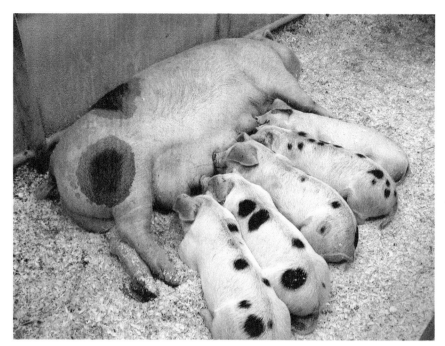

Figure 1.12 Gloucester Old Spot sow and litter.

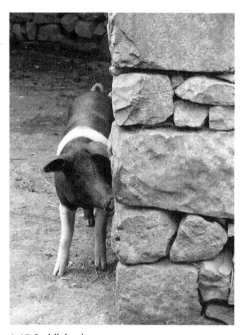

Figure 1.13 Saddleback.

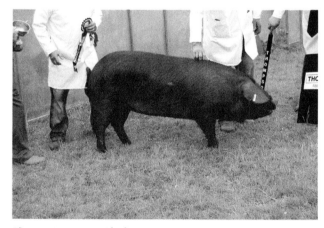

Figure 1.14 Large Black.

probably limit further development since pig welfare can be severely compromised if pigs are put on to sites where the rainfall exceeds 750 mm/year and the land is not free draining or relatively flat. In fact, much of the outdoor rearing of pigs has now ceased in the United Kingdom since farmers have discovered that the environmental conditions were too severe and too difficult to manage.

European Council Directive 91/630/EEC set out the 'minimum standards for the protection of pigs'.

This legislation was incorporated into UK law by SI 2126 'The Welfare of Livestock Regulations 1994'. However, the UK legislation not only implemented the European Directive but added the abolition of stalls and tethers by 1 January 1999. Some of the other European countries decided to address other aspects of production; for example, in the Netherlands, fully slatted flooring systems were phased out by 2006.

The imposition of legislation on production inevitably affects the way pigs are produced. European legislation has been passed in an attempt to reduce the environmental impact of agriculture: Integrated Pollution Prevention and Control Directive (IPPC Directive 96/61/EC) and the Nitrates Directive (Directive 91/676/EEC). The IPPC Directive aims to reduce all pollution emissions to air, water and soil and to make more efficient use of resources. The Nitrates Directive aims to prevent pollution of surface and groundwater by excess nitrate. Pig production in the future is likely to be even more tightly controlled by legislation as pressure from welfare and other lobbying bodies mounts on governments. This, plus the change in the way world trade is changing, will inevitably affect the economics of pig production and accordingly the size and structure of the UK pig industry. The breeds of pigs used and the husbandry procedures adopted will continue to evolve.

Pig meat production

In 2011, the EU produced 23 million tonnes of pig meat (FAOSTAT), and the United Kingdom produced around 1.3 million tonnes. When compared with other European countries, the UK consumer eats less pig meat, with the total consumption figures being 803 000 tonnes for pork and 488 000 tonnes for bacon. The UK pig industry is about 104% self-sufficient for pork but only 52% for bacon. The balance of bacon production comes from Denmark, Holland and France. The UK industry is unusual in that it produces pig meat from uncastrated males, which means that in order to avoid *boar taint*, pigs are slaughtered at lighter weights in that country. The average slaughter weight has however risen in recent years and is now over 80 kg (BPEX 2009). However, as a result, fat content as measured by P_2 has also increased. This has had a negative influence on grading, which in the United Kingdom is now done using the EU grades as follows:

Grade	Lean meat (%)
S	60 or more
E	55–59
U	50–54
R	45–49
O	40–44
P	<40
Z	Partially condemned or with soft fat or pale muscle
C	Poor conformation

Carcase dressing can be different in the United Kingdom when compared with the rest of Europe; in the United Kingdom, if the tongue, flare fat, kidneys and diaphragm remain with the carcase, adjustments to payment are made to take this into account. The lean meat percentage is calculated using the back fat measured at the P_1, P_2 and P_3 positions which are 4.5, 6.5 and 8 cm, respectively, from the dorsal midline, level with the head of the last rib. Payment is based on back fat at the P_2 position and on carcass weight.

Historically, pigs in the United Kingdom were sold as pork pigs, cutters, bacon pigs and heavy hogs. This classification has largely disappeared and been replaced by three weight bands. According to the MLC Yearbook 2006, in 2005, these weight bands, P_2 measurements and distribution of kill were:

Carcase weight (kg)	Average carcase weight (kg)	P_2	% of GB kill
<60	54.8	9.3	5.3
60–80	72.1	10.7	69.1
>80	84.8	12.0	25.6

Glossary of terms

The following definitions are those used in EU legislation:

Boar	A male pig after puberty, intended for breeding
Gilt	A female pig intended for breeding, after puberty and before farrowing
Pig	An animal of the porcine species of any age, kept for breeding or fattening
Piglet	A pig from birth to weaning
Rearing pig	A pig from 10 weeks to slaughter or service
Sow	A female pig after the first farrowing
Weaner	A pig from weaning to the age of 10 weeks

Additional facts

In Europe, piglets must not be weaned from the sow at an age of less than 4 weeks unless the welfare or health of the sow or piglets would otherwise be adversely affected. This is not the case in the United States where it is not unusual to find piglets weaned between 16 and 19 days of age.

On average, UK producers weaning at 4 weeks of age will achieve between 2.3 and 2.44 litters/sow/year, with between 22 and 25 piglets born/sow/year and in the region of 18–22 slaughter pigs sold per sow per year. Feed conversion is around 2.5:1. Producers using outdoor systems tend now to produce only one pig less per sow per year than those using indoor systems.

Goats

The principal goat-producing countries of the world are the following (in millions): India, 157; China, 142.2; Pakistan, 61.4; Bangladesh, 50.5; and Sudan, 43.4 (FAO, 2011).

Consumer demand for meat with a low saturated fat content and an alternative to traditional dairy products has seen an increase in the numbers of those species which are naturally lean and/or provide a source of milk other than cow's milk, for example, goats and deer. In the United Kingdom, there are now over 88 000 goats, with approximately 33 000 milk-producing goats in England and Wales (DEFRA 2003). Goat milk can be utilised in the production of many commercial products including hard and soft cheeses and yoghurt. Meat is a by-product, as are skins and goat hair. Steps were recently taken in Britain to produce home-bred mohair and cashmere from imported Angora goats.

Domesticated goats, descended from native breeds in the East, probably Iran, are found throughout the world, even in torrid and frigid zones where they are superior to cows for milk production. Besides milk, some breeds are kept for their hair, for example, Angora and Cashmere, while young goats are a source of kid leather. They are especially useful for small-scale milk production and can be maintained in buildings and on pasture where it would not be possible to keep cattle or sheep.

Breeds can be roughly classified into two main groups: Swiss, which are prick eared and include Alpine and Toggenburg; and Nubian, which are African in origin, chiefly Egyptian, and have long drooping ears and Roman noses, for example, Angora, Cashmere and Maltese.

While the market for goat meat in Britain has not yet assumed much importance, in France, there are now some 121 000 goat farmers. Many of these have developed broiler goat units in which 3–7-day-old kids are reared on high-vitamin milk powder to a live weight of 10 kg at 1 month of age, when they are slaughtered. The average carcase dead weight is 6.3 kg. The carcases are split and the meat is exported, mainly to Italy, skins being utilised for shoemaking.

Poultry

The main poultry-producing regions of the world include the following (in 1000 metric tonnes ready to cook equivalent, 2011): the United States, 17.11; China, 12.08; Brazil, 11; Mexico, 7.7; Russia, 2.9; India, 2.2; Turkey, 1.6; and the United Kingdom, 1.3 (FAOSTAT).

It is probably true to say that no other farm enterprise is as widespread throughout the world as is that of poultry farming. Certainly, no other farming activity has made such vast strides in recent years as the production of meat and eggs for table use. In many countries, it is regarded as the most important sector of the agricultural industry. While many farmers keep a few poultry for their own use to provide meat and eggs, the other extreme is represented by large commercial organisations in which thousands of birds are kept under the most modern systems of management. The major part of the poultry industry consists of domestic fowls, but turkeys, ducks, geese and guinea fowl are also reared, turkeys being especially common in the United States and Britain. While it is still not unusual for meat and egg production to go hand in hand on small enterprises, they are mostly separate activities with the larger concerns. Indeed, the early 1950s saw the commencement of the broiler industry, which in the United Kingdom now has an annual production of 820 million broilers and combines in most instances breeding, hatching, rearing, slaughter, processing, packing and marketing; efficiency and competition are the motivating forces. This operation is said to be 'vertically integrated'.

The rapid trend towards larger enterprises is exemplified by the broiler industry in the United Kingdom, where some 75% of the whole industry is controlled by six companies. While in the early years only a few hundred birds were reared on one holding, nowadays, it is not uncommon for 1 million birds to be housed on a single poultry farm, as many as 40 000 birds being kept in one house. In the United Kingdom, house size generally varies from 12 000 to 35 000 birds, and there may be 1–10 houses on each individual site rather than in huge integrated units, this trend being dictated by disease control and welfare considerations.

Concentrated efforts have been put into the breeding of poultry for both egg and meat production, not only to enhance productivity but also to control disease, which could be devastating to the industry. Instead of pure breeds, commercial poultry are now represented by hybrids.

Poultry meat production in the United Kingdom is provided in the main by broilers, turkeys and ducks, together with geese, poussins and end-of-lay hens, guinea fowl and some game species such as grouse, partridges, pheasants and quail. Ostrich farming for meat production and leather is a significant enterprise in South Africa.

Definitions

Broilers

Slaughtered normally at around 42 days at live weight of about 2.3 kg. Food conversion rate is 1.75:1 with a kill-out of 69%. Broilers are housed in environmentally controlled buildings.

Poussins

Young birds, 23–28 days old, with an average live weight of 0.5 kg. Oven-ready, they weigh 0.25–5 kg. Poussins are mainly sold to the retail trade.

End-of-lay hens

Birds at the end of their laying life, sometimes called boiling fowl, and weighing around 2 kg, form a substantial trade in meat for processing. Some live, fat hens are required for Halal slaughter in Britain.

Nearly all the broilers in the major production areas in the world are reared on deep litter on the floor. Using modern strains of fast-growing birds, the majority are raised until they are approximately 6 weeks of age, when they are harvested, that is, caught, crated, loaded and transported to the processing plant. Nowhere is intensivism more evident than in broiler production, where the health of the breeding stock and the growing birds is essential for economic and welfare reasons. Breeding flocks have a detailed vaccination programme which gives protection against respiratory diseases such as infectious bronchitis and Newcastle disease as well as Marek's disease, egg drop syndrome, avian epidemic tremor and infectious bursal disease (IBD). The broilers themselves may be vaccinated against Gumboro disease and other infections and in addition will have a coccidiostat in the ration to prevent coccidiosis.

The keeping of large numbers of birds together makes it essential that nutrition, ventilation and temperature, stocking densities and management are optimal. Very close supervision of the birds is essential, and correct treatment/management changes must be prompt. It is vital that detailed records are kept since it is usually from these that early signs of disease are detected, for example, water consumption, reduced food intake, weight gain and egg production in layers.

Two aspects of management help birds keep free from disease. Biosecurity – safety from transmissible infectious diseases, parasites and pests – is a term that embodies all the measures that can or should be taken to prevent viruses, bacteria, fungi, protozoa, parasites, insects, rodents and wild birds from entering or surviving and infecting or endangering the well-being of the poultry flock. An 'all-in/all-out' policy operates where the birds on a unit are approximately the same age and all are slaughtered; the unit is then thoroughly cleaned and disinfected prior to the arrival of a new batch of birds.

Turkeys are nowadays not confined to the Christmas period. A wide range of weights is produced, depending on the particular trade, and these may be as low as 4 kg and as high as 9 kg or more. Some large cocks can be as heavy as 18 kg. The popular weight of bird for the average family in Britain is between 5 and 6 kg.

Ducks are produced both oven-ready frozen – used mainly in the catering trade – and oven-ready fresh chilled – sold mainly retail – and are available in weights from 2 kg upwards. Table ducks can make very fast live weight gains, attaining 3.6 kg in 49 days at a food conversion of 2.3:1. The kill-out percentage is 72%. In the United Kingdom, 90% of ducks are Pekin. Small specialist producers use other breeds such as Barberi. Generally, Pekin ducks are considered a cold-weather duck and are predominant in northern Europe, and Barberi are predominant in southern Europe and warmer countries.

Compared with domestic fowls and turkeys, geese and ducks are of minor importance. Sales of *geese* are usually confined to the Christmas period. They are generally regarded as being a specialised product in that they have a high feed conversion ratio, 5:1, and are expensive to produce. A female can produce 50–60 offspring which are killed normally at 18–22 weeks weighing around 10 kg live weight with a kill-out of about 75%. Nowadays, owing to hybridisation, the meat content of the carcase is much higher. In Denmark, Germany, Austria, Poland and parts of France, commercial geese production is an important enterprise; in some instances, force-feeding with noodles or other foods is carried out to produce enlargement of the liver, from which the delicacy paté de foie gras is prepared.

In England, the keeping of geese and ducks is subject to the terms of the Welfare of Farmed Animals (England) Regulations 2007 and other legislations, as is all livestock farming, so that geese and ducks have the same welfare protection as other animals. Their force-feeding might, therefore, be regarded as causing unnecessary stress, depending on the professional assessment of the inspecting veterinary officer, and would not be allowed in the United Kingdom.

Guinea fowl can be reared intensively and kept indoors, the first part of their life under brooders. They are killed at 8–9 weeks of age and have a food conversion ratio of 3:1. France and Italy produce large numbers.

There is no doubt that poultry is Britain's favourite meat at the moment, its market continuing to grow at the expense of red meat. Chicken has a 78% share of the retail market, while turkey now stands at 19%. The major growth sector in the poultry industry in recent years has been that of value-added products, now estimated to be worth over £600 million for chicken. Altogether, poultry are worth some £2000 million. Most of the retail sales of chicken (87%) go to the multiples, only 6% going to butchers. The trade is divided into fresh chilled and frozen birds and portions.

Rabbits

Under commercial rabbit-rearing conditions in the United Kingdom, only 2 of the 40 breeds of rabbit are used for meat production. These are the Commercial White and Californian.

Rabbits have high fertility rates (some breeds can produce 60 offspring per year), fast growth rates (1.75 kg at 8 weeks of age) and a food conversion efficiency of 2.5:1. A killing-out percentage of around 50 head-off, hot carcase weight can be achieved. A measure of the potential of the rabbit as a meat-producing animal can be gauged by comparing it with a breeding ewe. A 70 kg ewe is capable of producing 40 kg of lamb carcase per year, whereas a 4.5 kg doe is able to produce 75 kg of rabbit meat in the same time.

Rabbit meat is low in fat (3.8%) and high in protein (20.7%), which compares favourably with chicken (2.5% fat and 21.5% protein), beef forequarter (18.9% fat and 18.3% protein), lamb leg (17.5% fat and 18.7% protein) and pork ham (19.6% fat and 19.7% protein).

Rearing is often a large-scale enterprise in Europe, where farms of several thousand does can be found, but rabbits are mainly kept on small farms where labour costs are low. The average size of a rabbit farm in the United Kingdom is a 40–50 doe unit. For the industry to be successful, it must develop on the same lines as the poultry industry, that is, highly organised with specialist attention to the cost of labour, food, equipment, breeding, nutrition, disease prevention and housing.

The optimum weight for slaughter lies around 2.7 kg, which is achieved at about 12–14 weeks of age, although this depends on factors such as breed, feeding systems and management but mainly the environment.

Rabbit-processing plants have to conform to EC standards. Integrated premises have facilities for rearing, slaughter, refrigeration and packing, the end products consisting of whole fresh rabbits, sausages and burgers, stewpacks and cooked and coated portions as in the poultry industry.

Stunning is by electricity, as opposed to home killing where animals are stunned by a blow to the head, which is immediately removed, or the spinal cord is broken in a manner similar to that for poultry.

Imports of Chinese rabbits have been a serious source of competition for the British industry, but they are not of the same standard as British supplies.

While the rabbit is an animal which can utilise many types of feedingstuffs unsuitable for human consumption, it is susceptible to certain conditions such as the enteritis complex, which may be a form of nutritional deficiency allied to an infection caused by microorganisms. Respiratory diseases are also common, and these, along with the above, represent important areas for research as well as good husbandry. Labour input is very high for rabbit breeding, and one person can only manage a maximum of 250–300 does.

Deer

The farming of red deer has now become firmly established in the United Kingdom and other European countries and on a much larger scale in New Zealand. In the latter country, the emphasis is on the production of antler in velvet for the lucrative oriental trade, a practice prohibited by law in the United Kingdom.

There are three different kinds of pasture land which, taken together with the system of livestock production practised, provide a basis for the classifying of farm units into hill farms, upland farms and lowland farms. Hill deer farms produce weaned calves which are sold to upland and lowland farms, where they grow much faster to breeding or slaughter live weights. Upland farms breed stags which may be suitable for use on hill farms and sell breeding stock and store calves to lowland farms; they can also produce prime venison. Some upland farms will also export breeding stock and import new bloodlines from abroad. *Lowland* farms sell breeding stags to the upland farmer and can import and export livestock as well as being a major producer of prime venison.

It was estimated by the British Deer Farmers Association from the Agricultural Census in 2005 that 300 deer farms operated within the United Kingdom farming 33 000 deer. Park deer are also increasingly being used for venison production. Estimates made in 2005 show that Scotland had at least 300 000 wild red deer with an estimate of approximately 500 000–600 000 roe deer across Britain.

While most of the deer farmed in Britain are red deer, smaller numbers of fallow, roe, sika and wapiti are also kept.

New Zealand's 1.5 million farmed deer graze on approximately 4000 farms. Average herd size is about 375, although the largest herds comprise several thousands. Deer are processed in specialist plants. Revenue from New Zealand venison exports is known to fluctuate widely with the amount of venison exported rising from 16 000 to 27 000 tonnes between 2002 and 2006; however, due to a reduction in price the value of these exports only increased marginally from US $210 to US $250 million (Deer and deer farming – Venison exports, Te Ara – The Encyclopaedia of New Zealand). The major market group was Europe, with Germany the main importer, followed by Scandinavia and France.

Consumer demand for lean meat is fully met in venison, which has a low fat content (5–10%) compared with levels of 25–40% found in some traditional cuts of beef and lamb.

Husbandry mainly centres round the red deer (*Cervus elaphus*) because of its ease of handling compared with

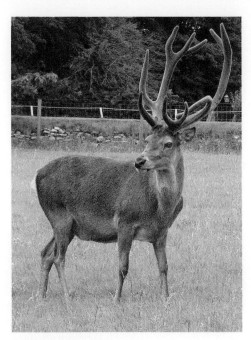

Figure 1.15 A red deer stag.

the other species, some of which can be aggressive, for example, wapiti (*Cervus canadensis*).

The calves are weaned in September. Housed calves appear to thrive much better than those out-wintered unless very good shelter is available. The principal problem in housing deer is bullying, and it is important to separate deer into groups of similar size and to quickly identify and remove either aggressive deer or those being bullied. Where there is abundant fenced rough pasture and forest to provide shelter, adult deer are best out-wintered because of bullying indoors.

The most suitable areas for deer farming are good, well-sheltered grassland with good fencing and shelter because of the lower subcutaneous fat content than in cattle and sheep and the consequent poorer insulation.

Rutting (the annual sexual display in the male) occurs in the autumn and is accompanied by increased aggression, vocalisation, testicular activity, shedding of velvet and a strong urine odour. The rut lasts for 2–5 weeks (late September to October) (Fig. 1.15).

Single calves are born in the spring (late May to June) after a gestation of 231 days. At birth, they weigh an average 8.5 kg and reach sexual maturity at 16 months. Farmed deer are slaughtered at various ages (8–30 months) and produce dressed carcase weights of 53–60 kg live weight. Some 33% of the carcase is regarded as first-class meat.

Stocking rates vary according to the type of land and pasture utilised, from 0.66/hectare on heather-dominant hills to 12–16 hinds with their calves, per hectare, on good lowland pasture.

Handling of deer

Because of their relatively sensitive nature, aggression at times and powers of agility, it is essential that they are handled efficiently and with care. Housing has been shown to be of value, especially for calves, but care has to be taken with dominant types (which must be removed) and to allow sufficient trough space.

Good handling systems are necessary for collection of deer for tuberculin testing, blood sampling, weighing, anthelmintic and other treatments, etc. Drugs such as etorphine hydrochloride (Immobilon) and diprenorphine (Revivon) are frequently used to immobilise animals humanely, projectile syringes being fired from rifles or blowpipes into the hindquarter or shoulder.

References

Department of Food and Rural Affairs (DEFRA). (2008) *United Kingdom Slaughter Statistics 2008*, https://statistics.defra.gov.uk/esg/slaughterns.htm (accessed 8 April 2014).

Dransfield, E., Nute, G.R., Hogg, B.W. and Walters, B.R. (1990) *Animal Production*, 50, 291.

Food and Agriculture Organisation of the United Nations (FAO) (2011) FAOSTAT, Statistics/Production/Livestock Primary/Cattle/Animals Slaughtered Products Quantity.

Living Costs and Food Survey (2011) *Department of the Environment, Food and Rural Affairs*, Office of National Statistics, London.

Orr, D.E. Jr. and Shen, Y. (2006). World pig production: opportunity or threat? Midwest Swine Nutrition Conference, 7 September 2006, Indianapolis.

Woods, V.B. and Fearon, A.M. (2009) *Livestock Science*, 126, 1–20.

Further reading

Universities Federation for Animal Welfare (1988) *The Management of Farm Animals*, Ballière-Tindall, London.

Alexander, T.L. and Buxton, D. (eds) (1994) *Management and Diseases of Deer*, Veterinary Deer Society, London.

Elblex Meat and Livestock UK Yearbook, 2011.

Farm Animal Welfare Council

Animal Welfare Act, 2006.

MLC Year Books Cattle, Pigs and Sheep.

Defra Codes of Practice.

Report on the Welfare of Broiler Chickens, 1992.

Report on the Welfare of Sheep, 1994.

Report on the Welfare of Turkeys, 1995.

Report on the Welfare of Pigs Kept Outdoors, 1996.

The Welfare of Farmed Animals (England) Regulations, 2007.

2

Anatomy

There are four main types of tissues in animal bodies:

1 Epithelial tissues are found on external and internal surfaces and also form specialised structures such as the liver.
2 Muscular tissues, constituting the flesh of animals, are of three main types: voluntary (striped, striated), involuntary (unstriped, unstriated, smooth) and cardiac (a special form of striated muscle found in the heart).
3 Connective tissues include the skeleton, which gives rigidity to the body. Blood is a specialised form of connective tissue although it is sometimes classified alone.
4 Nervous tissue is the most specialised of all the tissues. It transmits the nerve impulses of both sensation and movement.

The animal body is a highly developed multicellular organism, consisting of billions of cells specialised to form tissues. Each tissue has a special function; the tissues are further grouped together to form organs. An organ is a group of tissues arranged in a special manner to carry out a special task, for example, the heart, stomach, kidney and bone. Organs are again grouped to form systems, each of which performs essential body functions.

The systems of the body are 11 in number, as follows: osteology and arthrology (bones and joints), digestive, respiratory, circulatory, lymphatic, urogenital, nervous, endocrine, myology (muscles), sense organs (ear, eye, organ of smell and organ of taste) and common integument (skin and appendages).

Descriptive terms

Certain terms are used to describe the exact position and direction of the different body parts, assuming that the animal is in the standing position:

Dorsal, superior or upper structures or positions lie towards the back or dorsum of the body, head or tail.

Ventral, inferior or lower positions are directed towards the belly or venter.

The longitudinal median plane divides the body into two similar halves. Structures that are nearer than others to the median plane are said to be medial or internal, while those farther away from it are lateral or external. Planes parallel to the median plane are sagittal to it. Parts which lie towards the head are cranial or anterior, while those towards the tail are caudal or posterior.

In relation to the limbs, the terms proximal and distal are used, those lying towards the junction with the body being proximal and those at a greater distance away from the body being distal. Above the knee and hock, the terms cranial and caudal are used for front and rear positions, those below the knee and hock being dorsal and palmar and dorsal and plantar, respectively.

The terms superficial and deep denote relationships from the surface of the body, for example, superficial and deep flexor tendons of the legs.

Osteology and arthrology

Bones

The skeleton, composed of some 200 bones, acts as a support and protection for the soft tissues of the body and provides a system of levers for locomotion and body

Gracey's Meat Hygiene, Eleventh Edition. Edited by David S. Collins and Robert J. Huey.
© 2015 John Wiley & Sons, Ltd. Published 2015 by John Wiley & Sons, Ltd.

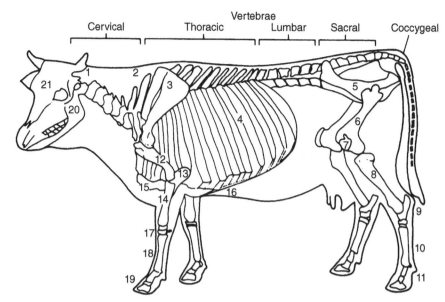

Figure 2.1 Skeleton of ox. 1, atlas; 2, 7th cervical vertebra; 3, scapula; 4, ribs; 5, pelvic girdle; 6, femur; 7, patella; 8, tibia; 9, tarsus; 10, metatarsus; 11, phalanges; 12, humerus; 13, ulna; 14, radius; 15, sternum; 16, xiphiod process; 17, carpus; 18, metacarpus; 19, phalanges; 20, mandible; 21, cranium (by courtesy of Sisson and Grossman, 1975).

movement (Fig. 2.1). It also acts as a blood-forming organ, producing red and white cells, haemoglobin and platelets.

The long bones of the very young animal are very long, slender and smooth, with their prominences less pronounced. With age, ossification of cartilage takes place and the bone becomes more rigid. In the very old animal, there is a decrease in bone organic matter, making the bone more brittle and liable to fracture.

The proportion of bone in the dressed carcase of beef, that is, the two sides, varies between 12 and 28%, according to breed and bodily condition, being about 15% in a good beef carcase and increasing with the age and weight of the animal. It is lowest in Aberdeen Angus cattle but is as high as 28% in second-quality cows. The average percentage of the bone in lamb is 17–35%, in bobby calves 50%, in veal calves 25%, in pork 12–20% and in poultry 8–17%.

The skeleton of the meat animals is divided into two parts: the axial skeleton comprising the vertebral column or the spine, ribs, sternum and skull and the appendicular skeleton representing the bones of the limbs. The foreleg contains the scapula, humerus, radius and ulna, carpus, metacarpus and digits which are composed of phalanges. The *hindleg* is made up of the pelvic girdle (ilium, pubis and ischium), femur, tibia and fibula, tarsus, metatarsus and digits.

The *vertebral column* or spine is divided into five regions – cervical (C), thoracic (T), lumbar (L), sacral (S) and coccygeal (Cy), representing the neck, chest or thorax, loins, sacrum (fused sacral vertebrae) and tail,

respectively. In meat animals, it consists of the number of individual vertebrae shown in Table 2.1.

The *sacrum* is in the shape of a pyramid and formed of three to five fused sacral vertebrae, except in the fowl in which 14 fused lumbar and sacral vertebrae form the synsacrum. The *sternum* or breast bone in mammals is composed of six to eight fused segments. In the fowl, the sacrum is a very large bone covering almost all of the ventral part of the body.

There are generally the same number of *ribs* as the thoracic vertebrae; they are divided into sternal or asternal ribs depending on whether or not they articulate with the sternum.

Carcase bones are valuable means of *identification* of the different species of food animals, for example, where substitution is suspected. Where the teeth of a bovine animal are unavailable for examination, the *age* can be estimated with reasonable accuracy by examination of the carcase bones. This estimation is based on the degree of ossification of certain parts of the skeletal system, the most valuable of which are the cartilaginous extensions of the spines of the first five dorsal vertebrae. Ossification in these spines develops as shown in Table 2.2.

In *cows*, these changes take place more rapidly and the cartilage has ossified after 3 years.

A further useful guide as to the *age* can also be obtained from the ischiopubic symphysis. In cattle up to 3 years of age, this can be cut with a knife, but after this age, a saw is necessary. Similarly, the red bone marrow of the vertebrae is gradually replaced by yellow bone marrow, and distinction can be drawn between

Table 2.1 Vertebrae of the spine

Ox	C7	T13	L6		S5	Cy 18–20
Sheep and goat	C7	T13	L6		S4	Cy 16–18
Horse	C7	T18	L6		S5	Cy 15–21
Pig	C7	T14–15	L6–7		S4	Cy 20–23
Rabbit	C7	T12	L7–8		S3–4	Cy 14–20
Chicken	C15–17	T7	L + S14 (fused synsacrum)			Cy 5–6 + pygostyle (fused caudal vertebrae)

Table 2.2 Ossification of the cartilaginous extensions of the spines of the first five dorsal vertebrae (bovines)

Age (years)	Ossification
1	The extension is entirely cartilaginous, soft, pearly white and sharply delineated from the bone, which is soft and red
2	Small red islets of bone appear in the cartilage
3	The cartilage is greyish, and red areas are more numerous
4–5	The area of ossification within the cartilage extends until the proportion of bone is greater than that of cartilage
6	The cartilage has ossified into compact bony tissue, though the line of junction between the cartilage and bone can still be defined

the soft vascular bones of the young animal with cartilage discernible at the joints and the hard, white, bleached appearance of bones in old cows. In young bovines, the cartilage is discernible between the individual segments of the sternum, but after 5 years of age, it begins to be replaced by bone; at 8 years, two or three cartilaginous divisions are still apparent, but at 10 years, the cut surface of the sternum presents a uniform bony structure.

In *sheep*, the break at the carpus, or knee joint, is a valuable guide as to the age. In *lambs*, the joint breaks in four well-marked ridges resembling the teeth of a saw, the ridges being smooth, moist and somewhat pink or congested. In older sheep, the surface of the joint is rough, porous and dry and lacks redness. The determination by X-ray of the amount of cartilage present at the epiphysis of a long bone in a joint of meat provides unassailable evidence in cases where there is dispute as to the age of the animal from which the meat was derived. The degree of ossification, determined by X-ray, in the ischial portion of the pubic symphysis enables a leg of lamb to be differentiated with certainty from that of an old sheep.

Digestive system

Tongue

Ox

In the ox tongue, the filiform papillae are horny and directed backwards; they have a rasp-like roughness which aids in the prehension of food. The posterior part of the dorsum, that is, the upper surface, is prominent and defined anteriorly by a transverse depression which is frequently the seat of erosions due to actinobacillosis. On either side of the midline on the prominent dorsum are 10–14 circumvallate papillae; the epiglottis, if left on the tongue, is oval in shape. Black pigmentation of the skin of the tongue is frequently observed but is quite normal and of no pathological significance.

Sheep and goat

The tongue is similar to that of cattle, but the centre of the tip is slightly grooved and the papillae are not horny. The sheep tongue may be differentiated from that of the calf by the fact that it is narrower, the dorsal eminence is more marked, the surface is smoother and the tip is more rounded. Black pigmentation of the surface of the tongue is common in black-skinned sheep.

Pig

The tongue is long and narrow and there is no dorsal ridge. One or possibly two circumvallate papillae are present on each side of the midline near the base of the tongue, and the surface is studded with fungiform papillae.

Horse

The tongue is long and flat with a spatulate end. There is no dorsal ridge, and only one circumvallate papilla is present on each side. The epiglottis is pointed. Pigmentation is never seen.

Stomach

Ox (Fig. 2.2, Fig. 2.3 and Fig. 2.4)

The *oesophagus* is comparatively short and wide, measuring about 1 m long and 5 cm wide. The voluntary muscle, which performs the reverse peristaltic action in rumination, weighs about 340 g.

The *stomach (paunch)* consists of four compartments: the rumen, the reticulum, the omasum and the abomasum, which is the true digestive stomach and secretes gastric juice. The *rumen* occupies 75% of the abdominal cavity; it is bounded on the left side by the abdominal wall, on the anterior extremity by the reticulum and part of the omasum and on the right side by the remainder of the omasum, the abomasum and the intestine. The *reticulum*, which is placed transversely between the anterior extremity of the rumen and the posterior surface of the diaphragm to which it is adherent, causes a depression on the posterior aspect of the thin, left lobe of the liver (Fig. 2.2). The omasum and abomasum are attached to the posterior surface of the liver by means of the *omentum* or *caul fat*, the root of this membrane being apparent on the posterior aspect of the liver to the left of the portal lymph nodes when the liver is removed from the carcase. The omentum, after connecting the liver and omasum, is continued to the lesser curvature of the abomasum and thence to the duodenum. The anatomical relations of the bovine stomach play an important part in the aetiology of traumatic pericarditis. The average capacity of the stomach is 150 l.

Mucous membranes

Rumen Brown or black in colour except on pillars or folds where it is pale and studded with large papillae

Reticulum Honeycomb-like appearance with four-, five- or six-sided cells

Omasum Prominent longitudinal folds, about 100 in number, and sometimes called the 'bible'

Abomasum Some 30 prominent oblique folds in the body of the abomasum but absent in the pyloric portion

A feature of the calf stomach is the relatively large size of the abomasum as compared with the small size of the rumen, which remains small until the animal is weaned. As the calf commences to take solid foods, the size of the rumen increases until in the adult animal it represents 80% of the total stomach capacity and the abomasum 7–8%.

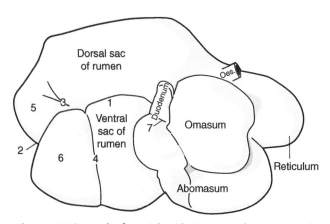

Figure 2.2 Stomach of ox, right side. Oes, oesophagus; 1, insula between right longitudinal groove below and accessory groove above; 2, caudal groove of rumen; 3 and 4, right dorsal and ventral coronary grooves; 5 and 6, caudodorsal and caudoventral blind sacs; 7, pylorus. The positions of the reticulum, omasum and abomasum have been altered by removal of the stomach from the abdominal cavity and inflation.

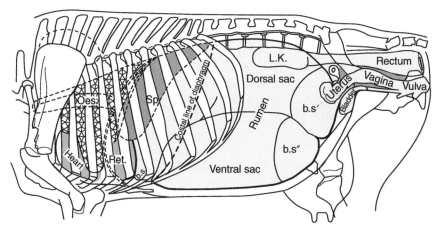

Figure 2.3 Projection of viscera of cow on body wall, left side. b.s., atrium of rumen; b.s.', b.s.", blind sacs of rumen; O, ovary; Oes, oesophagus; Ret., reticulum; Sp, spleen. The left kidney (L.K.) is concealed by the dorsal sac of the rumen and is indicated by dotted lines. The median line of the diaphragm is dotted.

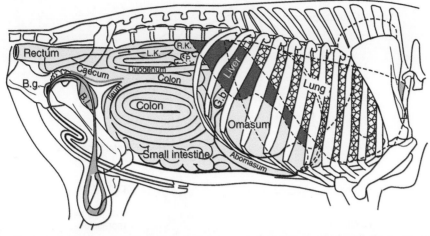

Figure 2.4 Projection of viscera of bull on body wall, right side. B.g., bulbourethral gland; B.l., urinary bladder; G.b., gall bladder; L.K., left kidney; P. (above duodenum), pancreas; P. (below G.b.), pylorus; R.K. right kidney; V.s., vesicular gland. Costal attachment and median line of diaphragm are indicated by dotted lines.

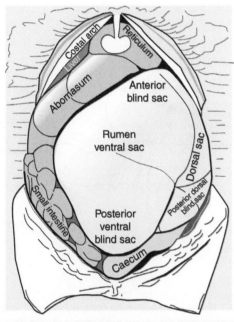

Figure 2.5 Abdominal viscera of sheep, ventral aspect. For 'anterior blind sac', read cranial end of ventral sac; for 'posterior ventral blind sac', read caudoventral blind sac; for 'posterior dorsal blind sac', read caudodorsal blind sac.

Sheep and goat (Fig. 2.5)

The stomach is similar in structure to that of the ox and has an average capacity of 18 l. The first and second stomachs together yield 0.9 kg of tripe; the fourth stomach is also sometimes used, but the third is often discarded. The sheep rumen is also used in Scotland as a container for haggis (cooked minced heart, liver and lungs, seasoned with salt, pepper, cayenne, nutmeg and grated onion mixed with oatmeal and shredded beef

Table 2.3 Length of intestines (m)

	Small intestine	Large intestine
Cattle	36.5	9
Horse	24.3	6
Sheep	25.6	6
Pig	17.1	4.8

suet). Mechanical methods for the cleaning of both ox and sheep stomachs are now operating satisfactorily in modern triperies.

Pig

The pig stomach is a simple one, semilunar in shape, with a small pocket or diverticulum at the cardiac (i.e. oesophageal) end. The mucous membrane of the cardiac end is pale grey, while the central fundic region is reddish brown, becoming paler and corrugated towards the pyloric end. The average capacity of the stomach is 6.5 l.

Horse

The horse stomach is a simple one; the mucous membrane of the whitish oesophageal portion is clearly distinguishable from the reddish, soft and vascular fundic and pyloric portions. The average capacity is 12 l.

Intestines

Small Duodenum, jejunum and ileum
Large Caecum, colon and rectum

The average length of the intestines is shown in Table 2.3. Thus, for practical purposes, the ratio of the length of the small intestine to the large intestine is 4:1.

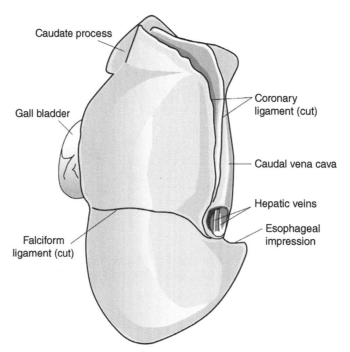

Figure 2.6 Liver of ox, diaphragmatic surface, hardened *in situ*.

Liver

With the exception of the horse, the livers of all the food animals are reddish brown in colour. The liver, the largest gland in the body, lies mainly to the right of the midline in all animals, its convex anterior surface conforming to the hollow of the diaphragm to which it is attached on its dorsal surface and its concave visceral surface (with portal vein, hepatic lymph nodes, gall bladder, common hepatic duct and hepatic artery) in contact with the pancreas, reticulum, omasum and abomasum with the caudal vena cava prominent on its dorsal border.

Ox (Fig. 2.6)

The liver is poorly divided into three lobes: a thin left, a thicker right, and a caudate lobe or thumb piece. The left and right lobes are divided by a slight notch, the umbilical fissure, which indicates the point of entry of the umbilical vein while the calf is *in utero*. In the cow, the left lobe of the liver is thin, elongated and often markedly cirrhotic. Running transversely across the upper border of the liver is the posterior vena cava, and on its posterior aspect, the liver shows the root of the omentum, gall bladder, portal vein and portal lymph nodes, the vein and lymph nodes being partly concealed by the pancreas.

The weight of the ox liver is about 5.4 kg, that is, about 1% of the live weight, although in feedlot cattle and heavier animals, the liver may weigh up to 6.3 kg. The calf liver, which is relatively larger than in the adult,

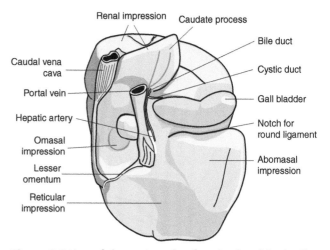

Figure 2.7 Liver of sheep, visceral surface, hardened *in situ*. The papilliary process is the round projection between the omasal impression and the left branch of the portal vein.

weighs 0.9–1.1 kg; its tenderness, its usual freedom from parasitic and other pathological conditions and its therapeutic value in the treatment of anaemia ensure the highest price.

Sheep (Fig. 2.7)

The liver is similar in shape to that of the ox, but the caudate lobe is more pointed and its edges are well defined. This is a useful distinguishing feature between the sheep and calf liver. The caudate lobe in the latter is more rounded and has a blunter extremity which frequently extends beyond the lower edge of the liver.

When the calf liver is laid on the table, anterior surface uppermost, the caudate lobe fits neatly into the liver like a carpenter's joint.

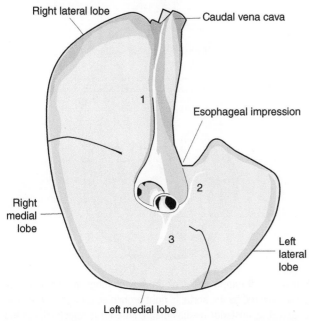

Figure 2.8 Liver of pig, parietal surface. 1, large hepatic veins opening into caudal vena cava; 2, coronary ligament; 3, falciform ligament.

An adult sheep's liver weighs 453–680 g but undergoes a marked hypertrophy in ewes approaching parturition.

Pig (Fig. 2.8)

Pig liver has five lobes, two smaller inner, two smaller outer and a caudate lobe. The oesophageal notch is prominent, but the identifying feature is the large amount of visible interlobular tissue which gives the surface of the organ its classical 'Morocco leather' appearance. The lobules are mapped out sharply and are polyhedral, and the organ, because of the amount of interlobular tissue, is less friable than in the other food animals.

Its weight varies from 0.9 kg in pork pigs to 2 kg in sows.

Horse (Fig. 2.9)

Horse liver has three distinct lobes and a thumb piece which terminates in a point. A notable feature is the absence of a gall bladder. The horse liver is purplish and weighs about 4.5 kg.

Pancreas (gut sweetbread)

The ox pancreas is reddish brown, loosely lobulated and roughly the shape of an oak leaf. It is attached to the back of the liver and is deeply notched to accommodate the portal vein. The average weights of the pancreas are as

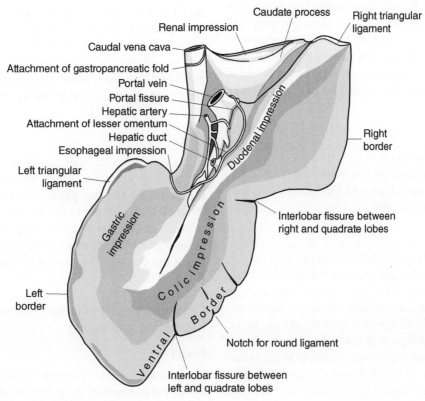

Figure 2.9 Liver of horse, visceral surface.

follows: cattle, 226–340 g; horse, 340 g; sheep, 85–142 g; and pig, 28–56 g.

Respiratory system

The much smaller thoracic cavity (containing the lungs, heart and associated large vessels) is separated from the abdominal cavity (in which all the other body organs are situated) by the strong musculomembranous *diaphragm* (convex in front and concave posteriorly).

The respiratory system comprises the nose, nasal cavity, part of the pharynx, larynx, trachea and lungs. Respiration allows an adequate intake of oxygen and the removal of carbon dioxide by bringing blood in the lungs into close proximity with the alveolar air.

The pleura lines the chest cavity and in the healthy animal is a smooth, glistening membrane divided into a right and left sac. Each sac covers the chest wall (the parietal pleura) and the lung (the visceral pleura). The two sacs (pleurae) join in the central mediastinal space in which are situated the mediastinal lymph nodes and which is traversed by the aorta, oesophagus and trachea.

Lungs

Ox (Fig. 2.10)

The cartilaginous rings of the ox trachea meet at an angle and form a distinct ridge along the dorsal aspect. The *left lung* has three lobes named, from before backwards, the apical, cardiac and diaphragmatic. The *right lung* has four or five lobes, its apical lobe receiving an accessory bronchus from the trachea. The lung lobulation is well marked by the large amount of interlobular tissue and is particularly evident in old cows. The pair of ox lungs weighs 2.2–3.0 kg.

Sheep

Sheep lungs resemble those of the ox in the division of the lobes, but their consistency is more dense and leathery, they are duller in colour, and the lobulation is less distinct. They weigh 340–907 g.

Pig

The number of lobes varies, with two to three on the left and three to four on the right, because the apical and cardiac lobes can be subdivided. The tissue is very spongy and compressible, and the surface lobulation is particularly well marked. Of all the food animals, the pig lungs show the greatest variations in colour, varying from red to light pink, but these variations are due to slight variations in the amount of blood left in the lungs after bleeding and are of no pathological significance. The pig lungs weigh 340–453 g.

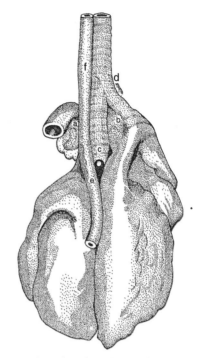

Figure 2.10 Lymph nodes of the bovine lungs. a, left bronchial partly covered by the aorta; b, right bronchial; c, middle bronchial; d, apical; e, posterior mediastinal; f, anterior mediastinal, related inferiorly to the oesophagus and trachea.

Horse

The lobar divisions are very indistinct in the horse; only two left lobes and three right lobes can be clearly distinguished. The horse lungs are long and may be further differentiated from those of the ox by the absence of surface lobulation and the absence of an accessory bronchus, while the ends of the cartilaginous rings of the trachea overlap like a piston ring. The horse lungs weigh 2.2–3.0 kg.

Pluck

In the pig, sheep and calf, the internal organs comprising the larynx, trachea, lungs, heart and liver constitute the *pluck*. In the pig pluck, the oesophagus remains attached and is related to the trachea, which is short and consists of 32 cartilaginous rings. In the sheep, the oesophagus is removed with the stomachs in the dressing of the carcase. The trachea is long and composed of about 50 rings.

Circulatory system (heart, arteries, capillaries and veins)

Heart

The heart, a hollow muscular organ acting as a pump, lies in the pericardial sac in the mid-mediastinal region of the thorax between the lungs. Its muscular portion, the *myocardium*, has a smooth lining, the *endocardium*, to its four cavities (left ventricle and atrium, right ventricle and atrium). Covering the cardiac muscle is the *epicardium*, the visceral layer of the pericardium.

In reality, the *circulation* consists of two pumps, the left and right sides, the former being involved with the systemic circulation and the latter the pulmonary circulation.

The heart is reddish brown in colour in all the food animals; the myocardium has a firm consistency, and the epicardium and endocardium are smooth and glistening. The right and left ventricles may be readily distinguished by palpation, the wall of the left ventricle being three times as thick as that of the right, while the mitral valve and its chordae tendineae are stronger than the tricuspid valve of the right side. A certain amount of blood clot is found normally in each of the ventricles after death.

Ox

The ox heart shows three ventricular furrows on its surface. Two *ossa cordis*, which are cartilaginous until 4 weeks after birth, develop at the base of the heart in the aortic wall. The ox heart weighs 1.8–2.2 kg. In pregnant cows and in those with a septic infection, it is frequently pale, flabby and friable.

Sheep

There are three ventricular furrows, while in later years, a small *os cordis* may develop on the right side. The heart weighs 85–113 g.

Pig

Only two ventricular furrows are normally present in the pig heart although a rudimentary posterior furrow may be present. The apex is more rounded than in sheep, and the heart cartilage ossified in older animals. The weight is 170–198 g.

Horse

The heart has two ventricular furrows, the aortic cartilage becoming partly ossified in older animals. The average weight is 2.7 kg, although much greater in racehorses; in the thoroughbred horse Eclipse, the heart weighs 6.3 kg.

Portal circulation

The portal circulation is important in the study of the spread of certain parasitic and bacterial infections throughout the body.

The portal vein is formed by two main branches, the gastrosplenic and mesenteric veins which drain the stomach and intestines. The veins also drain blood from the pancreas. Venous blood from these organs is conveyed by the portal vein to the liver. The liver is drained by the hepatic veins which enter the posterior vena cava, wherein the blood is conveyed to the heart.

Bacteria or parasites which gain entry to the portal vein may be arrested within the sinusoids of the liver, but this organ is an imperfect filter and organisms may pass through to the heart and thence to the lungs. For example, hydatid cysts may be found in the lungs and occasionally immature liver flukes in the lungs of cattle and older sheep but not in pigs.

Spleen (melt)

The spleen is not essential to life. In the foetus, it forms red and white cells, lymphocytes being produced during the life of the animal. It also acts as a storage for RBCs and for the destruction of old red cells and platelets. Antibodies are formed in the spleen, which, in certain diseases, for example, anthrax or trypanosomiasis, becomes very enlarged.

Ox (Fig. 2.11)

The spleen of the ox is related to the left dorsal side of the rumen and also to the diaphragm. In the young bovine, it is reddish brown, elongated and slightly convex with rounded edges; lymph follicles are apparent on the cut surface. In the cow, the organ is bluish and flat with sharp edges and rounded extremities; it weighs 0.9–1.3 kg.

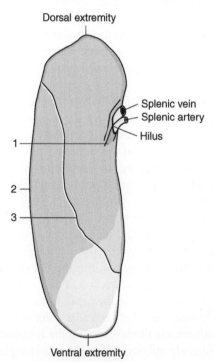

Figure 2.11 Spleen of ox, visceral surface. 1, area of attachment to rumen (non-peritoneal); 2, caudal border; 3, line of peritoneal reflection.

Sheep

The spleen is usually found attached to the pluck, being removed with it in the dressing of the carcase. It is oyster-shaped and soft or elastic to the touch and weighs 56–85 g. In both ox and sheep, the spleen is adherent to the rumen.

Pig

The pig spleen is connected to the greater curvature of the stomach by the serous membrane known as the gastrosplenic omentum. The organ is elongated, tongue-shaped and triangular in cross section, while its under-surface shows well-marked longitudinal ridge to which the omentum is attached; it weighs 113–425 g. The relatively loose attachment of the pig spleen to the stomach often leads to splenic rotation, resulting in torsion and acute swelling of the organ.

Horse

The equine spleen is flat, sickle-shaped and bluish and weighs 453–907 g.

Lymphatic system (Fig. 2.10 and Fig. 2.12)

Lymph is the medium by which oxygen and nutritive matter are transferred from the blood to the body tissues and waste products are removed. Although the blood capillaries approximate to the individual body cells, actual contact is through the lymph. The presence of lymph around the tissue cells is maintained by a slow exudation of fluid through the capillary walls and into the surrounding tissue; this fluid is similar to the plasma of the blood but is thinner, more watery and poorer in protein, which cannot pass readily through the capillary walls.

After the lymph has fulfilled its function of feeding the tissue cells, it is forced by the animal's muscular movements into the finewalled *lymphatics*, which arise as blind-ended vessels in the tissues. These are similar to veins but have thinner walls and more valves; when distended with lymph, they have a characteristic beaded appearance.

Practically, all lymph vessels discharge their contents into the *lymph nodes*, and with rare exceptions, all the lymph throughout the system passes through at least one lymph node before it returns into the blood circulatory system. In every case, the direction of flow of lymph in an organ is from the centre of the organ towards its surface. The lymph nodes consist of a reticular framework of elastic and smooth muscle fibres enclosing the lymphatic tissue which contains lymphocytes. The intestinal lymphatics are the route of absorption of fat from the digestive tract.

The lymphatic vessels conveying lymph to a lymph node are known as *afferent* lymphatics, and the area drained by the particular lymph node is known as its drainage area. An appreciation of the drainage system of lymph nodes is of particular value in the judgement of septic infections and of the tuberculous carcase (Fig. 2.12).

After passing through one or more lymph nodes, where some impurities are removed, the lymph is conveyed by *efferent* lymphatics to discharge eventually into larger lymph-collecting vessels, which all flow towards the heart. The largest of these lymph-collecting vessels is the *thoracic duct*, which commences as a thin-walled dilation about 19 mm in width and is known as the *receptaculum chyli*. This dilation is situated in the abdomen, lying above the aorta at the level of the last dorsal vertebra, and receives lymph from the lumbar and intestinal trunks; it is the main receptacle for the lymph from the posterior part of the body. The thoracic duct is about 6.3 mm in width, passes forwards through the diaphragm, traverses the thorax and opens into the anterior vena cava in the anterior thorax. Lymph from the anterior part of the body is carried towards the heart by two tracheal lymph ducts, which commence at the lateral retropharyngeal lymph nodes and pass down the neck on each side of the trachea and oesophagus; each duct discharges into the jugular vein of its own side.

The size of the lymph nodes varies from that of a pinhead to that of a walnut, though the posterior mediastinal lymph node of the ox may reach a length of 20 cm. Lymph nodes are generally round or oval and somewhat compressed; in the ruminant, they are large and few in number, but in the horse, they occur in large numbers and in clusters. The size of lymph nodes is relatively greater in the young growing animal than in the adult.

The colour of the lymph nodes shows considerable variation and may be white, greyish blue or almost black. The mesenteric lymph nodes of the ox are invariably black, but in the pig, the lymph nodes are lobulated and almost white, with the exception of those of the head and neck which are reddish.

The consistency of the lymph nodes varies in different parts of the body, the nodes of the abdomen being generally softer than those of the thorax. A physiological oedema of the supramammary and iliac lymph nodes will invariably be encountered in the lactating animal.

The response of a lymph node to an irritant is normally rapid, involving enlargement, congestion and possibly tissue breakdown; thus, the size, colour and consistency of the lymph nodes form a valuable guide in the estimation of disease processes in the animal body.

Haemal lymph nodes

These are deep red or almost black in colour, oval in shape and up to the size of a pea but differ from the lymph nodes in their anatomical structure and in the

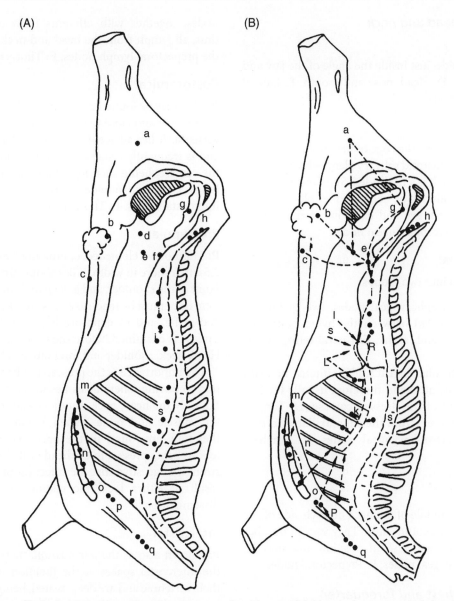

Figure 2.12 Carcase of bullock. (A) Position of lymph nodes: a, popliteal; b, superficial inguinal; c, precrural; d, deep inguinal; e, external iliac; f, internal iliac; g, ischiatic; h, sacral; i, lumbar; i″, renal; m, xiphoid; n, suprasternal; o, presternal; p, prepectoral; q, middle cervical; r, costocervical; s, intercostal. (B) Direction of the lymph flow: l, lymph from intestine; S, lymph from stomach; L, lymph from liver; R, receptaculum chyli; j, lymph from posterior mediastinal lymph node discharging into thoracic duct; k, lymph from bronchial lymph nodes; l, lymph from anterior mediastinal lymph nodes.

absence of afferent and efferent lymphatics. The haemal lymph nodes are supplied by arteries which break up in the gland substance and discharge their blood into tissue spaces; in this respect, these nodes bear a resemblance to the spleen and may, in fact, be described as accessory spleens. Like the spleen, they contain numerous white blood corpuscles together with red blood corpuscles in various stages of disintegration, hence the red colouration of the nodes.

Haemal lymph nodes are numerous in the ox and sheep but are not found in the horse or pig. In cattle, they occur especially along the course of the aorta and in the

subcutaneous fat, while in sheep and lambs, they are most common beneath the peritoneum in the sublumbar region, being larger and more numerous in animals suffering from anaemic and cachectic conditions. The red lymph nodes of the head and neck of the pig are frequently mistaken for the haemal lymph nodes.

Lymph nodes of the ox

P: Position. **D:** Drainage area. **E:** Destination of efferent lymph vessels of node. (Nomenclature varies in different texts, countries, etc.)

Nodes of the head and neck

Submaxillary

P: One on each side, just inside the angle of the jaw and embedded in fat. **D:** Head, nose and mouth. **E:** Lateral retropharyngeal nodes.

Parotid

P: One on each side, on the edge of the masseter muscle, and covered by the parotid salivary gland which must be incised to expose it. It is a flat node 7.5 cm long by 2.5 cm wide and should always be examined in old cows. **D:** Muscles of the head, eye and ear, tongue and cranial cavity. **E:** Lateral retropharyngeal nodes.

Retropharyngeal

These are divided into two groups:

1   The internal retropharyngeal nodes, two to four in number and situated between the hyoid bones. **D:** Pharynx, tongue and larynx. **E:** Lateral retropharyngeal nodes
2   The lateral retropharyngeal nodes situated beneath each wing of the atlas and therefore usually located at the neck end of the dressed carcase. **D:** Tongue and receive efferents from the submaxillary, parotid and internal retropharyngeal nodes. **E:** Tracheal lymph duct

Middle cervical

P: Situated in the middle of the neck on each side of the trachea and often absent in cattle. They vary in number from one to seven and also in position and size. **D:** Lateral retropharyngeal nodes. **E:** Prepectoral nodes.

Nodes of the chest and forequarter (Fig. 2.10 and Fig. 2.12)

Prepectoral

These are known also as the lower cervicals and may be considered anatomically as a continuation of the upper and middle cervical chain. The middle cervical group may, in fact, extend to the upper group or may reach back almost to the prepectorals. **P:** The prepectorals are two to four in number on each side and are embedded in fat along the anterior border of the first rib. The main node of this group is superficially situated about the middle of the first rib and just anterior to it; the haemal lymph nodes are usually present in the fat around this group. The second node of this group is on the same level and just anterior to the main node but is deep-seated and is exposed by making an incision 10 cm long and 5 cm deep through the triangular-shaped scalenus muscle. **D:** Efferents from upper and middle cervical nodes, together with efferents from the prescapular; thus, all lymph from the head and neck passes through the prepectoral lymph nodes. **E:** Thoracic duct.

Costocervical

P: This may be found on the inner side or just anterior to the first rib and close to its junction with the first dorsal vertebra. It lies adjacent to the oesophagus and trachea and is frequently removed with these in the dressing of the carcase, being then found anterior to the heart and lungs. **D:** Neck, shoulder, parietal pleura and first few intercostal nodes. **E:** Thoracic duct.

Prescapular

P: This node is elongated, commonly 7.5–10 cm long and 2.5 cm or more in width. It lies about 10 cm in front of the point of the shoulder, and a deep incision 15 cm long and 5 cm deep must be made to expose it. The node is embedded in fat, and its exposure is greatly facilitated if the carcase is examined before the onset of rigor mortis. **D:** Head, neck, shoulder and forelimb. **E:** Thoracic duct.

The importance of the prescapular lymph node in relation to bovine tuberculosis lies in the fact that it drains not only the head, neck, shoulder and forelimb but also the muscle and bone. When lesions of tuberculosis, therefore, are found in the prescapular node without lesions being present in the head or its lymph nodes, it is strongly suggestive that the infection of the node is the result of either local inoculation or haematogenous dissemination.

Intercostal

P: Known also as the *dorso-costal*, these are situated in the intercostal spaces at the junction of the ribs with their vertebrae and are deep-seated, being covered by the intercostal muscle. Most of these nodes are small, and not all of the spaces may contain nodes. **D:** Muscles of the dorsal region, intercostal muscles, ribs and parietal pleura. **E:** Mediastinal lymph nodes.

Subdorsal

P: This superficial group lies in the fat between the aorta and the dorsal vertebrae. The nodes are irregular in arrangement, varying in length from 12 to 25 mm, and are frequently removed with the lungs in the dressing of the carcase; they may then be found by incising the upper surface of the mediastinal fat between the lungs. In some areas, the thoracic portion of the posterior aorta is left attached, and the subdorsal lymph nodes, which run down on each side of the vessel wall, will then be found on the carcase. The more posterior nodes of the group, no matter how the carcase is dressed, usually remain on the forequarter and can be found by incising the fat below the dorsal vertebrae just anterior to the diaphragm. **D:** The same structures as the intercostals and also the mediastinum, pericardium, diaphragm and efferents from the intercostal lymph nodes. **E:** Thoracic duct.

Suprasternal

P: Known also as the sternocostal, these nodes lie between the costal cartilages and are covered by muscle. They may be exposed by an incision 7.5 cm from and parallel to the cut surface of the sternum and are found at the junction of the internal thoracic vein with a line continuing the posterior border of each rib. The node in the fourth intercostal space is large and readily exposed, but the nodes are not present in every intercostal space. The largest of this group, known as the *presternal* or anterior sternal node, is superficially placed and embedded in fat on the first segment of the sternum. **D:** Diaphragm, abdominal muscles, intercostal muscles, parietal and visceral pleura and peritoneum. **E:** Thoracic duct and prepectoral nodes.

Bronchial (Fig. 2.10)

P: There are two main bronchial nodes, the right and left, together with two smaller nodes. The left bronchial is 4 cm × 2.5 cm in size, often irregular in shape and found close to the left bronchus, being embedded deeply in fat and partly covered by the aorta. The right bronchial is related to the right bronchus, is usually smaller than the left and is partly hidden by the right lung; it is absent in 25% of cases, while in others, two nodes may be found. The middle bronchial node is situated in the middle line above the bifurcation of the trachea but is absent in 50% of cases; a further node, the *apical*, is placed on the accessory bronchus where it enters the apical lobe of the right lung. **D:** Lungs. **E:** The left bronchial node discharges into the thoracic duct, the right bronchial node into the posterior mediastinal node or thoracic duct, and the middle bronchial or apical into the anterior mediastinal nodes. When the right bronchial node is absent, the lymphatics of the diaphragmatic lobe of the right lung discharge into the posterior mediastinal and left bronchial node. A node known as the *inspector's node* is present in 75% of cases and is situated at the junction of the two cardiac lobes of the right lung.

Anterior mediastinal (Fig. 2.10)

P: These are numerous, lying in the mediastinal space anterior to the heart, and are related anatomically to the oesophagus, trachea and anterior aorta. **D:** Heart, pericardium, mediastinum and thoracic wall and receive efferents from the apical and middle bronchial lymph nodes. **E:** Thoracic duct.

Posterior mediastinal (Fig. 2.10)

These nodes are 8–12 in number and situated in the fat along the dorsal wall of the oesophagus. The largest and most posterior of these nodes lies posterior to the heart, being up to 20 cm long and extending almost to the diaphragm; in some cases, this large node is replaced by two smaller ones. **D:** Lungs, diaphragm and, via the diaphragm, the peritoneum, surface of the liver and spleen. They receive efferents from the right bronchial node. **E:** Thoracic duct.

Axillary

P: Known also as the brachial, this node is about 2.5 cm long, covered by the scapula and situated in the muscle external to and about midway along the second rib. **D:** Muscles of shoulder and forelimb. **E:** Prepectoral node.

Xiphoid (ventral mediastinal)

P: Found in the loose fat at the junction of the sternum and diaphragm at the level of the sixth rib and related anatomically to the apex of the heart. This node is absent in 50% of cases. **D:** Pleura, diaphragm and ribs. **E:** Suprasternal lymph nodes.

Nodes of the abdomen and hindquarter (Fig. 2.12)

The position of these nodes is described as if the hindquarters were suspended by the hock in the normal manner.

Lumbar

P: These are situated in the fat covering the lumbar muscles and are related anatomically to the aorta and posterior vena cava. Some of these nodes are superficial, others being embedded in the loin fat; the haemal lymph nodes are common in this region. **D:** Lumbar region and peritoneum. They receive efferent vessels from the internal and external iliac, sacral and popliteal nodes. **E:** Receptaculum chyli.

Portal

P: Known also as the hepatic, these form a group around the portal vein, hepatic artery and bile duct and are covered by the pancreas. Another group, which includes the lymph node draining the pancreas, lies between the edge of the pancreas and the caudate lobe of the liver. The portal nodes vary from 10 to 15 in number. **D:** Liver, pancreas and duodenum. **E:** Receptaculum chyli.

Renal

P: This node belongs in reality to the lumbar group and is found in the fat at the entrance to the kidney. In this position, a split blood vessel is found, and the node can be exposed by making an incision lengthwise through this vessel and continuing the incision 2.5 cm deep into the lumbar suet. **D:** Kidneys and adrenal body. **E:** Receptaculum chyli. The renal lymph nodes vary in size and number.

Mesenteric

P: These comprise a large number of elongated nodes which lie between the peritoneal folds of the mesentery and receive lymph from the intestines. These nodes may be divided into a small duodenal group which drains the duodenum, the efferent lymphatics passing to the portal nodes of the liver and a jejuno-ileal group ranging in number from 10 to 50 and 0.5–12 cm in length. The long nodes form the main chain parallel to and some 5 cm from the intestine, while the small nodes are scattered throughout the mesentery between the small intestine and the colon. **D:** The small intestine (jejunum and ilium). **E:** Receptaculum chyli.

Splenic

Splenic lymph nodes are absent in the ox and sheep. Lymph drained from the spleen passes to the gastric chain of the lymph nodes. Several splenic lymph nodes are present in the horse and pig.

Gastric

P: These are numerous and difficult to group satisfactorily; a number form a chain along the right and left longitudinal grooves of the rumen. **D:** Walls of stomach and spleen. **E:** Receptaculum chyli. The gastric group are rarely incised in meat inspection.

Iliacs

These are situated near the terminal branches of the aorta and are embedded in fat.

Internal iliac P: This may be exposed by an incision level with the junction of the sacrum and the last lumbar vertebrae. Several nodes are present, lying some 18 cm from the vertebrae and 1–5 cm in length. **D:** This node drains the muscle and pelvic viscera, including the muscles of the sublumbar region, pelvis and thigh; the femur, tibia, patella, tarsus and metatarsus; the male and female genital organs; and the kidneys. It receives efferent vessels from the external iliac, precrural, ischiatic and superficial inguinal nodes. **E:** Lumbar lymph nodes and receptaculum chyli.

External iliac P: A single or double node 1–2.5 cm in length and situated laterally to the internal iliac. It lies beneath the external angle of the ilium at the bifurcation of the circumflex iliac artery but is sometimes absent on one or both sides. **D:** Abdominal muscles, sublumbar area, posterior part of the peritoneum and some efferents from the popliteal node. **E:** Internal iliac and lumbar lymph nodes.

Superficial inguinal (male)

P: These lie in the mass of fat about the neck of the scrotum and behind the spermatic cord. **D:** External genitals and adjoining skin area. **E:** Deep inguinal when present or, failing this, the internal iliac.

Supramammary (female)

P: These lie above and behind the udder; there are usually two present on each side, one large and one small, the larger pair, about 7.5 cm in size, approximating to each other and the small pair being found above or in front of the larger pair and 0.5–1.5 cm in size. In the heifer, these nodes may be found on a straight line level with the cut pubic tubercle. **D:** Udder and external genitals. **E:** Deep inguinal when present or internal iliac.

Deep inguinal

P: In the inguinal canal and frequently absent; when absent, the internal iliac functions in its place. **D:** Hindlimb and abdominal wall. **E:** Internal iliac. According to some authors, the deep inguinals are part of the external iliacs.

Ischiatic

P: This lies on the outer aspect of the sacrosciatic ligament and is exposed by a deep incision on a vertical line midway between the posterior part of the ischium and the sacrum. **D:** Posterior pelvic organs and also receives efferents from popliteal node. **E:** Internal iliac.

In many countries in Africa, the ischiatic node is incised on routine post-mortem examination of beef carcases because the bites of the tick *Hyalomma rufipes*, which attaches itself to the perianal region, frequently cause abscess formation.

Sacral

P: These are not constantly present and are unimportant. If present, they are difficult to distinguish from the medial iliac lymph nodes.

Precrural (sub-iliac)

P: This node is known also as the prefemoral and is embedded in fat; it may be exposed by an incision at the edge of the tensor fascia lata, the incision being made about 18 cm down from the apex of this muscle. **D:** Skin, prepuce and superficial muscles. **E:** Internal iliac nodes.

The precrural nodes, draining the umbilicus, should always be palpated in calves and if necessary incised.

Popliteal

P: This is deeply seated in the round of beef and is exposed by a deep incision along the superficial seam or division which connects the ischium and os calcis, the node lying midway between these and 15 cm deep. **D:** Lower part of the leg and foot. **E:** Lumbar and iliac nodes and also ischiatic node.

Lymph nodes of the pig (Fig. 2.13)

Head and neck

The nodes of the head and neck are numerous and somewhat difficult to group satisfactorily. They include the following.

Submaxillary (mandibular)

These lie anterior to the submaxillary salivary gland near to the angle of the jaw and are covered by the lower part of the parotid salivary gland. There are commonly two nodes on each side, one large and one small.

Anterior or upper cervical

Known also as the accessory submaxillary or submandibular, these lie a short distance behind and above the preceding nodes, being separated from them by the submaxillary salivary gland.

Parotid

There are several nodes on each side, which are red in colour, one of the largest being situated just posterior to the masseter muscle of the lower jaw and partly covered by the parotid salivary gland. One or two nodes may be left on the inner side of the jaw after the head is removed.

Prescapular (superficial cervical)

On account of the short neck of the pig, these nodes lie close to the parotid salivary gland, being partly covered by its posterior border. They form an oblique chain which is directed downwards and backwards to the shoulder joint. This chain really includes all the superficial cervical nodes and is best exposed by a long incision, made on the inside of the carcase, from the nape of the neck to the lower border of the neck and just anterior to the shoulder joint. The prescapular lymph nodes in the pig receive lymph from the submaxillary, parotid and upper cervical nodes and thus may become tuberculous as a result of primary infection of the lymph nodes of the head. Enlargement of the prepectoral node in pigs may occur as a result of arthritic changes in the forelimbs.

Other nodes

Precrural (sub-iliac)

In adult pigs, this is up to 5 cm in length and 2.5 cm in width and is most easily exposed by an incision through the peritoneal aspect of the carcase deep into the fat and 2.5 cm in front of the stifle joint, the incision being made at right angles to the vertebral column.

Popliteal

When present, these are superficial but are absent in 50% of cases. A small subcutaneous node, known as the hock node or Hartenstein's gland, can constantly be found and is superficially placed on the posterior aspect of the limb about a hand's breadth above the tuber calcis.

Gastric

These and the pancreatic nodes are situated on the lesser curvature of the stomach.

Bronchial

In addition to the right and left bronchial, this group includes one on the bifurcation of the trachea and another at the apical bronchus of the right lung. The posterior mediastinal nodes are rudimentary or absent.

Portal

Several nodes are present about the portal vein, the largest being about 2.5 cm long. The portal lymph nodes may be removed during evisceration of the carcase and can then be found on the mesentery beneath the pancreas or in the fat attached to the lesser curvature of the stomach.

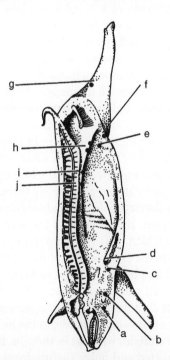

Figure 2.13 Side of pork showing position of lymph nodes: a, submaxillary; b, anterior or upper cervical; c, prepectoral; d, presternal; e, precrural; f, superficial inguinal; g, hock node; h, iliac; i, lumbar; j, renal.

Urogenital system

Urinary organs

Two kidneys, two ureters, bladder and urethra.

Genital organs

Female two ovaries, two uterine (fallopian) tubes, uterus, vagina, vulva, clitoris and mammary glands.

Male two testes and epididymes, two vasa deferentia, seminal glands, prostate, bulbourethral (Cowper's) glands, urethra and penis.

Kidney

In addition to their functions in the excretion of urine and in acid–base balance, the kidneys produce two hormones, renin and erythropoietic factor. Renin acts in the formation of a blood peptide which increases blood pressure and stimulates the secretion of aldosterone, a hormone controlling the reabsorption of sodium. The erythropoietic factor stimulates the formation of a protein which increases the red cell production in the bone marrow.

Ox (Fig. 2.14)

The kidneys are reddish brown and composed of 15–25 lobes which are fused at their deeper portions; each lobe terminates in a blunt process or papilla, visible when the kidney is split. When the rumen is empty, the left kidney lies to the left of the vertebral column, but as the rumen becomes filled, it propels the kidney towards the right side of the body, though injury due to pressure on the ureter is usually avoided. This orientation of the left kidney is rendered possible by its loose attachment to the lumbar region. The left kidney, by reason of its mobility, is roughly three-sided and of a somewhat twisted appearance, but the right kidney has a more regular, elliptical outline. The weight of each kidney is 283–340 g.

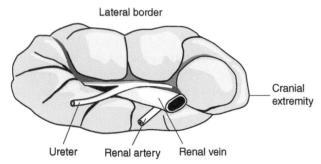

Lateral border

Cranial extremity

Ureter   Renal artery   Renal vein

Figure 2.14 Right kidney of ox, ventral surface. Organ hardened *in situ*. Fat has been removed from fissures between lobes.

Sheep and goat

The kidneys are dark brown, bean-shaped and unlobulated and possess a single renal papilla. As in the ox, the left kidney of the sheep and goat is freely movable. Each kidney weighs 56–85 g.

Pig (Fig. 2.15)

The kidneys are smooth, bean-shaped and reddish brown but thinner and flatter than in the other food animals; 10–12 renal papillae are present internally. The weight of each kidney is 85–170 g. In the pig, the bladder is large with a long neck; the ureters enter posteriorly in the neck region. This predisposes the animal to bilateral hydronephrosis, because, when full, the bladder hangs down into the abdominal cavity and the long neck presses against the pubis, thus closing the ureter openings and interfering with urination.

Horse

The right kidney is triangular- or heart-shaped, and the left is bean-shaped and longer than broad. The weight of each kidney is 680 g.

Reproductive system

Uterus (Fig. 2.16)

Cow

The uterus consists of a small body, less than 2.5 cm long, and two cornua or horns, about 38 cm long. The uterus of the cow and ewe has characteristic cotyledons on the mucous membrane of the body and uterine horns; these are oval prominences, about 100 in all, and in the non-gravid bovine uterus are about 1.5 × 0.5 cm. During pregnancy, and as the foetus develops, the cotyledons hypertrophy, becoming pitted or sponge-like, and then measure up to 10–12.5 cm in length and 4 cm in width. Evidence as to whether a slaughtered female is a heifer or a cow may be established by opening each uterine horn and cutting transversely through the wall, including the diameter of a cotyledon. Generally, in the uterus of a heifer, the cotyledons are surrounded by a shallow moat which usually disappears in the cow. The blood vessels in the exposed wall of the uterus of the cow are contorted and bulge from the surface. In the heifer, the blood vessels can be seen clearly but do not bulge and show little contortion. The blood vessels in the cotyledon are the most valuable guide; in the heifer, they are very fine and straight, whereas in the cow, they are very distinct, contorted and bulge slightly from the cut surface. This method assumes that the cotyledons enlarge

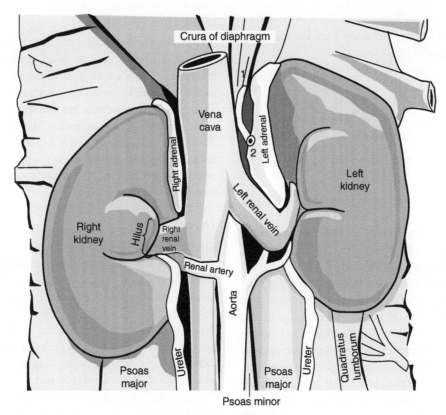

Figure 2.15 Kidneys of pig *in situ*, ventral view. 1, hepatic artery; 2, splenic artery.

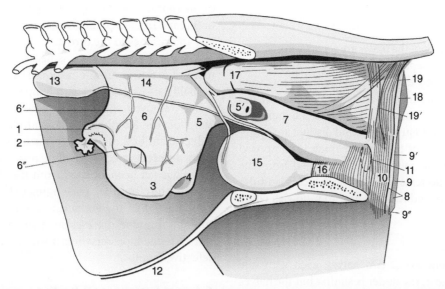

Figure 2.16 Lateral view of genital organs and adjacent structures of mare. 1, left ovary; 2, fallopian tube; 3, left horn of uterus; 4, right horn of uterus; 5, body of uterus [5′, cervix]; 6, broad ligament of uterus [6′ and 6″ show the extent of the broad ligament of the uterus]; 7, vagina; 8, vulva; 9, rim and commissures of vulva [9′ and 9″ show the extent of the rim and commissures of vulva]; 10, constrictor muscle of vulva; 11, vestibular bulb; 12, abdominal wall; 13, left kidney; 14, left ureter; 15, bladder; 16, urethra; 17, rectum; 18, anus; 19 and 19′ are the posterior and anterior of the anal sphincter muscle.

if the animal is in calf and regress in the non-pregnant uterus, that is, that the animal must have been at least 3½ months or longer in calf.

Ewe

The *uterine horns* are relatively long, the cotyledons being circular, pigmented and much smaller than in the cow, while in advanced pregnancy, the centre of each is cupped or umbilicated.

Gilt and sow

The *uterine horns* are very long and arranged in coils. The mucous membrane has no cotyledons but is arranged in numerous thin longitudinal folds. The *ovaries* are rounded with an irregularly lobulated surface. The sow and gilt carcase may be differentiated not only by the developmental condition of the udder and teats but also by examination of the uterine arteries. In the sow, the *udders* are enlarged, and in the broad ligaments of the uterine horns, the peripheral branches of the uterine middle arteries are torturous owing to pregnancy. In the gilt, these arterial vessels are less apparent and almost straight. Characteristic histological changes also take place in the uterine arteries during and after pregnancy; there is hyperplasia of the elastic fibres in the intima and media of the vessel wall, the intima is hypertrophied, and the internal elastic lamina is split into two or more layers. Similar changes can be observed in the arteries supplying the ovary.

Udder

Cow

The right and left sides of the udder are separated anatomically by a tendinous septum. Although a strong septum does not exist between the fore- and hindquarters of the same side, all four quarters are anatomically distinct, and injection of differently coloured fluids into the four teats shows that they each drain separate and distinct areas.

The smooth udder of the heifer, which is composed almost entirely of fat, must be distinguished from the pendulous fleshy udder of the cow in which glandular tissue predominates and which is grey to yellowish white in colour.

Ewe and goat

The udder is composed of two halves, each with one small teat. In the goat, the udder is similar but the halves are more pendulous and the teats are more strongly developed and directed forwards.

Sow

There are 10–16 mammary glands, arranged in two parallel rows; each possesses a flat triangular teat, and the glandular substance appears whitish red on section.

Endocrine system

The *endocrine* or *ductless glands* (thyroid, parathyroids thymus, adrenals and gonads, i.e. testes and ovaries) produce secretions or hormones which pass directly into the bloodstream to act on another organ or tissue. The liver and pancreas are both endocrine and exocrine glands, each possessing ducts, and are usually described with the digestive system. (*Exocrine* glands such as the sweat, mammary and lachrymal glands pass their secretions along ducts to the surface of the body.)

Thymus

The thymus is pinkish white and distinctly lobulated and constitutes the *true sweetbread*. It consists of two portions; the thoracic portion (heart bread) is rich in fat and roughly the shape of the palm of the hand in the ox and lies in the thoracic cavity, extending back to the third rib where it contacts the base of the heart; the second portion (neck bread) is poor in fat and consists of two lobes joined at their base and extending up the neck on either side of the trachea, diverging and diminishing in size as they pass up the neck and reaching almost to the thyroid gland.

In the *calf*, the thymus is at its largest at 5–6 weeks, when it weighs 453–680 g, but gradually atrophies. By the onset of sexual maturity, little of the cervical portion remains. It is very small in 3-year-old cattle, but a vestige of the thoracic portion may be seen in cows even after 8 or 9 years. In the *pig*, the thymus is large and greyish yellow and reaches to the throat.

In early life, the thymus is necessary for the development of certain immune responses and antibodies. It is probably also associated with lymphocyte production. If this is removed shortly after birth, the production of lymphocytes, lymphoid tissue and plasma cells is much reduced; antibodies are not formed; and skin grafts, even from different species, are not rejected. Since no hormone has yet been isolated from the thymus, it should probably be classified as belonging to the circulatory system rather than the endocrine system. In animals, certain autoimmune diseases such as haemolytic anaemia and systemic lupus erythematosus are associated with a defective thymus.

Adrenal (suprarenal) bodies

In the *ox*, the adrenal glands are related to the two kidneys and lie anterior to them. The left adrenal body is in contact with the dorsal sac of the rumen, though it does not rotate with the left kidney when the rumen is distended. After dressing of the carcase, portions of the right adrenal body may sometimes be found attached to the posterior aspect of the liver or sometimes to the central muscular portion of the diaphragm.

In the *sheep*, both the adrenals are bean-shaped, but the left is not in contact with its kidney. In the *pig*, the adrenals are long and narrow, each lying on the inner aspect of the kidney.

The adrenals are reddish brown in colour, and a section of them reveals a well-marked cortex and medulla.

Testicles (testes)

In the *bull*, the testes have an elongated oval outline; they are about 12.5 cm long and weigh 283–340 g. The epididymis is narrow but is closely attached to the testicle along its posterior border. In the *ram*, the testicles are large, pear-shaped, and more rounded than in the ox, being 10 cm long and 255–283 g in weight. In the *boar*, the testicles are very large and irregularly elliptical, while the epididymis is well developed and forms a blunt conical projection at both ends of the testicle.

The testes or male gonads have two functions: the production of spermatozoa and the production of *testosterone*, the main hormone responsible for the development of male secondary sexual characteristics.

Ovaries

The ovaries, in addition to producing ova, secrete three hormones: *oestradiol, progesterone* and *relaxin*. Oestradiol, formed in the ovarian follicles, promotes female secondary sexual characteristics and sexual behaviour. Progesterone is formed in the corpus luteum, and during pregnancy, it prevents ovulation by inhibiting the secretion of luteinising hormone. Relaxin, also produced by the corpus luteum, relaxes the pelvic ligaments during parturition. The ovaries also control cyclical changes in the reproductive system which ensure development of breeding seasons when weather conditions, temperature, food, etc. are suitable.

Collection and yield of glands (Table 2.4)

Although valuable pharmaceutical products are prepared from the ductless glands, it is only when there is a very large weekly kill that their collection becomes an economic proposition.

Successful utilisation of glands entails careful handling from the moment the animal is killed. The entire glands should be removed immediately, freed from surrounding fat or tissue and, according to the variety of gland, either frozen to a temperature of −10°C or placed in acetone. Cutting into the substance of a gland significantly reduces the hormone yield, and it should not be soaked in water. In the case of the pancreas, care must be taken to leave the gland whole and not to remove adjoining portions of the duodenum whereby trypsin might be liberated and the insulin destroyed.

Table 2.4 Yield of glands used in medicine

Gland	No. of animals required to produce 500 g of fresh material	No. of glands required per 500 g finished product
Pituitary, whole (cattle)	199	1 100
Ovary (cow)	39	210
Ovary (sow)	50	298
Parathyroid (cattle)	243	1 990
Suprarenal (cattle)	22	127
Pancreas (beef)	2	26 500
Pancreas (calf)	18	8 830
Pancreas (pig)	11	132 500
Testis (bull)	1.5	7
Thyroid (cattle)	22	100 110

Skin

The skin or common integument acts as a protective covering for the body and merges at the natural orifices with the mucous membranes of the digestive, respiratory and reproductive systems. With its covering of hair, wool, feathers, nails or horn, it acts also as a temperature-regulating mechanism, and since it contains many sensory nerve endings, it protects the body against injury and is thus an important sense organ.

Sweat (sudoriferous) and sebaceous glands are found in the skin, the former involved in temperature and tissue fluid regulation and the latter secreting sebum which prevents loss of fluid and in some species playing an important part in the sexual life of the animal.

The *mammary glands* are modified skin glands associated in function with the reproductive system.

Horns

Estimation of the age of cattle by means of the horns entails counting the number of rings on the animal's horns, but these rings must not be confused with the small wrinkles situated at the root of the horn which are an indication that the animal has been ill fed during its growth. The first ring appears at about 2 years, and thereafter, one ring is added annually so that the age in years in cattle equals the number of rings plus one. In cows, it is not unusual for the rings to be removed by scraping, and greater accuracy as to the age may be obtained by examination of the incisor teeth or carcase bones.

Muscular system

The muscular system is composed of skeletal (voluntary, striated), cardiac (involuntary, striated) and smooth (involuntary, non-striated) muscle. Smooth muscle is found in certain organs, glands and blood vessels and responds to the demands of the autonomic nervous system.

Skeletal muscle along with associated connective tissue and intermuscular fat forms the flesh or butcher meat and represents 25–45% of the animal's live weight.

There are some 300 muscles in the *animal* body which, despite vast differences in the size, shape and function of each, all possess the same basic structure. Muscles are made up of numerous tiny spindle-shaped multinucleated *muscle cells* or *fibres*, each encased in a thin membrane, the *sarcolemma*. Groups of muscle cells joined by a loose connective tissue (*endomysium*) form bundles sheathed in the connective tissue *perimysium* and fatty deposits. The connective tissue *epimysium* covers the complete muscle.

Connective tissue

Connective tissue is present in two forms in the animal body, white and yellow. A typical example of the white connective tissue is the *fascia* connecting the muscular bundles. The main constituent of the white connective tissue is *collagen*, which is converted into gelatin by boiling. The yellow connective tissue, as seen in the yellow fascia covering the abdominal muscles and in the *ligamentum nuchae*, consists of elastin, which cannot be softened by boiling.

Fat

Fat develops in connection with the connective tissue and has an important influence on both the odour and flavour of the different meats. It varies in consistency according to its composition, which is again controlled by the species, the feeding method and the site of the fat in the carcase.

On a commercial scale, edible fat is converted into oleo oil and oleo stearin for margarine manufacture; oleo stearin is also used for soap and candle manufacture and is mixed with cooking fats to harden them. Inedible fat is used for the production of lubricants, soap, candles and glycerine and as a binder for animal feed.

Determination of age by dentition

Determination of age and sex is important in the keeping of records of disease found on routine examination and also in the recognition of the carcase of the cow, ewe and sow, animals in which dangerous affections of a septic nature are most likely to occur. It is also of value where a system of mutual insurance of animals intended for slaughter exists and an inspector may be called upon to pass expert judgement as to the age and sex of any animal

Table 2.5 Dental formula for the ox, sheep and goat

Temporary (deciduous) teeth	
Upper	0 0 3
	2 (I C P) = 20
Lower	3 1 3
Permanent teeth	
Upper	0 0 3 3
	2 (I C P M) = 32
Lower	3 1 3 3

C, canine; I, Incisor; M, molar; P, premolar.

Table 2.6 Dental formula for the pig

Temporary (deciduous) teeth	
Upper	3 1 3
	2 (I C P) = 28
Lower	3 1 3
Permanent teeth	
Upper	3 1 4 3
	2 (I C P M) = 44
Lower	3 1 4 3

C, canine; I, Incisor; M, molar; P, premolar.

Table 2.7 Dental formula for the horse

Temporary (deciduous) teeth	
Upper	3 0 3
	2 (I C P) = 24
Lower	3 0 3
Permanent teeth	
Upper	3 1 3(4) 3
	2 (I C P M) = 40 (42)
Lower	3 1 3 3

C, canine; I, Incisor; M, molar; P, premolar.

in dispute. Where meat is supplied to public institutions, there is the possibility of the substitution of cow meat for that of bullocks or heifers or for the substitution of ewe mutton for that of lambs or young sheep. Here again, the judgement of the inspector will be of value.

In the food animals, age may be estimated with reasonable accuracy from the teeth (Table 2.5, Table 2.6, Table 2.7 and Table 2.8), from the horns of cattle or from the carcase bones.

Teeth

Ox

The age is estimated by the period at which the permanent incisor teeth erupt and come into wear; these periods are subject to variation, depending on sex, breed and method of feeding.

Table 2.8 Ages at which the permanent incisors appear

	First pair	Second pair	Third pair	Fourth pair
Ox	1½–2 years	2–2 years	3 years	3½–4 years
Sheep	1½–1½ years	1½–2 years	2½–3 years	3½–4 years
Pig	1 year	16–20 months	8–10 months	Canines 9–10 months
Horse	2½ years	3½ years	4½ years	Canines 4–5 years

The corner pair of permanent incisors is subject to the greatest variation in the time of eruption, and well-bred cattle or animals that are well fed and well housed tend to erupt their teeth earlier than scrub animals or those that are poorly fed and poorly housed. In pedigree cattle, the corner incisors may appear soon after completion of the 3rd year, and in bulls, they are not uncommonly present at 2 years and 10 months.

The dental formulae for the temporary and permanent teeth are shown in Table 2.5. The upper and lower figures correspond to the teeth of the upper and lower jaw. After the permanent incisor teeth have erupted, the degree of wear on their cutting surface and the amount of neck visible above the gums are a guide to the animal's age. The neck of the central pair of incisors is perceptible at the 6th year and that of the lateral centrals at 7 years, of the laterals at 8 years, and of the corner incisors at 9 years. Subsequent to this, the incisor teeth are small and much worn, and it is then possible to confuse an animal 1½ years of age, and therefore possessing all its milk incisors, with an animal of about 10 years, but this can be avoided by recognition of the exposure of the roots of the teeth in the older animal due to shrinkage of the gums and projection of the roots from the alveolar sockets.

Sheep

The milk incisors in sheep are all present at birth or shortly after and remain until the animal is 1 year old. Where sheep are fed on turnips, however, a number of the temporary incisors may be broken off before the animal is 1 year old.

A notch develops between the central pair of incisors at 6 years of age. The formula for the temporary and permanent dentition in sheep is identical with that in cattle.

Goat

It is generally accepted that up to 4 years of age, the goat is as many years old as it has pairs of permanent incisor teeth. Thus, a goat in which the last pair of permanent incisors has erupted may be estimated as 4 years old.

Pig

The period of eruption of temporary and permanent teeth in pigs is subject to considerable variation, and dentition is not a really satisfactory or accurate guide to the animal's age. Estimation of the age in pigs is only likely to be necessary in the case of show animals in connection with their eligibility for particular age classes. There is variation in the figures quoted by various authorities as to the ages at which the permanent incisors appear in the various animals. Sisson and Grossman (1975) give the figures shown in Table 2.8.

Determination of sex

Cattle

Differentiation may be established between the carcase of the bull, stag, bullock, heifer and cow.

Bull

The outstanding characteristic in the bull carcase is the massive development of the muscles of the neck and the shoulder, with the forequarter, except in well-bred animals, being better fleshed than the hindquarter. This development of the crest is diagnostic in bulls, and in some American packing houses, the funicular portion of the ligamentum nuchae is cut at its insertion to the dorsal vertebrae, the effect being to make the carcase approximate more in appearance to that of the bullock.

In the dressing of the bull carcase, the testicles and spermatic cord are removed, leaving an open external inguinal ring partly covered by scanty scrotal fat. The pelvic cavity is narrow and can be spanned with the hand, while the pelvic floor (ischiopubic symphysis) is angular and the pelvic tubercle strongly developed. The bulbocavernosus muscle, often referred to as the erector and retractor penis muscle, is well developed, and the cut adductor, or gracilis muscle, is triangular in shape; in young bulls, however, the posterior portion of this muscle is not covered with fat, and the gracilis muscle therefore appears bean-shaped. The muscle of young bulls is light or brick red in colour and similar to that of the bullock, but in older bulls, it is dark red, dry and poor in fat.

In some European countries and the northern countries of South America, cattle are rarely castrated, and it is the custom in dressing the carcase to leave the testicles attached to the hindquarters. These organs are much in demand by the population, many of whom regard them as an aphrodisiac.

Stag

If the male bovine is castrated later in life, at perhaps a year old, it will have developed certain bullish characteristics, the chief of which is the strong development of the muscles of the neck and shoulder. Such animals are known as stags and, except for the muscular development of the forequarter, differ little in appearance or quality from the normal bullock.

Bullock (steer)

The muscles of the neck and crest are not so strongly developed as in the bull, but fat is more evenly distributed over the carcase and is particularly abundant in the pelvic cavity; the scrotal fat is abundant and completely occludes the external inguinal ring. The pelvic cavity is narrow and can be spanned with the hand, but although the pelvic floor is angular and the pubic tubercle is prominent, these characteristics are not so marked as in the bull carcase.

The posterior or ischial portion of the gracilis muscle, which presents a triangular appearance, is covered with fascia and fat, while there is a well-marked bulbocavernosus muscle, though this is less strongly developed than in the bull. Bullock flesh is lighter in colour than bull flesh and has a brick red colour with a shiny, marbled appearance due to the presence of intermuscular fat.

Heifer

In the dressing of the heifer carcase, the udder remains on each side of beef and is characterised by its smooth and regular convexity and, on section, by the predominance of fat and lack of evidence of glandular tissue. The absence of bulbocavernosus muscle may be noted, and a useful feature in distinguishing the forequarter of the heifer or cow from that of the bullock is the enlargement at the end of the foreshank (radius). In the cow or heifer, the bone is slim and rather straight, but in the bullock, it is markedly enlarged. In the heifer or cow, remains of the broad ligament of the uterus are apparent on the inner abdominal wall, about a hand's breadth below the angle of the haunch.

Cow

The cow carcase is more slender and less symmetrical than that of the bull or bullock and shows a long tapering neck, a wide chest cavity, a curved back and prominent hips. The pelvic cavity is wide and can scarcely be spanned with the hand, while the pelvic floor is thin, only slightly arched, and the pubic tubercle is only slightly developed. The exposed gracilis muscle is crescentic or bean-shaped, but no bulbocavernosus muscle is present. The udder, except occasionally in animals which have had only one calf, is removed, leaving a triangular ragged space on the outer aspect of the abdominal wall. In the cow, both external fat and internal fat are irregularly distributed and yellowish in colour.

Calf

In the dressed bobby calf, the male may be recognised by the presence of testicles and the open external inguinal ring. A transverse cut with a knife just above the pubic tubercle will expose the root of the penis. In the heifer calf, the rudimentary udder remains on the carcase.

Sheep

Ram

The carcase has strong muscular development of the forequarter, the inguinal rings are open, and the scrotal or cod fat is sparse or absent.

Wether

The carcase is usually well proportioned with evenly distributed fat and abundant, lobulated cod fat. The root of the penis can be exposed by a transverse section with the knife above the pubic tubercle and in the wether is no thicker than an ordinary pencil.

Gimmer

The carcase is characterised by its symmetrical shape and the presence of a smooth convex udder.

Ewe

The carcase is angular in shape, with long thin neck and poor legs. The udder is brown and spongy and never sets; it is removed in dressing, leaving a roughened area on the outer abdominal wall, though portions of the supramammary lymph nodes frequently remain on the carcase.

Differentiating features of the carcases of the sheep and goat are shown in Table 2.9.

Table 2.9 Differentiation of carcases of sheep and goat

Feature	Sheep	Goat
Back and withers	Round and well fleshed	Sharp, little flesh
Thorax	Barrel-shaped	Flattened laterally
Tail	Fairly broad	Thin
Radius	1½ times length of metacarpus	Twice as long as metacarpus
Scapula	Short and broad. Superior spine, bent back and thickened	Possesses distinct neck. Spine straight and narrow
Sacrum	Lateral borders thickened in form of rolls	Lateral borders thin and sharp
Flesh	Pale red and fine in texture	Dark red coarse with goaty odour. Sticky subcutaneous tissue which may have adherent goat hairs

Pigs

Differentiation must be established between the carcase of the boar, hog, gilt and sow.

Boar

The boar possesses an oval, strongly developed area of cartilage over the shoulder region which may become calcified in old boars and is known as the *shield*. The scrotum is removed in the dressing of the carcase, the area of removal being apparent on the inside of the thigh. The cut gracilis muscle is triangular, while the root of the penis will be present on one of the sides when the carcase is split and a strongly developed bulbocavernosus muscle will then be apparent. Strong, curved canine teeth (the tusks) are present in the boar.

Castration of the adult boar produces an animal known as a *stag*, which is both heavier and fatter and commands a higher price than the boar carcase. Stag pigs show some reduction in the density of the shield as a result of castration, but as both boars and stags may be used only for manufacturing purposes, being skinned and boned out, this reduction of the shield is not of great importance, and the chief advantage is the diminution of the boar odour.

Hog

The differentiation of the hog and gilt carcases frequently presents difficulty, as teats are present in both male and female pigs, though in the male they are small and underdeveloped. Evidence of castration in the hog is seen as two puckered, depressed scars, and in both the hog and the boar, there is evidence of the removal of the preputial sac. The belly fat on one side of the abdominal incision is grooved, and on the floor of this incision, the retractor penis muscle can be seen, which is long, thin and pale red in colour. When the carcase is split, remains of the bulbocavernosus muscle can be seen, while the gracilis muscle is covered with connective and fatty tissue.

Gilt

In the gilt, the space left below the tail after removal of the anus and vulva is greater than in the hog, the abdominal incision is straight and uninterrupted, and the cut surface of the gracilis muscle is bean-shaped. In sows, there is greater development of the udders and teats, and though canine teeth are present in the female pig, they do not develop.

Horse and ox differentiation

Carcases of the horse and ox may be differentiated by the following details:

1 In the horse, the unusual length of the sides is noticeable, together with the great muscular development of the hindquarters.

2 The thoracic cavity is longer in the horse; this animal possesses 18 pairs of ribs, whereas the ox has 13 pairs.

3 The ribs in the horse are narrower but more markedly curved.

4 The superior spinous processes of the first six dorsal vertebrae are more markedly developed in the horse and are less inclined posteriorly.

5 In the forequarter, the ulna of the horse extends only half the length of the radius; in the ox, it is extended and articulates with the carpus.

6 In the hindquarter, the femur of the ox possesses no third trochanter; the fibula is only a small pointed projection, but in the horse, it extends two-thirds the length of the tibia.

7 In the horse, the last three lumbar transverse processes articulate with each other, the sixth articulating in a similar manner with the sacrum. They do not articulate in the ox.

8 The horse carcase shows considerable development of soft, yellow fat beneath the peritoneum, especially in the gelding and mare, but in the stallion, the fat is generally of a lighter colour and almost white. In the ox, the kidney fat is always firmer, whiter and more abundant than in the horse.

9 Horse flesh is dark bluish red, beef lacking the bluish tinge. Horse meat has a pronounced sweet taste and well-defined muscle fibres.

Debasement of food (adulteration and substitution)

The EU Standing Committee on the Food Chain and Animal Health was established following the adoption of Regulation (EC) No. 178/2002 which set out the general principals and requirements of food law in the EU.

The Food Standards Agency is responsible in the United Kingdom for food safety and standards under the Food Standards Act 1999.

Under the Food Safety Act 1990 (as amended), it is an offence to sell any food which is not of the nature or substance or quality demanded by the purchaser.

The term '*wholesome*' is defined as 'promoting or conducive to good health or well-being'. It was recognised many centuries ago that food must be sound and entirely fit for human consumption. Meat must be derived from healthy animals reared and slaughtered under high standards of welfare and hygiene, and their products processed with due attention to cleanliness.

Continuous control of operations from livestock production to the consumer's home is essential if a safe quality product is to be created and enjoyed. Regrettably, many opportunities exist from the farm to retail outlet for adulteration, accidental or malicious, and misrepresentation to occur.

The chief substitutions of inferior flesh for that which is more highly valued are those of horse for beef, goat for lamb, cat for rabbit and, previously, rabbit for poultry. Another form is the replacement of steer and heifer meat of high quality with lower-quality cow and bull beef. The use of *C. bovis*-infected meat which has been refrigerated to replace Grade A heifer and steer beef is not unknown, and the perennial use of the word 'lamb', when in fact mutton is being sold, is yet another form of substitution and deception.

In recent times, kangaroo meat has been imported from Australia into Britain and the United States and has been used in the United Kingdom in the manufacture of meat pies, pasties and beef burgers, on occasions along with the inclusion of condemned meat.

While substitution can, and does, occur at the carcase and meat cut stage, it is when meat is in a comminuted form that adulteration most often takes place. Using modern technology, production techniques are used to create debasement at a very sophisticated level. This pernicious practice creates great problems for the food analyst and enforcement agencies, besides being a health threat for the consuming public.

That it is not a new practice is illustrated by the introduction to a standard text on food law, Bell and O'Keefe's *Sale of Food and Drugs*, which states, 'The act of debasing a food or drug with the object of passing it off as genuine, of the substitution of an inferior article for a superior one to the detriment of the purchaser, whether done in fraud or negligence, appears to be as old as trade'.

The high price of meat, the wide range of proteins of an inferior nature which can be used, the processed form of the product, the analytical difficulties presented and the economic considerations all appeal to the unscrupulous manufacturer.

Ingredients used

Many different types of non-meat proteins and animal-based proteins are used in an attempt to disguise the true meat content on analysis. These ingredients are often referred to in the trade as 'meat extenders' or 'meat substitutes', which can, of course, be used legitimately. It is their illegal use which results in fraud.

Non-meat proteins include vegetable protein, for example, soya bean, which can be given a 'texture' simulating a meat appearance and cereal.

Cereal is an ingredient which is sometimes added to 'all-meat products' and has the ability to absorb water, giving the product a drier appearance more like its natural form, besides affecting the initial analytical determination, depending on the type of cereal used.

The consumption of certain forms of cereal adversely affects the health of persons suffering from coeliac disease, a condition in which the mucosa of the small intestine becomes abnormal owing to contact with dietary gluten, a reserve protein found in wheat, barley, rye and probably oats. The undeclared presence of cereal probably therefore has a serious relevance.

Animal-based proteins often include those parts of the carcase which are of low value and only some of which are legally defined as 'meat', for example, pork rind, bone protein, urea, dried blood and plasma. While there can be no objection to their inclusion, it is the excessive extent of usage, in amounts far in excess of that naturally associated with the type of meat involved, which constitutes abuse and fraud. On occasions, pork rind is incorporated into a product in which there is no pork flesh present.

Rind may be cooked with water, emulsified with milk protein or vegetable proteins or dehydrated, ground and rehydrated (using as much as four times its own weight of water) before being incorporated into a sausage or 'meat' product.

Bone protein or *ossein* is extracted from animal bones. Like rind, it is an incomplete protein but, hydrated with four parts of water, is used to replace a similar weight of proper meat, yet another disguise to the true meat content of the product.

Urea, a natural nitrogenous waste product found in the urine of animals and man, can also be manufactured from ammonia and carbon dioxide by heating under pressure. It has no nutritional value at all and is normally used as a fertiliser and animal feed additive. Very soluble in water, its presence in a meat product for human consumption adds nitrogen and thereby increases the 'protein' calculation.

Dried blood and plasma are normally used for animal feed, pet food or fertiliser or are discharged as effluent, only a small amount being consumed as black puddings. There can be no objection to the proper inclusion, after suitable treatment, of sterile blood and plasma in meat products, provided their presence is declared and they are not used in lieu of real meat. Rehydrated with water, blood and plasma have the effect of disguising the true meat content for the food analyst.

Water is a natural constituent of meat, varying in amount according to its age, method of handling, species, form of refrigeration, environmental factors, etc. In today's technology of curing, more pickle than is necessary to effect a proper cure is used. Increased water uptake of meat has been shown to be a property of the myofibrils (which are involved in muscle contraction), which make up about 70% of lean meat. In addition to excess cure, polyphosphate is also added to the curing solution and ensures that only minimal water loss occurs at the cooking stage. Tumbling or massaging of the cured meat enables the curing solution to be more thoroughly absorbed. The end result is a product (cooked ham or shoulder) which contains added water in the form of curing solution. While consumers probably on the whole prefer moist ham, there must obviously be a limit to the water content of cured meats.

Food tampering

Malicious tampering with food has become a major concern for food companies and authorities. The display of various kinds of products on supermarket and other shelves is an opportunity for the criminal to introduce deleterious materials on and into food, usually for purposes of extortion. Attacks have occurred on meat companies and butchers' shops, although the main forms of food product involved have been packaged entities other than meat. Nevertheless, the threat to meat and meat products is very real, mainly because of the animal connection. Even though most of the threats are bogus, panic and fear are created, and with media publicity involvement, there is a resulting loss of consumer confidence, institution of laboratory tests and recall and destruction of product, all of which entail much monetary loss.

Control measures include close liaison with police authorities, the creation of an emergency management team and plan, the establishment of a security system, alerting of all staff to this menace, the appointment of a public relations officer to deal with the media, formulation of a recall plan, liaison with independent laboratories and the use of tamper-proof packaging where appropriate.

Reference

Sisson, S. and Grossman, J.D. (1975) *Anatomy of the Domestic Animals*, 5th edn, W. B. Saunders, Philadelphia.

Further reading

Varman, A. and Sutherland, J.M. (1995) *Meat and Meat Products, Technology, Chemistry and Microbiology*, Chapman & Hall, London.

3

Meat establishment construction and equipment

Since the cost of providing and maintaining an abattoir is very high, it is essential at the outset to ensure that there is a need for a new establishment and that it will operate close to maximum throughput. It is a common mistake for farming entrepreneurs to assume that there is a ready profit available when they compare the price per kilogram paid by a slaughterhouse for a live animal to the retail price of meat and meat products.

The overall number and siting of abattoirs in any country should be geared closely to the demands of livestock production. This should be balanced with a desire to ensure animal transport times are kept to a minimum and with a requirement for facilities to deal with on-farm emergency slaughter animals.

Site

A suitable site for an abattoir should have the following facilities:

1 Mains water and electricity supply (daily usage of water can be in excess of 1000 l/tonne dressed carcase weight for cattle, 3000 for sheep, 6000 for pigs).
2 Mains sewerage.
3 Contiguity with uncongested transport systems, close to motorway access.
4 Proximity with public transport, for employees.
5 Proximity to supply of varied labour.
6 Freedom from pollution from other industries' odours, dust, smoke, ash, etc.
7 Ability to separate 'clean' and 'dirty' areas and access.
8 Remoteness from local housing and other development to avoid complaints about noise and smell.
9 Good availability of stock nearby.

10 Ground suitable for good foundations including piling and freedom from flooding.
11 Sufficient size for possible future expansion.

The actual site need not be a flat one. Indeed, slopes can provide suitable loading bays for stock and product and are of value when two or more floors are contemplated. In general, urban sites should be avoided; rural and nominated industrial sites are preferred.

Thought should be given at an early stage to hard and soft landscaping the site to limit the impact of the establishment on the surrounding environment.

Environmental statement

It will be important at a very early stage in the planning and design of a meat plant to consider the possible effects of the operation of the plant on the local and wider environment. Planning authorities will often require the production of an *environmental statement* (ES) which will be used in determining the suitability or otherwise of the proposed plant in the particular location.

Before an ES can be produced, an *environmental impact assessment* (EIA) must be carried out. The EIA is a process by which information about the environmental effects of a project is collated, assessed and taken into account by the Planning Service in reaching a decision about whether a proposed development should be approved. In the case of a meat plant, it is likely that the following would be considered:

• The characteristics of the development, including its size; cumulation with other developments; use of natural resources; production of waste; pollution and

Gracey's Meat Hygiene, Eleventh Edition. Edited by David S. Collins and Robert J. Huey.
© 2015 John Wiley & Sons, Ltd. Published 2015 by John Wiley & Sons, Ltd.

nuisance, for example, operational noise and odour; and the risk of accidents which could affect the environment

- The location of the development, for example, the existing land use, the abundance of natural resources in the area and whether it is intended for a sensitive location, for example, an area designated as being of Special Scientific Interest, Area of Outstanding Natural Beauty, etc.
- Effect of increased traffic movements in the locality
- Wastewater disposal

The ES will normally include the following elements:

- Justification of the need for the development
- Description of development comprising information on the site, design and size of the development
- Identification of outputs to the environment
- Report of established baseline data (ambient air quality levels, traffic flows, etc.)
- Anticipated environmental impacts at both construction and operational stages
- A description of the measures envisaged in order to avoid, reduce and, if possible, remedy significant adverse effects

The ES is likely to be a substantial document and will normally be accompanied by a non-technical summary for use by laypersons. These documents will be available to all interested parties and will be used by the planning authority in determining the outcome of *planning application* and possibly by review bodies in the event of any appeal or public enquiry.

Submission of plans

While there is no legal requirement to do so, it is wise to submit copies of any proposed site plans for a new establishment or, if any significant changes are to be made to the layout of an existing establishment, to the authority responsible for the eventual approval of the establishment and to any other body responsible for recommendation of approval. In addition, most authorities require a formal application procedure and the completion of a pro forma that details the proposed throughput of the facility, the class of livestock to be processed, the number of employees and the likely operating hours. The completion of such a pro forma frequently assists the applicant in clarifying, in his own mind, the proposed business model.

The *site plan* (scale 1:500) must show the complete premises, the outline of the curtilage of the site and the location in relation to roads, railways, waterways and adjoining properties and their function. Catch basins, water and sewer lines, storage tanks, etc. must also be shown. The *floor* plan (scale 1:50 or 1:100) relates to layout of walls, doorways, windows, partitions, rail systems, equipment, work stands or platforms, toilets, chutes, conveyors, staircases, hot and cold water connections, ventilation fans, work positions of operatives, etc. The position of drainage gutters and floor gradients must also be included.

The *plumbing* plan gives details of the drainage system, which must ensure that toilet and floor soil lines are separated until outside the building and that the former do not connect with grease traps.

Since specialised knowledge is required in the design and construction of a meat plant, it is vital that competent architects, veterinarians and engineers with years of experience are employed along with reputable contractors.

Flow lines

It is essential that the plans indicate the flow lines for product, waste, equipment, personnel and packaging in order to ensure the adequate separation of dirty from clean areas. A gradient of cleanliness exists in a slaughterhouse from the lairage and waste product areas through to the removal of the main sources of faecal contamination, the outer integument and the gastrointestinal tract. After final inspection, the carcase should be considered as clean. It is imperative that the layout of the establishment makes further contamination of the meat as difficult as possible so all movements of product or people against the hygiene gradient should be eliminated or minimised by design.

Area size

Careful consideration must be given to the size of the site, with allowance for the various buildings and traffic circulation. The maximum permitted dimensions of an articulated vehicle, with its container, are 2.55 m wide and 18.75 m long resulting in very large turning circles being necessary. Particular consideration should be given to the positioning of loading bays where the turning space required is increased when several vehicles are parked parallel to each other.

Completely separate routes for stock and meat vehicles should be provided. Approach roads should be at least 6.5 m for two-way traffic and 3.5 for one-way systems. When all the various buildings are considered, it will be realised that a large area is necessary.

Generally, a small abattoir (up to 30 000 units/year) will occupy 1–2 acres, a medium plant (50 000+ units/year) 2–4 acres, and a large meat plant handling over 100 000 units annually about 4–6 acres. (One adult bovine is equivalent to two pigs, three calves or five sheep.)

There must be an adequate partition between the clean and dirty sections, ideally with completely separate entrances and exits for traffic involved. If only one entrance is possible, such vehicles must be routed in different directions after entry.

Facilities

The following basic facilities are required for the slaughter of cattle, sheep, pigs, goats, solipeds and poultry (Fig. 3.1):

1 Adequate lairage or, climate-permitting, waiting pens for the animals.
2 Slaughter premises large enough for work to be carried out satisfactorily. Maximum slaughter rates for the different species should be specified.
3 A room for emptying and cleansing stomachs and intestines.
4 Rooms for dressing guts and tripe if this is carried out on the premises.

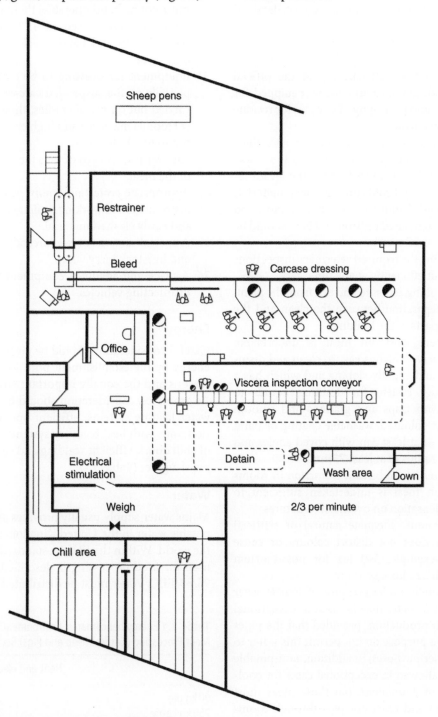

Figure 3.1 Floor layout of a sheep slaughter establishment.

5 Separate rooms for the storage of fat and hides, pig bristles, horns and hooves which are not removed on the day of slaughter.

6 A separate room for preparing and cleaning offal, including a separate place for storing heads if these operations are carried out but do not take place on the slaughter line.

7 Lockable premises reserved, respectively, for the accommodation of sick or suspect animals, the slaughter of such animals, the storage of detained meat and the storage of seized meat.

8 Sufficiently large chilling or refrigerating rooms.

9 An adequately equipped, lockable facility for the exclusive use of the staff carrying at the official controls. In addition, a room suitably equipped for the preparation and packaging of samples for residue and disease surveillance.

10 Changing rooms, washbasins, showers and flush lavatories that do not open directly onto the work-rooms. The washbasins must be near the lavatories and must have hot and cold running water, materials for cleansing and disinfecting the hands and hand towels which can be used only once. There should be a receptacle for used towels.

11 Facilities enabling the required veterinary inspections to be carried out efficiently at any time.

12 Means of controlling access to and exit from the plant.

13 An adequate separation between the clean and the contaminated parts of the building.

14 In rooms where work on meat is undertaken: waterproof *flooring* which is easy to clean and disinfect, rat-proof and slightly sloping and which has a suitable *drainage* system for draining liquids to drains fitted with traps and gratings and smooth walls with light-coloured, washable coating or paint up to a height of at least 3 m with coved angles and corners with a radius of at least 75 mm.

15 Adequate *ventilation* and *steam extraction* in rooms where work on meat is undertaken sufficient to eliminate condensation on overhead structures.

16 In the same rooms, adequate natural or artificial *lighting* which does not distort colours or cause shadows, for example, 540 lux for post-mortem inspection with 220 lux elsewhere.

17 An adequate supply, under pressure, of *potable water* only. *Non-potable water* may be used in exceptional cases for steam production, provided that the pipes installed for the purpose do not permit this water to be used for other purposes; in addition, non-potable water may be allowed in exceptional cases for cooling refrigeration equipment, but these pipes must be painted red and must not pass through rooms containing exposed meat.

18 An adequate supply of *hot potable water*.

19 A *wastewater disposal system* which meets hygiene requirements.

20 In the workrooms, adequate *equipment for cleansing and disinfecting hands and tools* and as near as possible to the workstations. However, in rooms in which meat is cut, centralised sterilisation of knives may be used. This has the benefit of reducing steam, and potentially condensation, in the workroom. Taps must not be hand operable; there must be hot water for hand wash mixed to 45°C, disinfecting non-scented soap and hand towels which can be used only once.

21 Equipment for dressing to be carried out as far as possible on the suspended carcase. Where flaying is carried out on metal cradles, these must be of non-corrodible materials and high enough for the carcase not to touch the floor.

22 An overhead system of rails for the further handling of the meat.

23 Appropriate *protection against pests*.

24 Instruments and working equipment of non-corrodible and easily cleaned material.

25 A special section for *manure*, adjacent to the lairage and livestock lorry wash.

26 A place and adequate equipment for cleansing and disinfecting vehicles.

Energy

Careful consideration should be given to efficient use of energy by the establishment both for obvious financial reasons and the equally important environmental ones. As examples, consideration should be given to efficient water heating systems, efficient operation of refrigeration units with heat recovery systems, automatic closing of chill doors, efficient scalding and singeing systems for pig slaughter (Table 3.1).

Water

Mains water supply usually provides an ample supply of potable water in the United Kingdom and most parts of the world. Within the EU, the standard for potable water used for food processing is described within Directive 98/83/EEC. Water must be distributed to all parts of the

Table 3.1 Energy benchmarks: Environment Agency, The Red Meat Processing (Cattle, Sheep and Pigs) Sector

	Heat and electricity (kWh/animal)
90 kg pig	30–125
250 kg cattle	70–300

plant under adequate pressure, which in the mains pipeline should be at least 20 psi. Hot and cold water are necessary, the hot, from a central heating system, distributed at 45°C for cleaning wash-hand basins and at 82°C for cleaning of equipment and tools. On-site water storage tanks holding at least one day's consumption are usual. Storage tanks must be covered to protect the water from contamination. Should contamination occur, it must be possible to completely drain, flush and sanitise the system (Table 3.2).

If non-potable water is used for steam production, refrigeration or fire control, it must be carried in separate lines and identified as such.

It is increasingly important that for environmental protection reasons water use in meat processing establishments should be minimised. The first step in this process is to carefully analyse water use, as is demonstrated for pig slaughter in Figure 3.2.

Drainage

Water must not be allowed to 'pool' on the floors of production areas. Floors in wet areas should slope uniformly to drains, the gradient being 1:50. As a general

Table 3.2 Benchmark water consumption: Environment Agency, The Red Meat Processing (Cattle, Sheep and Pigs) Sector

Cattle	700–1000 l/animal
Pigs	160–230 l/animal
Sheep	100–150 l/animal

rule, floor drains should be fitted at the rate of one drain for each 40 m² of floor area.

Where blood tends to collect, for example, under dressing rails, special provision must be made to supply drainage valleys which should slope to drains in the valleys at a gradient of at least 1:25. The valleys themselves should be 60 cm wide and should continue under dressing lines for the collection of all blood and bone dust. Blood and wastewater solids must be collected separately from the wastewater and dealt with in accordance with by-products legislation (see Chapter 8).

Catch basins for grease recovery and *traps* and *vents* on drains must also be provided, both to be properly sealed and easily cleanable and the latter to be effectively vented to outside the building.

Special arrangements have to be made for dealing with stomach and intestinal contents, the drains for bovine material to be at least 20 cm in diameter and for the smaller species 15 cm.

In the United Kingdom, by-products legislation requires that drains in cattle/sheep slaughterhalls be trapped with 4 mm screens, to prevent the possibility of contamination of the effluent with pieces of nervous tissue greater than 1 g – the possible infective dose of BSE. The material collected by this screening is then dealt with appropriately as specified risk material (SRM), Category 1 by-product.

Lighting

Adequate natural or artificial lighting must be provided throughout the meat plant. Natural lighting should take

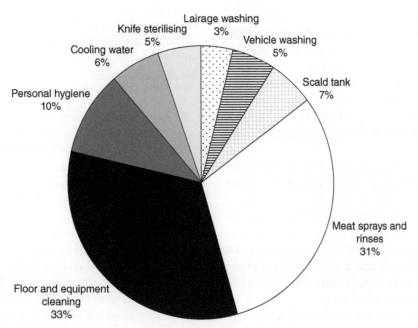

Figure 3.2 Typical water balance for areas in a pig abattoir: Environment Agency, The Red Meat Processing (Cattle, Sheep and Pigs) Sector.

the form of efficient north lights. North-facing windows will largely preclude solar gain, but frosted glass or glass fitted with solar film will also reduce solar radiation.

The type of lighting must not distort colours. It is generally recommended that the overall intensity should not be less than:

540 lux at all inspection points
220 lux in workrooms
110 lux in other areas

These intensities of light are usually taken at levels of 0.9 m from the floor, except in inspection areas where the height is 1.5 m. Protective shields must be fitted to lights in areas where fresh meat and offal are exposed to prevent contamination from shattered glass.

Ventilation

Adequate ventilation must be provided to prevent excessive heat, steam and condensation and to eliminate or reduce airborne pathogens which may present a health and safety risk to operatives or public health risk to consumers. Ventilation also prevents the accumulation of odours, dust, etc., but it should not cause draughts and thus another potential hazard to operatives. Particularly in multistorey plants, draughts arising from lift wells, stairways, chutes, etc. should be prevented. Opening ventilators and windows should be screened and internal window sills sloped.

Floor and wall finishes

All parts of the meat plant must be capable of being easily cleaned. This means that all floors and wall coverings or finishes should be non-toxic and non-absorbent, the floors also being non-slip. The floors of slaughterhalls, lairages, workrooms and chill rooms should be coved at wall junctions to assist effective cleaning.

It is recommended that walls should be faced with a smooth, durable, impermeable material with a light-coloured washable finish. Ceilings should also be smooth, hard and impervious and all overhead structures easily cleaned.

The types of operations encountered in abattoirs inevitably involve *impact damage*. Good design and layout can do much to prevent this, as can the employment of careful, skilful operatives. Surface materials should be capable of withstanding impact; doors should be wide enough to allow easy passage of personnel, carcases and offal on conveyorised lines and trucks; and their jambs should be protected with metal covers (they should be solid where necessary and self-closing.

Abattoir operations entail wet floors on which quantities of fat and blood are usually present. While floor finishes should be easily cleaned, they should also be non-slip. Operatives are required to wear easily cleaned, safety (non-slip) footwear, and no one should be allowed on a slaughterhall floor, in particular, without proper footwear. In certain places, it is wise to incorporate carborundum or aluminium oxide in order to provide a non-slip surface. Pin rolling or grooving of the surface also assists in preventing slipping.

Walls and floors may be made of concrete, granolithic concrete or tiles. Wall sheets are often used in the form of plastic laminates and stainless steel sheets. Although it is the most expensive, stainless steel is undoubtedly the most satisfactory; it is very strong, easily cleaned and completely non-corrosive and does not flake, cause discoloration or affect the taste of meat and offal.

Doors

These should be wide enough to allow passage of product without contact with the doorway. A width of 1.5 m is usually adequate. Doors must be constructed of rust-resistant material which is easily cleaned. Double-acting doors should have a glass (reinforced) panel at eye level. Plastic strip doors, because of difficulty of cleaning and their liability to scratch, crack or break, are unsuitable except where packaged product is moved.

Equipment design

Since mechanical handling systems and other types of equipment used in meat plants usually form the major part of the overall cost, it is wise to consider design aspects as well as operating efficiency, durability, etc. Within the EU, the requirements for hygienic design of equipment for foodstuffs are contained within the machinery directive, 2006/42/EC. These are translated into the food processing machinery standard, BS EN 1672-2+A1: 2009 or ISO 4159. Faults in construction and design include:

1 Use of wood for equipment and tools. Wood cannot be cleaned and disinfected with ease and is liable to deteriorate rapidly in moist surroundings.
2 Use of unsuitable fastenings which can work loose and contaminate the product.
3 Provision of ledges, ridges, crevices, joints and corners where meat, fat, etc. can lodge and cause bacterial build-up.
4 Badly recessed nuts, bolts and screws can also gather scraps and hinder cleansing.
5 Use of expanded metal for decks, walkways and staircases especially near conveyors. All these should be constructed from non-slip solid plate.
6 Metal joints which are rough. Joints should be welded and then ground to a smooth finish.
7 Fixed covers for conveyors that make cleaning difficult.

The design and location of equipment should be such as to allow for ease and efficiency of cleaning and disinfection.

Pest control

The ingress of birds, rats, mice and insects such as flies and cockroaches can cause serious problems since in addition to the dirt they create, they may carry food-poisoning organisms. *Birds*, especially sparrows, starlings, feral pigeons and gulls, inhabit areas where food and nesting material are available. They feed on meat scraps, dung, insects and animal feed.

In some food factories, sparrows have become an even greater problem than mice, defying air curtains and currents, netting, flashing lights, bird distress noises, anti-perch gel, etc. While these measures may be useful in some instances, avoidance depends on a high level of hygiene.

Rats and mice are also attracted by the presence of food and may gain entrance from adjoining properties or be transported into the plant in animal feed, etc. Mice have been known to be introduced into an abattoir in polystyrene insulation for use in chill rooms. Control is effected by ensuring cleanliness, absence of food scraps and the use of specialist pest control firms. A sketch plan of the premises indicating numbered bait points should be produced and a record of usage of each point noted, as well as dates of inspection and any structural defects. These should be inspected regularly, and if increased activity is seen, further control measures must be taken.

Insects are drawn into food premises mainly by the presence of pre-digested food, such as excreta, and by warmth. Nearby breeding grounds such as waste tips, stagnant ponds and sewage works may be responsible for the responsible for an increased population of flies. Plant location and design are important factors in prevention of fly infestation, for example, the manure bay must be sited away from meat areas.

Scrupulous cleanliness, the avoidance of direct sunlight in rooms, the use of air curtains with horizontal air draughts, strip door curtains, ultraviolet light, electrocutors, mesh screens, etc. are of value, especially cleanliness. Insecticidal sprays should be used with discretion and confined to non-meat sectors.

Small abattoir units

While larger meat plants are capable of greater throughputs per man, they have high fixed overheads which can be a problem for their operators. Under these circumstances, the smaller establishment has advantages, particularly in remote areas, by being sited close to production regions, thereby cutting transport costs.

The concept of a *mobile slaughter facility* has been developed in the United Kingdom by the Humane Slaughter Association and several Scandinavian countries. Fitted with a stunning box, it includes hoists, bleeding area, dressing cradles, chill room and storage for by-products, detained and effluent material. The unit operates from a home base and visits farms on request, the farms providing basic facilities of water, electricity, lairage pens, toilet and changing rooms. While the advantages in animal welfare are obvious, the organisation of official controls must be given careful attention (Fig. 3.3).

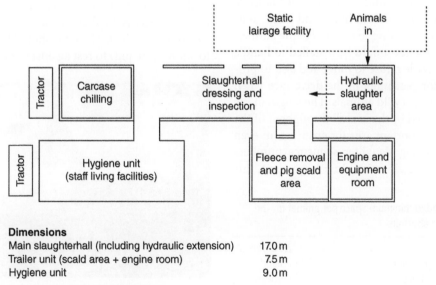

Dimensions

Main slaughterhall (including hydraulic extension)	17.0 m
Trailer unit (scald area + engine room)	7.5 m
Hygiene unit	9.0 m

Figure 3.3 General layout of the mobile slaughterhouse.

Lairage (see also Chapter 6)

A knowledge of animal behaviour is fundamental to lairage design. The importance of suitable lairage accommodation for animals awaiting slaughter cannot be overestimated, since good design can play a key role in ensuring that animals are unloaded and moved through the lairage with minimal intervention and therefore minimal stress. This not only ensures animal welfare but in addition assists in ensuring good eating quality.

Water must be made available to animals at all times in the lairage. The facility provided must be suitable for the type and numbers of livestock. Forage and feeding facilities must be made available if animals are to be kept in the lairage for more than 12 hours. A suitable sized store is therefore required for the storage of feed and forage and of bedding material where this is used.

An isolation pen, with solid walls and separate drainage, must be available for sick or 'suspect' animals.

Toilet and *hand-washing facilities* must be provided in the vicinity of the lairage. *Boot-washing equipment* is an essential component for farmers, buyers and lairage staff.

Points for connection for a power hose should be placed conveniently, so that all parts of the lairage can be reached by a sufficient supply of water for cleansing; an adequate estimate is 500l per adult bovine slaughtered. Whatever system of lairage is adopted, special emphasis must be placed on ease of cleansing, comfort for the animals and ease of handling them.

Cattle lairage (Table 3.3)

Cattle lairage pens may be constructed of solid rendered block wall or tubular galvanised steel and at least 1.8 m high. Tubular steel should be used rather than box metal as it is easier to clean with a power hose. While durable tubular fencing has been found satisfactory for holding pens, the final *drive races* should have solid sides, non-slip floor surfaces and lighting to encourage the animals to go forwards. Side gates should be installed to handle emergencies when cattle refuse to move and also to provide escape gates for personnel in the drive race when they are confronted with wild animals. The length of the final race is determined by the overall throughput of the meat plant. It is an important area for ensuring an even flow forwards, checking slaughter sequence numbers and other forms of identification. In a large plant, this race can be 36 m long, with stop gates to prevent the animals going backwards. Catwalks must be provided alongside the race to enable handlers to control stock movement, check identification, etc.

Gates should be 2.4 m wide gates (at the end of each pen) which can be used for the pens and/or closing the adjoining passageway. For cattle, pens may be 7.6 m × 6 m, large enough to hold 20–25 cattle.

Sheep lairage

Sheep pens should be 0.9 m high with passages 0.9 m wide between them. To prevent animals putting their heads through the lower rails of the pens, these rails should not be more than 15 cm apart. Double-hinged gates should be used in all sheep and pig pens, as they greatly facilitate entry and exit of stock; two adjoining pens can accommodate an overflow of animals if a sliding gate is provided between the pens. Since sheep drink quite freely after transport, sheep pens must be provided with water troughs, placed some 50 cm from the floor to prevent fouling. Hayracks should also be provided above the level of the sheep's heads (Fig. 3.4).

Straw should be provided for solid floors to help keep the sheep dry. Expanded metal floors will achieve the same purpose.

There is no objection to cattle and sheep lairages being provided in the same building, but while pigs and sheep may be housed together without detrimental effect, cattle do not appear to rest well in the company of pigs.

Pig lairage

Pig pens are preferably constructed with solid walls. If rails are used, they should be stronger than those required for the sheep lairage; the lower horizontal rails of the pen should not be more than 15 cm apart to prevent pigs putting their heads between the rails. The feeding troughs should be so designed that the pigs cannot gain access to them while the troughs are being cleansed and filled. The pens should be long and narrow to allow more pigs to rest against the walls.

Table 3.3 Recommended minimum space per animal for the housing of livestock in abattoirs

Cattle (loose)	2.3–2.8 m²/head
Pigs (bacon and small porkers)	0.6 m²/head
Heavy pigs, calves and sheep	0.75 m²/head

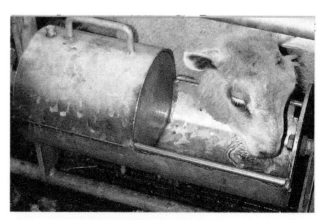

Figure 3.4 Well-designed sheep drinker.

A mechanical version of the 'pig board' used routinely to move pigs is employed in many pig lairages. A development of this *automatic lairage system* with pens divided into sections each holding a maximum of 15 pigs. Automatic filling and emptying of the pens is achieved using computer controlled lifting/driving gates. The system is said to improve welfare standards with reduction of damage due to fighting.

A fine water spray and/or litter in the lairage pens are useful means of reducing fighting among pigs, cooling them and reducing the incidence of pale, soft, exudative (PSE) pork.

Deer lairage

Although the majority of farmed deer in Britain are still slaughtered by shooting in the field, some are handled in special on-farm abattoirs and others in larger abattoirs. Because of the nervous nature of these animals, which are very subject to stress, it is essential that good facilities for holding and slaughter are provided. It is also vital that expert handlers are on hand.

The UK Farm Animal Welfare Council (FAWC) has recommended that the slaughter of deer should take place only in specially licensed premises and that deer should not be slaughtered while other species are being handled/slaughtered unless separated from those other activities by solid walls to exclude noise.

Reception areas for unloading and lairage pens should have smooth high-impact walls and a circular crush gate of 5 m maximum diameter with two solid swing gates, centrally hung at least 1.83 m (6 ft) high. Unlike the requirements for cattle and sheep, lighting should be subdued throughout the lairage and stunning areas, which should interconnect.

Clipping or cleaning of livestock

Although washing of animals, for example, cattle, bison, horses, etc., is practised in tropical and subtropical countries, it is contraindicated in temperate regions, for example, the United Kingdom, except possibly for pigs. Facilities usually consist of a footbath spray system or bath and an adequate draining area prior to slaughter. A system for recovering solids and a final potable water wash must be included.

In the United Kingdom, clipping of cattle and sheep in the lairage is a common method of reducing the level of faecal contamination of the hide or fleece prior to the dressing process. If it is intended to use pre-slaughter clipping as part of an overall hygiene management system, then suitable facilities need to be provided at the construction stage. For cattle, a holding facility which gives the handler good access to the animal while ensuring adequate controls for health and safety should be provided.

An alternative to pre-slaughter clipping is clipping after slaughter on the dressing line. This has the advantage of removing all animal welfare and handler health and safety concerns. However, the facility must be so designed as to eliminate all risk to the exposed carcase from dust created during the clipping process. This can be achieved by physical separation of the clipping from the exposed carcase by, for example, in a two-level slaughterhouse, clipping after the bleeding channel but before the carcase is elevated to the floor above for dressing, making use of air curtains or other physical barriers. The amount of dust can be reduced by using vacuum incorporated into the clipper mechanism.

Manure disposal

Considerable quantities of lairage waste in the form of bedding and dung require periodic removal, preferably a covered site near the lairage, from which it can be conveniently loaded for removal. It may be possible to load it directly onto a large trailer which can be removed as necessary. The digesta obtained from the stomachs and intestines of slaughtered animals requires separate treatment. It is sometimes used as compost for horticultural purposes and is sometimes spread on land without any further treatment.

The siting and operation of the store should minimise the hazard presented by flies which may accumulate especially in warm weather.

Slaughterhall

The transfer of animals from lairage to slaughterhall is easy if the abattoir is well designed. If an upper kill floor is used and the site is on a slope, the animals can be walked directly on the slaughter floor; using a ramp as necessary. Cattle and sheep can readily be driven up a ramp as steep as 1 in 6, though the ramp should be provided with battens and a catwalk.

The size and type of slaughterhall depends upon the species to be slaughter, the maximum possible capacity and the slaughter and dressing systems to be adopted. Sufficient space must be provided to allow hygienic processing, to avoid cross-contamination. Good lighting and ventilation must be provided.

Stunning area

The area in front of the stunning pen where the bovine animal falls should be at least 3 m in width to the opposing wall or bleeding trough and be fitted with upright bars 5 cm in diameter and 1.2 m high, spaced at 40 cm intervals, for safety purposes, should improperly stunned animals regain their feet. The floor of this area, usually called the dry landing area, must be properly drained and possess high-impact and non-slip properties to aid the work of the operative who must enter this high-risk area to apply a shackle for hoisting. Efficient shackling and hoisting is important to assist rapid bleeding especially if the animal has only been stunned rather than killed.

A raised sturdy frame of expanded metal onto which the animal is ejected aids cleanliness and reduces wetness. This is important since every animal slaughter comes into direct contact with this area. Consequently, one animal with a dirty hide has the potential to contaminate the hide of many subsequent animals.

Bleeding area

No meat plant should be built without careful consideration being given to the full utilisation of by-products, edible and inedible. Edible blood must be stored under refrigeration at a maximum temperature of 3°C.

The *bleeding trough* should be at least 1.5 m wide and possess a good gradient, side walls of the same height and two drains, one for blood only and the other for water when cleansing only. The length of the bleeding line will depend on the throughput and the system of conveying carcases but should be generous, since the majority of blood flow requires 6–8 minutes. The bleeding trough has two points for the reception of blood: one at the actual point of sticking where the greater volume of blood will be handled and thereafter a longer gradual slope that collects 'drip' blood classed as inedible. The overhead bleeding rail should be about 4.9 m above the floor of the dry landing area, dressing rails about 3.4 m high. The bleeding trough must have a smooth impervious surface, often a suitable grade of stainless steel. It should be fitted with a double drain – one opening for the blood to be pumped to a tanker for disposal and the other for wash water.

Various systems of hygienic bleeding of livestock, mostly cattle and pigs, are in use, and these may or may not be combined with an in-plant blood processing department. The specialised nature of blood processing, as with inedible by-product processing, means that it may be more satisfactory to collect these items efficiently and then consign them to an outside central plant for final processing.

Consideration should be given to the size and siting of the sticking knife wash and sterilising facility. The sticking operative must use one knife for the initial skin cut and another for severing the blood vessels in order to minimise the risk of introducing contamination.

For hygienic bleeding for edible purposes, *the stainless hollow knife* combined with cleanliness and a sodium citrate/phosphate anticoagulant is used. The knife is held in the wound by hand, by a rotating endless screw or by other means. For low throughput slaughter establishments, individual containers are used for holding the blood; with large throughputs and high rates of slaughter,

several blood draining knives (as many as 14) can be used in a 'carousel' which rotates synchronously with the bleeding conveyor. Arrangements must be made for routine sterilisation of the knives and adequate staff to man this additional operation.

The hollow knife is made of stainless steel in two sizes, for cattle and pigs. Various designs are available, but they usually consist of a tubular handle with a deflector plate and two blades set at right angles to each other. They are easy to strip for sharpening and cleaning and are combined with an anticoagulant dispensing tube. The broad blade should be directed in the longitudinal direction of the animal. A suitable form of tubing, for example, made of collagen, connects the knife to containers where the blood is cooled prior to collection.

A system which correlates each batch of blood to the carcase from which it originates must be operated so that if a carcase is subsequently condemned the blood from that animal may also be condemned.

The bleeding trough for sheep and pigs should preferably be enclosed on both sides as for cattle and have a width of 1.1–1.2 m with the overhead bleeding rail 2.7 m high, and dressing rails 2.3 m high for sheep and 3.4 m high in the case of pigs.

Cattle carcase dressing

Following bleeding, carcase dressing may commence only when the absence of signs of life of the animal has been verified (Council Regulation No. 1099/2009, Annex III, para 3.2). If the throughput for cattle slaughter is less than 10/hour, 'cradle dressing' may be the technique of choice. The cradle should be of high specification stainless steel construction, robust and easily cleaned with solid polyurethane wheels. However, in most modern slaughter facilities, some form of line dressing is the norm.

Hindleg, hide removal, evisceration, carcase splitting, inspection, kidney and channel fat removal and carcase washing stations must have platforms at suitable positions and heights for operatives and inspectors to work efficiently and without unnecessary stooping and labour (Chapter 14 for more detail on Health and Safety). Working platforms should be of corrosive-resistant metal, with ducted drainage from the floor and hand, apron washing and knife sterilising facilities. For safety reasons, the edge of the platform should be provided with upraised edges, toe bars and guard rails as required.

Of particular importance is the position of the *viscera inspection table*, especially for adult cattle, where the top of the moving-top table should be about 2.7 m from the top of the conveyor rail and the vertical centre of the carcase positioned at the edge of the viscera inspection table (1.5 m wide). A hydraulically powered skip arrangement may be required to dump the gut onto the viscera inspection table.

The carcase splitting saw station usually requires a 'rise and fall' platform equipped with a saw steriliser for use between carcases. It is important to attempt to contain the sawdust from the bandsaw by using a ceiling to floor stainless steel screen and a 'sock' to contain the effluent from the integrated saw blade wash.

On-the-rail dressing

The development of *line dressing* of carcases originally emanated from Canada. Essentially, the carcase is conveyed by gravity or power along an overhead rail; after stunning and bleeding, the process of dressing is divided up into various stages, each undertaken by a separate operator as the carcase reaches him. Although some establishments use the traditional one man–one job approach, a better approach is to allow one operative to follow the carcase through several operations. Besides reducing the labour load, this arrangement also makes for better job satisfaction and gives the opportunity to build in an apron, equipment wash and knife sterilisation step. A combination of several machines, tools and correlated items of equipment (brisket saw, hock cutters, hide puller, aitch bone cutter, etc.) enables complete dressing to be carried out at high rates of slaughter. Use of robotics, especially for pig slaughter, has been developed, but cost of installation and difficulties with the quality of dressing have hampered their widespread introduction.

Several systems of line dressing are in operation, the type depending mainly on the level of throughput, equipment design and species, being most complicated in cattle. Ideally, the dressing line should be as straight as possible so as to physically separate by a maximum distance the dirty hide on carcase from the clean dressed one. A straight line also permits the hygienic removal of waste and by-products to rooms located parallel to the slaughter line.

There are four main types of line dressing for cattle.

Gravity rail system

In this method, the carcases are suspended from a spreader and single-wheel trolley or runner, transferred by gravity to each station and stopped by a manually operated stop on the overhead rail.

The system is used for lower slaughter rates of 10–40 cattle/hour. It is probably the most compact and economical of the systems. Being the simplest in design, there is less chance of serious breakdowns with consequent loss of production. Various items of equipment may be used with the gravity rail, for example, a moving-top viscera inspection table or a paunch truck, but because throughput is small, a mechanical hide puller is rarely used. Adequate ceiling height is necessary because of the pitch of the rail to gravitate the carcases.

Intermittent powered system

This system can be used for rates of 10–75 cattle/hour. It involves the mechanical moving of the carcases suspended on a spreader (gambrel) and trolley along a level rail at intervals by means of a variable timing device which can be pre-set to suit the slaughter rate.

Continuous powered system

In this method, the dressing line is in continuous motion and is used for higher rates of kill, 40–120 cattle/hour. More sophisticated equipment is associated with this slaughter line, for example, mechanical hide puller and moving-top inspection table as with the 'Canpak' system.

The carcase can be revolved a full 360° while on the rail, allowing the operator to work all sides from one position. Associated with all line systems are platforms which can be varied in height and position, enabling the operator to carry out his task more efficiently.

'Canpak' system

This is a continuous conveyorised method in which the carcases are suspended by heavy beef trolleys or runners from the overhead rail; no spreader or gambrel is used. Developed and patented by Canada Packers Ltd., Toronto, Canada, it is probably the most common form of line system now used in large modern meat plants. Rates of slaughter from 50 to 150 cattle or more per hour can be achieved depending on the type and extent of associated equipment and the number of operators.

A typical sequence of operations on a modern line system is shown in the beef slaughter flow chart in Figure 3.5. In the United Kingdom, a number of additional tasks are carried out to remove the bovine specified offals and to check their removal.

Advantages of line dressing

1 Since carcases are conveyed to each dressing station, there is no need for operatives to be idle while carcases are being hoisted or positioned.
2 The line system is said to be safer for operatives than traditional slaughter systems.
3 Because carcases do not touch the floor and their dressing is more conveniently carried out, 'on-the-rail' dressing is hygienic.
4 Elimination of the handling of heavy shackles, trolleys and spreaders; the use of comfortable platform position for personnel; and the use of mechanical tools reduce tedious labour.
5 An efficient line system increases throughput and may enhance the value of the carcase, hide and offal because of superior workmanship.

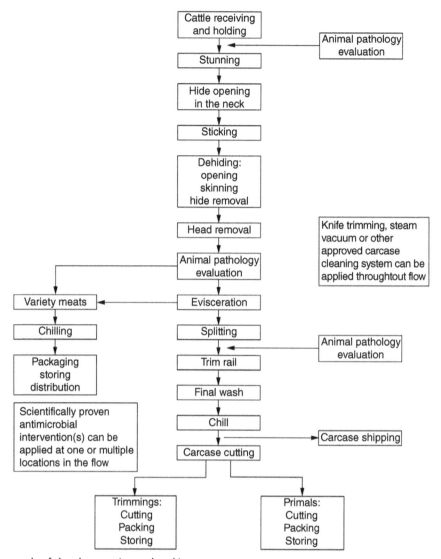

Figure 3.5 Flow diagram: beef slaughter, cutting and packing.

Possible disadvantages

The line system, however, being mechanically complex, demands a high standard of engineering maintenance, and when breakdowns do occur, production ceases completely. The repetitive nature of the work can be largely offset by job rotation if personnel are so trained. Meat inspection is sometimes said to be made more difficult and possibly less efficient. An efficient system of meat inspection on a line system requires good lighting (540 lux that does not distort colours); proper carcase and offal conveyor synchronisation; a good identification system; adequate, efficient and conscientious inspection staff; proper inspection points with ability to co-ordinate findings; an efficient recording setup; and adequate *time* for the examination of each carcase. At the higher rates of slaughter, separate recording staff should be uti-

lised, particularly for detailed information. Unimpeded movement between inspection points is essential if an inspector needs to cover more than one inspection point.

For new beef installations, consideration should be given to the performance of *hot boning* subsequent to the dressing line. This practice allows for the preparation and chilling of cuts without the problem of cold shortening.

Sheep slaughterhall

Though larger installations are best served by retaining the cattle slaughterhall for cattle only, in smaller establishments where cattle and sheep killing are not likely to take place at the same time, a portion of the cattle hall can be adapted for slaughter and dressing of sheep, usually by the installation of a parallel line.

The following is an example of a slaughter line for sheep which requires 17 operatives with a potential production of 150 sheep/hour:

1   Pen sheep and stun
2   Shackle and hoist
3   Stick
4   De-elevate to crutch conveyor
5–9   Conveyor dressing (remove feet, commence fleece removal, saw brisket)
10   Elevate to overhead rail
11   Clear tail and commence backing
12   Back and chute fleece
13   Remove head
14   Eviscerate abdomen
15   Wash
16   Eviscerate thorax
17   Weigh and tag
18   Final wash

The feet should be removed with a special instrument, avoiding the usual practice of individual removal with the skinning knife and the all-too-frequent littering of the floor with these parts.

The New Zealand Meat Industry Research Institute (MIRINZ), in the 1980s, developed a method of *automatic pelt removal* to produce blemish-free and hygienic carcases with the minimum of labour which is now widely used. The valuable hindquarter is completely untouched, and there is no stretching of the pelt. Termed the 'inverted' method, the carcase is suspended by the forelegs or in a near-horizontal position on twin conveyors. A 'Y' cut is made from forelegs to throat releasing the 'vee' flap, which is fed into the brisket skinner to clear the foreleg pockets. The two shoulder flaps are then pulled down, and the 'vee' flap is split by hand. The head is removed and discarded under veterinary control. The pelt is further prepared for automatic removal by skinning the belly and groin. The carcase is now ready for the operation of two pelting machines – the shoulder puller and the final puller, the former drawing the shoulder flaps in a downward/backward direction, while the latter (a hydraulically operated arm and clamp) grips the fleece centrally and strips it downwards off the hindquarter and shanks. The fleece is then released through a floor chute to the pelt room.

Pig slaughterhall

A pig slaughter line built to handle pork pigs is generally not suitable for sows and boars. This should be borne in mind at the planning stage.

The scalding, depilation, scraping and singeing of pig carcases are inherently dirty processes. This usually makes it necessary to physically separate these processes from evisceration in order to ensure hygienic operation.

Scalded, depilation, scraping and singeing take place immediately after bleeding is complete. In the smaller abattoirs, scraping is done by hand, but in large abattoirs and bacon factories, a mechanical dehairing machine is used. It is estimated that if there is a regular throughput of some 200 pigs on 2–3 days/week, a dehairing plant is necessary. An extraction system, which removes steam from the canopies over the scalding tanks and keeps the temperature of the steam raised by heated air, serves to prevent condensation and fogginess.

A typical pig slaughter operation of up to 650 pigs/hour would consist of the operations shown in the pork slaughter flow chart in Figure 3.6.

Scalding and dehairing

The factors to be considered relating to scalding and dehairing are hourly rate of slaughter, size of pig to be handled, ease of operation of the machines, efficiency of cleansing and corrosion.

A typical scalding tank is maintained at 60–62°C; effective scalding requires 6 minutes at 60°C, 5 minutes at 61°C. It is important to contain the steam as completely as possible and to remove it by efficient extraction in order to prevent condensation. Consideration should be given in the design as to the rapid removal of carcases from the tank in the event of mechanical breakdown or a carcase becoming stuck in the equipment as the carcase will quickly cook, particularly the loin/tenderloin, and will be considered unfit for food.

In the scald tank, before operations begin, there can be as many as 40 000 bacteria/ml in the tank, rising to 45–800 million organisms/ml after the scalding of 600 pigs. Among these were aerobic and anaerobic spore-forming bacteria, cocci and organisms belonging to the coli–proteus groups; of 220 samples of scalding water, *Salmonella paratyphi* and *S. typhimurium* were isolated on one occasion. It has been discovered that developmental types of *Salmonella* could occur in the sludge of the scalding water and that a deep infection of the pig meat can arise from the bacterial flora on the surface. In addition to micro-organisms, parasites such as *Ascaris suum* and whipworm (*Trichuris trichiura*), hair, epithelial cells, *Balantidium coli* and moulds such as *Aspergillus* and *Mucor* may be found. Many of these can gain entrance to the lungs and to the area of the stab wound.

Vertical scalding

Vertical scalding of pig carcases involves the use of a double-walled tunnel in which steam, generated from a water bath in its bottom, is blown over the carcases and through a ventilator located over the condenser. The temperature in the tunnel is controlled by a thermostat at 61–64°C. The cooling water from the condenser in

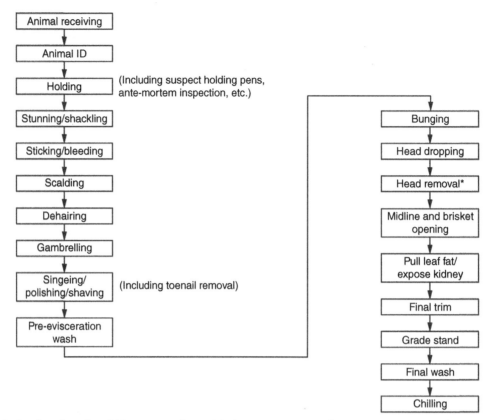

Figure 3.6 Pork slaughter flow chart (skin on carcase). Asterisk denotes two options for processing carcases: skin on or skinned.

the tunnel is used to flush the pig carcases during the dehairing process. Before entry into the tunnel, the carcase should hang for 3 minutes and then lie on its side for 2 minutes. The pig carcases are then transported to the tunnel on a rising rail so that the head is lower than the other parts of the body during the whole scalding process, which lasts 6 minutes. Trimming and singeing take place afterwards. Vertical scalding is claimed to greatly improve the bacteriological standard of the pig meat, produce bacteria-free lungs and reduce muscular degeneration. This reduced incidence of PSE (pale, soft, exudative muscle) is said to be due to the fact that vertical scalding does not produce a rise in body temperature to above 41°C as in normal scalding operations. Dehairing is also said to be better with this method, and operating costs are also claimed to be reduced (Fig. 3.7).

Singeing and scraping

Immediately after mechanical dehairing, the pig carcase may pass through a machine containing rubber whip-like fingers which remove any loose hair before entering an oil- or gas-powered singer typically at 800–900°C for 9–12 seconds. This chars the outer epidermis black, which is then removed by passing the carcase through a series of stainless steel scrapers and nylon brushes.

Screening must be provided to control the water spray and detritus generated by this process.

Refrigeration accommodation

EU Regulation No. 853/2004, Annex III, Chapter VII, requires the operator to ensure that, unless other specific provisions provide otherwise, post-mortem inspection must be followed immediately by chilling in the slaughterhouse to ensure a temperature throughout the meat of not more than 3°C for offal and 7°C for other meat along a chilling curve that ensures a continuous decrease of temperature. Importantly, the temperature decrease having been attained, it must be maintained and ventilation must be sufficient to prevent condensation on the surface of the meat.

In order to achieve these legal requirements, and those of good practice, all but the smallest slaughterhouse will require two chills for carcases. This is necessary to avoid hot carcases from the slaughterhall being mixed with chilled meat with a resultant increase in temperature of the surface of the chilled carcase and condensation. The number and size of the chills must be such as to match the throughput of the facility, the species to be slaughtered, whether beef carcases are to be suspended by the Achilles tendon or aitch bone and the carcase maturation regime to be implemented. Consideration should

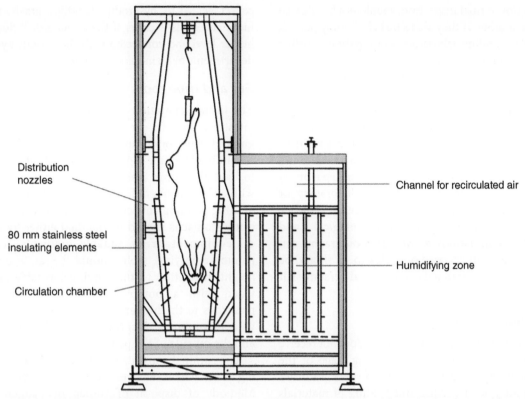

Figure 3.7 Vertical scalding of pigs showing, cross section of humidifying chamber, channel for recirculated air and humidifying zone (by courtesy of SFK AmbA, Copenhagen, Denmark).

Distribution nozzles

80 mm stainless steel insulating elements

Circulation chamber

Channel for recirculated air

Humidifying zone

also be given to the capacity of each chamber to permit optimal energy use and the implementation of an effective cleaning schedule.

In addition, offal on trays and A-frames can be chilled in the same chill as the carcases. However, boxed meat may not be stored in the same chill as exposed meat, so if the intention is to package and store the offal prior to dispatch, a separate chill will be required.

The carcases must be hung in such a way as to allow free movement of cold air around them; rail spacing should be 0.9 m for beef, 0.7 m for pigs and 0.5 m for lambs. Theoretically, the minimum space between carcases on rails should be 0.3–0.4 m. However, pig carcases in particular may be packed much tighter in the chill, often touching, without significant 'hot spots' being subsequently detected.

The positioning of the chiller unit within each chill room is important to ensure efficient operation and hygienic operation. Poor positioning of the unit with, for example, the steel beams supporting the rail system interfering with airflow or drip water or condensate falling onto carcases, particularly during defrosting cycles, should be avoided. The effectiveness of the unit's system to remove condensate from the evaporator via a drip tray and pipes is important and usually requires these to be well insulated and may incorporate a heater.

It is essential to record temperatures in order to control the chilling process, preferably on a continuous basis using charts or computer-generated records. The recording of relative humidity is also of value as is the occasional checking of air speed.

Internal finishes of chills should be durable and impervious, with good insulation and floor drainage. Areas of walls where contact with carcases may occur, for example, on loading, should be protected with stainless steel or plastic sheeting.

It is vital that chill and freezer doors be close fitting and that they be provided with an internal opening device to avoid personnel being closed in the rooms.

Detained meat room

Carcases detained for further examination should be routed by a special rail to the *detained meat room*, which should be located adjacent to the main slaughterhall inspection points in order to achieve close liaison over disease findings. All parts of the carcase must be identifiable pending the final decisions. From this detained meat room, the overhead rail must reconnect with the main slaughter line for direction of carcases either to the chill rooms or to the condemned meat room. It is important that there should be ample space for the examination of carcases which, being hot at this stage and prior to final inspection, should not be allowed to touch each other. If they are to be held for any period, for example, pending laboratory examination, chilling accommodation is necessary.

Good lighting which does not distort colours and is of an intensity of not less than 540 lux is required. The normal facilities of good drainage, easily cleaned surfaces and adequate sterilisation and recording equipment are also necessary. A 'rise and fall' platform or elevated stand is required for detailed examination and trimming of beef carcases. If this particular department is situated adjacent to the meat plant laboratory or sample storage room, this is an added advantage, since microbiological, pathological, parasitological and biochemical examinations, as well as photography, can be more conveniently carried out. This room should be enclosed and entry restricted to authorised personnel. It must be lockable.

Condemned meat room

All too often, the condemned meat room does not receive the attention it deserves at the planning stage of the establishment, especially with regard to space. In order to arrange for proper sorting and holding of materials unfit for human consumption prior to dispatch into their correct animal by-product category, adequate space, refrigeration and drainage along with the supply of durable and lockable containers and weighing facilities are essential. A suitable rail linkage with the detained meat room and other means of handling materials complete this important area, which must have lockable doors. The condemned meat room should be so positioned as to minimise the risk of cross-contamination by the material having to cross through or under the slaughter line.

Hide and skin store

Although primarily intended for the stacking and cooling of hides and sheep skins awaiting collection, the hide and skin store can conveniently be used for the reception of cattle and sheep feet. Again, consideration needs to be given at the planning stage to whether hides and feet are to be considered edible or inedible. Cattle hides can be used for the extraction of collagen, and feet may be scalded, depilated, singed and marketed fit for food following inspection.

Generally 'edible' hides are chilled, and inedible salted.

Careful thought should be given at the planning stage to suitable arrangements for all areas where by-products are held pending dispatch, not only in relation to their position, size, layout, chute system with slaughterhall floor, etc. but also in connection with the facilities for easy loading onto vehicles. A system of handling hides and skins in palletised containers is of value, as is gravity feeding of vehicles which

collect feet. As for by-product handling, gravity feeding of hides and skins is easier if the slaughterhall floor is on a higher level and connected with the various by-products departments by stainless steel chutes.

Gut and tripe room

The initial separation and emptying of stomachs and intestines must be carried out in a separate room, the gut and tripe room, unless hygienic operations can be maintained by time separation. Usually, it is convenient to have this room associated with moving-top tables, with an arrangement for discharging to a macerator or holding pending collection for composting, etc. Heavy cattle stomachs should be handled either by mechanical equipment or by suitable gradients. The cattle paunch-emptying table should be at a convenient height in relation to the moving-top table or be provided with a power-operated hoist for elevating paunches to the higher level. The table must be fitted with an 'umbrella' of spray rods for cleaning the inside and the outside of the paunches.

The ruminal contents may be transferred via a rotating screw, which removes most of the water, into a skip. Methods of disposal of rumen or paunch contents include the following:

1 Landfill, which is an undesirable and uneconomic approach and is becoming less common.
2 Spreading of untreated raw paunch manure directly onto agricultural land is environmentally questionable but still a quite common approach.
3 Use of ensilaged/silaged paunch manure as a feed for livestock has cost implications and the unfavourable perception of feeding waste to animals.
4 Burning, which is not cost-effective.
5 Composting of paunch waste into an organic fertiliser. This method of disposal is simple and part of the natural cycle of life, but it requires special equipment and ample space to produce compost commercially.

Ruminal contents should not be discharged to the effluent collection system. In addition to the high oxygen demand (COD > 100 000 mg/l), undigested solids are not easily degraded in biological systems and tend to build up as sludge in the system, thus reducing treatment efficiency.

Subsequent processing of stomachs and intestines should take place in a separate unit.

Red offal room

Offal such as liver, lungs and kidneys should be trimmed and then placed in a chill or freezing room depending on the ultimate system of disposal. Offal for edible purposes should be held at a temperature not exceeding 3°C.

The edible fat room

This is a completely separate holding room, usually situated near the gut room and where edible fat is held pending dispatch.

Cutting rooms

EU legislation states that within a slaughterhouse, a carcase may only be cut into half carcases or quarters and that half carcases may only be cut into no more than three wholesale cuts. Further processing must be carried out in a specifically approved cutting establishment which may be integrated with a slaughter establishment or stand alone.

Building services, equipment and hygiene conditions are similar to those applying to abattoirs.

During the cutting process, the temperature of the building should not exceed 12°C, and the rooms should have sufficient refrigeration accommodation to keep meat at an internal temperature of not more than 7°C, offal 3°C. There must also be a temperature recording system installed in the cutting room (Fig. 3.8).

It is usual for carcase hygiene and compliance checks to be carried out in an area immediately prior to the cutting room. This may include some trimming, for example, removal of the official hygiene stamps, a check for the presence of SRM, a check for rail grease or detritus which the carcase may have obtained during storage and a check of the carcase temperature and pH. In addition, carcases may be weighed and traceability and batch code details recorded. Facilities will need to be provided for these checks.

Rooms must be provided for the hygienic storage of plastic trays and cartons. The storage of plastic trays which are to contain meat outside is unacceptable even if the trays are to be washed and lined. Exposed meat must be kept separate from cardboard because of the risk of cardboard dust contaminating meat. Conveyers which carry cardboard cartons must be guarded to contain the dust but be easy to dismantle for cleaning.

Equipment wash

A properly designed equipment wash adjacent to workrooms is essential to avoid buggies, bins and other equipment being washed in workrooms, corridors or other inappropriate places. There should be a one-way system through the wash room, to avoid the mixing of clean and dirty equipment, good drainage and, most importantly, good steam extraction.

Fresh meat dispatch area

The fresh meat dispatch area must be sited away from the dirty part and access to it restricted to vehicles associated with meat and offal for human consumption. If at all possible, the floor level of the loading bay should be at vehicle floor height, and the whole area should be roofed so that personnel can work in inclement weather conditions. A system whereby the meat plant rails co-ordinate with those of the meat transport vehicles is of great value in efficiently and hygienically loading meat for delivery. There must be protection against pests of various kinds as well as stops to prevent damage to plant walls. This is best achieved by a docking system whereby there is no air movement from outside the premises into the dispatch area or vehicle.

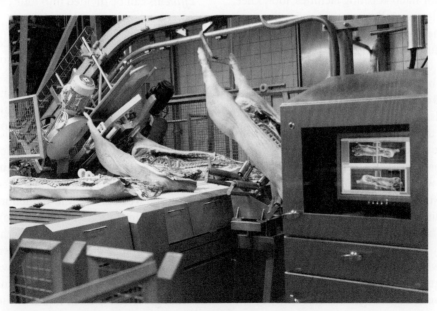

Figure 3.8 Automated pig carcase splitting (Reproduced with permission from Henning).

Vehicle washing

An often neglected facility is that for the cleaning of meat transport and animal transport vehicles.

The former should be provided in the clean side of the establishment and have adequate high-pressure hoses with hot water and detergent along with good drainage for vehicles and wash area. For livestock vehicles lorries, it is sufficient to provide a supply of cold water under pressure along with appropriate disinfectant. As for the meat vehicle wash area, suitable floor gradients are necessary in the plant dirty section. It is not unreasonable, in view of the great importance of having clean vehicles, to insist on the cleaning of all meat vehicles before loading and all stock lorries after unloading.

General amenities for personnel

The ideal layout for amenities is one which forces operatives to follow hygienic practice by design. The entrance lobby should open into a room containing lockers for street clothes which opens into the slush room, or hygiene lobby, containing boot wash, hand wash, apron wash and hanging area before entering into the processing room. Toilets and canteen should be placed on the entrance lobby side of the changing rooms forcing the operate to disrobe completely into street clothes before visiting either.

A sufficient number of flush lavatories, showers and wash-hand basins must be provided. One lavatory for every 15 employees is recommended. It is recognised that showers are rarely used by operatives under normal circumstances so their number should only be sufficient to fulfil the requirements of the competent authority. Non-contact taps for hand-washing facilities, foot, knee, elbow or photo-electric cell operation must be used. Hand towels are the preferred method for drying hands. Separate units must be provided if both sexes are employed.

Lockers should be of metal construction with sloping tops and placed 40 cm above the floor in order to facilitate cleaning. A plastic, stainless steel or wooden bench along the front of the lockers at this level completes the furniture. Separate lockers should be provided for each employee's personal and work clothing, if alternative means of storing work clothing and equipment is not provided. Soiled working clothing should not be stored in lockers but be directed to the laundry.

Urinals should be installed in toilet rooms for male personnel.

It is well worthwhile giving close consideration to the layout and design of changing facilities for staff. Ventilation in these areas is of great importance, as is a code of practice for their use.

The efficient operation of a meat plant depends greatly on the well-being of its personnel. Although a fully trained *industrial nurse and* a well-appointed *first-aid room* are considered beneficial, especially for the larger premises, not only to deal with cuts and other problems associated with slaughtering operations but also to assist materially in raising hygiene standards and preventing the onset of zoonoses, they have mostly been replaced by a trained first-aider.

A *laundry* and conveniently sited *car park* are necessary departments of the modern meat plant and a comprehensive *system of internal communication* and adequate *security arrangements*.

Veterinary office

An adequately equipped lockable facility, preferably a room, for the exclusive use of the veterinary service is essential. The rooms should be provided with hand-washing and shower facilities and lockers for clothing (work and personal) and meat inspection equipment. A convenient means of cleaning footwear before entry into changing rooms is an advantage.

Treatment of effluent

The processing of carcases and the resultant by-products give rise to large amounts of highly polluting wastewaters, semi-solids and solids, which must be separated and treated before being discharged into the environment.

The objective of effluent treatment is to produce a product that can be safely discharged into a waterway or sewer in compliance with the recommended limits for discharge.

Effluents can be divided into four categories:

1 Non-toxic and not directly pollutant but liable to disturb the physical nature of the receiving water
2 Non-toxic and pollutant load to organic matter content of high oxygen demand
3 Toxic – containing highly poisonous materials
4 Toxic and pollutant due to organic matter of high oxygen demand and toxic in addition

The most effective way to reduce cost of wastewater treatment through capital expenditures or operating expenses is through reduction at source of the volume of waste to be treated. Volume reduction can be achieved through minimisation of water usage and spillages and also through good housekeeping within the processing facility. The first priorities at the effluent treatment plant are to separate effluent from storm water, to lessen the quantity of material requiring treatment, to physically separate gross solids from liquid effluent and to reduce the amount of biological treatment required.

This can be achieved by the use of grilles over drains, fat traps, grit settlement and other preliminary treatments, along with continuous dry cleaning or 'clean as you go' during the operation of the plant and at breaks in production.

Pollution parameters

Biochemical oxygen demand (BOD) is a measure of the readily biodegradable material in a wastewater. It is obtained by measuring the oxygen consumed by aerobic organisms, when a known volume of the effluent is added to a known volume of oxygen-saturated water and incubated at 20°C for 5 days. It is generally used to express the concentration of pollutant within a wastewater.

Chemical oxygen demand (COD) is a measure of the oxygen required for the oxidation of all oxidisable organic and inorganic matter in a known volume of effluent, using a standard technique. The COD is often used as a faster and more accurate means of determining the oxygen requirements of an effluent before treatment. A ratio between BOD and COD can be established for a particular wastewater. COD measurement can be used as a predictive measurement of BOD.

BOD and COD values vary greatly in the various food processing operations (Table 3.4). BOD can cause oxygen depletion to waterways into which it is discharged, whereas COD may not but may contain inhibitors or toxins that could also have detrimental effect on flora and fauna.

Chloride (Cl) is a measure of salinity.

Dry matter (DM) or *total solids* (TS) is the final weight of solids derived from a known amount of effluent that has been dried to a constant weight at 105°C over 24 hours. It is measured in gram per litre or milligram per litre.

Grease, fat and oil are a group of substances having common properties of immiscibility with water and a lower specific gravity, which cause them to float. Concentrations are measured by the amount of solvent required for the effluent to become soluble. Some water authorities in the United Kingdom will accept a level of 100 mg/l. The substances tend to coat treatment systems,

clogging pipes, pumping systems and screens. They reduce oxygen transfer and can seriously reduce the efficiency of aerobic treatment systems. They also lead to odour problems as accumulated grease or fat becomes rancid.

pH is a measure of the acidity or alkalinity of an aqueous solution. Pure water has a pH value of 7.0. Biological wastewater treatment processes work best at a pH value of 7.0 (neutral).

Total nitrogen (N) occurs in three forms in effluents: organic nitrogen, inorganic nitrogen and free ammonia and nitrites. *Ammonia* in solution is toxic to aquatic life; the maximum discharge to sewers is 40 mg/l. High nitrate concentrations in natural waters encourage algae and other plant growth, thus blocking water courses. The maximum level permissible in potable water is 0.5 mg/l. Levels of 0.5 mg/l or greater in chlorinated water lead to taste and odour complaints and also to the development of THMs or trihalomethanes which are bio-cumulative and carcinogenic.

Pathogenic bacteria: Potable water should not contain any coliform organisms.

Suspended solids (SS) refer to matter which is insoluble and is suspended in the water. It consists of both organic and inorganic components. The organic material will eventually be degraded.

Temperature should not be more than a few degrees above the temperature of the receiving water in order not to disturb the natural biocycle.

Turbidity and colour: Effluent should be clear and colourless.

Volatile solids (VS) are used as a measure of biogas production (not applicable to aeration tanks, only useful in the context of anaerobic digestion).

Treatment

Chemical and microbial standards are set for the discharge of effluent, and these will depend on the volume and strength of the effluent and dilution properties of the receiving watercourse or public sewer to which it is being discharged.

Air pollution with regard to odours is measured subjectively and is related to the effect the odour has on the public, that is, the degree of 'nuisance'.

Preliminary treatment: Screening, solids and grit removal

Preliminary treatment is based on the removal of solids, and this is best done by letting all water pass through one or more screens. These screens should be non-clogging and self-cleaning, adaptable to variable water flows, easy to clean automatically or manually (when required), odourless and noiseless. The resultant screenings may

Table 3.4 Average BOD values for some food processing operations

Source	BOD (mg/l)
Poultry meat plant	1000–1200
Pig meat plant	1500–2000
Cattle/sheep meat plant	1400–3200
Fish processing	1000–3000
Dairy (washings)	600–1300

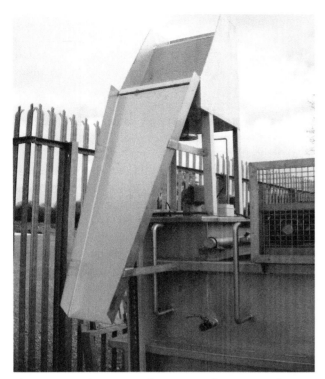

Figure 3.9 Wedge wire rundown screen (by courtesy of Enisca, Cookstown, Northern Ireland).

need the organic content to be reduced by washing. After the removal of coarse solids, the effluent stream still contains finely SS, fats and grease. Further screening may be required. Coarse screening generally will be 10–25 mm with fine screening reducing to 5–6 mm. For small quantities of low-grade material, a simple fat trap is all that is required. This is in the form of a minimum-turbulence, flow-through tank generally consisting of a number of stages. Settleable solids can remain long enough to settle out on the bottom of the tank, while grease and fine solids rise to the surface. Continuous sludge removal and skimming of the surface to remove scum are essential (Fig. 3.9).

Dissolved air flotation (DAF) is a successful method of removing SS, fats, grease, and BOD and is particularly useful to provide partial treatment for discharge to a sewer. It causes a physical separation of suspended matter, fats and grease by the production of micro-bubbles of air that attach themselves to the suspended material, lifting it to the surface to form scum, which is removed by a continuous scraper mechanism, while the supernatant liquor is discharged continuously either to a sewer or for further biological treatment. The addition of chemicals that aid flocculation results in a higher removal efficiency of BOD, SS and fat. A large range of flocculants is available, for example, ferric chloride/sulphate, ferrous sulphate, aluminium sulphate (alum), sodium carbonate (soda ash), calcium carbonate (lime),

polyelectrolytes and others. Each flocculant works at an optimal pH range. The pH of the effluent has to be adjusted and varies depending on the flocculant used. Typically, the addition of caustic soda or hydrochloric acid is used to control the effluent pH (Fig. 3.10).

Balancing tanks may be required when strict control of hourly and daily flow rates is required or when production is cyclical throughout a 24-hour period. Balancing tanks should be aerated to maintain a fresh wastewater and avoid odour generation.

Secondary treatment

Secondary treatment is carried out using various types of *biological treatment systems*, which involve maintaining under controlled conditions a mixed culture of micro-organisms which utilise the continuous supply of organic matter present in the effluent to synthesise new cells.

Anaerobic digestion is carried out in totally enclosed systems to prevent the entry of air. It will result in a fast reduction of organic material with the production of biogas. With a BOD higher than 2000 mg/l, it becomes advantageous. The system operates as a two-stage fermentation process in which the stages occur simultaneously within the digester.

During the first stage, bacteria break down complex organic substances into simpler compounds, the most important being volatile fatty acids (VFA). In the second stage, methanogenic organisms utilise the VFA to yield methane and carbon dioxide. Maintaining the pH at around 7.0–7.2 is very important. Overproduction of VFA will lower the pH and stop the process, which can be difficult to re-start. This is very much a 'living' process, and the addition of a balanced effluent is essential. Too much protein can destroy the process, and therefore, blood must not be introduced. There is a high capital cost, the operatives require extensive training, and the surplus treated effluent requires further aerobic treatment before it can be discharged into water courses.

Activated sludge process

Aerobic digestion is less sensitive to shock loading; the retention time is shorter, and therefore, the tanks are smaller and cheaper. Air is added via low-pressure air blowers in combination with fine bubble air diffusers or by using surface aerators powered by geared motors (Fig. 3.11).

The factors which affect the degree of aeration required by the reactor are concentration of dissolved oxygen, the hydraulic retention time and substrate-loading rate, pH, temperature, presence of toxic substances, nutrient content and discharge consent requirement.

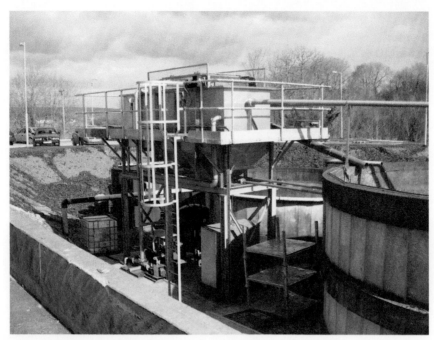

Figure 3.10 Typical DAF installation (by courtesy of Enisca, Cookstown, Northern Ireland).

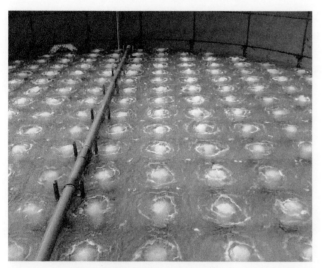

Figure 3.11 Fine bubble diffused air systems (by courtesy of Enisca, Cookstown, Northern Ireland).

The dissolved organic matter, colloidal residues and fine solids are oxidised to carbon dioxide and water. Proteins are broken down into nitrates and sulphates by a mixed culture of micro-organisms in the reactor. The major product of the process is new cells (biomass). The biomass, together with material which has resisted biodegradation, is separated out from the treated effluent in settling tanks (clarifiers). The supernatant liquor from the clarifier is discharged over a weir for disposal or further treatment, if required. A proportion of sludge

(return activated sludge) which settles out at the base of the clarifier is returned to the reactor vessel to maintain the critical concentration of biomass. The remainder (waste activated sludge) is drawn off to be concentrated and may require further treatment before disposal. Where sludges are to be applied to land which is fallow or is to be seed-bed for arable crops, the application is unlikely to become a problem unless the land is close to urban development, when odours may cause a nuisance. Low-trajectory agricultural slurry spreaders can be used. When sludges are to be applied to grassland, there is a greater risk of grazing stock ingesting any pathogens present. In the United Kingdom, a minimum holding period of 4–6 weeks is required for animal slurries. However, in some EU member states, a period of 6 months is mandatory. Alternatively, sludge can be injected into the soil; application rates will vary with soil type, field capacity and type of crop. Rates in excess of $120\,m^3$/ha are most likely to lead to run-off by leaching or via land drains.

Further reading

Food and Agriculture Organization (FAO) Standard design for small scale modular slaughterhouses, www.fao.org/docrep/003/t0034e/T0034E01.htm (accessed on 9 April 2014).

MLC Industry Consulting, Slaughterhouse Design Manual, March 2007.

Recommended Animal Handling Guidelines and Audit Guide, 2007 Edition, American Meat Institute Foundation.

4

Preservation of meat

The primary purpose of food preservation is to prevent food spoilage. Whether food spoilage is mild or extreme, the primary cause is the action of micro-organisms – bacteria, moulds or yeasts – aided by enzymes. As living organisms, they can survive and develop only under particular environmental conditions; under unfavourable conditions, they die or at least fail to develop.

The underlying principle of all food preserving methods, therefore, is the creation of conditions unfavourable to the growth or survival of spoilage organisms by, for example, extreme heat or cold, deprivation of water and sometimes oxygen, excess of saltiness or increased acidity. The methods by which meat foods may be preserved are drying, curing, cold, heat, chemicals, irradiation and high pressure.

Preservation by *chemicals* may be achieved by, for example, the addition of sulphur dioxide to foodstuffs such as fresh sausage, but this and the use of other chemicals are greatly restricted by food regulations in most countries, although research continues to find an acceptable chemical means of preservation.

Chemical preservation can also be achieved by smoking of meat and fish usually as an adjuvant to commercial salting and pickling.

Physical changes in stored meat

Meat undergoes certain superficial changes as a result of storage, chief of which are shrinkage, sweating and loss of bloom.

Shrinkage

Shrinkage or loss of weight occurs as a result of *evaporation* of water from the meat surface; carcases cut into quarters dissipate water vapour rapidly and continuously and retail joints even more so. On the other hand, evaporation is inhibited by membranes such as the pleura and peritoneum and, in carcases of well-nourished animals, by the solidification of the superficial fat and drying of the connective tissue. A freshly killed carcase dissipates body weight slowly, losing 1.5–2.0% of weight by evaporation during the first 24 hours of hanging. Further loss of weight during storage depends on the humidity of the storage room: the drier the air the greater the amount of evaporation. The high-velocity cold air system (TurboChill) reduces body heat of freshly killed animals by increasing the rate of heat removal from the surface of the carcase and hence reduces surface temperature quickly. Avoidance of all evaporative weight losses by high humidity facilitates the formation of moulds, so an accurate balance between temperature and humidity must be maintained; the dry, impervious film on the carcase surface is perhaps the best protection against the growth of spoilage organisms.

Sweating

This denotes the *condensation* of water vapour on meat brought from a cold store into ordinary room temperature. The condensation occurs because the refrigerated carcase lowers the temperature of the air to below the dew point. In the winter months in Britain, the dew point is generally below 4.5°C, and sweating is unlikely to occur, but in the summer, the dew point is always over 7°C, and moisture will be deposited on the carcase. If the quarter or side is cut up immediately after removal from the chilling room, sweating will be extended to the individual joints.

Gracey's Meat Hygiene, Eleventh Edition. Edited by David S. Collins and Robert J. Huey.
© 2015 John Wiley & Sons, Ltd. Published 2015 by John Wiley & Sons, Ltd.

Loss of bloom

Bloom is defined as the colour and general appearance of a carcase surface when viewed through the semi-transparent layers of connective tissue, muscle and fat which form the carcase surface. If these tissues become moist, the collagen fibres in the connective tissue swell and become opaque and the meat surface assumes a dull, lifeless appearance. Loss of surface bloom in beef carcases may also be caused by dehydration or undue oxidation, but it may be prevented by avoiding temperature fluctuations that permit alternate drying and dampening of the carcase surface. It is also important to keep the relative humidity of cooling chambers high and ensure free circulation of air. Muscular tissue also tends to become brownish on exposure to air as myohaemoglobin changes to the brown pigment methaemoglobin, but the actual amount of exposed muscle in a side of beef is so small that this is of little or no consequence. Refrigeration has little effect on the carcase fat except in the case of frozen meat which has undergone a prolonged period of storage, in which case rancidity may develop.

Chemical changes in stored meat

The chemical changes that take place after slaughter are indicative of a slight degree of breakdown in protein, due either to endogenous enzymes or to those of micro-organisms. The odour of the meat becomes progressively more marked but never undesirable; the flavour may be described as stale, rendering the meat unpalatable but not repulsive.

The storage life of meat is more dependent on the chemical changes that take place in fat rather than in muscle, for fat rancidity, even if only slight, is objectionable. The condition of the fat therefore determines the length of storage, for while the lean muscle of a carcase may be still improving in flavour, the changes in fat may render the meat repugnant and unmarketable.

Drying

Although drying as such plays only a minor role in preservation today, the whole vast process of refrigeration is largely based on the principle of drying, that is, the removal of water available for microbial growth. Again, salting largely owes its preservation action to the extraction of water by osmosis.

It is essential that as little water as possible is put on sheep and cattle carcases during dressing.

Water activity or water availability (a_w)

Water activity or water availability, a_w, is a measure of the partial vapour pressure of the foodstuffs compared to that of pure water at its surface. Water molecules are loosely orientated in pure liquid water and can easily rearrange. When solutes are introduced, these orient the water molecules around them and make them much less available for use by micro-organisms. With the exception of *Staphylococcus aureus* and most moulds, micro-organisms are poor at competing with solutes for the water molecules.

The a_w varies little with temperature over the normal growth range of micro-organisms. Pure water has the highest a_w possible (1.0), and the a_w decreases with the addition of solute (always <1).

Various NaCl solutions will give the following a_w.

%NaCl (w/v)	a_w
0.9	0.995
3.5	0.98
7.0	0.96
16.0	0.90
22.0	0.86

The a_w may greatly affect the ability of an organism to survive heat. The thermal death time (D_{60}) for *Salmonella typhimurium* at 60°C is 0.18 minutes at an a_w of 0.94.

The a_w stated for an organism is usually the minimum at which growth will take place, but growth will increase with increasing a_w. Lower than minimal a_w will not necessarily kill the organisms, and they will remain infectious. It is difficult to standardise an a_w for a specific food as this may vary depending on the source, the age of the food and even different parts of the food.

Meat curing

While curing may be applied to all kinds of meat, it is best adapted to those with a high fat content, for example, pork or fine-fibred beef intermixed with fat, and it is for this reason that brisket and flank of beef make high-quality pickled meat. On the other hand, lean beef, veal or mutton becomes dry and unpalatable on pickling.

Salt

Salt is the principal preserving material used in curing on a commercial scale, though it appears to have little directly harmful effect on bacteria; large quantities of salt or sugar produce the same result as would be obtained by the extraction of water. Indeed, the osmotic pressure of the strong salt or sugar solution removes the water necessary for bacterial growth from the meat. Halophilic (salt-loving) bacteria require salt for optimum growth and are not affected; they are, however, slower growing than non-halophilic bacteria.

Distinction must be made between salted meats (beef, pork) and cured meats (bacon, ham, corned beef). In salted meats, the dry salt first dissolves in the surface

Table 4.1 Curing salts and additives

Ingredient	Level in curing brine	Function
Sodium chloride	15–30%	Preservative, improves texture
Sodium nitrate[a]	0.15–1.5%	A source of nitrite
Sodium nitrite[a]	500–1000 ppm	Preservative, reduced by meat enzymes to NO, which combined with myoglobin (the uncured meat pigment) forms nitrosomyoglobin, the cured meat pigment
Polyphosphates	2–4%	Reduce cooking losses, for example, during smoking, improve texture
Sugars, for example, sucrose, maple syrup	1–4%	Improves flavour by masking the harshness of the salt
Liquid smoke	ca. 1%	Flavouring agent
Sodium ascorbate[b]	0.2–1.0%	Reducing agent. Improves colour formation and stability by effecting rapid reduction of NO_2 and NO_3 in the meat

[a] In the United Kingdom, levels must not exceed 500 ppm $NaNO_3$ and 200 ppm $NaNO_2$ in the final product.
[b] Varies considerably; refer to manufacturer's instructions.

fluid and then passes slowly inwards until it is evenly distributed throughout the meat substance. A considerable amount of the moisture is removed when the salt draws to the surface some of the fluid in which it dissolves. Microscopically, salted meat, compared with fresh meat, shows a diminution in the size of the intercellular spaces as a result of loss of water.

Curing may be defined as the addition of *salt* (NaCl) and *nitrate/nitrite* or *nitric oxide* to the meat, which results in a conversion of the meat pigments, predominantly myoglobin, to the nitroso or cured form. Myoglobin in freshly cut uncured meat is in the reduced form (purple), which in contact with air is rapidly oxygenated to oxymyoglobin, which is bright red and responsible for familiar colour of freshly cut meat. If oxidised, these pigments are converted to metamyoglobin, which is unattractive and gives a brown or grey colour. Under suitable conditions, these pigments can be converted to the nitroso form (nitrosomyoglobin) by the addition of nitric oxide. During the curing process, nitric oxide is formed by reduction of nitrites formed by bacteria from nitrates. Nitrosomyoglobin gives freshly cut cured meat its bright red colour but is unstable and rapidly oxidises to the brown and grey forms. However, on heating, the nitrosomyoglobin is converted to nitrosohaemochrome, a pink colour (e.g. of cooked ham or corned beef) as distinct from the grey and brown of the cooked uncured meat (e.g. roast beef).

Ingredients used in curing

Basically to produce a cured meat, only *sodium chloride* and a source of *nitric oxide* (*nitrate* or *nitrite*) are required. However, with a demand by consumers for a greater variety of cured meats in relation to saltiness and other flavour components, a wide range of substances can be used (Table 4.1). Each ingredient has a specific function and is used accordingly.

Production of bacon and ham

Pork may be cured by either salting or pickling. Dry salting gives a less consistent product and takes longer and is therefore more expensive.

The raw material in the United Kingdom and Ireland, an 80–100 kg live weight pig, is slaughtered and eviscerated to produce an 80 kg carcase. Slaughter weights have increased by 10 kg over the last decade to come closer to the EU average of around a 90 kg carcase, Italy killing the oldest and heaviest pigs producing a 125 kg carcase for Parma ham production.

White-skinned pigs have traditionally been preferred as the bacon rind has a more attractive appearance. A pig with light shoulders; long, level back; and deep and level flanks with broad hams is most likely to yield a carcase well endowed in the region of the most valuable bacon cuts, for in a side of bacon the collar and foreleg together should not weigh more than 25% of the whole side.

After *stunning* and *bleeding* for at least 6 minutes, most pig carcases in the British Isles are *scalded*, *dehaired*, *singed* and *scraped* in preparation for bacon production rather than being skinned. The scalding water may contain different types of bacteria originating from the pig's skin and gastrointestinal tract, including *Salmonella*. The temperature of the water in the drag-through scalding tank at 60°C is generally sufficient to reduce vegetative growth. The skins of scalded pigs have low numbers of both enteric pathogens and spoilage bacteria, but the subsequent dehairing process recontaminates the skin. The bacterial content of the muscle and viscera does, however, appear to be affected by the type of scalding equipment. Vertical scalding of pigs on the line in a 'steam cabinet' reduces the opportunity for contamination of the carcase via the stick wound. After dehairing, the carcase is hoisted onto a greased skid rail and transferred to a singeing plant, which consists of two vertical half-cylinders lined with heatproof bricks. The carcase is *singed* by a fired combination of oil and air or by gas burners at a temperature of 1300°C. Temperatures on the skin surface vary, but thermal imaging studies have demonstrated a range of carcase surface temperatures immediate after full body singeing between 100 and 200°C.

Singeing colours the skin brown, removes any hairs still remaining, hardens the subcutaneous fat, enhances the keeping quality of the meat and sterilises the external surface of the pig so that following effective singeing the bacterial load on the carcase surface has been completely removed Berends *et al.* (1997). On leaving the furnace, the carcases are sprayed with cold water and scraped and polished in a tunnel containing banks of stainless steel scrapers and nylon brushes until the burnt brown epidermis has been removed and the pig appears white. These procedures, however, recontaminate the surface of the carcase to the order of 10^4 bacteria/cm^2. Bolton *et al.* (2002) suggested the process could result in an overall reduction of contamination of the order of 3 log units/cm^2.

The majority of these are spoilage bacteria, predominantly *acinetobacteria*, *moraxellae* and *pseudomonads*, with enteric organisms such as *E. coli* and *Campylobacter* at single figures per cm^2.

The carcases are then ready for evisceration, inspection, weighing and grading followed by immediate transfer via overhead rails to the chills where they are chilled to <4°C within 24 hours.

Cutting

Under modern systems, very few Wiltshires (full sides of bacon) are produced, it being more common to reduce the side to individual primal cuts before curing. The butchery processes vary but generally commence on removal from the chillers with the removal of the head and forelegs while the pig is still suspended on the overhead rail. This produces two sides which are dropped onto a moving steel conveyor, before the removal of the jaw flap from the fore. The hindleg is cut midway through the hock, and the fore-end is removed by a bandsaw at the level of the third and fourth rib. The fillet (also known as the tenderloin) runs from the third most posterior rib back along the dorsal surface of the abdominal cavity to the gammon. This is carefully removed, and any loose pieces of meat, for example, the diaphragm, are trimmed off the side. The gammon, the hindleg, is removed by a bandsaw, midway between the head of the femur and a part of the sacrum known as the oyster bone. The pelvic bones are removed and the gammon is trimmed.

The spinal column, or chine bones, is removed using a circular saw, and the middle is slit into belly and back cuts. The ribs may be removed individually, by a process known as single ribbing, or in sheets. Finally, excess fat is trimmed off, and in most cases, the rind is removed.

Application of the pickle

Salt for the cure may be kept in a large silo through which water filters to produce a saturated salt solution. This is chilled to −2 or −3°C and *nitrite* added to a concentration not exceeding 150 mg/kg. Usually, nitrate is not used as a constituent of the pickle. This is because nitrate is only effective in so far as it is converted into nitrite by bacteria present in the cover brine. *Sodium ascorbate* is added as a source of ascorbic acid, a reducing agent, which aids the formation of nitrosomyoglobin and hence ensures that the bacon or ham has good colour formation and stability. In a maple cure, sugar, maple crystals and seasoning give the bacon a unique flavour. *Polyphosphates* aid water retention in the cured meat during the cooking process, so reducing shrinkage during cooking, making the hams more succulent and improving the texture of smoked product.

The amount of curing salts which can be used is regulated in the United Kingdom by the Miscellaneous Food Additives and Sweeteners in Food Regulations 2007, implementing recommendations from EFSA 2003. The legislation restricted the amount of sodium nitrite that can be used as an input to 150 mg/kg, which is equivalent to 178 mg/kg of potassium nitrate. For sterilised meat product, the input is reduced to a level of 100 mg/kg of sodium nitrite equivalent to 123 mg/kg potassium nitrate. Exceptions are made for some traditional processes, such as traditional immersion-cured products, including Wiltshire hams, and traditional dry-cured meat products. Permitted levels for these products vary and are based on levels of residue rather than input levels. As an example, the maximum residue limit for Wiltshire bacon or ham is 250 mg/kg of nitrate.

This was in recognition that nitrites can react with secondary and tertiary amines to form nitrosamines, which are carcinogenic. Earlier methods of curing, by hand injection of pumping brine (called stitching) followed by immersion of the sides in cover brine for at least 4 days, have largely been superseded. The brine or pickle is now introduced into all sides of the prepared cuts by automatic pumping machines which introduce pickle under pressure through needles approximately 2 cm apart. The addition of pickle increases the weight of the piece by approximately 10%.

Immediately after pumping, the middle cuts, back and belly, are vac packed and heat sealed. They are held in cellars at a temperature below 4°C for at least 48 hours before going for blast freezing (−6°C for 5 hours), slicing and packing. The freezing process suspends curing and assists high-speed slicing.

The gammons, after pumping, are immersed in traditional tiled or stainless steel tanks of cover brine for 3 days. The cover brine is used for approximately 3 weeks before it is discarded and is constantly monitored bacteriologically. In former times, cover brine was used indefinitely and was thought to impart unique flavours to the product.

Production of cooked hams

Reformed cooked hams are produced from defatted lean cuts. Following pickle injection, these are tumbled in a machine that looks like a cement mixer with sharp stainless steel blades in a rotating drum or massaged in a 'Bel Lagan' massager. In general, small pieces of meat are *tumbled*, while large pieces are *massaged*. The machines rotate for 7 minutes in every hour for 18 hours, moving the meat around and ensuring that a uniform cure and colour are attained. The physical action also tenderises the muscle and aids fast penetration of the curing agent, thus saving on curing time. The process releases the albuminous protein myosin from the meat, leaving its surface in a gelatinous state. When cooked, the meat binds together, the myosin acting as a seal, aiding water retention.

When removed from the tumbling or massaging process, the product may be allowed to rest for up to 24 hours, or it may be immediately further processed.

Large pieces are manually packed into pots with pressure lids and cooked for 14 hours to a core temperature of 70°C. Smaller pieces are automatically fed into presses which extrude the pork into pre-soaked fibrous casings. These are semi-cooked for 4–5 hours to a core temperature of 42°C in preparation for slicing and vacuum packing.

To ensure consistently high quality, a mid-process analysis is carried out. A random sample of product, selected from different cuts, is analysed for levels of nitrite, salt and added water. There is a standard declaration of not more than 10% added water for middles, backs and streak. Massaged or tumbled product is allowed up to 20% added water.

Traditional dry-cured bacon

Although described as dry cure, some brine is injected by hand into the eye muscle of the back and deep into the gammon. Both cuts are then sprinkled with the dry-cured mixture, which contains nitrite, before being covered in salt. The middles are stacked, cut surface up, for 5 days, after which excess salt is shaken off and the sides are turned rind up, and left for 2–3 weeks. The gammons are packed into tanks with salt for 4 weeks. On removal, all cuts are washed down to remove some of the salt. They are then hung on racks and singed with a blowtorch to remove any slime on the surface and dried overnight, in a room with circulating air at 10–20°C. The bacon produced may then be smoked, if required, and prepared for dispatch by trimming the gammons and rolling and placing the middles in stockinette.

Alternative dry cure

An alternative type of dry curing entails placing fresh rindless pork backs on racks, freezing, pressing into shape, allowing to temper and slicing. As it comes to the end of the slicing line, the product is sprayed on both sides with salt and nitrite solution and then packaged. Curing takes place in the bag, there being not more than 3½% salt in the final product.

Smoking

Smoking of cured pork improves its keeping properties further, as well as imparting an appetising colour and flavour. Traditionally, smoking was carried out over several days in a brick oven with smouldering oak, hickory or hardwood sawdust and hot ash piled on the floor.

It is now more common to use an insulated steel cabinet enclosing a heat-exchanger system. The cuts to be smoked are hung on racks and placed in the cabinet, and the temperature is raised to approximately 32°C for 30 minutes. Smoke, produced by a smoke generator consisting of a hopper which automatically feeds dry hardwood sawdust onto a cast iron hotplate, is drawn into the cabinet for 1–2 hours. It is important to ensure that the temperature does not rise above 37°C or the fat may melt.

The chief bacteriostatic and bactericidal substance in woodsmoke is formaldehyde. The combination of heat and smoke usually causes a significant reduction in the surface bacterial population. In addition, a physical barrier is provided by superficial dehydration, coagulation of protein and the absorption of resinous substances.

Common defects in cured meat

1 *Fiery red areas* are caused by lack of available nitrite – miscure. This may occur in deep meat cuts.
2 *Jelly pockets* are caused by injection of brine into connective tissue, which it denatures.

3 *Areas of discolouration* may be caused by bruising or blood splashing. This can be very obvious in the cooked product.
4 *Rancidity in frozen bacon* may be identified by pronounced yellowing of the fat. Although all bacterial growth stops when bacon is frozen, certain chemical reactions can proceed at −8°C.
5 *Browning.* The cured meat pigment nitrosomyoglobin changes to the brown metamyoglobin owing to dehydration caused by low humidity, high temperature and oxidation caused by prolonged exposure to air, excessive nitrate and poor packaging.
6 *Greening* may be caused by excessive nitrate and by bacterial contamination.

Micro-organisms on cured product

The most common form of spoilage found on cured meats is mouldiness, which may be due to *Aspergillus, Alternaria, Fusarium, Mucor, Rhizopus, Penicillium, Cladosporium* and other moulds.

Micrococci are resistant to salt and consequently are most common where salt levels are high, especially the fat. *Lactobacilli* are less resistant to salt but more resistant to smoke. These, together with *Acinetobacter, Bacillus, Pseudomonas* and *Proteus*, may result in the fermentation of sugars in the product to produce *sours* of various types. Pickling cannot be relied upon to destroy parasitic infections, for example, *cysticerci* in beef or pork.

Refrigeration

The modern meat industry is based on efficient refrigeration. Carcases of freshly slaughtered animals have surfaces that are warm and wet and thus provide a perfect substrate for the growth of pathogenic and spoilage organisms. Chilling immediately post-slaughter reduces the surface temperature to a value below the minimum growth temperature for many pathogens. The combination of low temperatures and surface drying inhibits the growth of spoilage bacteria. To provide a long, safe, high-quality shelf life, the temperature of the meat needs to be kept at a temperature close to its initial freezing point. Combining a high standard of hygiene and packaging with a temperature of −1 to +0.5°C during storage, transport and display can routinely extend shelf life to 12 weeks. If longer periods are required, then freezing the meat will extend the storage period into years. Scientific studies show that freezing has little if any effect on the eating quality of red meat. Overall, the studies indicate that the meat may be slightly more tender after freezing. Freezing does increase the ultimate amount of drip from meat, and this makes the meat less attractive. However, the increased drip does not influence the eating quality after cooking.

In the process of refrigeration, heat is extracted from the carcase in the chill rooms, two basic laws of physics being involved in this process. First, the boiling point of a liquid – the temperature at which it is turned into vapour – depends on the pressure. At normal atmospheric pressure (1 atm = 760 mm Hg; 29.92, 1013.25 N/m² at sea level), water boils at 100°C, but at a pressure of 0.1 atm, it boils at 46°C. Conversely, water vapour at 50°C and 0.1 atm can be condensed back to water by increasing the pressure to 1 atm. When a liquid passes into a vapour, it absorbs heat which is given off again when it condenses.

Refrigerants are liquids or liquefied gases with low boiling points, for example, ammonia or hydrofluorocarbons (HFCs), which, in the refrigeration cycle, extract heat at low temperature when evaporated and give off this heat to the outside air when recondensed.

The preservative action of refrigeration is based on the prevention of multiplication of harmful bacteria, yeasts and moulds by the artificial lowering of the temperature. The failure of bacteria to grow at or below freezing depends mainly on the removal of the available water as ice; about 70% is removed at −3.5°C and 94% at −10°C. A further factor is the inhibition of the life processes of spoilage organisms at low temperatures, though the actual lethal effect is small. At a temperature of −8°C, the multiplication of all micro-organisms stops and only resumes when the temperature is raised later to a suitable level. Neither fast (cryogenic) nor slow (blast) freezing completely destroys all the bacteria commonly found in beef carcases; frozen meat which is thawed yields an abundant supply of water and forms an excellent medium for bacterial growth. In addition, the pH of muscle, which remains constant while the meat is frozen, falls rapidly after thawing but then rises rapidly to create an environment which favours bacterial multiplication.

The surface growth of *mould* on meat is controlled not only by the temperature but by the relative humidity of the atmosphere. Some moulds are capable of growing on the surface of meat at several degrees below freezing point, but they require the presence of water in the surrounding atmosphere as otherwise they lose water by evaporation and wither. For the prevention of mould, the temperature and relative humidity must therefore be kept as low as possible.

Mechanical refrigeration

Carbon dioxide and sulphur dioxide were at one time commonly used as cooling liquids (refrigerants), but carbon dioxide is uneconomical, and sulphur dioxide is corrosive and toxic.

Legislation

Currently, legislation on refrigeration tends to concentrate on the desired outcome of maintaining the cold chain in order to minimise the growth of pathogens or spoilage micro-organisms. This is key to the operators' responsibility to maintain a food safety management system incorporating 'pre-requisites' and implementing the principles of HACCP. Temperature controls are often considered to be part of a HACCP pre-requisite programme. These requirements encompass not only effective refrigeration equipment in rooms handling, storing and transporting fresh meat but also a requirement to ensure sufficient airflow and ventilation to reduce humidity and facilities that are sufficiently large to prevent overloading particularly during peak production periods.

Regulation No. 853/2004 requires red meat to be reduced from a muscle temperature of 35–40°C at slaughter to an internal temperature of 7°C, white meat to 4°C and offal to 3°C, progressively.

The legislation also requires the refrigeration system to be fitted with recording equipment which can monitor and control the temperatures of the storage or working environment so as to monitor and adjust the equipment to achieve the desired effect. Automatic monitoring system should be fitted with an audible and visible alarm. Most alarm systems now have the capability to be viewed remotely through mobile communication devices.

Regular recalibration of monitoring equipment is essential.

Ammonia, first introduced in 1876, is still used extensively today, although it is somewhat corrosive and has a penetrating odour so that leaks can affect stored products. There is a revival of interest in ammonia as a refrigerant for larger plants because of the lesser effect on the ozone layer. Today, the chlorofluorocarbons (CFCs) – primarily the freons – are being replaced by hydrofluro-carbons (HFC), again because of the lower ozone depletion potential, this time due to the absence of chlorine.

The temperature utilised in refrigerating chambers falls into two main categories according to whether the meat is *chilled* or *frozen*, but whichever method is employed, the important points are constant temperature, good air circulation and right humidity.

Chilling of meat

Chilling scarcely affects the flavour, appearance or nutritional value of meat and is particularly useful for short-term preserving. The meat is maintained at about +1°C and preferably in the dark, for light accelerates the oxidation of fat with the liberation of free fatty acids and the production of rancidity. The atmosphere is kept dry to hinder the formation of moulds, which are more likely to attack chilled meat than frozen.

In recent years, emphasis has been placed on shorter chilling cycles and lower temperatures – 'quick chilling' – for the following reasons:

1 Both time and building space are saved, and higher rates of product handling are achieved. Overheads in labour are reduced and capital investment in buildings is minimised.
2 The meat is said to have a better keeping quality because lower air temperatures (usually below −3°C initially) retard the rate of growth of bacteria on the surface of carcases where their concentration is most pronounced.
3 Shrinkage of meat is reduced substantially – an important economic factor.
4 The 'bloom' is said to be enhanced by quick chilling.

In order to achieve the aforementioned objectives, different time/temperature schedules exist for the different kinds of carcases. Surface discolouration and freezing of the carcase must be avoided.

Prior to the second half of the twentieth century, it was customary to hang beef carcases at ambient temperatures for 24 hours before placing them in chill rooms. (Indeed, in many abattoirs at that time, refrigeration was non-existent.) Chilling times of 36–48 hours for lowering the deep round temperature of beef carcases to 7°C are still common.

Quick chilling refers to a rapid lowering of carcase temperature starting not later than 1 hour after slaughter and avoiding freezing.

Low temperatures and high air speeds incur a risk of cold shortening. Pig carcases, however, should be cooled as quickly as is economically feasible as they are less susceptible to cold shortening.

The phenomenon of *cold shortening* was first encountered in New Zealand when rapid cooling schedules for lamb freezing were first introduced. Toughness of the meat occurred owing to extreme contraction of muscles subjected to temperatures of around 10°C before the muscles were in normal rigour, that is, while the pH was still above 6.2 and adenosine triphosphate (ATP) was still present. Cold shortening can also occur with beef carcases and even in parts of the carcase, for example, the loin, with fairly slow chilling. It can be avoided by delaying the start of chilling, for example, for 10–12 hours when the pH will be below 6.2 and rigour will have taken place with the complete disappearance of ATP from the muscle, or not chilling to below 10°C in less than 10 hours. Cold shortening can also be prevented by the use of electrical stimulation, which advances the onset of rigour (see also Chapter 6).

Various schedules are in operation for the chilling of meat, but many of these pay little attention to the time required for heat to be extracted from the centre of heavy muscle and dispersed at the surface. Important issues are the velocity of air over the carcases, the uniform airflow throughout the chill room (although this depends also on the evenness of carcase hanging), temperature and relative humidity. Higher temperatures and air velocities and low relative humidity increase the weight loss due to drying out. The Meat Research Institute in Britain estimated that beef carcases stored in chill rooms can lose as much as 0.1%/day, while lambs can lose 0.5% in a relative humidity of 90%. Smaller items of meat lose relatively more because of their relatively larger surface area. On the other hand, high relative humidity increases spoilage. A relative humidity of about 90% appears to be suitable for commercial chilling and for retail purposes.

Air circulation rates are high in quick-chilling operations, often 70–110 times the room volume per hour. The carcase is initially warm and wet but evaporation from the surface is rapid. In order to minimise loss of carcase weight while maintaining a short chilling cycle, high air circulation rates are necessary to lower the carcase temperature and carcase surface-water vapour pressure as quickly as possible. Later, when the carcase temperature has been sufficiently lowered, slower air circulation rates are more beneficial (Table 4.2).

Table 4.2 Chilled shrinkage of a pig carcase – 60 kg dressed weight

	Air temperature (°C)	Air speed (m/s)	Chilling shrinkage (%)	
			A	B
Quick chilling	0.5	0.25	1.9	1.5
Rapid chilling	−7	2	1.4	1.0

Source: Cooper, R. (1970) Proceedings of the International Institute of Refrigeration, Leningrad.
A, 24 hours after slaughter; B, 1 hour after slaughter.

The Food Safety and Inspection Service of the US Department of Agriculture advises that for carcase-chilling coolers, rails should be placed at least 0.6 m from refrigerating equipment, walls and other fixed parts of the building and 0.9 m (especially for header and traffic rails) from walls in order to promote cleanliness and protect walls from damage. The top of the chill rails should be at least 3.3 m for beef sides from the floor level, 2.7 m for headless pigs and calves, 2.2 m for beef quarters and 2 m for sheep and goats (Fig. 4.1).

It is necessary to have several chill units, rather than one large chill room, with dimensions 18–30 m long (maximum), 7.6–15 m wide and 4.8 m high (minimum). Refrigeration requirements for the aforementioned cycle would be approximately 755–880 kcal/hour per carcase of 290 kg weight (dry) with about 9.9–11.3 m³/min of air circulated per carcase.

Pork carcases, because of their smaller size, the presence of a skin and relatively greater fat content, can tolerate much lower air temperatures and consequently shorter quick-chilling cycles, even as short as 4–7 hours, but most British abattoirs produce pork, like beef and lamb, during a 24-hour cycle, the carcases usually being chilled in air at 4°C and at an air speed of 0.5 m/s. Work at the British Meat Research Institute showed that *ultrarapid chilling of pork* in air at −30°C and 1 m/s for 4 hours resulted in complete loss of heat in this short time with a 1% saving in evaporative weight loss compared with the control carcases handled in the traditional manner. Similar work carried out under practical conditions on beef carcases in Australia used initial air temperatures of −15°C and an air velocity of 3 m/s for 5 hours, resulting in a reduction of shrinkage from 1.2 to 0.6%.

(a)

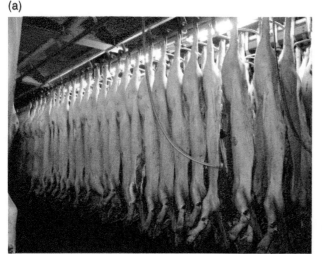

(b)

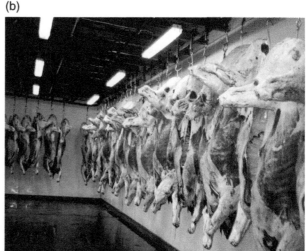

Figure 4.1 (a) Pig carcases suspended in a chiller (Reproduced with permission from David Armstrong). (b) Beef carcases suspended by the 'aitchbone' for chilling (Reproduced with permission from John Hood).

In high-throughput establishments, the most efficient protocol is to chill carcases initially in a 'pre-chiller' using a high rate of heat exchange to remove much of the heat at the surface rapidly, before transfer of the carcases to the main chillers with a lower rate of heat exchange.

Freezing of meat

The chief types of meat foods preserved by *freezing*, as distinct from chilling, are mutton, lamb, pork and rabbit, but there are rather wide differences of opinion as to the proper freezing temperature. In Germany, the temperature is maintained at −6°C and in Australia −11°C. In South America, much lower temperatures may be used in what are termed *sharp freezers*; for example, pork may be stored at −18°C, which prevents oxidation and resultant rancidity. During sea transport, a temperature of −9 to −8°C is maintained in the holds, while the air is kept dry and in circulation.

In the United Kingdom, it has been customary to hold meat in *cold stores* at temperatures of −20°C. It is now generally recognised that lower temperatures are more satisfactory since they reduce deterioration of carcase meat, and temperatures no higher than −18°C, even −30°C, are now being advocated. It was believed that very low temperatures resulted in excessive dehydration; this is now considered to be incorrect.

Current EU legislation does not specify temperatures at which meat should be stored but rather simply states that it should be frozen without delay and that time should be allowed to allow the temperature of the meat to stabilise. Previous legislation stated that this stabilisation should permit *beef* quarters should be accepted for freezing at a temperature not above +7°C and frozen within 36 hours to an internal temperature of −7°C or below. The acceptance temperature of *pig* sides is below +4°C; they must be frozen at −30°C and held in the freezer until all the meat is at −15°C or below. Frozen storage for beef must be at a temperature of −17°C and at −20°C for pig meat.

Such low temperatures can be attained only in special *blast freezers* with air temperatures of around −34°C, air speeds of about 3–5 m/s and holding times of up to 25 hours. The form of wrapping greatly affects the freezing time; if it is loose, the pockets of air or cartons act as insulation and thereby increase freezing times. Wrapping in moisture-proof packaging, or traditionally in stockinette, can offset water loss.

Cold stores are designed to hold frozen meat and other foods at a required temperature, although various temperatures and air speeds are used in different premises. While the meat trade in Britain is resistant to the use of very low temperatures for cold storage, work at the UK Meat Research Institute at Bristol has shown that at −10°C weight losses of meat are much greater than

Table 4.3 Practical Storage Life (PSL) at different storage temperatures

	PSL (months)		
	−12°C	−18°C	−24°C
Beef carcases	8	15	24
Lamb carcases	18	24	>24
Pork carcases	6	10	15
Edible offals	4	1–2	18

Source: Refrigeration and Process Engineering Research Centre, University of Bristol, Churchill Building, Langford, Bristol, UK.

at −30°C because the amount of water vapour that air can hold before it becomes saturated increases as temperature rises.

The commonly held belief that frozen meat will keep indefinitely is not true. The practical storage life (PSL) of frozen carcase meat is given in Table 4.3.

For *optimum results in chilling and freezing* and the prevention of growth of spoilage and food-poisoning bacteria, the following criteria should be adopted:

1 Initial design of refrigeration space must consider product tenderness, weight loss, possibility of spoilage, size of individual units, space required, rail height and floor and wall surfaces.
2 Temperatures must be checked regularly.
3 Overloading must be avoided and carcases must not touch each other.
4 Door opening and closing must be kept to a minimum.
5 Adequate airflow around carcases is essential.
6 Carcases of different species must not occupy the same area.
7 Cold shortening must be avoided by not chilling below 10°C in less than 10 hours.

Liquid nitrogen

This refrigerant is increasingly being used in the food industry, especially for freezing and automated production lines. A moving belt carries the food through a tunnel and under a liquid nitrogen spray at the outlet. The food is frozen and the vaporised nitrogen is extracted by fans and discharged to the atmosphere. The liquid nitrogen is stored in vacuum-insulated tanks.

This form of *cryogenic freezing* is said to produce less dehydration (usually <0.3%) and better flavour, colour, aroma, texture and nutritive value in the food than the conventional types which utilise large volumes of cold air on the product. Higher operating efficiency and low running and maintenance costs are also claimed. Being constructed in stainless steel and capable of being quickly stripped down, the freezer tunnel can be rapidly and thoroughly cleaned.

Mobile meat containers are now nitrogen cooled using either the gas, at −196°C from a tanker via a towed distribution unit, or the liquid as a coolant. The latter can reduce the temperature of the container more quickly but requires heavy storage vessels to be carried and is thus relatively expensive. There is also a tendency towards discolouration of the carcase and condensation on unloading; exposure to the air may restore the colour, while the use of loading hatches with an awning can reduce condensation. The cost, however, is some four times that of mechanical refrigeration.

Freeze-drying or lyophilisation

This is the process of removing water from frozen foods. The food products must be in comminuted form (sliced or diced), and packaging must be completely moisture-proof since the dried products are hygroscopic. At the present time, beef, pork, chicken, shellfish and other foods such as mushrooms, fruits, peas and vegetables are preserved by this process. Since meat has a relatively high moisture content, it is relatively expensive to preserve by freeze-drying methods, which at this stage of development can be regarded only as a supplement to traditional methods of refrigeration.

Storage of fresh meat

Meat cutting in supermarkets is labour consuming, and as the cost of labour continues to increase, means to reduce these costs are being sought. Deboned and trimmed meat, in the unfrozen state, offers cost savings in labour and transportation and requires less energy for storage than does frozen meat. This has resulted in a shift to more centralised meat cutting at packing plants where the carcase is reduced to smaller sections called *primal* and *subprimal cuts*. These cuts are vacuum packed in high-barrier bags placed in cartons or baskets for shipment to retailers or processors, where they are further reduced to retail-sized cuts or products.

Vacuum packing

This is a process in which primal cuts of meat are placed in a gas-impermeable form of plastic (polythene, nylon/polythene, polyester/polythene) laminate bags at 2–4°C and a pH of 5.5–5.8. Two basic systems are used: (1) 'Cryovac', in which the air is sucked out and then the pack is passed through either a water dip or a hot air tunnel, and (2) drawing a vacuum without heat shrinkage. The advantage of (1) is that drip is reduced and there is less possibility of the package being torn. The packs are stored at between −18 and 1°C. The residual oxygen is consumed by tissue respiration, and carbon dioxide

accumulates. In the absence of water and air, bacterial multiplication is significantly reduced, and shelf life can be maintained for up to 3 months, provided that the meat is of good microbiological standard. In the absence of air, the meat assumes a bluish discolouration of myoglobin but on re-exposure to air regains its normal red colour on oxygenation to oxymyoglobin.

Modified atmosphere packing

Packing meat in a *modified atmosphere packaging* (MAP) which utilises sealed high-barrier packages in which the air has been replaced with a mixture of gases which reduces the rate of deterioration of the meat and permits the preparation of packs for retail centrally. Most often, these gases include 10–50% carbon dioxide, which inhibits the growth of many micro-organisms that cause spoilage of refrigerated meats. For fresh red meats, the gas mixture often contains 20–50% oxygen so that the myoglobin will be in the oxygenated cherry-red form. The meats must be sealed in high-barrier films which will keep the air out and prevent the modified atmosphere from escaping.

The process depends on the ability of carbon dioxide gas, when present in high concentration, to prevent the growth of moulds. Facultative bacteria may or may not be suppressed by carbon dioxide, while lactic acid bacteria and anaerobes are virtually unaffected. On the other hand, the highly aerobic bacteria and yeasts and moulds are selectively inhibited by carbon dioxide, and the storage of meat in an appropriate concentration of this gas will therefore retard surface decomposition, though it will not prevent deep-seated anaerobic spoilage. Mould growth can be arrested completely at 0°C if 40% CO_2 is used, but any concentration over 20% rapidly produces methaemoglobin on the exposed muscle and fat, and the bloom is lost. Experiments have shown that in 10% CO_2, the storage life of meat at 0°C is double that of meat stored in ordinary air at a similar temperature, and in this way, the storage life of chilled meat can be extended to 60–70 days.

Refrigerated meat transport and storage

Depending on the type of trade and length of journey, meat may be transported by road in properly insulated and refrigerated (mechanical or liquid nitrogen) vehicles or insulated or non-insulated non-refrigerated vehicles. Only refrigerated transport can be considered adequate; all other modes are totally ineffective, especially the non-insulated type, particularly for chilled meat.

A well-designed *refrigerated road vehicle* should have the following qualities: high standard of insulation, good internal lining, airtight door seals, watertight flooring, rigidity of construction, efficient refrigeration unit, provision of temperature indicators in the driving cab and properly spaced overhead rails. In addition, it should be economical, lightweight and noiseless.

The maintenance of the internal temperature is influenced by the difference between the inside and outside temperatures, insulation, the number of times the doors are opened and closed, loading temperature of the cargo, capacity rating of the refrigeration system, respiration rate of the product, etc. Vehicles left standing with doors wide open in high summer temperatures attract not only heat but also undesirable arthropods.

An efficient insulating medium is provided by urethane foam sprayed between inner and outer linings. This material expands to fill all crevices and has a low heat loss factor, a low water absorption rating and a density of 23–38 kg/cubic metre. Lining materials must be smooth, impermeable, durable, easily cleaned and able to withstand detergents and hot water. They must also be non-toxic and as far as possible free from seams. Typical lining materials are glass fibre-reinforced panels, special non-marking aluminium (bare aluminium can mark fresh unwrapped hanging meat) and plastic-coated and stainless steel sheeting.

Floors should be very durable, watertight and easily cleaned. There should be no crevices or sharp corners throughout the inside of the vehicle which would hinder cleaning.

While construction of transport vehicles is normally suitable for hanging quarters of beef, lamb carcases, packaged meat, etc., the same does not hold for offal which is not in cartons. It is important that for the retail delivery of meat and offal, there should be good handling facilities; it must not be placed in an unwrapped state on the floor. Loading should be effected into a previously chilled vehicle which has its own refrigeration unit and is well insulated, should be direct from the cold store into the vehicle and, whenever possible, should be made using an enclosed loading bay. This prevents temperature increase during the loading operation. The vehicle temperature during transit should be monitored and recorded.

When the vehicle is unloaded, either into a transit cold store or at its final delivery point, product temperature should be checked before unloading, and transfer to the chilled storage should be immediate.

Changes in frozen meat

Two outstanding and unfavourable changes take place as a result of the freezing of meat:

1 The physical state of the muscle plasm (globulin and albumen proteins) is considerably altered. When meat is frozen below −2°C, the formation of ice crystals so raises the concentration of these proteins that they become insoluble and do not regain their solubility when the meat is thawed. A similar irreversible change may be observed if eggs are frozen.

2 The freezing point of meat lies between −1 and −1.5°C, when crystals begin to form: at −1.5°C, 35.5% of the muscle water is ice; at −5°C, 82% is ice; and at −10°C, 94% is ice. During freezing, the water present in the muscle fibres diffuses from the muscle plasm to form crystals of ice. In the past, it has been believed that the speed of freezing has an important bearing on the size of the ice crystals and the future quality of the product. It has previously been postulated that when meat is frozen *slowly*, the largest crystals are formed between the temperatures of −0.5 and −4°C and are largely located outside the muscle fibres; this temperature range is known as the *zone of maximum ice formation*, and where meat is subsequently stored within this range, the ice crystals continue to grow in size during storage. It has also been surmised that if meat is frozen *rapidly* to a temperature lower than −4°C, the ice crystals are small and lie mainly within the muscle fibres; if lowering of the temperature is sufficiently fast, many of the crystals are ultramicroscopic in size, and all of them are smaller than the cells in which they are formed. Doubt is now being cast on this theory as the *rate of freezing* appears to have minimal effect on thawing drip loss. *Quick freezing of meat* has made rapid strides and is applied to lambs, calves, pigs, poultry, fish and various wholesale cuts, the latter being distributed wrapped in cellophane or a latex rubber container base. The temperature of a food may be reduced by quick freezing to as low as −46°C by contact with metal against which streams of brine at very low temperatures are directed; some methods use atomised sprays of cold brine, which produce no distortion of the muscle cells and practically no 'drip' on thawing. It is, however, unlikely that the quick freezing of whole quarters of beef will become a commercial proposition, for a temperature of −275°C would be required to quick-freeze a quarter of beef in 30 minutes.

'Weeping' or 'drip'

Weeping denotes the presence of a watery, bloodstained fluid which escapes from frozen meat when it is thawed and consists mainly of water, together with salts, protein and damaged blood corpuscles. The latter are responsible for the pink colouration of the fluid and are readily recognisable on microscopical examination. Weeping is an undesirable feature and is caused partly by the rupture of the muscle cells and tissues by crystals of ice and partly by irreversible changes in the muscle plasm. The amount of drip is greater in beef than in mutton, lamb or pork, but the better the original quality of a beef carcase, the less on average will be the drip from the meat after thawing. Quarters of frozen beef defrosted at 10°C for 3 days and cut into large wholesale joints lose about 1–2% of their weight during the following day, while smaller joints of the retail trade lose 1.5–2.5%.

It is claimed that drip is minimised if thawing is very slow. One method employed for beef is to subject the meat to a temperature of 0°C with 70% humidity, gradually increasing the temperature to 10°C and the humidity to 90%; the forequarter requires 65 hours for complete thawing and the hindquarter 80 hours. The major effect on drip is the final temperature on thawing.

It is known that the faster the rate of breakdown of ATP in muscle, the more rapid is the onset of *rigor mortis* and the greater the release of fluid from the muscles. If the rate of breakdown of ATP could be slowed, that is, rigor mortis delayed, less free fluid would be available for drip formation on subsequent freezing and thawing.

Durability of frozen meat

Frozen meat stored too long becomes dry, rancid and less palatable, the most important change being the breaking down of the fat into glycerine and free fatty acids, with the production of *rancidity*. The better the quality of meat, the less trouble one encounters in its storage. The storage temperature, the degree of fluctuation in the storage temperature and the type of wrapping (packaging) in which the meat is stored are generally thought to have the main influence on frozen storage life.

Temperature fluctuation is of limited importance when the product is left at a temperature below −18°C and the variation in temperature is only 1–2°C. Well-packed products and those that are tightly packed in palletised cartons are also less likely to show quality loss. However, poorly packed items are severely affected by temperature changes.

Freezer burn

This occurs on the outer surface of frozen offals, particularly the liver, hearts and kidneys, and is caused by loss of moisture from the outer tissues. It may sometimes be seen where a carcase is stored, unwrapped, close to the opening of a cold air duct. The meat or offals have a brown, withered discolouration. This can be prevented by using suitable packaging or cryogenic freezing.

Effect of freezing on pathogenic micro-organisms and parasites

Some bacteria are destroyed by freezing, but low temperatures merely inhibit the growth and multiplication of most until conditions favourable to their growth appear. Freezing is therefore of no great value in rendering a carcase affected with pathogenic bacteria safe for human consumption, nor are the bacteria commonly found on beef carcases destroyed by slow or sharp freezing. Anthrax bacilli can withstand a temperature of −130°C, while *Salmonella* can withstand exposure to −175°C for 3 days, and tubercle bacilli have been found alive after 2 years in carcases frozen at −10°C. The virus of foot-and-mouth disease can remain viable for 76 days if carcases of animals slaughtered during the incubative stage of the disease are chilled or frozen immediately afterwards. Under similar conditions, the virus of swine fever may remain infective in the bone marrow for at least 73 days and has also been shown to be viable in frozen pork for 1500 days. Freezing is, however, a valuable method for the treatment of meat affected with certain *parasitic infections*. For example, pork affected with *Cysticercus cellulosae* can be rendered safe if held for 4 days at −10.5 to −8°C as can beef with *Cysticercus bovis* by holding for 3 weeks at a temperature not exceeding −6.5°C or for 2 weeks at a temperature not higher than −10.5°C. *Trichinella* cysts in pork are destroyed by holding the carcase for 10 days at −25°C, but this is unreliable if the pork is more than 15 cm thick.

Heat: Thermal processing

The underlying principle of all food preserving methods is either the creation of unfavourable environmental conditions under which spoilage organisms cannot grow or the destruction of such organisms. In commercial canning, carefully selected and prepared foods contained in a permanently sealed container are subjected to heat for a definite period of time and then cooled. In most canning processes, the heat destroys nearly all spoilage organisms, and the permanent sealing of the container prevents reinfection.

Aseptic canning, involves the use of high temperatures for short periods. The food is sterilised at 120°C for 6 seconds to 6 minutes depending on the food, before it enters a sterilised can which is then closed with a sterilised lid. This method is said to improve the flavour and the vitamin content of the canned product.

Aluminium or coated aluminium may be used as alternatives to mild steel and tin in the fabrication of *cans*. While it has the advantage of lightness (and thereby lower transport costs) and freedom from sulphiding and rust, it buckles fairly easily. Efforts are being made to produce an alloy strong enough to withstand the stresses of processing, packing and transport.

Flexible *pouches* made from laminates of thermoplastic and aluminium foil are widely used. They will not, however, withstand the high internal pressure developed during processing and must therefore be sterilised in media (water or steam and air) capable of providing an external pressure sufficient to balance the internal one.

For the thermal processing of the open or sanitary can, flame sterilisation, for example, the Tarax flame steriliser developed in Australia, combined with rotation of the can, is now used for certain products. This system has the advantage of being relatively cheap and is capable of providing very efficient heat transfer in those products with some liquid.

Future forms of thermal processing may involve the use of microwave energy, hydrostatic sterilisers using high-efficiency steam and fluidised-bed systems.

Traditional canning methodology

As a food container, the metal can – first developed by Nicolas Appert in France in 1795 – has certain virtues possessed by no other type of container for heat-processed foods (Fig. 4.2). It has a high conductivity, which is of importance during processing; it cannot easily be broken; and being opaque, any possible deleterious effects of light on the foodstuff are avoided.

There are currently three main methods of can manufacture, the most common being the traditional *three-piece food can*. Constant research and development are in operation to improve techniques and designs. Over the years, the amount of metal in cans has been reduced, and soldering, which involved the use of lead, has long been discarded. The process of can manufacture begins with sheets of tinplated steel (Fig. 4.3) (1). Some of these may be coated with lacquer and dried in ovens for 15–20 minutes. Lacquers are used to prevent contact between food and tinplate and vary in type according to the class of food to be canned – acid foods like fruit, high-protein foods such as meat, etc. The lacquer-coated sheets are cut into lengths and widths for specific can sizes (2, 3). Individual strips are then rolled into cylinders (4), and the two edges of the cylinder drawn together with an overlap which is *electrically welded* (5). At this stage, the cylinders are given a further coat of lacquer on the seams and dried in an oven. A lip is next formed on each end of the cylinder (6). Separate ends (lids and bases) (7) are made in a different area, and the rims of these ends are curled, and a sealing compound is injected into the curl (8). The base is next joined to the cylinder body, the sealing compound forming an airtight seal. The cans, with their separate lids, are now ready for use by the food processor.

The *two-piece drawn and wall-ironed can* (DWI) consists of two pieces of tinplate, the body and base being formed from one piece of metal and the lid from another.

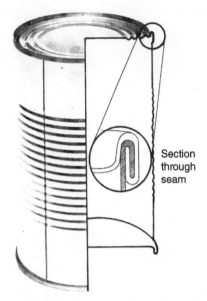

Figure 4.2 Modern food can showing section through seam (by courtesy of Metal Box Ltd).

The body and base are shaped from a thick piece of tinplate which is drawn up, ironed and ridged for strength and then given a coat of lacquer.

The *drawn and redrawn* (DRD) can is manufactured from two pieces of tinplate, the body being made from a disc-shaped piece, lacquered on both sides and drawn up to form a shallow cup and then redrawn a second and third time to make a deep cup.

Although the term *tin can* is applied to currently used containers, this is something of a misnomer as they are constructed of mild steel with a thin coating of pure tin representing about 1.5% of the can's weight. Coating of the steel plate is necessary to prevent corrosion, and in some foodstuffs, such as fish or fruit, a fish or fruit lacquer is used. Unsightly staining of the surface of certain foodstuff, known as *sulphiding*, may also occur and is avoided by use of a phenolic meat lacquer or a sulphur-resistant lacquer. An alternative method of avoiding sulphiding is now being extensively employed for meat packs and consists of chemical treatment of the inside of the can to form an invisible film, the solution used being a strong alkali bath containing phosphates and chromates.

Treatment of food to be canned

The food to be canned must be clean and of good quality; the use of any material showing obvious signs of spoilage will result in deterioration in quality of the product. Many foods, particularly fruits and vegetables, are scalded or blanched before treatment, to cleanse the product, to produce shrinkage which permits adequate

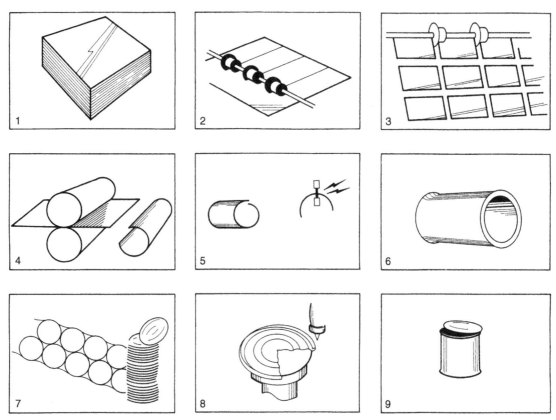

Figure 4.3 Stages of can manufacture (by courtesy of Metal Box Ltd).

filling of the can, to remove gases and to prevent oxidative changes which might cause deterioration. A firm, dry pack is required for meat foods without any excess of free liquor in the can; the moisture content of meat is therefore reduced by parboiling in steam-heated water, which produces up to 40% shrinkage in corned beef, 32% in ox tongues and 30% in pork tongues. Highly fattened animals are unsuitable for corned beef, as the meat is too fat and the finished product has an objectionable taste and appearance. The meat is therefore obtained from cattle which are older and leaner than those furnishing the supply of chilled or frozen beef.

After meats have been parboiled, they are taken to the trimming table where inedible parts such as bones, cartilage and tendons, together with surplus fats, are removed.

Canning operations

Cans may be filled either by hand or by automatic machinery, the next process being exhaustion or removal of air from the can before it is sealed. When meat with gravy is being canned, it is important to put the gravy in first in order to ensure freedom from air bubbles, which could aid bacterial growth. It is essential to make sure the cans are not being overfilled.

Filling

It is important that the correct weight is filled into each can. Overfilling can result in underprocessing and distortion of the can's seams. Underfilling may result in air pockets within the product which may interfere with the transfer of heat by conduction during processing. Any delay between filling and processing may allow bacterial growth with a resulting loss of quality.

Exhausting

Exhaustion is necessary for the following reasons: to prevent expansion of the contents during processing, which may force the seams; to produce concave can ends so that any internal pressure may be readily detected and warrant rejection of the can; to lower the amount of oxygen in the can and prevent discolouration of the food surface; and, in fruit packs, to reduce chemical action between the food and container and to avoid hydrogen swells. Although the production of a vacuum probably has little effect on micro-organisms, experience has shown that tins containing a vacuum keep better than those with air in.

Exhaustion of a can may be carried out in two ways:

1 *Heat exhausting*, in which the contents are filled cold into the can, which is then passed through a steam-heated

chamber before sealing. The ends of the can are loosely attached to permit the escape of air, sealing being completed when the cans leave the exhauster.

2 *Vacuumising*, in which the cold material is filled into the can, which is then closed in a vacuum-closing machine, the can being subjected to a high vacuum during the sealing operation.

Following closure, the cans are usually washed, before processing, in water at 80–85°C, containing a non-ionic detergent.

Processing

With the exception of such foods as sweetened condensed milk or jam, all canned foods are processed, that is, given final heating, after hermetic sealing. The term 'processing' is an exact one; it is not sterilisation since certain canned foods after processing may still contain living organisms. Although canned foods will keep with certainty if sterilised, they are then liable to alteration in colour and texture. Food to be canned is threatened on the one hand by bacterial spoilage and on the other by danger of overheating. The canner therefore chooses a middle course, the minimum heat employed in processing being controlled by the nature of the food in the can and the types and number of bacteria likely to be present.

During processing, heat penetrates to the centre of the can by conduction and by convection currents. In solid meat packs, the heat diffuses by *conduction* only, and the process is therefore slow; the *convection* currents in loosely packed foodstuffs transfer heat faster. Solids loosely packed in a liquid will, therefore, heat more rapidly than those that are tightly packed. Canned ham, being the largest and most solid pack of all the canned foods, requires very careful processing.

In non-acid foods, such as meat, the destruction of bacterial spores is slow; temperatures of about 115°C are required for adequate processing within a practical time limit. In commercial practice, the cans are placed in metal baskets in closed retorts and processed by pressurised steam.

The amount of heat used is based on that required to destroy the spores of *Clostridium botulinum*, the so-called botulinum cook. It is quantified as the *D-value*, which is a measure of the time taken to achieve a 10-fold reduction in the bacterial numbers at a given temperature. The accepted standard for a safe heat treatment is the time/temperature combination which will achieve a reduction in *Cl. botulinum* by a factor of 10, otherwise expressed as 10D. Monitoring of this critical control point must ensure that the time/temperature and pressure parameters are measured continuously and automatically to ensure all cans receive the correct

'cook'. The system must also ensure that processed and non-processed cans cannot be mixed.

Cooling

Prompt cooling after processing is important, as it checks the action of heat and prevents undue change in texture and colour. In addition, cooling reduces the considerable internal pressure of the cans which builds up during processing. The cans may be placed under cold water showers, immersed in a cold water tank or pressure cooled in the retort. The standard of the cooling water should be that acceptable for public drinking water supply, that is, it should be clean and wholesome. Reliance cannot be placed on chlorination alone, which has little effect on any organisms if organic matter is present; river water will require sedimentation and filtration before final chlorination. The amount of chlorine added to cooling water should be enough to produce, after 30 minutes contact time, a free residual chlorine content of 0.5 ppm or more, and a chlorinated water supply should show no coliform bacteria in 100 ml water, a standard readily obtained by effective treatment. In commercial practice, cans are water cooled to 38°C, and the residual heat dries the exterior and prevents corrosion.

Can washing

Cans that have just been cooled are dirty and greasy on the outside and are therefore washed in a bath with soap or saturated with fatty alcohols and rinsed to facilitate subsequent handling, lacquering and labelling.

Outside lacquering

Commercial lacquer or enamel is a colour varnish containing vegetable or synthetic resin. Lacquer may be applied to the outside of the tin to prevent external corrosion, particularly when the cans are destined for humid climates. Although external lacquering is not common in the canning of vegetables and fruits, it is almost universal in the salmon canning industry, not only because the UK market insists on shipments finished in this way but also because the loss through rusting would otherwise be enormous.

Container handling

The contents of hot wet cans may be infected if the cans are subjected to mechanical abuse and exposed to excessive concentrations of micro-organisms around the seam or seal areas, for example, from operatives' hands. Thus, manual handling of hot wet cans must be avoided, and it is wise to discard cans manually handled while, for example, clearing runway blockages. Surfaces coming into direct contact with cans must be checked for efficiency of cleaning ($<10\,\mathrm{cfu/cm^2}$).

Canning of meats

Corned beef is perhaps the best known of the canned meat products, although considerable quantities of canned ham, ox, sheep and pig tongues and spiced hams are now manufactured. The preparation of corned beef will illustrate the procedure normally adopted in the preparation of canned meats.

Corned beef

Corned beef is prepared from beef pickled in salt, nitrite and sugar; boiled for 1 hour; and then trimmed of soft fats, tendons, bones and cartilage. The texture and the fat content depend on the taste of the country for which it is intended, some countries preferring a lean corned beef and others a higher fat content; that for the UK market generally contains about 10% fat. Pickling is essential, for without it the meat after processing would be very much shrunken and dark in colour, while the can would contain liquid and dripping. The meat is machine cut and packed automatically into cans. The shrinkage from original fresh boneless meat to its weight when finally packed is 40–45%. The cans are then capped with the vent open and sealed under a vacuum. In some cases, exhaustion is carried out, with the vent open, in a process retort for 45 minutes at 104.6°C; the can is then removed, and the vent is closed as soon as it ceases blowing.

Subsequent processing varies in different plants. In some cases, the cans are put into retorts and processed at a pressure of 0.632 kgf/cm² for 2½ hours or more, depending on the size of the can. A 450 g tin of corned beef requires 21½ hours at 104.6°C, a 2.5 kg tin 5 hours at 105.5°C, and a 6.3 kg tin 6 hours at 108.3°C. In other cases, the cans are immersed in boiling water for 3½–4 hours. Processing is followed by cooling, degreasing and lacquering.

Canned hams

Hams are boned by hand and forced into a pressure mould to produce the required shape. The metal container for hams is double seamed, though without a rubber gasket, sealing being done by hand soldering followed by exhausting and soldering of the vent hole. The hams are finally cooked without pressure at 93.5°C for several hours. Cooking at a higher temperature for a shorter time in a pressure retort is contraindicated, as it produces deleterious changes in the ham texture and heavy weight loss due to exudation of fat and gelatin. An increase of only 10 minutes in cooking at these higher temperatures can increase the overall cooking loss to 5%. Large hams 1.4–7 kg would be unpalatable if cooked at normal canning temperatures and should be subjected to 80°C for up to 60 minutes. This produces a 'pasteurised'

ham which will have potentially a greater bacterial flora. The cans should be stored at 0°C.

Foods packed in glass

A great variety of foods is packed in hermetically sealed glass containers, and though the treatment of these differs somewhat from foods packed in cans, the principles of preservation are the same. The disadvantages of the glass container are that its greater weight, fragility, lessened output for the same amount of equipment and labour, together with the extra expense in packing, limit its use for the higher-grade products. On the other hand, it is less susceptible to attack by the product it contains and the contents may be readily inspected. The metal caps of glass containers are usually lacquered tinplate, with a paper liner inside to prevent discolouration resulting from corrosion of the metal. The cap is held firmly against a rubber gasket on the rim of the glass container and thus forms a hermetic seal.

Glass-packed foods are processed for a longer period than canned foods but at a lower temperature, as there is risk of fracture of the glass, and both heating and cooling must therefore be carried out more slowly. The modern method is to process in pressurised steam-heated water. At the conclusion of processing, the steam is shut off and cold water is slowly admitted to the retort, but the air pressure is still maintained to prevent the cap from being blown off by the internal pressure which develops in the container.

Spoilage in canned foods

It was at one time thought that the keeping qualities of canned goods depended upon the complete exclusion of air. Later, it was suggested that the heating destroyed all micro-organisms, while the sealing of the can prevented the entry of others, and that decomposition, when it occurred, was due to faulty sterilisation or to the entry of bacteria through a fault in the can. Neither of these views expresses the whole truth because living bacteria can often be found in sound and wholesome food, and bacteriological methods show that any canned meats or meat products contain living organisms, even after modern processing methods. The mere presence of living organisms is of little or no significance in assessing the soundness of canned goods.

The organisms responsible for *spoilage* in canned goods may be spore forming and therefore resistant to commercial processing, or they may be non-sporing organisms which gain access via leakages after processing. Aerobic spore-forming bacteria may be present in sound samples of canned goods. Spores probably remain dormant under the anaerobic conditions of a properly sealed can but, if supplied with air through faulty sealing, may develop and produce enzymes which decompose the foodstuff.

Non-sporing proteolytic or fermenting bacteria, for example, *Proteus* and *E. coli*, may cause decomposition of canned foods; no single type of organism is responsible for microbial spoilage. The problem of spoilage in canned goods is not the simple one of the presence or absence of such bacteria, but why in some cans bacteria of this type decompose the contents, while in others they remain inactive. Though *yeasts* and *moulds* are of great importance as causes of unsoundness in acid substances containing sugars, for example, canned fruits, they are of less importance in canned meats and marine products. The presence of yeasts, moulds and non-sporing bacteria in canned meat foods is evidence of leakage after sealing and can make the food unsound. Canned goods which, on opening, show such evidence should be condemned.

Types of spoilage

Canned goods are classified as spoiled when the food has undergone a deleterious change or when the condition of the container renders such change possible. Spoiled cans may show obvious abnormalities such as distortion, blowing, concave ends or slightly constricted sides; or they may present a perfectly normal external appearance.

A can with its ends bulged by positive internal pressure due to gas generated by microbial or chemical activity is termed a *swell* or *blower*. A *flipper* has a normal appearance, and though one end flips out when the can is struck against a solid object, it snaps back to normal under light pressure. A *springer* is a can in which one end is bulged but can be forced back into normal position, whereupon the opposite end bulges. All blown cans pass successively through the *flipper* and *springer* stages, and these two conditions must be regarded as suspicious of early spoilage of the can contents. A change in the appearance of the gelatin surrounding meat packs is usually associated with the formation of gas, the gelatin being discoloured and more liquid in consistency. It should be remembered, however, that in hot weather the gelatin of meat packs is likely to be of a more fluid nature. These abnormal cans are brought about by imperfect canning operations such as inadequate exhaustion of air before sealing, overfilling and the so-called nitrate swell which arises during thermal processing and is recognised during subsequent cooling, but whose nature is not fully understood.

A *leaker* is a can with a hole through which air or infection may enter or its contents escape. An *overfilled can* is one in which the ends are convex due to overfilling, but filling by weight or accurate measurement has done much to obviate this condition, and most tins classified as overfilled are actually in the early stage of blowing. Though an overfilled can cannot properly be regarded as a spoiled can, it must be differentiated from

a blower, and it emits a dull sound when struck, whereas a blown tin emits a resonant note. The term *slack caps* denotes a can which has a movement of one of the ends similar to that of a can in the early stages of blowing but is now rarely, if ever, encountered, and the great majority of cans classed as slack caps are blown and should be treated as such.

Spoilage of canned goods may be of microbial origin or chemical origin due to deleterious influences such as rust or damage.

Microbial spoilage

Bacteria of the decomposing or fermenting type are the most important as regards canned foods, while spore-forming bacteria are the most resistant. There are three main types of spore-forming organisms which can resist normal processing and may cause spoilage in canned foods: gas-producing anaerobic and aerobic organisms with an optimum growth temperature of 37°C, gas-producing anaerobic organisms growing at an optimum temperature of 55°C and non-gas-producing aerobic or facultative anaerobic spore-forming organisms with an optimum growth temperature of about 55°C, which produce *flat sours*.

Processing is not a substitute for cleanliness and will destroy a small number of bacteria rather more easily than a large number. Bacteria subjected to heat or other harmful influences are destroyed in accordance with a definite law which prescribes that where two different suspensions of the same organism are subjected to heat under uniform conditions, the number of bacteria will be reduced by the same *percentage* over equal periods of time.

Insufficient processing is a cause of unsoundness of canned goods, though not the all-important factor generally assumed.

The bacteria found in canned meat or fish are nearly always secondary invaders gaining access through a leak. Microbial spoilage may thus result from underprocessing or from *leakage* through the seam. Leakers may be detected by the disappearance of the vacuum from the sides and ends of the can, and bubbles appear if the can is held under water and squeezed. Another test for leakage is to heat the can to 38°C in the interior and allow it to cool slowly; if a leak is present, there will be no concavity of the sides or ends. The detection of leakers by striking the suspect can with a mallet has little value in industrial practice. The most common form of leaking occurs at the seams and may sometimes be detected by liquid or stain on the can surface. Mould formation on the surface of canned meats is also indicative of leakage, but cannot be detected until the can is opened.

Flat souring in canned goods produces a sour odour of the foodstuff but the can is not blown. Canned foods susceptible to flat souring are those containing sugar or starches and meat products such as sausages or pastes containing cereal. True flat sours are caused by thermophilic organisms (*B. coagulans, B. stearothermophilus, B. circulans*) which are exceptionally heat resistant and attack carbohydrates, producing acid but not gas. Sourness in canned foods may also arise due to leaking cans, or it may have developed in the foodstuff before processing. This latter form of spoilage is most likely in packs cold filled in warm weather, particularly if the cans are open for even short periods prior to processing.

Flat souring of canned goods due to thermophilic spore-forming organisms cannot be detected until the can is opened and its contents are examined, but is unlikely to occur in temperate climates unless storage conditions have been exceptionally hot; it is, however, comparatively common in tropical and subtropical countries or in cans imported from them.

Ham spoilage may be caused by faecal streptococci, for example, *Streptococcus faecalis var. liquefaciens*, which may liquefy jelly and cause off-colour, off-flavour souring.

Chemical spoilage

Hydrogen swell may occur quite independently of fermentation or bacterial decomposition and is associated with the formation of hydrogen gas in the can following *internal corrosion*. Imperfections or scratches on the inner tin coating may expose small areas of steel, and, where the contents are acid, an electric couple may result, the reaction producing hydrogen gas. Electrolytic action is accelerated by oxygen and by the colouring matter (anthocyanins) of red fruit. Cracks in the inner lining of lacquer serve to concentrate electrolytic action on the areas of steel exposed and increase the rate of hydrogen release. Cans affected with hydrogen swell may show varying degrees of bulging from flipping to blowing. If the tin is punctured, there is emission of hydrogen gas, which is colourless and burns on the application of a flame. The condition is chiefly associated with foods containing organic acids such as *fruits*, particularly plums, cherries, raspberries, blackcurrants and loganberries.

The *range of acidity* most favourable to the production of hydrogen swell lies between pH 3.5 and 4.5, and the less acid fruits therefore give more trouble than those of higher acidity, but with proper precautions, there should be very little trouble from hydrogen swells in commercially packed English fruits for at least a year after canning. The condition is seldom encountered in canned vegetables and is practically unknown in canned meat foods, but it is sometimes seen in tinned sardines. Although the contents of a can in hydrogen swell may be

quite harmless, the routine methods employed in the examination of canned goods render it impossible to distinguish between tins blown owing to hydrogen swell and those blown as a result of deleterious changes due to bacteria or yeasts. All blown tins, whether fruits, meats, vegetables or condensed milk, must be regarded as unfit for food, and leakers, springers and flat sours, together with tins whose contents show evidence of mould, should likewise be condemned.

Purple staining on the inner surface of cans in which sulphur-containing foods are packed may occur with all fish and meat products, especially the liver, kidneys and tongue. It is due to the breakdown of sulphur-containing proteins in high-temperature processing by the thermophilic *Clostridium nigrificans* ('sulphur stinker'); hydrogen sulphide is liberated, and a thin layer of tin sulphide is formed on the inside of the can. This discolouration does not involve the foodstuff itself and varies from a light pink to a dark purple, but it may be accompanied by a blackening of both the inside of the can and the surface of the foodstuff if the hydrogen sulphide attacks the steel base-forming iron sulphide. It is of more serious import than the deposition of tin sulphide, as it may lead to pitting of the steel and disfigurement of the surface of the meat pack. Discolourations of both types may be prevented by a sulphur-resisting lacquer, the basis of which is copal gum dissolved in a suitable solvent to which are added substances capable of uniting with the volatile sulphur gases released while the food is being processed.

Rust or damage

Cans showing external *rust* require careful consideration. It is a condition particularly liable to occur beneath can labels when the adhesive contains hygroscopic substances. Cans in which the external surface is slightly rusted without noticeable pitting of the iron may be released for immediate sale and consumption, but if the rust is removed with a knife and inspection with a hand lens reveals the iron plate to be definitely pitted, there is danger of early perforation and the cans should be condemned. Minute perforations of the tinplate, known as *pinholing*, permit the entrance of air and lead to spoilage of the can contents. Pinholing may originate from the outside but also from the inside of the can where the tinplating is imperfect or has been fractured during seaming, and in this case, lacquer lining aggravates the trouble, as the cracks that occur in the lacquer aid in concentrating the chemical action on a small area. A can which is a leaker or pinholed may occasionally seal itself by blocking of the holes with the contained foodstuffs and may then proceed to blow; such self-sealing cans may blow at any period of their storage life, whereas an underprocessed can will blow early in its life, generally within the first few months. Where unfilled cans are stored and allowed to rust internally before being filled, the can edges may become rusted, with the result that during processing a chemical action may take place between the rust and meat juices and give rise to an unsightly grey precipitate of iron phosphate in the meat jelly.

Considerable significance should be attached to cans *damaged* by rough handling, the important factor in their judgement being the extent and location of the damage. Marked deformation of the can seam is attended by considerable risk of leakage, and such cans should be condemned. Slight indentations on the can body are permissible, but severe dents on the body may cause seam distortion, and such cans should be rejected; any can having a dent at one end should also be rejected for it is possible to reduce a springer to normal, at any rate temporarily, by hitting it upon the corner of a box. Nail holes in cans caused during the closing of packing cases may also be encountered, and such cans should be rejected even if the contained foodstuff appears perfectly normal. It is important to reject any can which is in the least suspicious or which shows lack of concavity of the ends.

The public health aspect of canned foods

Improvements in the canning industry during recent years, together with greater appreciation of its hygienic requirements, have done much to remove the public prejudice against canned foods, which were thought to cause food poisoning. Food poisoning is usually the result of improper handling of food during preparation or storage, and with the exception of botulism, food-poisoning outbreaks are nearly always caused by bacteria which would be destroyed during processing. *Salmonellae* are destroyed with certainty by the temperatures attained in commercial processing. The minimum standard of processing now universally recognised by reputable canners ensures the destruction of *Cl. botulinum* spores in low- and medium-acid foods. A lower processing temperature is, however, permissible in cases such as cured meats, in which the curing salts have an inhibitory effect on the growth of the organism and the production of toxin.

Staphylococci, and more rarely streptococci, are now recognised as a cause of food poisoning mainly in prepared or unheated foods, such as cheese, salad, milk or ice cream. These organisms are ubiquitous in nature, but their main source is the human or animal body, where they are normally present on the skin, in the intestine and in the respiratory tract. Staphylococci, however, are relatively susceptible to heat, and even the more resistant staphylococcal enterotoxin, which may withstand a temperature of 100°C for 30 minutes, is destroyed during commercial processing. Cans may occasionally become infected by these organisms through a leak, and in the

absence of accompanying gas-forming bacteria, there will be no 'blow' and the can will appear normal. Most cases of food poisoning now associated with canned foods are the result of contamination after the can is opened, but a number of cases of typhoid fever associated with canned foods have occurred in Britain. The outbreak in Aberdeen in 1964, in which there were over 400 confirmed cases, was attributed to the post-processing entry of contaminated cooling water in a 2.7 kg tin of corned beef of South American origin.

Viewing the question as a whole, canned foods are considerably less likely to be a source of food poisoning than ordinary fresh foods. The possibility of secondary contamination of canned foods with pathogenic bacteria also raises the question of the wisdom of leaving food in a can after it has been opened. From the public health standpoint, there is no reason why an open can, properly stored, should not be used as a food container; it should, however, be covered to prevent contamination and kept cool.

Microbiological examination of canned meats

Where suspected outbreaks of food poisoning attributed to canned food occur, the normal laboratory procedures for isolation of the responsible organism (*Salmonella, Staphylococcus, Clostridium*, etc.) are adopted, care being taken in the sampling, transport, identification, handling, etc. of the suspect food.

In order to ensure the safety and stability of large consignments of hermetically sealed containers of meat products, attention should be directed at the standards of *methods used at the point of production* (quality assurance), namely, hygiene levels, temperatures for heat treatment, water supply, etc., which should supply more important information than the microbiological testing of numerous containers, which would not only be wasteful but would be unlikely to detect entities such as botulism.

Examination of the *quality of containers* is important to ensure that there are no damaged, rusty, blown, etc. cans. If there is reason to suspect that a consignment of meat products in hermetically sealed containers is unsatisfactory, sampling and inspection procedures should be adopted along the lines recommended by the Codex Alimentarius Commission (see 'Further reading'). The number of samples to be taken is assessed according to the expected hazard and the laboratory facilities available in the case of shelf-stable canned products. For non-shelf-stable products, five containers are examined visually and their contents examined microbiologically. Both *aerobic* and *anaerobic* microbiological techniques are undertaken, decisions as to rejection or approval being based on bacterial plate counts (Sampling and Inspection Procedures for Microbiological Examination of Meat

Products in Hermetically Sealed Containers, Codex Alimentarius Commission of FAO/WHO).

Other methods of meat preservation

Antioxidants

An *antioxidant* is defined in the UK Miscellaneous Food Additives Regulations 1995 No. 3187 (as amended in 1997) as 'any substance which prolongs the shelf-life of a food by protecting it against deterioration caused by oxidation, including fat rancidity and colour changes'.

Antioxidants often improve flavour in cooked meat and some prevent colour changes.

Preservatives

A *preservative* is defined in the aforementioned regulations as any substance which prolongs the shelf life of a food by protecting it against deterioration caused by micro-organisms.

Schedule 2 of the 1995 regulations gives a list of permitted preservatives and antioxidants.

In the assessment of any additive for use in a food, three criteria have to be considered:

1 Benefit or need accruing to the food industry, retailers and customers
2 Safety in use
3 Satisfactory standard of purity of the chemical

Other substances are added to foods for specific purposes, for example, emulsifiers, stabilisers, acids, non-stick agents, air excluders, phosphates, humectants, sequestrants, firming agents, anti-foam agents, colouring agents, flavours and solvents, in addition to nutritive substances such as vitamins A, B_1 (thiamin), C and D, nicotinic acid and calcium. While some of these additives contribute to the shelf life, they are not normally regarded as true preservatives.

See also Food Additive Legislation, Guidance Notes (www.food.gov.uk/multimedia/pdfs/guidance.pdf).

Irradiation

Electromagnetic radiation is known to inhibit the growth of micro-organisms, and a considerable amount of work has been expended in an attempt to use it for the sterilisation of foods. Close attention has been paid to the effect on the nutritional value of the treated foods, as well as the possible production of carcinogens and induced radioactivity.

Infrared radiation

Infrared rays have been mainly used to dry fruits and vegetables and for heat blanching in the same way as high-frequency radiation. Infrared rays have a wavelength of 3×10^{-4} cm.

Ultraviolet radiation

Ultraviolet rays occur at wavelengths of radiation between 100 and 3000 Å and are invisible (the angstrom, Å, is a unit of length equal to 10^{-10} m or 0.1 nm). They have a bactericidal action which is especially valuable for destroying airborne bacteria and are utilised in storage vats and other tanks to destroy micro-organisms on or above the surface of foods. The penetrating effects of the rays are generally considered to be low and are influenced by factors such as the length of exposure, temperature, pH, relative humidity, light intensity and degree of contamination.

The wavelength for maximum bactericidal activity of ultraviolet rays is about 2500Å, which can be produced by mercury-vapour lamps. As would be expected, spores and moulds are more resistant than vegetative organisms, yeasts being only slightly more resistant.

Ultraviolet rays are currently used in the *ageing of meat* at relatively high temperatures to control the growth of surface organisms. The bactericidal effect is also due to shorter wavelengths which convert atmospheric oxygen to ozone, an additional bactericide.

Ionising radiation

Irradiation of food can be achieved by using either gamma-rays produced by a radionuclide, usually cobalt-60, or high-energy machines.

Both gamma-rays and electrons produce ions which induce a sequence of chemical changes in the food, thus causing the particular effect for which the irradiation was applied, for example, the killing of bacteria. These chemical changes are not unique to irradiation but are also produced by other conventional processing methods such as heating and cooking.

Although the two sources of ionising radiation produce similar reactions in a food, they may not be equally suitable for all food applications because of their different penetrating powers. High-energy electrons are less penetrating than gamma-rays, the extent of penetration being influenced by the energy (maximum permitted level is 10 MeV (mega-electron volt)) and density of the product.

Double-sided irradiation allows an increase in the effective thickness of a package, but electrons are not suitable for treating large bulk packages although they can be used for thin packs or for surface irradiation. With gamma-irradiation, pallets of up to 1 m thickness can be used.

The main features of an irradiation plant are the irradiation room, which contains the source of ionising radiation, and an automatic conveyor system, which transports the food into and out of the room. Around this room is approximately 2 m of concrete. In the case of a gamma-irradiator, the radionuclide continuously emits radiation and when not in use must be stored in a water pool, whereas machines producing high-energy electrons can be switched off and on. This naturally influences the financial feasibility, and a plant needs to be in continuous operation.

Uses

Some of the uses of ionising radiation are as follows:

1 Decontamination of food ingredients such as spices
2 Reduction in of the numbers pathogenic micro-organisms such as *Salmonella, Campylobacter* and *Listeria* in, for example, meat and meat-type products
3 Extension of shelf life of fruits, vegetables, meat and meat products
4 Insect disinfestation of grain, grain products and tropical fruits
5 Inhibition of sprouting in potatoes, onions and garlic

Effectiveness

The effectiveness of the process depends on the quality of the raw material, dose applied, temperature during irradiation, type of packing and storage conditions before and after irradiation.

Pathogens such as *Salmonella* and *Campylobacter* are sensitive to fairly low levels of ionising radiation. As the radiation dose increases, more micro-organisms are affected, but a higher dose may simultaneously introduce organoleptic changes, and there needs to be a balance between the optimum dose required to achieve a desired objective and that which will minimise any organoleptic changes. With *fresh poultry* carcases, an irradiation dose of 2.5 kGy (kilogray) will virtually eliminate *Salmonella* and extend the shelf life of the food by a factor of about 2 if the storage temperature post-irradiation is maintained below 5°C. (The gray is the SI unit of absorbed radiation dose, equivalent to transfer of 1 J of energy per kg of product being treated (1 J/kg).) Irradiation of poultry was approved in the United States in 1990.

Organoleptic changes

Higher doses will give an even greater reduction in the numbers of micro-organisms, but at doses of about 5 kGy or above, odour and flavour changes may be produced in the food during storage which will render it unacceptable. These are caused by the formation of volatile sulphur-containing substances – hydrogen sulphide, carbonyls, amines, etc. Hydrogen sulphide odour is lost on subsequent storage, and different odours develop. While beef is especially susceptible to the development of these unpleasant odours and flavours, pork is much less affected.

Irradiation doses up to 10 kGy can be applied to frozen poultry (−18°C) without causing any unacceptable organoleptic changes because in the frozen state the chemical reactions that bring about the desired effects of irradiation are hindered and a higher dose is necessary to achieve the same objective.

When treating *frozen* products, time in the irradiator should be kept to a minimum so that any temperature rise is not significant. Similar considerations regarding dose and irradiation conditions also apply to other products such as frogs' legs and shellfish.

Other requirements

The benefit to be gained from using irradiation, whether, for example, to control food-poisoning micro-organisms or to disinfect grain, will only be achieved if the food being treated is of excellent quality and is stored under suitable conditions before and after irradiation. This often involves chilled or even frozen storage, and, depending on the product, humidity control may also be necessary. The need to combine irradiation with suitable storage highlights the point that irradiation is not a technology that can stand alone. It is one technology among many others which in some cases may have advantages over the more conventional food preservation methods.

The Food Irradiation Regulations 2009 require licensing of premises which can carry out irradiation. The seven permitted descriptions of food are fruits, vegetables, cereals, bulbs and tubers, spices and condiments, fish and shellfish and poultry (see also 'Further reading').

High pressure

An interesting development, currently attracting a great deal of worldwide interest, is the use of high pressure. The pressures involved are immense, greater than at the bottom of the deepest ocean, which is over 6.5 tonnes per square inch. Work in Australia has shown that the cooked tenderness of meat can be improved by such treatment, either before or after rigor mortis, and Japanese workers have demonstrated that the time required for conditioning can be decreased. The microbiological quality of comminuted meat products can be improved, offering potentially increased shelf life. The water binding of beef patties is increased. However, all of this work is very much in its infancy and is likely to involve further capital investment and many hours of development to bring high-pressure-treated meat and meat products into the marketplace.

References

Berends, B.R., Van Knapen, F., Snijders, J.M.A., et al. (1997) *International Journal of Food Microbiology*, 36, 199–206.

Bolton, D.J., Pearce, R.A., Sheridan, J.J., et al. (2002) *Journal of Applied Microbiology*, 92, 893–902.

Further reading

The International Institute of Refrigeration, Rapid Carcase Chilling Plants Compared to Conventional Systems, Bowater, F.J., FJB Systems, www.fjb.co.uk/wpcontent/themes/fjp/publications (accessed 29 April 2014).

FAO, Codex Alimentarius, Canning/Sterilisation of Meat Products, www.fao.org/docrep/010/ai407e22.htm (accessed 29 April 2014).

Irradiated Food, www.food.gov.uk/policy-advice.irradfood/#.UdrcQmB (accessed 29 April 2014).

EFSA statement summarising the conclusions and recommendations from the opinions on the safety of irradiation of food adopted by the BIOHAZ and CEF Panels, www.efsa.europe.eu/en/efsajournal/pub/2107.htm (accessed 29 April 2014).

5

Plant sanitation

C.F. Loughney and S.R. Brown

Reasons for cleaning and disinfecting plant

It can never be assumed that the reasons for cleaning and disinfecting meat plants are sufficiently obvious to those responsible for practical plant hygiene or indeed that the procedures are simple enough to dispense with planning and training. The technology of plant cleaning and disinfection is a complex and changing mix of engineering, chemistry and microbiology, with many details to be understood and actions to be taken. Furthermore, this technology mix alone will not deliver effective and consistent open plant hygiene. That can only be realised by well-trained people working to procedures that are validated, documented and monitored; in short, professional management is also a key ingredient. It is therefore essential that the importance of plant hygiene be recognised at all levels within a meat/food plant organisation and that the scientific principles and professional management techniques are understood and employed by all concerned.

Food plants are cleaned for many reasons:

- To meet national and EU legislation (Council Regulation (EC) No 852/2004 and 853/2004) and the associated inspections by the relevant authorities
- To reduce the risk of litigation in relation to food poisoning and foreign body contamination
- To engender and maintain a general quality ethos within the entire organisation
- To meet retail customers' and consumers' quality expectations
- To satisfy the increasing number of standardised retail customer audits, for example, IFS (International Food

Standard, 2007) and BRC Audit (British Retail Consortium, 2011)
- To allow maximum plant productivity
- To project a hygienic visual image
- To ensure the safety of operatives and maintenance staff
- To help secure the shelf life of the products
- To avoid pest infestation
- To protect marketplace reputation

Although perhaps it is the most subjective reason of all, the *visual image* that a factory projects to a visitor can strongly influence securing or losing a customer contract or a competent authority approval. Additionally, it has a direct bearing on employee morale and the development of a total quality ethos. For these reasons, visual cleanliness and the absence of visible deposits and corrosion in the plant are goals as important as the control of microbiological and foreign body risks.

Cleaning unavoidably incurs costs and time and thus, from a production or finance manager's point of view, it is often seen as a necessary but unproductive evil. It is however rare to find these costs being fully analysed and controlled in a meat plant or indeed a link made to the benefits. Often, the obvious elements only, such as consumable hygiene chemicals, are stressed rather than the complete context of the hygiene budget. Full hygiene budgeting should properly include a factor relating to the possible catastrophic effects of hygiene failure and the protection of investment made in plant and brand image. Only with a full analysis of the business risk of poor hygiene (impact × probability) can the direct costs of hygiene be seen in their genuine context.

Gracey's Meat Hygiene, Eleventh Edition. Edited by David S. Collins and Robert J. Huey.
© 2015 John Wiley & Sons, Ltd. Published 2015 by John Wiley & Sons, Ltd.

Typical running costs for Cleaning Open Plant (COP)[1] in a modern meat plant break down as follows:

Labour and supervision	65%
Water supply, treatment, purchase	2%
Water heating	8%
Cleaning equipment depreciation	8%
Chemicals	7%
Corrosion	2%
Monitoring	5%
Effluent	3%
Downtime	+?[a]

[a] The cost of downtime is very dependent on the nature of the production process and the shift patterns. In round-the-clock production environments, reducing downtime can be critical to profitability.

Often, cost pressures on the large labour element are brought to bear upon cleaning teams, whether contracted or in-house staff. The first effect is on the wages, staff selection and training of the cleaning team. In some plants, hygiene operatives are wrongly seen as requiring a lower skill/educational level when compared to production staff. Direct management pressures on hygiene teams themselves may encourage individuals to cut corners or leave out individual steps in the cleaning sequence. This action may appear to save money in terms of the cleaning costs alone. However, it may easily lead to increased indirect costs in terms of the shelf life and safety of the food product, the hygienic image of the factory and the security of its customer contracts. All of these factors could seriously affect the viability and profitability of the meat plant.

Water costs (purchase, heating, treatment and disposal) can be significant, but it is important to understand the overall cleaning programme and the related effects of changing these variables, for example, by reducing water temperature, cost may go down, but will the surface hygiene results remain the same? Hygiene chemicals and equipment have a cost too, if badly managed and poorly controlled in use they can contribute to an unnecessary additional cost. Of course that is not to say that the overall costs of hygiene cannot be managed to a sensible budget, that is good management practice and absolutely essential particularly when one considers the rising cost of buying, heating and treating water. The main objective is to create a hygiene management system, inclusive of all the necessary inputs, actions and controls that will meet an agreed overall hygiene budget while delivering consistent hygiene to the required standard.

Over the last 10–15 years, under pressure from commercial quality factors and legislation, the average standards of design of food plants and their maintenance and cleaning have risen markedly. However, it is still the case

that the standards maintained and the professionalism with which hygiene is managed can vary greatly between different sectors of the food industry, between different plants in the same sector and between countries.

EU legislation has had and will continue to have an important effect on the design of new meat plants or the refurbishment of older plants. EU directives also have something to say about the requirement for routine cleaning and disinfection of food plants. Legislation requires that the local competent authority carry out audits of good hygiene practice (GHP), which shall verify among other issues training in hygiene and procedures, personal hygiene practices and pre-operational, operational and post-operational hygiene. The most recent set of EU regulations (Council Regulation (EC) No 852/2004 and 853/2004) came into force in 2005/2006. This is the most significant revision of EU hygiene legislation to date and effectively consolidates and simplifies previous and numerous regulations. The new regulations take an inclusive 'farm-to-fork' approach to the management of food safety and firmly place the responsibility for the production of safe food with the manufacturer. In addition, the regulations require that Guides to Good Practice are made available specifically to support the application of hazard analysis and critical control points (HACCP) and GHP. It is true that poorly designed, outdated and badly run plants should and can be closed down owing to failure to meet the legislative requirements. Any food company 'worth its salt', however, will see legislation as a bare minimum set of standards and will, through a total quality ethos and good manufacturing practice, aim for a consistent level of hygiene well above this minimum.

'Scotoma effect' or 'factory-blindness'

It is well known that any person working routinely in an environment such as a meat plant can gradually become mentally 'blind' to hygiene standards and potential problems in their plant. This 'scotoma' effect can be surprisingly powerful and can mean that visitors to the plant, for example, EU or competent authority inspectors or customers, will often see serious hygiene inadequacies missed by the plant personnel themselves. The 'scotoma' effect can only be overcome by constant vigilance, training, systematic monitoring inspection and internal auditing procedures. Outside assistance from specialist hygiene service companies and third-party auditors will also assist in reducing the negative impacts of this effect.

The chemistry of cleaning

Cleaning is essentially a physicochemical process involving a wide range of reactions, which depend greatly on a number of variables, which we will now consider.

The soil

In a meat plant, the most common 'soils' or deposits originate from the animals themselves and from any other ancillary additives or components used in the manufacturing process. These product-derived soils include the following:

Fats, oils and greases

These are often triglycerides of fatty acids and can vary from waxy solids to liquids. They are insoluble in water and can vary in their structure and properties, depending on their origin, differing between different body parts of the same animal species, between animals of different age and between different species. Poultry evisceration fats are very waxy and difficult to remove, for example, compared to beef tallow. Fats, oils and greases can change when exposed to air for some time (particularly those containing unsaturated fatty acids) and may oxidise or polymerise to become harder and more closely bonded to the surface. Exposure to very high temperatures, such as in ovens, will cause fats to carbonise and bond tightly even to stainless steel surfaces. Fatty or greasy deposits can be recognised by their greasy feel and water repellence, and when aged and oxidised to a moderate degree, they take on a cheesy opaque nature, which can be scraped easily with a fingernail. Fully polymerised oils can become almost plastic in feel and hardness. This effect is utilised when linseed oil is applied to cricket bats.

Proteins

These complex, large molecules are normally too large to dissolve easily in water. They have a specific shape that may change when exposed to high temperatures, a process known as denaturation, usually making them harder and insoluble. The best-known example of this is the changes seen in heating the white of an egg. This property of proteins is important in the processing of foods and in the selection of rinse water temperature used to remove protein deposits. In meat plants, bile and other gut-based soils may give rise to a green or yellow tenacious deposit on evisceration equipment. In pig-dehairing equipment, heavy, hard protein deposits are common. Blood proteins in abattoirs can create particular problems on porous surfaces, often giving rise to a green/brown, very resistant staining. Aged protein deposits can be quite hard, normally not scraping off easily with a fingernail.

Carbohydrates and starches

These, too, are large molecules, which may be insoluble, especially after exposure to heat. Their source is usually plant-derived materials used in producing sauces and coatings. Carbohydrate deposits can vary from soft and powdery to quite hard.

Miscellaneous deposits

Other soils may originate not from the food production process itself but from water, surface corrosion, vehicles and other outside materials. Such deposits include:

- *Limescale* from water drips and leaks or in hot water systems, tanks, cooking kettles, etc.
- *Corrosion deposits* of steel, zinc, aluminium, brass, etc.
- *Rubber marks* from forklift trucks
- *Adhesives* from labels
- *Inks and dyes* from stamps
- *Algae* in moist areas with high condensation
- *Fungi* in cold moist areas, especially near chills and freezers and in silicon sealants throughout the plant

These deposits may or may not present hygiene risks in themselves but are at least unsightly and at worst can act as absorbent and supportive substrates for other soils or micro-organisms. Chemically, they are very different from each other and may therefore need very different cleaning approaches. This is especially true because multiple types of soil are found frequently in the same plant, often combined in the same deposits. Physically, this usually makes them harder, more adherent and more difficult to remove. Just like sand and gravel, they reinforce cement to make concrete. It is important, therefore, to identify the soils present in each plant area by their origins and by their appearance. Only then is it possible to design the correct cleaning regime.

The substrate: Materials of construction

Many different materials may be found in meat plants, and while none is perfect, they do vary considerably in their ease of cleaning and their resistance to abrasion and to corrosion, either by the factory environment itself or by contact with cleaning chemicals. Smooth, impervious, abrasion-resistant, non-toxic surfaces are ideal and required by law (Council Regulation (EC) No 852/2004 and 853/2004), and industry guidelines have also been developed (EHEDG, 2004).

Stainless steel, of a high grade, is the best choice for many surfaces but, especially in its cheaper forms, is liable to pitting corrosion in the presence of chlorine and stress corrosion/cracking at elevated temperatures.

Mild steel will rust rapidly in moist and salty environments and should normally be avoided in meat plants.

Zinc (as a sacrificial coating on steel) and *aluminium* are both commonly found but are problematical because of their susceptibility to attack by strong alkalis, acids and some process fluids. At worst, they can be heavily corroded, embrittled or encrusted, none of which is helpful in maintaining hygienic surfaces. As a rule, they should be avoided where the nature of the production or cleaning process poses a corrosion risk.

Terrazzo and *concrete* may both become porous and cracked if mistreated and are liable to damage by acids.

Paints and other similar coatings can vary enormously in their resistance to attack by chemicals and hot or pressurised water and, once flaking, present a risk of foreign body contamination to the food. Chemical-resistant resins are available, but it is important to match the coating to the production and cleaning environment expected.

Plastics and *rubbers* also vary greatly. At their worst, they can swell on contact with some detergents, which may affect smooth running of machinery if present in gaskets, bearings, etc., or become embrittled by heat, light or chlorine. Some are surprisingly absorbent of soils, especially colourings, mineral oils, smoke, etc., and may even play the generous host to moulds.

The main point to look for in choosing surface material type is compatibility with the production environment, both physical and chemical, and with the cleaning regime. Compatibility with each other is also very important, particularly when two different metals such as mild and stainless steel are in contact in a moist environment. *Galvanic corrosion* invariably takes place, causing the 'lower' metal to corrode rapidly. This will also occur in welds which are poorly executed or where the choice of welding rod is incorrect.

Energies of cleaning

A principle of prime importance is that every cleaning process, of whatever kind, always involves a combination of four factors:

1 *Thermal energy*, in the form of hot water or steam. As a rough guide, an increase in temperature by 10°C in a detergent solution *doubles* the rate of the chemical reactions involved in cleaning.
2 *Mechanical energy*, in the form of brushes, water jets, turbulent flow in pipes or even the micro-agitation produced by the bursting of foam bubbles. In cleaning-in-place (CIP) of pipe systems, a flow rate of about 2 m/s is needed to ensure turbulence and avoid laminar flow, discussed in more detail later.
3 *Chemical energy*, which depends on the nature and concentration of the detergent used.
4 *Time*, which varies from hours in the case of soak cleaning to seconds in the case of tray or crate cleaning in industrial washing machines.

It is essential to understand the interrelation between these factors. Failure to do so will often lead to very poor cleaning results. While it is impossible, because of the complexity of the cleaning reactions, to be mathematical about it, there must be a balance between the four factors.

If one or more factors are limited by the cleaning conditions, for example, mild chemicals must be used to avoid corrosion of a surface and/or contact time is very limited, then one or more of the other factors must be raised to compensate, for example, water pressure and/or temperature.

Chemical and physical reactions of cleaning

Detergency involves many different reactions, physical and chemical, which depend on the nature of the soils to be removed and the nature of the detergent employed to remove them.

Physical reactions

The primary physical reactions are the following:

Wetting Wetting is defined as the displacement of one fluid from a solid surface by another. The displaced fluid may be air or some liquid or semi-liquid such as grease. The fluid displacing it is, for the purpose of our discussions, water or a detergent solution. Water alone is not sufficiently wet to displace many types of soils or even to displace air from water-repellent or 'hydrophobic' surfaces, for example, water droplets on a Teflon frying pan. In these cases, the water curls up under its own surface tension into droplets. Lack of wetting will prevent cleaning taking place.

To achieve wetting of such surfaces, chemical agents that have particular surface properties are employed: 'surfactants' or 'wetting agents'. These are organic molecules, which are different at each end. One end is essentially hydrocarbon in nature and closely resembles grease, oil or fat, that is, 'hydrophobic'. The other end is either ionised to give a positive or negative charge or consists of oxygen-containing groups. In either case, this end strongly attracts water, that is, it is 'hydrophilic'. The result is a dual-nature molecule, which concentrates itself at the interface between the water and the surface and allows wetting to take place as shown in Figure 5.1.

The nature of the surfactant – whether it foams or defoams, how it wets different surfaces and emulsifies different fats or how biodegradable it is – depends upon its exact design. There are many hundreds commercially available, which may be used in detergents and disinfectants, either alone or in combination.

Penetration Wetting is the first essential step in the removal of the soil. As wetting agents allow the detergent to displace air from surfaces, detergents are able to penetrate deep into porous dry deposits much faster than water alone. In doing so, the other active components of the detergent are enabled to react with soil components deep in the deposit at a much earlier stage.

Decreasing surface tension Wetting, spreading and angle of contact

◢ The effect varies depending on the nature of the surfactant

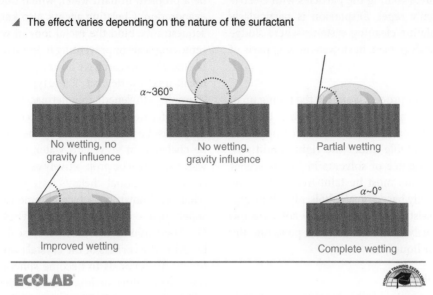

ECOLAB

Figure 5.1 Showing progressive wetting of a solid surface (Reproduced with permission from Ecolab. © Ecolab).

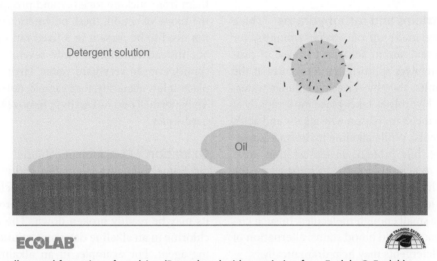

ECOLAB

Figure 5.2 Wetting, roll-up and formation of emulsion (Reproduced with permission from Ecolab. © Ecolab).

Emulsification Emulsions are suspensions of small droplets of one fluid in another. Milk, for example, is an emulsion of milk fats and proteins in water, stabilised by other molecules and ions present in the milk. Fats, oils and greases will not naturally disperse in water. First, the oil needs to be released from the surface it is resting on. Wetting is the first stage in this as the detergent undermines the oil–surface attraction and starts to displace the oil, which starts to roll up into droplets. This is accelerated if the temperature is high enough to soften or fully liquefy the oil or grease and/or if mechanical energy is applied to the soil. The oil droplets break away from the surface and float freely. Unless prevented from doing so, these droplets would coalesce as they contacted each

other at random and would eventually become large enough to re-deposit elsewhere. To prevent the coalescence, surfactants, either those involved in the wetting or other specialist emulsifiers, coat the surface of the oil droplets and stabilise the emulsion (Fig. 5.2).

Dispersion This is similar to emulsification except that it involves the breaking up and suspension of solid particles rather than fluid droplets. Dispersion is often carried out in a detergent by components other than surfactants, usually inorganic materials such as carbonates, silicates or phosphates or, in more advanced formulations, by special water-soluble charged polymers. The mechanism of maintaining a stable dispersion, thus allowing the soil particles to be rinsed freely away without re-deposition, involves coating the particles with electric charges that mutually repel. Dispersion is particularly important in circulating cleaning systems where sludge can build up, unless dispersed, in slower-moving parts of the system.

Solubilisation   This process is simply the taking up of soil components into a true solution, rather than an emulsion or a dispersion. While some soil components are naturally water-soluble under the right conditions, others need the assistance of solvents in the detergent solution. These solvents must be taint-free and of low toxicity and are usually based on alcohols, glycols or glycol ethers. They assist most where greasy soils are too hard to emulsify easily. Here, the solvents penetrate the grease and soften or liquefy it.

Chemical reactions

The most important chemical reactions include the following:

Hydrolysis of proteins and carbohydrates   These large molecules are made up of smaller subunits, for example, peptides and amino acids in the case of proteins. Hydrolysis involves splitting the molecules at the joints of the subunits, thereby releasing smaller water-soluble molecules. Hydrolysis takes place most rapidly at extreme pH and is the main reason why alkalis and acids are used in detergents. While alkaline hydrolysis is usually more effective, bile proteins in evisceration areas respond very well to acid hydrolysis. In some cases, the acid and alkaline hydrolyses may snip the larger molecule in different locations, neither of which alone is enough to produce small enough molecules. In such circumstances, for example, old blood stains, alternation of alkaline and acid detergents may help dramatically.

Saponification of fats, oils and greases   This is a particular form of hydrolysis in which an alkali reacts with triglyceride fat molecules, cutting the molecule in three places to give glycerol and soap, both water-soluble. In practice, the formation of the soap can be either helpful, because it acts as a wetting and emulsification agent in its own right, or harmful, because it produces unwanted foam in machine or circulation cleaning. In hard water, the foam is less of a problem, but formation of scum, that is, calcium soaps, may make the clean less efficient.

Chelation   Chelation of insoluble metal ions such as calcium, magnesium and iron. These ions may be present in scale already formed on a surface, where they provide anchorage for soil deposits and may become incorporated in the matrix of the deposit itself. Alternatively, they may be a problem in hard water, which undergoes heating or evaporation. Chelating agents, also known as chelants or sequestrants, bind the metal ions in water-soluble cages, removing scale or preventing it. In mixed scale/soil deposits, the chelates can have a very pronounced effect on the break-up of the deposit. These typical chelating agents, for example, ethylenediaminetetraacetic acid (EDTA) and gluconate, are restricted in their economy by the fact that they must be present in ratio to the metal ions needing to be chelated. In very hard water, or in large volumes of water, this may be prohibitively expensive. In recent years, these conventional chelants have been supplemented by what are known as substoichiometric chelants, usually water-soluble charged polymers. These act in two ways: (1) They inhibit the growth of scale microcrystals by blocking the corners of the crystals where growth occurs, forcing the crystals to become spherical. Any scale that does form is thus made soft and powdery and non-adherent to surfaces. (2) They act as dispersants, stringing microcrystals like pearls on a necklace and preventing them from sticking together and precipitating. Whatever the mode of action, these polymeric chelating agents do not need to be present in a fixed ratio to the metal ions, but instead function at only several parts per million (ppm), even in very hard water. Their main action takes place at low alkalinity, for example, during the rinse stage. They normally do not actively remove previously formed hard scales.

Oxidation   Oxidation of coloured materials, starches, etc. Some soil components respond well to chlorine, in the form of alkaline sodium hypochlorite. Coloured deposits may be bleached and some protein or fat deposits may be readily broken down. The main function of chlorine in an alkaline detergent solution is as an oxidising agent. For example, in an alkaline chlorine foam detergent, the alkalinity and the soluble chlorine molecules like the hypochlorite ion are <u>both</u> required to remove complex soiling made up of protein and fat. Periodic use of nitric acid-based detergents is common in some CIP applications. The treatment is primarily to achieve removal of inorganic scales, but it also has an oxidising effect on residual protein molecules not removed by the routine cleaning cycle.

Corrosion inhibition   Certain chemical components may inhibit the corrosion which normally takes place when aluminium and to a lesser degree zinc come into contact with detergents at very high or low pH. Silicates, for example, in the presence of caustic soda, can render the latter practically non-corrosive on aluminium although this is usually associated with a less effective clean and the increased risk of depositing an insoluble calcium silicate scale.

Enzymolysis   Protease, lipase or amylase enzymes may find use in specialist detergents where they can be quite effective at mild pH conditions. They split the large organic molecules with the same objective as alkaline or acid hydrolysis though enzymes can be more thorough in their effect. They are generally more difficult to formulate in a stable product.

Detergents: Design and choice

It can be seen, from the physical and chemical tasks needed for detergents to remove deposits, that the design of a detergent may be quite complex. In general, the more complex and varied the soil, the more different components need to be employed in the detergent. Other critical variables are the water hardness, the temperature and method of application, the safety considerations for operators and plant surfaces and the possible effects on the effluent system. To meet these varying requirements, the detergent manufacturers will have a range of different formulations. The main components, which may or may not be jointly present, include:

- Alkalis: caustic soda, caustic potash, carbonate, silicate and phosphate
- Acids: phosphoric, nitric, citric, glycolic, sulphamic and hydrochloric
- Chelating agents: EDTA, gluconate, glucoheptonate, citrate and polymers
- Solvents: isopropanol, propylene glycol, butyl diglycol and ethers
- Surfactants: anionic, cationic, non-ionic and amphoteric (many different types exist)
- Corrosion inhibitors: organic and inorganic
- Enzymes: protease, lipase and amylase
- Oxidising agents: hypochlorite, isocyanurates and peracids
- Stabilisers
- Viscosity modifiers

Any one detergent formulation may contain as little as 2 or even >15 individual components, blended carefully to the application and all its variables. Perfumes, such as pine, should not be incorporated in food plant cleaning chemicals as they can severely taint meat, even without direct physical contact.

In order to cover all the needs of the food and beverage industry, a detergent manufacturer's product range may comprise several hundred different formulations, but for any one plant, the choice is usually narrowed down to 2–10 products. The skill of the user, in conjunction with the hygiene chemical supplier, is in choosing which of the

many products to use. In meat plants, the biggest single volume of detergent used is normally an alkaline foam cleaner of some sort, with non-foaming crate wash detergent, manual neutral detergents and acidic foam descalers also finding use. Depending on the degree of further processing, other specialist products may be needed. As a rule, when choosing products for particular applications, the mildest, safest, least corrosive options should be tried first, with the 'heavier guns' being brought in as needed.

Detergent formulations may vary substantially in their effectiveness; failure to perform is usually not a question of a 'poor' product (though active ingredient levels can be inadequate in some cases) but rather of the choice of the wrong product, applied and controlled in an inappropriate fashion.

While a 'detergent' is designed to remove soils, another term – 'sanitiser' – is often used for some products of a similar type. In Europe, the term 'sanitiser' is taken to mean a combined detergent–disinfectant, while 'disinfectant' means a product designed to kill microbes but without deliberately employing a soil-removal effect.

Principles of disinfection

Soil deposits in a food plant would be bad enough if the problem was simply their rather unsightly appearance. However, the fact that they harbour, nourish and protect spoilage or pathogenic micro-organisms that are invisible to the naked eye makes the job somewhat harder. The soil must of course be removed as completely as possible by effective cleaning using the detergents discussed earlier. Typically, the reduction in the total viable bacterial count achieved by cleaning is of the order of 3–4 logs/cm^2. If the initial loading was $10^6\,CFU/cm^2$, which is frequently the case and higher in meat processing, there will remain counts of 10^2–$10^3/cm^2$ after cleaning. It is then necessary to reduce the bacterial numbers further, by the process of *disinfection*, to levels of less than a few hundreds. Complete *sterilisation*, the elimination of all life, is neither practical nor necessary in the disinfection of food plant surfaces. The reduction of microbes between the cleaning steps and the disinfection steps is variable, affected by the plant surfaces, soil type/level, cleaning programme and of course the chosen measurement of cleaning success. For instance, a study of cleaning techniques on the removal of biofilms described lower orders of effect during both the cleaning and disinfectant stages (Gibson *et al.*, 1999).

Biocidal active components

The class of hygiene chemicals known as *disinfectants* shares some components with detergents, but other aspects of the formulations are very different. Their

Mode of action of disinfectants

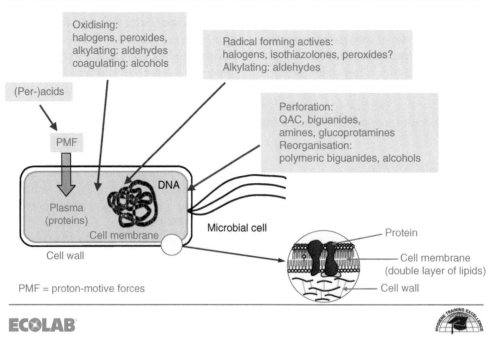

Figure 5.3 Action of biocides on bacteria (Reproduced with permission from Ecolab. © Ecolab).

function is to kill bacteria and other micro-organisms that are left on the surface after cleaning. They can kill microbes by several different methods, depending on which components are used in the disinfectant. Some affect the integrity of the cell wall, while others interfere with critical metabolic reactions inside the cell (Fig. 5.3). Scientific understanding of the mechanisms of action is well described and gaining focus driven by the need to understand the phenomenon of resistance (Maillard, 2002; McDonnell and Russell, 1999).

Some disinfectants are *oxidising* and will tend to react with most organic material, whether meat residues or bacteria. These oxidising disinfectants include *chlorine*, *iodophors* and *peracids*. These agents are usually rapid acting and broad spectrum in terms of the organisms they can kill inclusive of their spores, but they typically lack a residual effect. They may not be stable in hot water and may be corrosive on a range of metals and other surfaces, but they are usually low foaming.

It is sometimes wrongly assumed that a chlorine foam can act *fully* as a cleaner and a disinfectant and that subsequent disinfection is not needed. This is partly a false assumption, based on the perception of chlorine as a disinfectant. Depending on the pH, there is an equilibrium in chlorine solutions between the hypochlorous acid (HOCl) molecule and the hypochlorite ion (OCl⁻). The main active biocide in chlorine release agents is the hypochlorous acid molecule HOCl; it is uncharged and for this reason is thought to penetrate the cell walls

of microbes more easily. In chlorine foam cleaners, the application solution is usually around pH 10–11. The chlorine is therefore mostly present as the hypochlorite ion OCl⁻, which acts principally as a detergent and oxidising agent, helping with the removal of proteins and grease and the bleaching of some coloured substances. This pH effect and lack of free HOCl makes the disinfectant properties of alkaline chlorine solutions much weaker (up to a hundred times) than a straight hypochlorite disinfectant solution without alkalis. The better cleaning performance of the chlorine foam physically removes much of the bacterial load along with the dirt, but in areas where a very low surface bacterial count is desired, a separate disinfection stage is needed. This should normally not be a hypochlorite solution because of the risk of corrosion (even on stainless steel) from the breakdown products of the hypochlorite and product taint from poorly rinsed surfaces. The lack of heat and light stability of the chlorine can mean that no residual bactericidal effect is maintained after a relatively short time.

Non-oxidising disinfectants are typically based on quaternary ammonium compounds or 'quats' – a class of cationic surfactants and amphoterics – another class of surfactants with twin positive and negative charges, alcohols, biguanides or aldehydes. The non-oxidising agents are usually heat stable and less corrosive and have a residual biocidal or biostatic effect if left on surfaces. The surfactant-based disinfectants are often foaming, which can be a disadvantage if excessive rinsing is required or an advantage for reasons of visibility and procedural monitoring. The foam level can easily be controlled in a multi-injector satellite station (described in a later section) so this feature can be used as required.

Disinfectants: Design and choice

The method of kill and the point of attack on the defences of micro-organisms may be different in each case. Unless carefully formulated, disinfectants could have weaknesses at lower temperatures or against some more difficult-to-kill bacteria such as *pseudomonads*. This could be critical, for example, when disinfecting a chill.

Well-formulated disinfectants may employ several different biocidal components, often with surfactants and other agents to help in the killing action. This also helps eliminate the possibility of adaptation or even resistance developing among the population of micro-organisms. Development of resistance to antibiotics is well documented and increasingly observed in the medical and veterinary fields (Soonthornchaikul *et al.*, 2005). To date, a similar resistance pattern to biocides and disinfectants is not readily seen in industrial applications such as food plant disinfection. However, different susceptibilities have been described for culturable and viable non-culturable (VNC) forms of *Campylobacter*, against disinfectants at low in-use levels (Rowe *et al.*, 1998). There is increasing work in this area particularly looking for evidence of antibiotic-induced cross-resistance to standard disinfectants and vice versa, both in clinical practice (Russell, 2002) and in the food production system (Doyle *et al.*, 2006).

Disinfectants can be affected by residues of detergents left on surfaces, perhaps owing to inadequate rinsing. Anionic surfactants in the detergent may neutralise the cationic surfactant of 'quats', rendering them ineffective.

Disinfectants should be chosen in conjunction with the supplier, taking into full account the surface materials to be disinfected; the soil residues likely to be present after cleaning; the safety to operators and product; the specific organisms, if any, to be controlled; the ambient and solution temperature; and the timescale (rapid or residual) required. Cleaning and disinfection for some applications may be adequately combined into one operation using a sanitiser, which has the action of both a detergent and a disinfectant. Usually, this is a quat- or amphoteric-based neutral or mildly alkaline product for manual use. However, the one-stage product approach, while time-saving, does not give as consistent or as effective a final result as the two stages executed separately.

Under no circumstances should phenolic, pine or other highly perfumed disinfectants be used in a food plant, even in the offices. The risk of taint is high, even from very small airborne concentrations and especially in fatty foods. The risk is compounded by the presence of chlorine, even at low levels in factory water. Chlorocresols and chlorophenols may be formed which can taint meat at low levels, parts per billion (ppb).

Considering all of the information in this section on disinfection, the important points for industry at present are to:

- Select the right product type for a particular application
- Use freshly diluted product (if the product type demands an aqueous solution)
- Ensure the correct concentration can be routinely achieved and validate it
- Apply the product at the right point within the total hygiene procedure
- Ensure sufficient contact time (determined by product type/standard required)

Disinfectant kill rates can be routinely assessed via standard European Norm (EN) disinfection assessment tests, and although they 'mimic' the real environment, they are a controlled and standardised way of showing differences between disinfectant products (BS EN 1276, 2009; Maillard, 2005). Accordingly, they can be used as part of the selection criteria earlier.

Disinfection assessment tests are a good source of information about the basic efficacy of a biocidal molecule or formulated disinfectant product within certain test parameters. These tests measure kill rate (a mathematical log reduction of the viable members of a microbial population of known origin and size) while taking into account performance-limiting factors within the proposed use environment such as low temperatures and residual soiling. The effective in-use concentrations are then usually established at hundreds or thousands of ppm of biocidal molecules. This approach ensures that the final recommended in-use concentration of a disinfectant product is significantly above (often ×10 or ×20) the known minimum inhibitory concentration (MIC) of the individual biocidal molecules or disinfectant formulation. The MIC is the value of a standard laboratory test at which an antimicrobial agent will <u>prevent</u> growth of a specific micro-organism.

All of these points together are designed, in respect of current understanding, to ensure that the targeted micro-organisms are removed/killed and reduce the risk of temporary adaptation or even permanent resistance within a species or population.

Hygiene equipment and application methods

Detergents and disinfectants can be applied in a number of different ways, dictated by the nature of the cleaning task.

Manual cleaning

The agents may be applied manually, using cloth, mop, squeegee, brush, green pad, etc. This is usually reserved for small pieces of machinery or specific areas on larger machinery that is non-waterproof or which needs dismantling. It is labour intensive, can be dangerous when used on sharp or heavy equipment and usually requires safe, neutral chemicals. Detergents or sanitisers (combination detergents–disinfectants) may be used in this way, but not normally disinfectants, as the repeated immersion of the brush, pad or cloth in the solution after contact with the surface would tend to reduce the disinfectant efficacy. Manual cleaning varies significantly with the skill, commitment and time available to the operator. While once common, it is not normally used today for cleaning large plant areas.

Foam cleaning

This is the established method for COP consisting of large or intricate equipment and is the standard procedure in the vast majority of meat, poultry and other food and beverage plants worldwide. A foam blanket, created using a wide range of available equipment (see later), is projected from a nozzle, and allowed to act on the soil for typically 15–30 minutes, after which it is rinsed off with the released deposits. Large areas such as floors, walls, stands, conveyors and tables and intricate machinery such as fillers, defeatherers, blackscrapers, etc. are normally suitable for foam cleaning.

The foam itself is merely the carrier for the detergent to enable it physically to function. The quality of the foam may differ greatly, the best being creamy in consistency rather than either too dry or too wet. The foam should be applied as a thin, uniform layer. Coverage rates are quite rapid and overall economy is good as manual scrubbing is unnecessary and a little detergent concentrate generates a lot of foam (up to 500-fold). Only specially designed hygiene chemicals are suitable for foam cleaning. The foam itself is created by a special surfactant system that is present in the product in addition to the actual cleaning components. Normal detergents, which at first may appear quite foamy, will give a rapidly collapsing foam and should not be used for this purpose. Many speciality foam detergents and foam sanitisers are available, from caustic through neutral to acid, plus chlorine or quat, if needed. Recently developed advanced foams give a much improved cling to smooth vertical surfaces and can remain in contact with complete coverage for 20–30 minutes or more. Less well-designed formulations can often collapse rapidly and slide off before the cleaning action is complete.

Foam and disinfectant application equipment

This can be classified as mobile, centralised or satellite, although there is some overlap. In addition, a satellite foam application system is often part of the central rinsing system and additionally may facilitate disinfectant application, described later.

Mobile foamers may be based on air-driven pumps with tank or venturi injectors attached to medium- or high-pressure mobile washers. Advantages include lower capital cost and versatility, supporting the use of different hygiene chemicals in different areas. Disadvantages include potential lack of chemical solution strength control, maintenance problems due to abuse/wear and tear related to mobility, waste of unused chemical solution and preparation and put-away time. The once popular pressurised mobile tank is now subject to EU regulations on the routine safety testing of pressure vessels and has been largely replaced by the other technologies; examples are shown in Figure 5.4.

Centralised foam systems are based on an automatic chemical dilution tank and pump station, which pumps the solution, as a liquid under low pressure, to numerous outlets on a pipe work system throughout the factory. Compressed air is injected into the outlet 'foam boxes' to create the foam of the desired flow rate and air content. Advantages include consistent chemical strength throughout the plant with single-point control, no handling of concentrated chemical and the avoidance of drums of chemical in the factory production areas. The elimination of preparation and put-away time is also of benefit, saving about 30 minutes/operator/day. Chemical usage is typically 10–20% lower than with tank mobiles owing to reduction of waste. Disadvantages may include requirement for a capital budget, deterioration of the diluted detergent solution within the system due to water

(a)   (b)

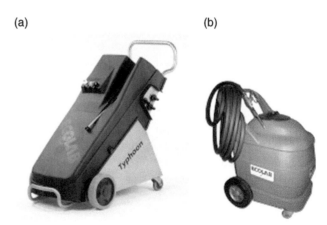

Figure 5.4 Showing mobile unit for foam/disinfection/rinse applications (a) and mobile unit for foam only applications (b) (Reproduced with permission from Ecolab. © Ecolab).

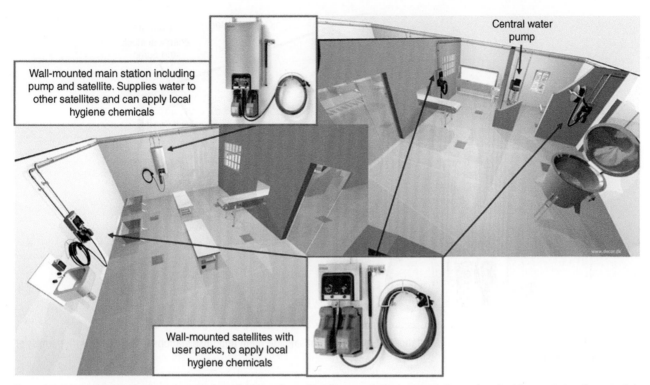

Figure 5.5 Demonstration room showing installations of satellite foam and rinse stations (Reproduced with permission from Ecolab. © Ecolab).

quality changes and/or poorly specified pipe work and reduction of hygiene chemical choice. However, the latter point can be remedied by using hybrid centralised/satellite foam boxes at chosen locations (see Fig. 5.6).

Satellite foam and disinfection systems are normally driven by centralised rinse systems using wall-mounted or trolley-mounted foam boxes equipped with venturi injectors at each outlet. In low- and medium-pressure rinse systems (circa 20–40 bar water pressure) utilising multi-injector satellite stations, compressed air can be selectively applied at each injector to create detergent foam and disinfectant spray or foam (Fig. 5.5). It is possible to have up to four different hygiene chemicals available for use at one station. In high-pressure rinse systems (>70 bar), atmospheric air alone can be drawn in using special venturi foam lances. High-pressure fixed systems have become less common over the last 10 years; the issues are discussed later under rinsing. Advantages of low- to medium-pressure satellite foam systems include the possibility for lower upfront and running costs (dependent on existing systems), complete versatility of chemical choice/concentration at each outlet and user safety and comfort. Disadvantages can include chemical drums in the production area, though the advent of satellite integrated hygiene chemical user packs has reduced this hazard and facilitated removal during production.

The development of direct concentrate dosing into satellite injectors has enabled the central provision of the main hygiene chemical of choice, a similar concept to the traditional central foam system described previously, but the chemical is not pre-diluted. This allows configuration of a hybrid central/satellite system which combines all the advantages of the two systems (see Fig. 5.6).

Gels

Gel cleaning uses special chemicals and spray equipment to give a thick, viscous layer of detergent that clings strongly even on vertical surfaces. This is normally confined to small areas where very long contact time of several hours is needed for burnt-on or otherwise very stubborn deposits. Gel chemicals may sometimes be foamed with certain types of foam equipment, but the high viscosity of the gel is effectively increased within the foam even further. This can lead to a slowing down of the cleaning reactions, which depend greatly on diffusion of detergent components into the soil and of soil components out of the deposit. For this reason, gels are not always economical for routine general cleaning of large factory areas, where time constraints usually dictate contact times of 15–30 minutes. Ensuring complete rinsing of gels can sometimes be difficult, depending on the design of the gel and its viscosity change on dilution.

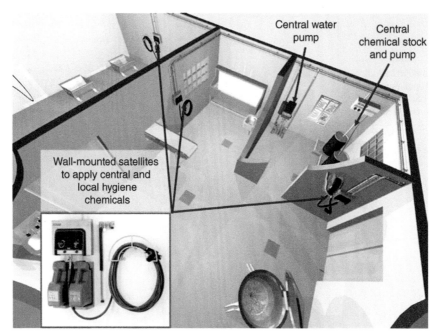

Figure 5.6 Demonstration room showing installations of hybrid central/satellite foam and rinse stations (Reproduced with permission from Ecolab. © Ecolab).

Spray

Prior to the advent of foam cleaning technology, this method was widely in use; however, it is now seldom used for the application of detergents. Spray cleaning uses a gun and/or lance linked to a pressurised water system; hygiene chemical induction is via an injector. This may be achieved using satellite foam and rinse equipment, mobile equipment or more simply via a backpack sprayer of diluted product. Using this method for cleaning is wasteful, it is difficult to see the application, it is often repeated unnecessarily, and the hygiene chemical runs off rapidly from vertical surfaces. It is slower and inferior in performance to foam cleaning. Conversely, it is the usual method of application for disinfectants, though as discussed earlier disinfectants can be applied as foams. The subtle difference in the case of disinfection is that this application is routinely concerned with food contact surfaces, it is a faster application than foaming and dependent on area and equipment to be treated and spraying via a satellite injector system or a backpack sprayer can both provide efficient outcomes.

Fogging

Aerial fogging uses compressed air or other equipment to generate a fine mist of disinfectant solution, which should hang in the air long enough to fill the room volume before settling on walls and difficult-to-reach surfaces. Fogging is primarily focused on complete surface disinfection in a defined enclosed area, though it is possible to reduce airborne micro-organisms associated with aerosols (debris and water droplets). Fogging systems can be small portable devices or built-in automatic central systems. Fogging is only worthwhile if the rest of the hygiene programme is properly carried out. The important parameters for effective fogging are the matching of the volume of liquid being fogged to the volume of the room, the temperature, the relative humidity and the rate of air change. Ideally, saturation of the air, with very fine droplets (10–20 μm) which stay suspended for a long time, gives the best results. Failure to create the correct fog droplet size and volume can mean that only the uppermost surfaces of the plant receive the disinfectant as it rains down and the air itself may remain largely unaffected.

Knife and cutting tool disinfection during processing

The EU hygiene regulations have over many years demanded that knives and cutting tools used in animal slaughter/processing be disinfected in hot water at 82°C (Council Directives, 64/433/EEC, 92/116/EEC, 95/68/EEC). It has been known for some years that this method has some significant drawbacks (SCVPH, 2001); some are listed below:

- The cost of producing the hot water
- The maintenance of steriliser boxes, particularly of heating elements
- Low comfort of the operator
- Creation of considerable volumes of water vapour and associated condensate

- Cooking protein onto blades forming and promoting biofilms
- Blunting of knives
- Poor microbiological status of the steriliser
- Creation of scale in hard-water areas
- Via a combination of the aforementioned factors, loss of cross-contamination control between animals

As discussed under Reasons for cleaning and disinfecting plant, there have been significant changes to EU legislation over recent years. One of the key changes in animal processing was in the procedure covering 'in-process' cutting tool disinfection (Council Regulation (EC) No 853/2004). The wording of this legislation changed as follows, to allow alternative means of disinfection:

> …They (slaughter houses and cutting plants) must have facilities for disinfecting tools with hot water supplied at not less than 82°C, or an alternative system having an equivalent effect…

Following this legislative change, alternatives have been proposed in order to establish in-process knife and cutting tool disinfection via chemical means. The selection of chemical disinfectant type is critical, as equivalent effect should be understood as (i) achieving at least the same microbiological control level on knives and (ii) maintaining the general food safety status of the product. This latter point is important when using chemical rather than heat disinfection since the change procedure introduces a potential food contaminant into the process, not

previously present using 82C potable water. Therefore, safe chemistry, effective dose and control methods, professional monitoring and management become a significant part of this new strategy for knives and cutting tools. Alternatives that provide equivalent effect need to be acceptable to and understood by the local competent authority and their infield team of meat hygiene inspectors and veterinarians because importantly, the disinfection of cutting tools remains a legal control point.

This new concept is still gaining ground in the EU, but it has been shown to be at least equivalent in a number of long-term trials with significant additional benefits, for example:

- Improvements to overall plant hygiene performance
- Reduced quality/safety incidences through more consistent knife treatment
- Cleaner working place
- Reduced levels of condensation which impacts positively on problematic microbial growth
- Improved working processes related to knife hygiene, soak time decreases and reduced blunting of knives (Fig. 5.7)
- Increased operator comfort through removing hot water/steam
- Cost savings in water and energy
- Sustainable and environmentally friendly application

A common theme for FBOs when considering alternatives to 82C would appear to be financial and sustainability drivers, assuming of course that the alternative

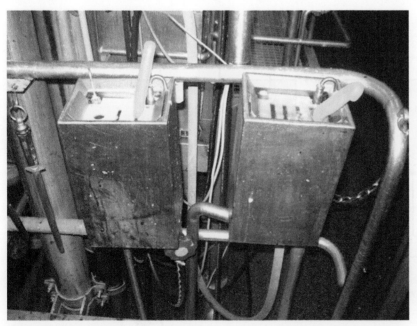
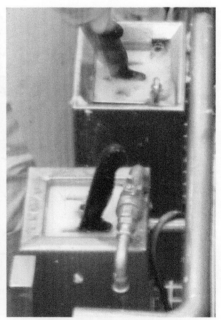

Figure 5.7 The visual effect of replacing 82C water with Inspexx disinfectant solution, picture on the right (Reproduced with permission from Ecolab. © Ecolab).

provides an equivalent food safety result. Turning off the steam or electrical elements in traditional knife disinfection baths can contribute significantly to the reduction of a plant's carbon footprint while also gaining other benefits for operators and product.

Machine washing

Industrial machine washing is typically done with an automatic or semi-automatic continuous tray wash or buggy wash machine with spray nozzles arrayed on booms in separate chambers of the machine or in separate cycles for detergent, rinse and sometimes disinfectant. An alternative machine design uses submersion tanks or flumes, through which the trays are slowly pulled. A less effective design is the circular carousel, which runs the risk of contamination of clean trays by dirty ones as there is only one entry/exit point. Other machines, especially for buggies and racks, may wash each item individually in a batch process. All machine types represent an expensive capital investment and are critical to the hygiene of direct food contact surfaces. Wash machines generally are large consumers of water, especially if not properly maintained and controlled. Filters should be cleaned regularly and blocked nozzles cleared. Prevention of liquid carry-over from one chamber to the next is also important. Tray wash machines can also be a contamination risk to the rest of the factory as they can produce large quantities of fine, contaminated aerosols, which may drift with natural airflows into critical areas. Chemicals used in these machines must be low foam or even actively de-foaming and should

be automatically controlled and dosed by conductivity probe, with the probe being cleaned regularly and the concentration checked. Location of the probe is important in obtaining representative readings. Machines should be set up for individual tray type; in this respect, nozzle positions, angles and spray patterns are crucial to obtaining a consistent hygiene result. If tray type and shape change significantly, the machine will need to be reset in order to maintain the required efficacy.

Cleaning-in-place (CIP)

CIP is used extensively for the interior cleaning of pipes, vessels, tankers, heat exchangers, fillers, etc. commonly found in breweries and dairies for the processing of liquid products. This approach is used in meat and poultry plants where giblets or other materials such as basting oils may be automatically transferred through pipe systems. The most recent adoption of CIP in food manufacturing is in the convenience foods department where sauces or marinades may be made. CIP involves a programmed cycle, including timed pre-rinse, cleaning and rinsing stages, and is nowadays usually automated or semi-automated with a system of valves, pumps and detergent tanks, often controlled by microprocessor (Lorenzen, 2005) (Fig. 5.8).

The main points to consider include the following:

Flow velocity – It should be sufficient all parts of the system to cause turbulent flow. This is generally around 1.5–2 m/s. Where pipe diameters vary in the one system, the largest pipe should have this flow rate. Failure to comply with this flow rate means smooth 'laminar' flow

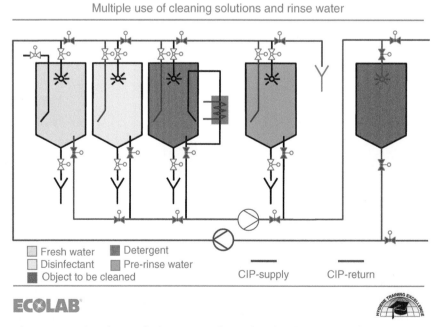

Figure 5.8 Diagrammatic representation of a standard CIP system (Reproduced with permission from Ecolab. © Ecolab).

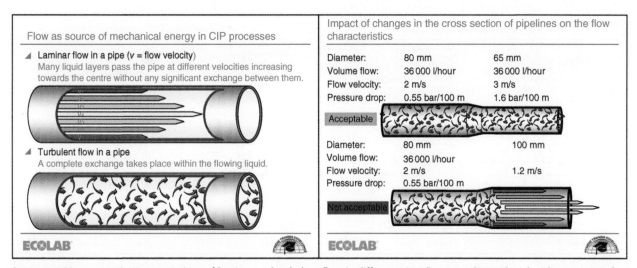

Figure 5.9 Diagrammatic representations of laminar and turbulent flow in different pipe diameters (Reproduced with permission from Ecolab. © Ecolab).

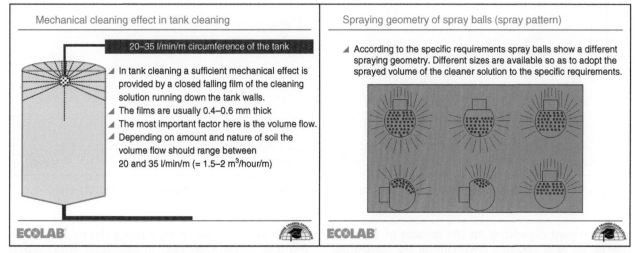

Figure 5.10 Spray ball types and mechanical cleaning effects in tank cleaning (Reproduced with permission from Ecolab. © Ecolab).

at the boundary layer close to the pipe surface, with little or no mechanical energy to help the cleaning (Fig. 5.9).

Spray pressure and pattern – Spray balls or rotating jets are used for the interiors of large tankers or vessels. Again, if impingement is too gentle or blind spots are protected from the impact of the spray, there will be insufficient energy to have an effective clean. Typical pressures are 1–3 bar for low-pressure systems and 6 bar for high-pressure systems. Flow rates of approximately 20–35 l/min/m circumference of the vessel are normally needed to achieve the desired results (Fig. 5.10).

Temperature – Generally, temperatures of 70–85°C are used which has a high bearing on the rate of the cleaning reaction.

Detergent control – Typically driven by a temperature-compensated conductivity probe and pump. Conductivity closely follows free caustic levels in CIP solutions and

allows for fully automatic control. Manual dosing, in contrast, runs the risk of chemical strength being too high or too low.

Chemical energy and foam control – The main detergent in CIP is normally an alkali, frequently caustic based. The additional components, such as surfactants for preventing foam and aiding wetting and chelating agents for removing scales such as calcium phosphate, may be included in the detergent formulation as supplied; this is called a built detergent. The additional components may also be supplied separately as a specialist additive product. For formulation reasons, additives are technically superior and more economical but require parallel dosing pumps for caustic and additive.

Recycling – Detergent solutions may be used more than once; it is economical and environmentally friendly and reduces the loading on effluent plants. Solutions

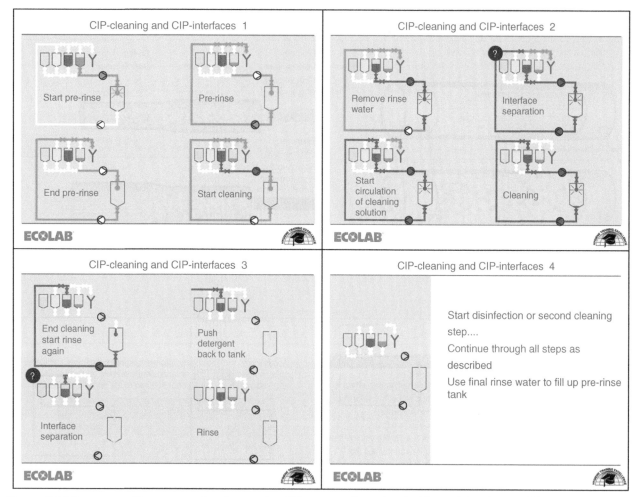

Figure 5.11 Shows a graphic representation of a complete CIP sequence (Reproduced with permission from Ecolab. © Ecolab).

may be reused depending on the amount of dirt they pick up on each cleaning cycle and on the suspension and chelating power of the detergent. If too heavily loaded, detergent solutions may re-deposit old soil or scale in slower-moving parts of the system. Filtration or centrifugation can sometimes be used to extend the life of the solution (Fig. 5.11).

Rinse systems

Meat plants need effective rinse systems for washing down the plant before and after the foam application and in some cases for generating the foam itself and applying disinfectant. A number of different systems are possible. The rule governing them all is that the cleaning impact of a water jet on a surface is proportional both to the pressure of the liquid at the point of contact and to the volume of liquid per second in the jet.

Traditional *steam hoses*, which mixed live steam with cold water, are now out of favour for a number of reasons, principally cost, safety, humidity and condensation. Although it may be thought that the very high

temperature of a steam hose had a disinfecting effect, this is in fact not the case, as expansion at the nozzle causes rapid cooling even at short distances, while conduction of heat away from the point of impact by the surface (usually a metal) means that sufficiently high biocidal temperatures on the surface itself are never reached. Live steam can also carry corrosion products from pipelines or carry-over of boiler treatment chemicals, neither of which is desirable hygienically.

Similarly, *low-pressure* (around mains pressure or <10 bar) water systems are inadequate for rinsing meat or poultry plants, because the water jet lacks sufficient energy to assist in the cleaning process.

At the other extreme, *high-pressure* rinse systems, based on either mobile pressure washers or built-in pump systems, have been widely used. Their use has been in decline for a number of safety, maintenance and hygiene reasons. These systems typically function at 60–120 bar, using piston- or plunger-type pumps. They create a vibration in plumbed-in systems, which can affect the life of the pipe work, which is narrow bore and expensive. The design of these positive displacement pumps causes pressure in the system to drop precipitously if the maximum flow rate is exceeded, for example, if one person too many uses an outlet simultaneously or if one nozzle is missing or worn out. The high velocity of the water from the nozzles causes the jet to break up at a distance of about 1 m into a fine mist, which has lost virtually all its momentum and impact. Rinsing of surfaces therefore needs to be carried out at close range. This is time-consuming for the operators and in addition causes the soil deposit to be broken up violently, creating contaminating aerosols. High-pressure water is also dangerous and may penetrate the skin or damage the eyes.

Medium-pressure rinse systems (20–40 bar) are a compromise option balancing both pressure and volume. Using multistage centrifugal pumps and wider-bore, medium-pressure-rated pipe work, these systems are vibration-free. Additionally, the latest technology utilises frequency-controlled motors to prevent start-up 'shock' and false starts and remove flow variations as different numbers of users come on to the system. The nozzles used may be individually selected for foam, disinfection and rinse (when satellites are in use) with the latter available in rotating versions and adjustable spray patterns. As the water velocity is lower and the volume per second higher, the jet retains most of its impact even at several metres distance. This means that rinsing can be faster, with a better sluicing-away effect. The extra water consumption per second is usually compensated for by a shorter rinse time. Water consumption in total, compared to a high-pressure system, is more or less equivalent, but labour savings (in the most time-consuming stage of the cleaning sequence) can be significant.

Water temperatures

Although the EU regulations call for 82°C water to be used for knife sterilisation, such high temperatures are impractical for most plant cleaning operations (with the main exception of CIP) for a number of reasons:

- The steam, humidity and condensation obscure vision and encourage microbial growth.
- Proteins are denatured on the surfaces and hard-water scale formation is increased.
- The load on the extraction and cooling systems is increased.
- Thermal shock can damage surfaces owing to differential expansion.
- Pipe work lifetime is reduced.
- The lances are too hot to hold and the water jet is dangerous.
- Energy costs are too high.
- Foam quality deteriorates at very high temperatures.

The temperature that gives the best compromise between effectiveness and economy is 50–65°C, which is enough to soften the fats encountered in meat plants, without the drawbacks shown earlier. In fish processing plants, because of the low denaturation temperature of the proteins, rinse water at circa 35°C is used. There are new developments looking at the possibility of reducing pre-rinse temperatures for more economical COP and CIP.

Contamination and re-contamination

Meat plant surfaces will be exposed to microbial contamination by direct contact with the exterior of the animal prior to and after slaughter and to the gut contents during and after evisceration. The dressing process and subsequent production stages are designed to reduce further direct contamination of food product with these micro-organisms. While viscera are kept physically separate from edible materials, plant surfaces in evisceration areas will have high bacterial counts. Personnel and external material such as pallets, vehicles, etc. also bring micro-organisms into the plant, especially onto the floors and into the air. The dispersal of micro-organisms within a plant is generally well reviewed and has been previously described (Board, 1983, chap. 3, pp. 57–68).

During cleaning, these micro-organisms, whether spoilage, pathogenic or harmless, may be disturbed in such a way as to be transmitted, perhaps directly onto food product itself or onto previously cleaned surfaces. This accidental *re-contamination* is carried by a number of possible *vectors*, which, unless understood and controlled, can nullify the effectiveness of the cleaning procedure.

Air

Air can carry dust from hide-pullers, fleeces, feathers, etc., especially in dry weather. This dust is likely to contain faecal bacteria, among others. Air can also carry aerosols (usually a combination of water, soil and microbes) that have been created, during rinsing, by washing machines, during boot washing and even during hand washing, though the last two produce less dense lower mobility aerosols than the first two. Aerosols that contain a high concentration of small particles (<20 μm) can easily move around the factory via local air currents and are generally recognised as a significant causal agent of re-contamination and/or cross-contamination (Burfoot, 2005). *Pseudomonas* spp., *Listeria* spp., *E. coli* and *Salmonella* spp. are frequently found on floors and drains, which makes the rinsing of these potentially problematic. Hot water or steam can also create aerosols, which condense on cold overhead surfaces, later to drip onto unprotected foodstuffs positioned below. For these reasons, great care must be taken to ensure that all product is removed from areas being cleaned. Differential air pressures must cause air to move from clean to dirty areas and not vice versa. Rinse hoses, even under low pressure, must not be inserted into drains.

Water

Water collecting in hollows on the floor or in blocked drain openings can quickly become highly contaminated. Splashes caused by people or vehicles going through the puddles can directly contaminate surfaces and raise local aerosols. Water used in washing the plant may be stored in holding tanks feeding the pumps. These may also become contaminated and, with warm water driving off the chlorine reserve, the rinse water itself may become a source of re-contamination.

People

Personnel are the biggest single source of contamination risk in a plant, from dirty protective clothing, inadequate hand washing, hair, jewellery, sneezes, coughs, cuts and sores. All plant personnel must be trained in hygiene and the proper clean protective work wear supplied. Hand-washing facilities must be conveniently located close to production stations and entrances. Bactericidal, non-perfumed soaps must be supplied, together with alcohol-based hand disinfectant in high-risk areas.

Surfaces

Surfaces, which are inadequately cleaned, may re-contaminate entire pieces of equipment. For example, one badly cleaned roller on an otherwise spotless conveyor belt can, in one rotation of the belt, smear it with grease and dirt. Similarly, cutting blades in saws, slicers, dicers, etc. must be very effectively cleaned.

Cleaning procedures

The previous sections on soil, substrate, detergents, equipment, methods and re-contamination should demonstrate that the cleaning of a meat plant is a complex job. Only with systematic procedures can a consistently hygienic plant be maintained. These procedures form part of the *cleaning schedule*, a working reference document that defines standards, methods, frequencies and materials for all cleaning and disinfecting operations in the plant. The schedule should form part of the Quality Manual of the plant and be available for consultation or inspection. Simplified extracts of the schedule, employing pictograms, may be used as wall charts for individual plant areas. Hygiene service suppliers often assist in the preparation, upkeep and training of the hygiene procedures.

To secure a due diligence defence in the case of prosecution, it would normally be necessary to show that a properly designed cleaning schedule was in place and was being followed. Under the new EU regulations, a HACCP or similar approach is mandatory for the management of food safety and GHP is mandatory and will be audited. These requirements are also clearly defined in other industry food safety standards (BS EN ISO 22000: 2005; International Food Standard, 2007; British Retail Consortium, 2011).

As mentioned earlier, cost pressures may encourage the cleaners to combine or leave out individual steps in the cleaning sequence. This should be avoided. Anyone responsible for food industry hygiene, and in particular in the methodology of cleaning, should have a clear understanding of what methods are correct for the cleaning of food plants and the dangers of incorrect or inadequate cleaning procedures.

The cleaning sequence

The optimal sequence for general routine surface cleaning of a food plant is:

1 Gross clean/preparation
2 Pre-rinsing
3 Detergent application
4 Post-rinsing
5 Disinfection
6 Terminal rinsing

Some of these steps may sometimes be skipped or combined (perhaps where the nature and quantity of the soil is light or during brief intermediate cleaning in production breaks), but for systematic daily cleaning, the sequence is very important. We will now look at each step in more detail.

Gross clean/preparation

This is the step that is most often incorrectly carried out or completely ignored. Food residue that is left on the equipment, surfaces and floors has many negative effects on the cleaning performance:

- It protects surfaces and the bacteria on them from the attack of the detergent.
- It reacts with and consumes the detergent so that its function is weakened or chemical wasted.
- It holds bacteria (often at very high levels) which can re-contaminate surfaces at a later stage in the cleaning, especially during the rinsing stage.
- It can directly re-contaminate surfaces with grease and protein which can act as nutrient for micro-organisms and as a barrier to disinfectant. This is particularly true on moving machinery such as conveyors.

- It can end up washed into the drainage system, either causing blockage in traps or high solids/biological oxygen demand (BOD) in the effluent.
- It encourages the cleaning team to miss areas, not to check their work, and to cut other corners.

A poor gross clean is the single biggest reason for poor or inconsistent bacterial counts on surfaces and for high bacterial contamination in aerosols caused by rinsing.

In a properly managed cleaning programme, all pieces of food product, meat, etc. which are larger than a fingernail are removed before application of detergent. Where possible, this should be carried out dry by hand-picking, scraping and shovelling. All rubbish/waste collected should be put in bags/bins and removed entirely from the area. It should be understood that all edible foodstuffs and product packaging should be removed before this stage. (It is a constant source of amazement how often this simple fact is ignored.)

Pre-rinsing

The purpose of pre-rinsing is to remove deposits, which cannot easily be removed by picking/scraping/shovelling, for example, blood, manure, small meat pieces and particles, etc. The rinse water should not be used as a brush for chasing large amounts of pieces around the floor and towards the drain. This would result in waste of water and time, blockage of drains, loading of effluent water with high volume and BOD/chemical oxygen demand (COD) and unnecessarily high humidity.

Pre-rinsing is particularly important in the case of cutting boards, where the thick deposits of grease would make true cleaning of the surface grooves and crevices impossible. Where fresh blood is a problem, the rinse temperature should be below 50°C to avoid coagulation.

After pre-rinsing, it is important to remove any water that may be lying in pools on flat surfaces as these would dilute the detergent solution and make it less effective. Any squeegee used to scrape off the excess water must be used only for food contact surfaces and not for floors.

Detergent application

The purpose of a detergent is to remove the thin tenacious layers of protein, grease, etc. that are still on surfaces which may already look clean. Detergents are not designed for removing large pieces of meat or thick layers of fat. Although they may seem to help in the removal of such large quantities, they will usually fail to remove the last residues actually bonded to the surface if these residues are protected by the thicker layers above them. It is in these thin residues that many bacteria can easily survive and grow and they can make any disinfectant, which is applied later, ineffective.

Foaming should be methodical and thorough, and the operator should check to see that all surfaces have been covered in the foam, both top and bottom. Foam concentration, dryness, thickness of application and contact time (15–30 minutes) are all very important in ensuring the correct results at a controlled, optimised cost.

Post-rinsing

Post-rinsing is again a very important stage. Care should be taken to minimise the amount of splash and aerosol formed, which may re-contaminate previously cleaned surfaces or blast particles of dirt high up on walls and ventilation socks. After post-rinsing, the surfaces should be free of all visible particles, layers of soiling and residues of detergent and should be 'visibly clean'. The soil and detergent residues and any soaps formed by alkaline hydrolysis of fats will tend to neutralise the disinfectant properties of quats. It is important to check the efficacy of the rinse, especially where parallel production lines are cleaned in sequence and splash could re-contaminate previously cleaned surfaces. The rollers of conveyors are particularly important. After rinsing, any pools of water should be removed from surfaces and vessels, whether disinfection is to follow or not.

Disinfection

Disinfection should only be carried out on a visually clean, well-rinsed surface, free of residual surface water. Direct food contact surfaces should be disinfected at least daily, with other surfaces (such as walls, doors, etc.) disinfected on a regular basis. The concentration of the disinfectant and its contact time (ideally >20 minutes) are both very important.

Terminal rinsing

Some disinfectants are suitable to leave on surfaces without final rinsing. The residual disinfectant often helps maintain a low microbial count for a considerable time after the cleaning sequence is finished, particularly important in dealing with any 'settling' aerosols. In addition, it provides more time for the surfaces to dry completely compared to carrying out a terminal rinse, which sets the drying time back again. The law surrounding terminal disinfection is currently different in many EU member states. Some have no official control requirements, while others have long-standing approval processes. The new EU directives, as previous versions, are not very descriptive about cleaning and disinfection procedures. There is of course an absolute requirement to clean and disinfect as appropriate, provide personnel hygiene facilities and ensure factory design that is suited to cleaning. There is no specific instruction about rinsing of terminal disinfectants other than the linked requirement that the business owner has a duty to carry out safe processing. It will eventually fall to the already running EU Biocidal Products Directive (Directive (EC) No 98/8) to license officially a biocidal product (circa 2008 onwards) for use in defined applications, inclusive of its manufacturer's 'in-use' claims and technical/toxicological supporting data. It is then envisaged that registered products with the right credentials can then be fully integrated into individual risk assessments. This legislation does not prevent any EU member states from applying additional requirements as they see fit.

If terminal rinsing is required, it should be done in time to allow surfaces to dry before production begins, but not so early that disinfectant is removed prior to the achievement of the surface hygiene target for residual micro-organisms.

Terminal rinsing should be much quicker than the pre-rinsing and post-rinsing stages as no contaminating particles of soil should be present and the surface area to be rinsed is smaller since routinely it is only direct food contact surfaces that are treated with terminal disinfectant. The microbiological quality of the water is very important. It must be potable or else it can be a source of re-contamination itself.

Monitoring of hygiene

Monitoring of cleaning and disinfection effectiveness is partly a matter of trained *visual assessment* and partly of *surface analysis and microbiology*. A plant that is not visually clean always presents a risk regarding the microbial contamination of food. The control and avoidance of food safety risks are, as mentioned earlier, best achieved using a HACCP approach. Legislation strongly recommends the use of HACCP principles to secure a due diligence defence. It is an ongoing discussion whether cleaning and disinfection activities could/should be used as critical control points (CCPs) in a HACCP system. This is certainly not a new idea and has been proposed for high-care areas (e.g. post-cooking/pasteurisation) where, for example, a dirty process surface (hazard) is a significant food safety risk (likely to be realised) to a ready-to-eat product processed on it (Harrigan and Park, 1991, pp. 156–158).

The new ISO food safety standard allows hygiene procedures to be designated operational pre-requisite programmes (OPRPs) when they are critical to food safety. These activities are treated like CCPs, and though they must not have critical limits assigned to them, they must be monitored (BS EN ISO 22000, 2005). Similarly, the recent BRC global standard (British Retail Consortium, 2011) refers to the fact that pre-requisite programmes have needed a much clearer role in HACCP programmes,

and the new BRC standard gives greater prominence to them.

It states that:

> …Where control is achieved through existing prerequisite programmes, this shall be stated and the adequacy of the programme to control the hazard validated … procedures of verification shall be established to confirm that the HACCP plan, including controls managed by prerequisite programmes, are effective…

Clearly, these standards are pushing for the elevation of some aspects of GHP/pre-requisite programmes to a higher level within the food safety management system, and if they are critical to the control of a known food hazard, they should be treated almost like CCPs in the HACCP system. If cleaning and disinfection (both CIP and COP) are to be classed in this way for some areas or types of process, then this means validation, verification and monitoring will be necessary to ensure adequate control is in place.

In order to monitor C&D procedures, a simple logical approach is possible in practice. Critical points in the cleaning and disinfection programme should be identified and monitoring protocols set up. Some of the points will be readily measurable, for example, the solution concentration of a detergent or disinfectant, while others may involve checking the procedure itself, for example, was foam coverage complete and for the required residence time. After each stage in the cleaning procedure, the operator should check for effectiveness and thoroughness. This check should be backed up by the hygiene supervisor, who, if not satisfied, should ask for a repeat of the stage. Quality assurance and/or production personnel should also check the plant regularly, looking in particular for old soil deposits not removed at the last clean, a build-up of fungi and corrosion/scale deposits. The hygiene supervisor and his/her team should also be periodically audited to ensure that the cleaning and disinfection procedures are being followed. If procedures are being followed but routine inspections provide evidence of short- and long-term surface hygiene issues, then cleaning procedures and frequencies must be reviewed and validated again. Chemical solution strengths should be regularly checked by titration, test kit or conductivity metre. This information should be used to validate the dilution method in use (injector, proportional pump, etc.), thus ensuring consistent performance every day. Internal monitoring can be usefully supplemented by audits from external experts, such as hygiene service suppliers, consultants, etc.

There is another way to approach HACCP and the possible requirement to elevate and include pre-requisite programmes that are critical to hazard control. If we consider the whole C&D procedure and its intended effect (a clean surface) as the CCP, then we require an assessment of surface hygiene in real process time in order to keep control of the process and make relevant decisions. The availability of rapid surface hygiene tests has meant that monitoring results are available in real time and an immediate decision can be made to clean again if hygiene procedures have failed. Most rapid systems are used daily to monitor the overall effectiveness of cleaning in critical areas; this permits re-cleaning to occur prior to production (Griffith, 2005; Griffith *et al.*, 1997). Such tests are usually based on the measurement of adenosine triphosphate (ATP), life's energy molecule which functions in many enzyme-catalysed reactions in all animals and plants, acting as a carrier of energy within cells and organisms. Food residues are rich in ATP, and when it is brought into contact with luciferin–luciferase, via swabs and reagents, a reaction takes place, which emits light – a process known as bioluminescence (Griffith, 2005).

Commercially available luminometers measure the intensity of emitted light, which is directly related to the concentration of ATP and thus the level of micro-organisms and food residues on the surface (Fig. 5.12). The fact that ATP test kits do not (unless a special stage is included) differentiate between somatic (meat/food product derived) cells and microbial cells is largely irrelevant, as the result is a measure of overall 'cleanliness' and either actual or potential microbial contamination. Currently, a human operator does these tests, and therefore, the monitoring activity, like the cleaning and disinfection process itself, is not wholly within the 'running production process' as for traditional CCPs identified within a HACCP system.

Rapid hygiene tests can also be used in tandem with microbiological tests during the validation of a cleaning procedure (Dillon and Griffith, 1999, pp. 75–76). The subsequent monitoring programme would then revert mainly to the rapid method only. Techniques such as ATP monitoring can be used to optimise cleaning protocols and evaluate different chemicals, solution concentrations and rinsing water temperatures. Statistical analysis of results over a period can identify trends more meaningfully than simply observing daily variations.

Microbiological assessment of surfaces is necessary to provide data and information about plant microbial populations and their sources and prevalence. This information is important for the control of pathogenic (food poisoning) and spoilage micro-organisms. Sampling should be carried out on representative and random points using skilled personnel (Griffith, 2005). Results

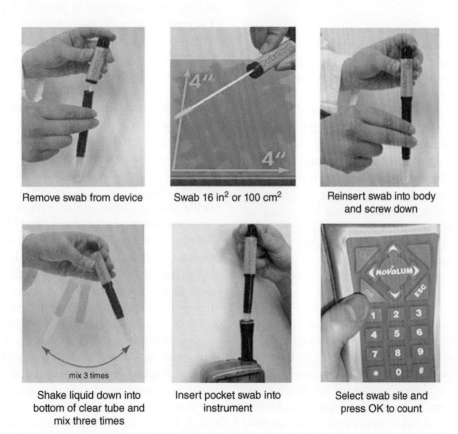

Remove swab from device   Swab 16 in² or 100 cm²   Reinsert swab into body and screw down

Shake liquid down into bottom of clear tube and mix three times   Insert pocket swab into instrument   Select swab site and press OK to count

Figure 5.12 Rapid hygiene monitoring using ATP-based bioluminescence (Reproduced with permission from Ecolab. © Ecolab).

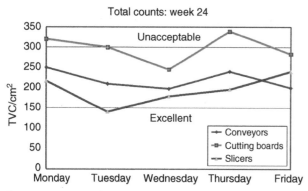

Figure 5.13 Example graph showing trend analysis of total counts over time for sample points on different surfaces (Reproduced with permission from Ecolab. © Ecolab).

should be reported regularly to management and fed back to the cleaning team for remedial action. In relation to surface hygiene, microbiological methods are useful for validating cleaning and disinfection procedures, but they do not provide useful data for daily real-time monitoring; however, they are used for long-term monitoring of surface population trends. Figure 5.13 shows the information that may be gained from monitoring over time; the limits in the graph are not meant to be representative of any particular process type.

Training

Training of all operatives and managers involved in plant cleaning is *critically important*. It helps develop and maintain a high self-esteem and status in the cleaning team (too often seen, wrongly, as less skilled than production workers) and a problem-solving, self-assessing quality attitude to the job. Training should cover the theoretical background in sufficient depth, particularly the microscopic 'enemy', the risks of re-contamination, the importance of procedures and the safe use of chemicals and equipment. Practical, on-the-job training should be continuous, especially when new plant or equipment is introduced or procedures are changed. For protection of due diligence, training should be recorded on the personnel records of those trained.

Safety

Industrial detergents and disinfectants are generally, because of the nature of the job they are designed to do, more concentrated and extreme in pH than domestic products. They should always be applied using the correct protective wear: gloves, goggles (or full-face protector), apron, boots, etc. In areas where high aerosol levels may be created, with a risk of heavy microbial contamination, a suitable facemask should be worn. Different

chemicals must not be mixed with each other unless under the express instructions of a competent person. All chemical containers must be clearly labelled with product-specific identification and safety information as per EU standards. Hygiene chemicals should be stored safely and systematically; dilution and dosing should where possible be automated. Automation has the dual advantage of reducing risk and contributing to validation and consistency. Safety data sheets on all chemicals must be available which conform to EU legislation. All equipment must be properly maintained.

Effluent and external odour control

It is beyond the scope of this discussion to deal in depth with these two complex hygiene-related issues. A number of general points, however, may be usefully made.

Effluent systems in meat plants may be affected by the misuse of some detergents and disinfectants. If 'high-volume slugs' of concentrate chemicals are left to drain that have very high or low pH, they may (if not neutralised in the balance tank) upset the balance within the microbiological population in biological treatment plants. The same is true for chlorine, quats and some other disinfectants. If a treatment plant is undersized for the effluent it receives at peak periods, especially the balance tank section, it is possible for 'breakthrough' of organics and surfactants to occur. This means that instead of being fully biodegraded in the plant, molecules survive to give possible foaming problems (especially where aeration occurs), high COD/BOD and increased suspended and dissolved solids. This may result in higher charges from the water authorities or possible penalties.

It is important in the factory pre-clean to remove as much organic matter as possible, for example, food residues, from production areas before detergents are applied. These larger pieces of organic material are not readily biodegradable and may block or blind the biological treatment plant. No bio-plant likes varying BOD loadings. Steady conditions are preferred if 'shedding' of filamentous growth is to be avoided. In activated sludge plants, the sudden ingress of high-COD material will result in low dissolved oxygen levels, thus potentially turning the plant anaerobic (with resulting malodours) or, by increasing the potential for filamentous growth, causing settlement problems in the final clarifier.

By definition, cleaning chemicals will dissolve, emulsify and disperse organic materials and carry perhaps excessive amounts to the effluent plant. It is also important not to discharge sudden, very large quantities of heavily loaded water, such as from scald tanks or cooking kettles. The risk is even higher if the water is hot, as fats and oils may be temporarily emulsified by the heat and may pass unhindered through the grease trap prior to the effluent system.

The biodegradability of the detergents and disinfectants themselves is also important, but not because they themselves contribute greatly to the total COD/BOD of the plant effluent. Their contribution, in comparison to that of the food process effluent and residual soil carried away by cleaning, is minor. There are some surfactants, previously common in many detergents and disinfectants, which are now known to partly biodegrade to slightly simpler, but more environmentally damaging, molecules. One group in particular, the alkylphenol ethoxylates (APEOs), is believed to have oestrogenic effects in river waters, possibly affecting the reproduction of aquatic organisms. They are banned in detergent and disinfectant formulations, as are other non-biodegradable surfactants (Council Regulation (EC) No 658/2004). The chemical supplier should be asked to supply chemicals, backed up by specific product data, which conform to the latest EU environmental regulations.

Odour control may be particularly important if the factory is situated close to residential areas. Odour may arise from the effluent plant itself, if aeration is inadequate, loading is excessive (see earlier) and anaerobic bacteria are flourishing. Such problems may be helped by improving aeration and reducing the COD/BOD loading to the plant. Other methods to assist the breakdown of proteins and other organics include the addition of *enzyme* preparations in the effluent stream as it leaves the plant or even in the factory drain system. The enzymes begin the biodegradation process early and assist the main treatment plant in handling its burden. Other odours may arise from exhausts from rendering plants and from waste skips. The most common chemical treatments used here involve 'scrubbing' the exhaust gases with fine showers containing oxidising disinfectants such as chlorine dioxide or peracetic acid or spraying the disinfectant into the skips themselves. These chemicals act to oxidise and break down the malodorous molecules (which are usually relatively small volatile molecules containing sulphur). An alternative approach is to use essential-oil-based sprays to destroy the molecules. Attempting to mask the malodour with a perfumed agent is usually not successful.

Conclusion

Plant cleaning and disinfection have deservedly earned a much higher profile than they had previously attained. While legislation has provided some of the impetus, the real driver for any food processing operation wishing to prosper is the need to keep its reputation intact, major retail customers happy and consumers confident in the brand and quality of its products. Particularly when food safety issues come to light and are taken up by the media, the damage can be to individual businesses or a whole food industry sector; it is vital for companies to maintain explicitly the highest hygiene standards. Profit margins are often very tight and cost pressures on one side, versus legislative and quality pressures on the other, contrive to make the meat plant hygienist's job more demanding and the cost of failure higher. It cannot be that we drive for a good and consistent hygiene performance at any cost; to be clear, that cost is in essence financial, but it breaks down to resources such as people, plant downtime, water and energy. That would not be prudent business practice, but importantly, it is also not a sustainable approach considering the present and future availability and increasing cost of water and energy. The achievement of a consistently good hygiene performance at a sustainable cost, in the broadest terms, that will always come from a professionally managed and well-controlled operation.

All persons involved in plant hygiene, from top management down, must appreciate that plant sanitation is a vital, skilled and multidiscipline task. It requires consistently effective management to ensure that the general methods and the fine details are kept under constant attention and that potential problems are highlighted and dealt with early enough to avoid them becoming real and damaging. Some companies choose to outsource their plant sanitation to specialist contract cleaners. If professionally resourced, trained and managed, contract cleaners are an effective solution.

However, some food companies prefer to keep this pre-requisite programme within the remit of their factory management to ensure more direct control, accountability and timely corrective action. Whatever choice is made, the fact remains that the food plant management must maintain a close interest in and understanding of plant hygiene and sanitation. Suppliers of hygiene equipment and materials, if selected for their quality and professionalism, can also be a major asset to the food plant hygiene manager, but the most important support that he or she can have is that of the senior management team in giving hygiene a status equal to that of production.

Note

1 COP is used throughout this text to mean Cleaning Open Plant. It is not a globally standardised abbreviation. It is used in the United States for Cleaning Out of Place where equipment is dismantled and moved to a cleaning room, and also Open Plant Cleaning (OPC) is in use in Europe.

References

Board, R.G. (1983) *A Modern Introduction to Food Microbiology*, Blackwell Scientific Publications, Oxford.

British Retail Consortium (2011) *Global Standard for Food Safety* (Issue 6), The Stationery Office, London.

BS EN 1276 (2009) Chemical Disinfectants and Antiseptics – Quantitative Suspension Test for the Evaluation of Bactericidal Activity of Chemical Disinfectants and Antiseptics Used in Food, Industrial, Domestic and Institutional Areas (Phase 2, Step 1), British Standards Institute, London.

BS EN ISO 22000 (2005) *Food Safety Management Systems: Requirements for Any Organisation in the Food Chain*, British Standards Institute, London.

Burfoot, D. (2005) *Handbook of Hygiene Control in the Food Industry* (eds H.L.M. Lelieveld, M.A. Mostert and J. Holah), Woodhead Publishing Limited, Cambridge/London, pp. 93–101.

Council Directive 64/433/EEC of 26 June 1964 on health problems affecting intra community trade in fresh meat. *Official Journal*, 121, 2012–2032.

Council Directive 92/116/EEC of 17 December 1992 amending and updating Directive 71/118/EEC on health problems affecting trade in fresh poultry meat. *Official Journal*, L062, 0001–0037.

Council Directive 95/68/EEC of 22 December 1995 amending Directive 77/99/EEC on health problems affecting the production and marketing of meat products and certain other products of animal origin. *Official Journal*, L332, 0010–0014.

Council Regulation (EC) No 658/2004 of 31 March 2004 on detergents. *Official Journal*, L104, 1–35.

Council Regulation (EC) No 852/2004 of 29 April 2004 on the hygiene of foodstuffs. *Official Journal*, L226, 3–21.

Council Regulation (EC) No 853/2004 of 29 April 2004 laying down specific hygiene rules for food of animal origin. *Official Journal*, L226, 22–82.

Dillon, M. and Griffith, C.J. (1999) *How to Clean*, MD Associates, Grimsby.

Directive (EC) No 98/8 of 16 February 1998 of the European parliament and of the council concerning the placing of biocidal products on the market. *Official Journal*, L123, 1.

Doyle, P.M., Busta, F., Cords, B.R. *et al* (2006) *Comprehensive Reviews in Food Science and Food Safety*, 5, 71–137.

EHEDG Document No. 8 (2004) *Hygienic Equipment Design Criteria*, 2nd edn, CCFRA Technology Ltd., Chipping Campden.

Gibson, H., Taylor, J.H., Hall, K.E. and Holah, J.T. (1999) *Journal of Applied Microbiology*, 87, 41–48.

Griffith, C.J., Davidson, C.A., Peters, A.C. and Fielding, L.M. (1997) *Food Science and Technology Today*, 11 (1), 15–24.

Griffith, C. (2005) *Handbook of Hygiene Control in the Food Industry* (eds H.L.M. Lelieveld, M.A. Mostert and J. Holah), Woodhead Publishing, Cambridge/London, pp. 588–616.

Harrigan, W.F. and Park, R.W.A. (1991) *Making Safe Food: A Management Guide to Microbiological Quality*, Academic Press, London.

International Food Standard (2007) *Standard for Auditing Retailer and Wholesaler Branded Food Products* (version 5), HDE Trade Services GmbH, Berlin.

Lorenzen, K. (2005) *Handbook of Hygiene Control in the Food Industry* (eds H.L.M. Lelieveld, M.A. Mostert and J. Holah), Woodhead Publishing, Cambridge/London, pp. 425–444.

Maillard, J.-Y. (2002) *Journal of Applied Microbiology Symposium Supplement*, 92, 16S–27S.

Maillard, J.-Y. (2005) *Handbook of Hygiene Control in the Food Industry* (eds H.L.M. Lelieveld, M.A. Mostert and J. Holah), Woodhead Publishing, Cambridge/London, pp. 641–665.

McDonnell, G. and Russell, A.D. (1999) *Clinical Microbiology Reviews*, 12, 147–179.

Rowe, M.T., Dunstall, G., Kirk, R. *et al* (1998) *Food Microbiology*, 15, 491–498.

Russell, A.D. (2002) *Journal of Applied Microbiology Symposium Supplement*, 92, 121S–135S.

SCVPH (2001) Opinion of the scientific committee on veterinary measures relating to public health: the Cleaning and Disinfection of Knives in the Meat and Poultry Industry, http://ec.europa.eu/food/fs/sc/scv/out43_en.pdf (accessed 10 April 2014).

Soonthornchaikul, N., Garelick, H., Jones, H., *et al.* (2005) *International Journal of Antimicrobial Agents*, 27, 125–130.

6

From farm to slaughter

Meat hygiene safety management systems should endeavour to take into consideration the entire process of production and processing involved in producing meat or meat products as food from farm animals. Only by ensuring the animals on the farm are managed in a responsible manner with respect to quality and integrity of feed provided, animal remedy use, husbandry and welfare can the high standards demanded by the consumer be assured. These demands have changed over recent decades in the Western developed countries from the immediate post-war call for cheap meat to the present requirement for a traceable, guaranteed safe and wholesome, environmental and animal welfare-friendly product.

Production of clean, healthy livestock (see Fig. 6.1 and Fig. 6.2)

The monitoring of all aspects of husbandry practices on the farm should be the first step in a longitudinally integrated meat hygiene management system. As long ago as 1990, the Richmond Committee on the Microbiological Safety of Food (Part II) concluded that 'farmers can contribute to food safety by producing healthy, clean and unstressed animals for slaughter, and we believe that this simple truth should be borne in mind by livestock producers and stressed by all who provide them with advice'.

EU Council Regulation 853/2004 emphasised the importance the primary producer has to play in ensuring the safety of their produce by introducing a requirement for appropriate hygienic controls on farm and making the producer of a food legislatively responsible for its safety.

The definition of food in EU Regulation 178/2004, Article 2 is 'any substance or product, whether processed or unprocessed, intended to be, or reasonably expected to be ingested by humans. Food shall not include (i) feed; (ii) live animals unless they are prepared for placing on the market for human consumption (iii) residues or contaminants'. The live domestic farm animal, being prepared for human consumption, is therefore food.

In addition, within the EU, the reform of the Common Agricultural Policy (CAP) in 2003 broke the link between financial support payments to farmers and the volume of production and introduced instead requirements for environmental protection and high standards in animal health and animal welfare. These requirements vary in detail in different member states and are usually described in national guides or codes of practice for good farming practice.

Regulation (EC) 852/2004 also encourages member states to develop national guides on good hygiene practice for control of hazards in primary production and associated operations (Part B, Annex I). Examples given of such hazards and measures may include:

1. The control of contamination such as mycotoxins, heavy metals and radioactive material
2. The use of water, organic waste and fertilisers
3. The correct and appropriate use of plant protection products and biocides and their traceability
4. The correct and appropriate use of veterinary medicinal products and feed additives and their traceability
5. The preparation, storage use and traceability of feed
6. The proper disposal of dead animals, waste and litter

Gracey's Meat Hygiene, Eleventh Edition. Edited by David S. Collins and Robert J. Huey.
© 2015 John Wiley & Sons, Ltd. Published 2015 by John Wiley & Sons, Ltd.

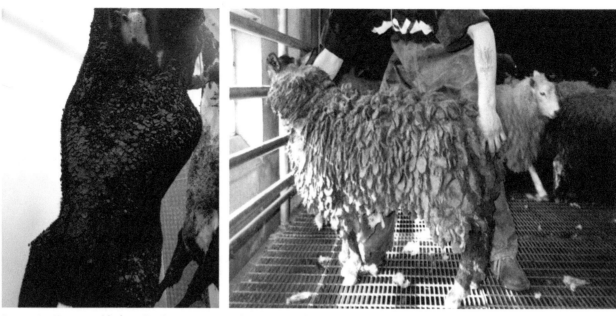

Figure 6.1 Unacceptable faecal/soil contamination (by courtesy of J.A. Ross MRCVS).

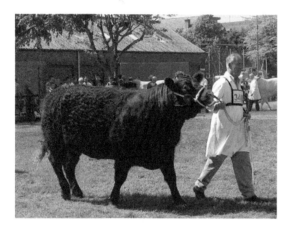
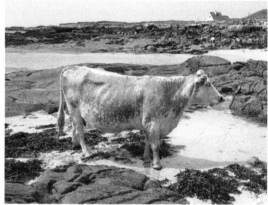
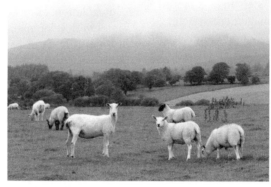

Figure 6.2 Excellent standards of animal cleanliness.

7 Protective measures to prevent the introduction of contagious diseases transmissible to humans through food and any obligations to notify the competent authority

8 Procedures, practices and methods to ensure that food is produced, handled, packed, stored and transported under appropriate hygienic conditions, including effective cleaning and pest control

9 Measures relating to the cleanliness of slaughter and production animals

10 Measures relating to record keeping

The starting point for the production of a national guide should consider the hazards described within the OIE guide to good farming practices for animal production food safety: www.oie.int/eng/publicat/rt/2502/review25-2BR/25-berlingueri823-836.pdf.

Clean livestock (see Chapter 8)

Some idea of the level of contamination of cattle hides with manure can be gained from the excellent surveys carried out by the British Leather Centre in their Hide Improvement Project. Their 1996 survey (Stosic, 1996), which covered the whole of the British Isles, showed the following main findings – Table 6.1 and Table 6.2.

There were significant variations between the different regions of the British Isles due, at least in part, to weather and husbandry systems. The worst month for the Irish and Scottish hides was February, while the peak for England and Wales was in April. It is significant that a wet climate, grass-based diet and slatted floor housing of finishing cattle are common features of livestock production systems in the two regions with the most hide contamination.

The average weight (3.7 kg) of cattle hide faecal contamination may be compared with that recorded by the former author (JFG) in February 1965 of 4 kg, an indication that there had not been much improvement over a period of over 30 years.

In addition to conveying the various food-poisoning pathogens (*E. coli* O157:H7, *Salmonella*, *Campylobacter*, *Yersinia*, *Giardia*, *Listeria*, etc.), faecal contamination of hides and fleeces is responsible for damage to hides and eventually leather ('coarsened grain') by excoriating the surface layers of the skin and exposing sensory nerve endings, causing pain, thereby making this a serious *welfare* problem. *Hazards* are also created for operatives engaged in carcase dressing through knife slips. The entire problem is costing the meat industry many millions of pounds annually and deserves immediate attention at farm (mainly), transport and meat plant levels.

Causes of dirty livestock

Under typical weather conditions in the British Isles, the production of clean cattle and sheep for slaughter is relatively easy where animals are at grass during the warm summer months. However, in wet winter weather, cattle and sheep all too frequently arrive at the meat plant in a very dirty condition. This is especially the case in those countries in the more northerly latitudes where livestock are housed during the winter months.

A survey carried out in Northern Ireland (Ingram, 1972) showed that the problem of dirty cattle was mainly related to bedded houses with or without open yards. The principal cause was found to be lack of bedding, aggravated by high stocking densities, poor ventilation causing condensation, poor drainage, inadequate floor gradients and infrequent removal of slurry. In some instances, deficiencies included incorrect cubicle size, improperly positioned or overflowing water bowls or troughs, blocked slats due to non-removal of slurry and cattle lying outside the cubicle or bedded area. The problem appeared to be worse on farms where heavier cattle were housed and fed silage. The growth of long hair during the winter months contributed greatly to the accumulation of muck on the cattle.

The following points should be given due attention by farmers producing stock for slaughter:

1 *Housing structure and layout*. Defects in design, layout, cubicle size and design, drainage, water bowls, slats, ventilation, etc. should be corrected. Regular maintenance is essential.
2 *Bedding*. Adequate bedding is essential. It is best to commence with a deep layer and subsequently to bed with larger amounts at regular intervals. A concrete area that is frequently scraped will serve to reduce bedding requirements. Regular and frequent removal of slurry is essential.
3 *Housing density*. Either over-crowding or understocking of pens can lead to cattle becoming dirty. If there are insufficient cattle in a slatted pen, the manure will not get tramped through and will accumulate.
4 *Clipping*. It is good practice to clip the bellies, briskets and flanks of cattle before housing to prevent the accumulation of matted muck on the hair. The practice of clipping the backs of cattle cosmetically for sale purposes is a waste of time and should be replaced by *brisket, belly and hip clipping for slaughter stock*.
5 *Management*. A high level of stockmanship, especially when animals are first housed, is essential. Individual animals that do not settle in a particular system should

Table 6.1 Summary of main findings of Hide Improvement Project

Total number of hides inspected	15 268
Average amount of dung per hide	3.7 kg
Percentage of hides affected	73%
Percentage of hides with over 4.5 kg dung	36%
Largest amount of dung/hide recorded	16 kg

Table 6.2 Hide contamination in different regions of Britain and Ireland

Scotland	1.85 kg
England and Wales	2.42 kg
Northern Ireland	4.32 kg
Republic of Ireland	5.57 kg

be removed if possible. It is often necessary to encourage or train cattle to lie in cubicles.

6 *Internal parasitism.* A veterinary-audited anthelmintic programme should be followed to prevent outbreaks of parasitic gastroenteritis in housed cattle. Attention should be paid especially to the risk of type II ostertagiasis in cattle.

7 *Transport and abattoir lairages.* Animals should leave the farm in a clean condition and be transported under conditions which allow them to arrive at the abattoir clean. In New Zealand, the use of trucks with expanded-metal floors with a 5 cm clearance over solid bases for all of the decks means that the lambs are standing clean and dry during transit.

Internal parasitism can also cause severe problems in *sheep*, with staining and clumping of the wool in the perineal region. Sheep folded on root crops, especially during inclement weather, can become heavily contaminated with soil, making hygienic dressing of the carcase difficult. *Sheep for slaughter should be given a ventral clip at least 16 cm wide from the neck to the anus.* Those folded on root crops should be put on clean grass for at least 1 week before dispatch for slaughter. Sheep suffering from scour, from whatever cause, should not be sent for slaughter until cured. There can also be a potentially serious problem where sheep arrive dirty but dry, from clouds of dust which are produced during the removal of the fleece. To counteract this, it is normal practice in New Zealand to pass sheep through a plunge dip as they enter the lairage. It has been demonstrated, however, that although this practice results in carcases with less visible contamination, there is in fact an increase in the total aerobic bacterial and *E. coli* count (Biss and Hathaway, 1996).

In Finland, the problem of excessively dirty cattle being presented for slaughter was greatly reduced by the application of a series of rules agreed by meat inspection veterinarians, farmers, the meat industry, the leather industry and the state veterinary department. Under this agreement, excessively dirty animals are detained to be slaughtered separately after the clean animals. The scheme has resulted in a decrease in the numbers of excessively dirty cattle by 85% (Ridell and Korkeala, 1993).

The text of the Finnish Agreement (which is combined with detailed advice given to all parties through education, instruction and the press) is as follows:

1 All the parties aim at a situation where animals offered for transport to slaughterhouses are as clean as possible.

2 If, however, excessively dirty animals are offered for transportation, the owner of the animals is requested to clean them. Animals are transported after cleaning when the next opportunity arises.

3 However, if excessively dirty animals must be received for transportation to a slaughterhouse, the procedure is as follows:

  a If dung can be removed through cleaning, animals will be cleaned before slaughter.

  b If dung cannot be removed through cleaning (solid dung layer), the animals must be slaughtered in the sanitary slaughter department. If this is not possible, the animals may be slaughtered in the common slaughterhall after clean animals have been slaughtered. All the slaughter facilities and equipment must be cleaned thoroughly afterwards according to the instructions of the inspection veterinarian.

  c The extra reasonable costs caused by the treatment and slaughtering of the excessively dirty animals are billed to the vendor/producer of the animals.

4 The inspection veterinarian on duty at the slaughterhouse decides which animals have to be slaughtered in the sanitary slaughter department or in the common slaughter room after the slaughter of the clean animals.

5 The slaughterhouse takes care that the animals do not get unreasonably dirty during transportation or in the lairage of the slaughterhouse.

In the United Kingdom and Ireland, the Clean Livestock Policy was introduced during 1996. This initiative was reinforced by the Pennington Report (1998) into the potential causes of the fatal *E. coli* O157:H7 outbreak in Scotland, which highlighted the need to tackle the problem of filthy hides or fleeces before they reached the slaughterhouse. Cattle and sheep considered by the official veterinarian to be dirty are rejected for slaughter during ante-mortem inspection. Guidelines were drawn up and agreed as to what would be considered too dirty – see UK Food Standards Agency and the Food Safety Authority of Ireland web sites at http://www.food.gov.uk/foodindustry/farmingfood/cleancattleandmeatsafety/ and http://www.fsai.ie/publications/index.asp#farm.

Throughout the EU, current food safety legislation emphasises the importance of hygiene on farm, the clean livestock for slaughter and the responsibility of the farmer. The EU guidance on Regulation 852/2004, Annex I, Part A, Point II. 4(c) states that 'farmers must take adequate measures to ensure the cleanliness of the animals going for slaughter'. In addition, 'slaughterhouse operators must ensure that animals are clean (annex III, section I, chapter IV, point 4 of Regulation (EC) No 853/2004)' and 'the official veterinarian is to verify compliance with the requirement to ensure that animals that have such hide, skin or fleece conditions that there is an unacceptable risk of contamination of the meat during slaughter are not slaughtered unless they are cleaned beforehand (annex I, section II, chapter III, point 3 of Regulation (EC) No 854/2004)'.

The effect of this legislation is that within the EU the clean livestock policies introduced by competent authorities are largely redundant since it is the slaughter-house operator who decides what is clean enough to be slaughtered within the context of their 'food safety management system'. The official veterinarian's role is to verify that the slaughterhouse operators follow whatever procedures they have decided are appropriate to deal with animals that are not clean.

Healthy livestock

The connection between animal and public health, while known for decades, has become popularised over the last few years since avian and swine influenza have been identified as the cause of deaths in the human population worldwide. This concept of 'one health' extends to food where the transmission of bovine spongiform encephalopathy, *E. coli* O157:H7, *Salmonella* and *Campylobacter* through meat to humans emphasises the link between animal production and public health. A number of incidents across Europe where animal feed contamination with dioxins has led to widespread product withdrawal and consumer concern only emphasise the links. An *ethos of good husbandry and stockmanship* on the farm is therefore essential if healthy animals are to be produced consistently for slaughter. This is particularly so where animals are cared for under intensive systems of agriculture, where attention to nutritional balance and preventive medicine programmes entailing the use of vaccines, anthelmintics and feed additives are of particular importance.

The use by farmers of veterinary herd health programmes to establish potential animal and public health hazards on farm and control them is essential under these circumstances but useful in all. While veterinary led, these schemes should involve a multidisciplinary team in their development, require the farmer to be actively engaged and should be regularly reviewed and updated.

Safe use of animal medicines

Careless and unhygienic use of the *hypodermic syringe* is responsible for much unnecessary pain in animals and for considerable damage to carcases and consequent partial condemnation due to the production of *abscesses*, and in some cases *necrosis*, at the site of injection. If animals are injected outdoors, a dry day should be selected and the injections should be made on clean animals. It is imperative that needles are changed frequently, for example, every 6 cattle or 25 sheep, and when there is a break in the work. A survey in the United States (Dexter *et al.*, 1994) recorded the incidence of injection-site blemishes in top sirloin butts to be 10.87 and 2.99%. The average weight per blemish was 123.39 and 5.48 g.

The *site* of the injection has to be selected carefully and must not be an area which is associated with the more expensive cuts. It is imperative, for example, that piglets are not injected with iron into the ham and that the hindleg is avoided when injecting lambs with antibiotics. Subcutaneous and intramuscular injections should be given either high up on the neck or on the lower rib cage. In sheep, the fold of wool-less skin behind the foreleg is a useful site. Sharp needles, with a metal rather than a plastic mount, are less likely to break during the injecting process. A 16 gauge needle is recommended for use in adult cattle and sheep.

Some anthelmintics which are injected subcutaneously in cattle and sheep can cause a very severe reaction and staining at the site of injection. This makes it imperative not only that sterile technique is observed but that the very long withdrawal period, of 60 days in some cases, is adhered to.

With the usual multidose injectors, it is impossible for the needle to be disinfected between each injection. However, a sleeve attachment is available which can sanitise the needle, by passing it through a polypropylene cap containing a biocide-impregnated foam, each time the needle is pushed through the animal's skin and withdrawn. The system works well for pigs where injections are made with the syringe at right angles to the surface of the skin, but less well in cattle and sheep where subcutaneous injections require the needle to pass through the skin at an acute angle.

The use of anthelmintics and feed additives requires the producer to be vigilant with regard to *withdrawal periods*. The keeping of good drugs records is both a practical necessity and a legal requirement. The improper use of *drenching guns* may lead to damage to the oral cavity and subsequent abscess formation in the mouth and throat.

Safe disposal of animal waste

An aspect of good management which is worthy of discussion on its own merit is the correct and safe disposal of animal waste. Incorrect disposal of farm animal excreta can present a potential hazard to public health, animal health and the environment. In recent years, the quantity of slurry in particular produced by intensive systems of agriculture has become, in some cases, the limiting factor to the further expansion of production. This is particularly so with the pig industry in the Netherlands, where it has been suggested that the country is in danger of disappearing beneath a sea of slurry (Table 6.3).

Slurry may be applied to the pasture or arable ground by tanker spreader, rain gun or injection. The production of aerosols by the first two of these methods has been demonstrated as spreading bacteria in a high concentration for at least 5 miles (Jones, 1980). For this reason, as well as for reasons of odour control and contamination of rivers

Table 6.3 Quantities of excreta, as slurry, produced by livestock

Type of livestock	Output of livestock (faeces and urine)
Dairy cow	41 kg/day
Pigs (fatteners)[a]	4.5 kg/day
Poultry (1000 laying hens)	800 kg/week

[a] Pigs fed dry. Use of swill or whey may increase this to 14–17 kg/day.

by surface run-off, slurry injection must be the method of choice for application.

The survival of potentially pathogenic micro-organisms in farmyard manure or slurry is dependent on several factors including the following:

1 *The micro-organism.* Some strains or serotypes of a micro-organism, for example, salmonellas, survive longer in the environment than others. Some can assume resistant forms which may survive for several years, for example, anthrax.
2 *pH.* The pH of fresh slurry and farmyard manure varies from 6.2 to 8.0 depending upon the species of origin and the constituents. In the case of slurry, the pH drops to below 6.5 within the first 4 weeks of storage and then gradually returns to zero. As a result, the majority of micro-organisms, in the case of *Salmonella* over 90%, are destroyed in the first month of storage. The low pH of peat and acid soils creates unfavourable conditions for the survival of many pathogens. Attempts have been made to sterilise slurry by altering the pH. This has been achieved by the addition of lime, formalin, ammonium persulphate and formic acid, but the expense of the procedure makes these techniques suitable only for situations where there has been an outbreak of a serious disease. Slaked lime is used to reduce the infectivity of slurry following serious *Brucella* outbreaks in Northern Ireland.
3 *Sunlight.* Ultraviolet light can have a bactericidal effect.
4 *Temperature.* The rise in temperature which occurs during composting of farmyard manure is generally sufficient to destroy all bacterial and viral pathogens except for bacterial spores. Shepherd *et al.* (2007) demonstrated that while composting, with periodic heap turning, was a practical approach to inactivating *E. coli* O157:H7 in cattle wastes on farm, the organisms could survive for months at the heap surface if it was not turned. However, since there is no discernible temperature increase within stored slurry, microbiological survival times are generally much longer.

The survival of pathogenic micro-organisms in soil is in addition influenced by the initial number of organisms, the available moisture and the presence of competitive bacteria. On pasture, the length of grass is important, organisms surviving longer at the base of the grass than at the top of the leaf. Although salmonellas, for example, have been reported as surviving for many months in soil, it is unusual for them to survive for more than 14 days on grass (Findlay, 1972). *E. coli* have been shown to survive for more than 11 weeks in slurry but for only 7–8 days on the pasture (Rankin and Taylor, 1969).

Comparison of survival times for different organisms is difficult, however, owing to the number of variables to be considered and differences between experimental design and measurement technique.

Experiments have shown that under normal farming conditions, infection of adult grazing animals from contaminated slurry on pasture is unlikely. However, if pasture which has been spread with fresh slurry is grazed within a few days by young or stressed susceptible animals, infection may occur.

On the basis of current knowledge, the following recommendations can be made:

1 Slurry should be stored for at least 60 days prior to spreading on land.
2 Any disease hazard can be virtually eliminated by spreading slurry or farmyard manure on arable land or grassland used for conservation.
3 Pasture treated with slurry should not be grazed for at least 30 days after spreading.
4 Since young animals are generally more susceptible to disease, they should graze treated pasture only after a prolonged period following application.
5 Utilisation of slurry should be related to the plant nutrient requirements.
6 Slurry, manure and digested sewage sludge should be ploughed in *immediately after application*. Slurry and raw liquid sludge can be injected to a depth of 50–80 mm in grooves 200–300 mm apart.
7 Ground treated with slurry/manure should preferably be ploughed immediately.

Sewage sludge

The solid material from human sewage sedimentation tanks is available for agricultural use in raw and dry digested forms. Raw sludge contains potentially harmful bacteria and, on occasions, the eggs of tapeworms such as *Taenia saginata*. In addition, sludge can contain many undesirable heavy metals such as cadmium.

In Great Britain, the application of wastes from off-farm sources on agricultural land is controlled by the Control of Pollution (Silage, Slurry and Agricultural Fuel Oil) Regulations 1991 and the Collection and Disposal of Waste Regulations 1988, which allow their use, without licensing, provided that they fertilise, or otherwise benefit, the land. The use of sludge is governed by the Sludge

(Use in Agriculture) Regulations 1989, implementing Council Directive 86/287/EEC. The aim of these regulations is to prevent the build-up of potentially toxic substances in the soil, the contamination of watercourses, the spread of disease and the creation of noxious odours.

Despite these regulations and associated codes of practice, pollution of watercourses is a regular occurrence, as is the stocking of land with farm animals, especially cattle and sheep, after organic wastes have been applied.

Animal welfare on the farm

The welfare of an animal is its state as regards its attempt to cope with its environment Broom (1986). Welfare therefore includes the extent of failure to cope, which may lead to disease or injury, but also the ease of coping or difficulty of coping. Hence, the welfare of an animal is related to its health.

Increased concern as to the welfare of animals within Europe, led in 1997 to an amendment to the European treaty, contained within the Treaty of Amsterdam, to define animals as 'sentient' rather than merely as agricultural products.

An animal's welfare, whether on farm, in transit, at market or at a place of slaughter, should be considered in terms of the 'five freedoms'. These freedoms define ideal states rather than standards for acceptable welfare. They form a logical and comprehensive framework for analysis of welfare within any system together with the steps and compromises necessary to safeguard and improve welfare within the proper constraints of an effective livestock industry:

1 Freedom from hunger and thirst
   By ready access to fresh water and a diet to maintain full health and vigour
2 Freedom from discomfort
   By providing an appropriate environment including shelter and a comfortable environment
3 Freedom from pain, injury and disease
   By prevention or rapid diagnosis and treatment
4 Freedom to express normal behaviour
   By providing sufficient space, proper facilities and company of the animal's own kind
5 Freedom from fear and distress
   By ensuring conditions and treatment which avoid mental suffering

Some intensive systems of agriculture make the attainment of these goals impossible in the short term, but national and European regulations on animal welfare are gradually moving to make them a legal requirement. The banning of all dry sow stall and tethering systems, which restrict the 'freedom to display most normal patterns of behaviour' by January 1999 in the United Kingdom and in Europe by 2013, was a move in this direction. However, many pig farmers suggest that keeping sows in groups may, in fact, be more stressful on the animals than a stall system

by introducing the animals to a competitive environment, the possibility of bullying and fighting and an introduction, therefore, of 'fear'. It should be possible, however, to measure up any husbandry system against the principles expressed in the five basic needs. Any animal housing system, for example, should provide the following:

1 Readily accessible fresh water and nutritionally adequate food as required.
2 Adequate ventilation, to control humidity, irritant gas concentrations and dust and a suitable environmental temperature. (In controlled-environment houses, e.g. broiler and intensive pig houses, there must be a warning system for electrical failure and a back-up system.)
3 Sufficient light for inspection purposes. Pigs should not be kept in permanent darkness.
4 A dry lying area.
5 A flooring, whether slats or solid, which neither harms the animal nor causes undue strain, injury or distress.
6 The correct stocking density. Both over-crowding and understocking can cause problems.
7 Internal surfaces and fittings of buildings and pens with no sharp edges or projections.
8 Internal surfaces of housing and pens which can be cleaned and disinfected effectively.

Intensive methods of husbandry, which involve automatic feeding systems, and slatted houses, which require little daily cleaning, greatly reduce contact between people and the animal. This increases the stress on the animal when it has to be handled for marketing, loading and transport. Hauliers report that pigs collected for slaughter from some large birth-to-bacon units are much more difficult to drive and load than those from finisher units where the pigs will have changed premises one or more times. Thought should be given to enriching the pigs' environment by introducing toys, such as rubber balls or chains, or walking through the pens regularly to increase their contact with humans. It has been suggested that leaving a radio on in a pig-finishing house accustoms the animals to human voices and makes them easier to handle.

Good stockmanship is the single most important factor in ensuring the welfare of livestock on farm. A management system may be acceptable in principle, but without competent, diligent stockmanship, the welfare of animals cannot be adequately safeguarded.

Assessment of an animal's welfare

The most obvious indication of poor welfare is behavioural changes which indicate that the individual animal is failing to cope with its environment. Interpretation of behavioural signs is fraught with difficulty as different species, type and individual animals may react differently to a given situation. For example, while pigs may vocalise when injured, sheep will remain dumb. However, Bradshaw, Hall and

The role of advisory bodies and charities

1 European Food Safety Authority

The European Food Safety Authority (EFSA) was set up in January 2002, following a series of food crises in the late 1990s, as an independent source of scientific advice and communication on risks associated with the food chain.

EFSA's remit covers not only food and feed safety but also nutrition, animal health and welfare, plant protection and plant health. In all these fields, EFSA's most critical commitment is to provide objective and independent science-based advice and clear communication grounded in the most up-to-date scientific information and knowledge.

EFSA's independent scientific advice underpins European food safety legislation. In the field of animal welfare, the Animal Health and Welfare Panel have produced comprehensive and detailed opinions summarising current scientific knowledge on welfare at slaughter.

http://www.efsa.eu.int/EFSA/ScientificPanels/efsa_locale-1178620753812_AHAW.htm

2 The World Organisation for Animal Health – (OIE)

Animal welfare was first identified as a priority in the OIE Strategic Plan 2001–2005. OIE Member Countries and Territories mandated the organisation to take the lead internationally on animal welfare and, as the international reference organisation for animal health, to elaborate recommendations and guidelines covering animal welfare practices, reaffirming that animal health is a key component of animal welfare.

The Permanent Animal Welfare Working Group was inaugurated in May 2002 and the first recommendations of the Working Group were adopted 1 year later. The OIE Guiding Principles on animal welfare were included in the OIE *Terrestrial Animal Health Code* (*Terrestrial Code*) in 2004.

The OIE convened a First Global Conference on Animal Welfare in February 2004 with a second during October 2008. As well as the Veterinary Services in OIE Member Countries and Territories, the Conference targeted livestock producers and actors in the meat sector, veterinary practitioners and international non-governmental organisations (NGOs) working in animal welfare. The main objective of the Conference was to raise awareness of, and to explain, the OIE's animal welfare initiative.

OIE have adopted five animal welfare standards to be included in the OIE *Terrestrial Code*. These cover:

a the transport of animals by land
b the transport of animals by sea
c the transport of animal by air
d the slaughter of animals for human consumption
e the killing of animals for disease control purposes.

http://www.oie.int/eng/bien_etre/en_introduction.htm

3 Council of Europe

The Council of Europe was founded in 1949 with the aim of achieving a greater unity amongst its 47 member countries.

The Council of Europe's work on animal protection was started in the 1960s. There are two reasons for this. First of all, respect for animals counts among the ideals and principles which are the common heritage of its member States as one of the obligations upon which human dignity is based. Secondly, in all Member States animal protection has become a topical subject on which governments have agreed to the necessity of concerted action. Five Conventions have been drawn up – on animals during international transport (ETS 65, 1968); animals kept for farming purposes (ETS 87, 1976); animals for slaughter (ETS 102, 1979); vertebrate animals used for experimental and other scientific purposes (ETS 123, 1986); and pet animals (ETS 125, 1987). All of these conventions are based on the principle that 'for his own well-being, man may, and sometimes must, make use of animals, but that he has a moral obligation to ensure, within reasonable limits, that the animal's health and welfare is in each case not unnecessarily put at risk'.

Scientific developments and intensification of practices were sources of important changes in the use of animals, in agriculture and food production, as well as in research and experimentation. The Conventions on the protection of animals elaborated at the Council of Europe were the first international legal instruments laying down ethical principles for the transport, farming and slaughtering of animals as well as for their use for experimental purposes and as pet. They have been used as a basis for and continue to influence all the relevant legislation in Europe.

The European Convention for the protection of animals kept for farming purposes (ETS 87, 1976) is a 'framework convention' which gives principles for the keeping, care and housing of animals, in particular in intensive breeding systems. A Standing Committee (T-AP) composed of Representatives of the Parties to the Convention, is responsible for the elaboration and adoption of more detailed recommendations to the Parties concerning the different species of animals for the implementation of the principles set out in the Convention. Details of the various conventions are to be found at: http://www.coe.int/t/e/legal_affairs/legal_co-operation/biological_safety%2C_use_of_animals/Farming/

4 Eurogroup for Animal Welfare

The Eurogroup for Animal Welfare was formed in 1980 as a confederation of non-governmental organisations with an interest in animal welfare.

Its function is to produce policy papers on animal welfare issues and to lobby the European Institutions. http://www.eurogroupforanimals.org/about/about.htm

5 Federation of Veterinarians of Europe

The Federation of Veterinarians of Europe (FVE) is a federation of veterinary association from 38 European countries representing the views of over 200 000 veterinarians. The welfare of animals is a key concern of the organisation.

Through working groups, the Federation has produced a number of opinions and policy documents which it uses to lobby the European Commission and Parliament.

Documents can be viewed at: www.fve.org

6 Farm Animal Welfare Council – United Kingdom

The Farm Animal Welfare Council (FAWC) is an advisory body established by the UK Government in 1979. Its terms of reference are to keep under review the welfare of farm animals on agricultural land, at market, in transit and at the place of slaughter; and to advise the Government of any legislative or other changes that may be necessary.

The Council can:

a investigate any topic falling within its remit.
b communicate freely with outside bodies, the European Commission and the public.
c publish its advice independently

Its reports on various animal welfare issues can be viewed at http://www.fawc.org.uk/reports.htm

7 Farm Animal Welfare Advisory Council

In Ireland, the Minister for Agriculture and Food appoints 18 members from the government Departments, the farming industry, welfare bodies and from veterinary groups to form the Farm Animal Welfare Advisory Council.

The Council has as its terms of reference:

a To identify ways in which the welfare of farm animals can be further improved and to prioritise areas requiring attention.
b At the request of the Minister/Department, to consider and advise on proposals for EU and national legislation relating to farm animals.
c To consider ways of increasing public awareness and development and dissemination of information relating to welfare of farm animals at home and abroad.
d To provide any other advice relevant to the welfare of farm animals as the Minister may seek from time to time.

Guidelines produced for various sectors of the livestock farming industry and for welfare of animals during transport can be found at: http://www.agriculture.gov.ie/fawac/index.jsp?file=publications.xml

8 Humane Slaughter Association

The Humane Slaughter Association (HSA) is the only registered charity that works, in the UK and internationally, through educational, scientific and technical advances, exclusively towards the highest worldwide standards of welfare for food animals during transport, marketing and slaughter.

The Association produces

a Up-to-date technical information and advice on all aspects of animal handling, transport and slaughter.
b Training in humane methods of handling and slaughter of livestock for farmers, vets, abattoir staff and students.

c Educational and technical videos, CD-ROMs, DVDs, and printed publications.

d Independent advice to governments, other welfare organisations and the food industry, both in the UK and worldwide.

e Regular visits to markets and slaughterhouses recommending and advising on improvements where necessary.

f Funding for essential research projects through grants and awards. Development and application of appropriate scientific advances into the working practices of the meat industry.

g Grants towards the improvement of animal handling facilities in markets and slaughterhouses.

Many of their publications are available on http://www.hsa.org.uk/

8 Compassion in World Farming

Compassion in World Farming is an international animal welfare organisation which was formed in 1967 to campaign against 'factory farming'.

Their publications are a useful resource.

http://www.ciwf.org.uk/resources/publications/default.aspx

Broom (1996) demonstrated that the number of pigs that remain standing during transport is a relevant measure of welfare in relation to the 'roughness' of the journey.

Assessment of welfare using physiological or biochemical measures is also difficult as these may fluctuate normally, for example, cortisone levels in most species tend to be higher during the morning than in the afternoon. However experimentally, measurement of heart rate, respiratory rate and blood hormone level has been shown to be useful.

As described later in this chapter, mortality, injury and carcase damage such as skin damage in pigs or bruising are often the most reliable indicators that an animal's welfare has been compromised.

Transportation of livestock

Having produced healthy livestock in good conditions, and as clean as possible, it is necessary to keep them free from contamination during the subsequent movement to the point of slaughter. It is of equal importance that they be kept free from injury, stress, loss of weight and disease during the journey. For all these reasons, it is essential that *livestock be slaughtered as close as possible to the point of production* in order to avoid long journeys. The humanitarian aspects of the transportation of animals are intimately linked with the economic ones, and these are of particular consequence in the case of young stock, pregnant stock and casualty animals. Work by Warriss and Bevis (1986) and Warriss, Bevis and Young (1990) in the south of England showed that the average lamb, at two meat plants, spent over 4½ hours in transit and travelled a distance of more than 200 km. Within the United Kingdom, Warriss, Bevis and Young (1990) estimated that 94% of slaughtered sheep spend less than 10 hours in transit. A survey conducted in 1985 found that although three-quarters of all pigs were killed within 10 hours of leaving the farm, over 22% were killed after 8 hours and some not for 32 hours.

Loading and unloading

Loading and unloading are often the most stressful parts of the transport process, for both animals and handlers. For sheep and pigs, most authorities consider that with good transport conditions, the stress of loading gradually dissipates over the first few hours of transport as the animals become habituated to the transport.

It is imperative that proper thought and planning be given to the procedure before commencing, to avoid the need to use excessive force. For pigs in particular, a proper loading ramp, especially if a lorry is being used, is essential. However, very steep ramps are undesirable because they distress the pigs, may lead to injuries through falling and by increasing the need for coercion tend to encourage the use of unacceptable force or electric goads.

Work carried out by Warriss *et al.* (1991), on 40–70 kg live weight pigs, indicates that *ramp angles* up to 20° appear to present few problems to pigs whether ascending or descending. Above 20°, there is a progressive increase in the time and thus, by inference, the difficulty with which the ramps are negotiated. Slopes of 30° and above are, from a subjective point of view, obviously difficult for some individuals to ascend and, particularly, to descend. When steep ramps are used, the spacing of the cleats may become critical. If it is too wide, the ability of the pigs to ascend may be particularly impaired. Philips, Thompson and Fraser (1988) suggested that a ramp sloped at 20–24° with cleats of 10–40 mm, spaced at a distance of 50–100 mm, was a feasible design.

Lapworth (1990) describes minimum design standards applicable to cattle loading and unloading facilities in Australia. He recommends that ramp floors should be stepped or cleated. Stepped floors should be of concrete with 100 mm rises and 500 mm treads. Cleats on wooden or concrete floors should be 50 mm wide, 50 mm high and 300 mm apart. A maximum slope of 20° is again recommended.

The journey to slaughter

One of the most important variables affecting the welfare of animals during transport is the behaviour of the people who load and unload the animals or drive the vehicle (Lambooij *et al.* 1999). The technique of the driver is particularly important especially the avoidance of fast cornering, violent acceleration or deceleration. While training is essential, evidence suggests that drivers who receive bonuses based on, for example, the meat quality after transport meets a certain standard, or deductions for failure to meet 'dead on arrival' targets or levels of bruising, can have a dramatic improvement in animal welfare.

In order to meet current legislative requirements for long-distance transport and to reduce some of the stress on pigs in particular, water is provided via a pipeline and spring-loaded bite drinkers at two foot intervals on each deck. The pipelines are rotated manually by a lockable lever at the rear of the vehicle, allowing nipples to be stowed out of harm's way in a vertical position during travel. Some lorries have also been fitted with cooling sprinklers.

EU transport legislation

All those who transport livestock in connection with an *economic* activity must do so in accordance with the requirements of EU Regulation 1/2005. The following general conditions apply to all livestock.

Protection during transport

Anyone engaged in the handling and transport of animals must be trained or competent to do so in a way that does not, or is not likely to, cause unnecessary fear, injury or suffering. All necessary arrangements should be made in advance to minimise the length of the journey and meet the animals' needs during the journey.

Animals must be fit for the intended journey.

Means of transport

The means of transport used must be designed, constructed, maintained and operated so as to avoid injury and suffering and ensure the safety of the animals (Fig. 6.3).

This includes requirements for:

- Cleaning and disinfection
- The provision of anti-slip floors
- Adequate lighting

Space allowances

Sufficient floor space and height must be provided for the animals appropriate to their height and the intended journey. This should be calculated using a formula that considers the animals' size in comparison to their weight. In most cases, internal height of the compartment in the road vehicle is important.

Duties of transporters

The welfare of animals must not be compromised by insufficient co-ordination of the different parts of the journey and weather conditions must be taken into account. For journeys over 65 km, a qualified attendant (i.e. one holding a certificate of competence) must accompany the consignment, except:

- Where the animals are transported in suitable containers with enough food and water (in dispensers which cannot be tipped over), for a journey of twice the anticipated journey time
- Where the driver performs the functions of an attendant (the driver must hold a certificate of competence)

Feed, water and rest periods

Water, feed and rest must be offered to the animals at suitable intervals and must be appropriate in quality

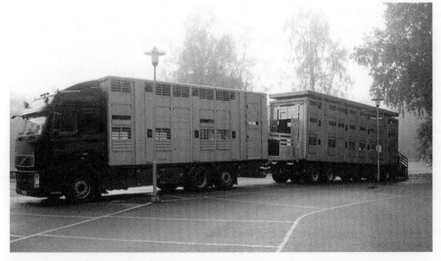
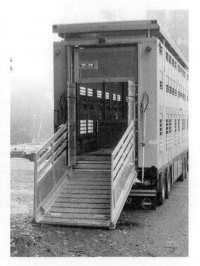

Figure 6.3 Swedish transport lorry.

and quantity with regard to the animals' species, age and size.

Livestock must not be transported for more than 8 hours, unless the additional requirements for vehicles carrying out long journeys have been met.

Pigs may be transported for a maximum period of 24 hours during which they must be offered water at appropriate intervals.

Cattle, sheep and goats may travel for 14 hours before being given a rest period of at least 1 hour during which time they are offered water and if necessary fed. After this rest period, they may be transported for a further 14 hours.

Horses may be transported for a maximum period of 24 hours during which they must be offered water and if necessary fed every 8 hours.

If after these journey times animals have not reached their destination, they must be unloaded, fed and watered and rested for 24 hours at an EU-approved 'control post'. After a 24 hours of rest, they may be transported again for a maximum journey time, after which a 48 hour rest must be taken, and the remainder of the journey treated as a new journey.

For poultry, suitable food and water shall be available in adequate quantities, except in the case of a journey lasting less than 12 hours or 24 hours for chicks provided the journey is completed within 72 hours of hatching.

Treatment of sick animals

When animals fall ill or are injured during transportation, action should be taken to prevent further suffering. They should, where possible, be separated from other animals and be provided with adequate space and bedding to lie down. They should either be given appropriate veterinary treatment as soon as possible or, if treatment is inappropriate, undergo emergency slaughter or killing in a way that does not cause them unnecessary suffering.

Farmers transporting their own livestock in their own vehicles for a distance less than 50 km from their holdings only have to comply with the general conditions, outlined in article 3 of the Regulation.

Travel documentation

On all journeys transporting livestock over 8 hours between EU member states or between EU member states and third countries, a **Journey Log** is required. The log lays out the detailed journey plan, is authorised before travel by the competent authority, completed by the transporter during the journey, signed by the keeper or official veterinarian at the destination and returned to the originating competent authority.

Journey Logs may be used by the competent authority to carry out random or targeted compliance checks.

All journeys not requiring 'Journey Logs' or qualifying for the farmer's exclusion for transporting their own livestock for a distance of less than 50 km from their holdings must have an **Animal Transport Certificate**.

An Animal Transport Certificate must carry the following information:

- Origin and ownership of the animals
- Place of departure and destination
- Date and time of departure
- Expected duration of the journey

In addition to the aforementioned requirements, all animals transported over 65 km and for up to 8 hours require **short journey transporter authorisation**, issued by their competent authority. To obtain authorisation:

- The transporter must be established in that member state.
- The transporter must have appropriate equipment and operational procedures in place.
- All staff must be trained and competent.

Anyone involved in the transport of animals must not have been convicted of a serious animal welfare offence in the 3 years preceding the submission of the application.

Those transporting animals for more than 8 hours require **long journey transporter authorisation** and a **Vehicle Approval Certificate** (not required for poultry). The vehicles must have been inspected and found to comply with the following technical requirements:

- An insulated roof.
- Mechanical ventilation.
- Temperature and data monitoring equipment.
- Satellite navigation.
- Ramps no steeper than 20° for pigs, calves and horses and no steeper than 26° 34 minutes for sheep and cattle.
- Ramps with a slope greater than 10° must have foot battens or other aids to grip and be fitted.
- Safety barriers must be fitted to lorries with more than one floor to prevent animals from falling or escaping during loading or unloading.

Loss of weight during transport

All animals transported to slaughter will suffer some loss of live weight during the journey. This loss is greater than that which would be lost solely by fasting for a similar period and is due mainly to a loss of water by sweating and respiration and waste materials in the urine and faeces. The factors affecting this loss are bodily condition, state of repletion, season and journey time. Pigs will lose 2.2–5.4 kg of their live weight (4–6% of body weight) during 24 hours' transport Lambrooij (2007); sheep lose 0.9–1.8 kg if kept in a lairage for 24 hours and up to 3.6 kg during transport; a calf of 149.6 kg live weight loses 4 kg during its first day of travel and 1.8 kg on the second day; and a bullock weighing 610 kg will lose 30–40 kg during the first day of travel but only 5–6 kg on subsequent days. Studies indicate that it takes 5 days for cattle to recover this loss.

However, it should be pointed out that there is evidence that feeding pigs up to the time of collection leads to higher transport mortality (Warriss 1995) and that pigs as monogastrics can suffer from travel sickness due to vehicle vibration which can be accentuated by poor roads and poor driving.

Studies in New Zealand indicate that in lambs the loss in carcase weight over the first 24 hours in transit is small. However, if the period without food extends beyond 24 hours, the loss of carcase weight becomes significant, amounting to approximately 0.5 kg/animal/day.

With bacon pigs, the loss in actual carcase weight is about 0.9 kg for every day of their journey, and it is probable that both muscular and fatty tissues are affected, with an abnormal loss of water from the muscular tissues. The effect of overexertion, excitement and strange surroundings on pigs during transit may also cause a loss of 6–7% in the weight of the liver.

The amount of weight loss in pigs increases with a rise in temperature and decrease in relative humidity. When Large White pigs were sprayed with fine sprays of cold water in an uncovered lorry which travelled 80 km, the weight loss was reduced by 50%. Pigs also lose weight when transported during very cold weather. Relative humidity and temperature also appear to be involved in the development of dark, firm and dry (DFD) meat in cattle, the incidence of which, at least in Britain, seems to be greatest during cold, muggy days of November.

In the United States, cattle transported by rail are stated to lose 1.48% of carcase weight on journeys of up to 161 km and 2.1% on journeys of 402–482 km. Tissue shrinkage begins during the early part of a journey, continues at a relatively uniform rate for 90 hours and then tends to diminish. Some shrinkage occurs even if animals receive food and water during transport but is less if these are provided during long journeys. In the past, cattle from the northern parts of Australia lost so much weight on their long overland trek to the slaughterhouses that they were placed on pastures for up to a year to regain the weight and quality needed to meet export demands.

From work in Australia, Thompson *et al.* (1987) report that in a 35 kg lamb of fat score 3, the losses of hot carcase weight were in the order of 4 and 6% after 24 and 48 hours' fasting, respectively, compared to mean losses in 27–32 kg lambs of 2 and 4%.

In relation to *weight loss* suffered during transit, it is possible in many cases to restore some, if not all, of this loss with adequate rest. Cattle transported by rail for

136 km in Zimbabwe and sustaining a total live weight loss of 12.88% (1.7% tissue loss) regained much of the tissue loss in 24 hours after resting and drinking water, but not eating. Even after rail transport for 4 days in South Africa during mid-summer, cattle recovered rapidly if rested with food and water. In the same country, the resting of adult Merino sheep for 24 hours with feed and water after rail transport for more than 3 days had a beneficial effect on carcase yield. Much of the weight loss in pigs during transport is believed to be due to loss of water, so it is important for these animals to have access to water before and after transport. However, it has been shown in Poland that resting pigs for 24 hours after transport does not help them to recover unless they are fed, and even feeding restores the condition of the muscles and liver but not the loss of carcase weight.

In the case of *farmed deer*, it was found that after a journey of 160 km lasting 3 hours, a group of 5 hinds lost 1.09% of their pre-transport weight when weighed within 90 minutes of slaughter. Three similar groups held in a lairage with *ad libitum* food and water for 3, 6 and 18 hours lost 1.93, 3.19 and 6.22% of their body weight, respectively. Although live weight loss increased with lairage time, hot carcase weight was unaffected (Grigor *et al.*, 1997).

Transport mortality

Death during transport is a measurement indicating a severe level of distress in transit. A mortality rate above zero must always be considered unacceptable from a welfare perspective. All those involved in the transport of animals must strive to achieve this ideal goal, especially faced with increased consumer awareness of the ethics of food, animal production and transport.

Deaths occur in all classes of livestock during transportation, although in most countries the incidence is less than 0.5%. In a survey of mortality rates in 2.9 million slaughter pigs throughout England, Warriss and Brown (1994) indicated that 0.061% died during transit, while 0.011% died in the lairage. Kephart, Harper and Raines (2010) reported a mortality rate of 0.06% in pigs irrespective of journey length, compared with a study by Abbott *et al.* (1995), who found a death rate during transport of 0.11%. These figures are very similar to those reported in the 1970s by Smith and Allen (1976), suggesting that the position has remained fairly stable over that 40-year period.

Extremes of *temperature*, especially heat, can be responsible for many losses in livestock, particularly pigs. At 32°C, death rates are twice that recorded at 16°C. More animals die when it is hotter, particularly above 16°C (Allen and Smith, 1974), and when animals are left in a stationary vehicle. It has been noted that in summer, pigs transported in the early morning fare better than those transported in the afternoon.

The National Livestock Safety Committee of the US Livestock Conservation Inc. has developed a *livestock weather safety index chart* which, in relation to current temperature and *relative humidity*, indicates in hot weather how safe stock in transit may be. They have also devised for low-temperature conditions a *wind chill chart* giving the relationship between actual temperatures and the wind speed, which is particularly important if animals are not sufficiently protected in moving vehicles.

The *post-mortem findings* in *pigs which have died in transit* are usually those of acute cardiac dilation and acute pulmonary hyperaemia. The left ventricle of the heart is no longer conical but more oval, while the papillary muscles and muscular ridges, normally apparent on the endocardium as prominent projections, are much flattened. Pericardial fluid is increased and there is, in severe cases, a diffuse skeletal muscle degeneration. The lungs are heavy and firmer than normal, finger impressions remain on palpation, and a frothy fluid oozes from the cut surface. Acute passive hyperaemia of the liver and spleen may be observed.

Lairage construction (see also Chapter 3)

During the rest period in lairages, animals must be kept under conditions which prevent any further contamination of feet, hides, fleeces or skins. Most lairages have solid non-slip floors, suitably sloped to adequate drains. Slatted floors have also been considered for cattle, but while contamination is reduced in most cases, there are problems in manure removal and disinfection, for example, after outbreaks of anthrax and salmonellosis, or where tuberculosis or brucellosis reactors are routinely slaughtered.

Movable slats, and especially expanded-metal floors, are particularly useful for sheep, where circulation of air below the floor can be useful for drying wet fleeces. Straw-bedded pens also provide a satisfactory environment for sheep, as long as there is good ventilation and drainage, while solid floors with no bedding, combined with regular hosing and good drainage, provide satisfactory conditions for cattle and pigs. Adequate hose points conveniently placed and providing sufficient volume and pressure of water are absolutely essential. So also are hoses with nozzles giving a fishtail spray which can quickly remove soil. The provision of pens with gates which can be used for closing pens and passageways assists the handling of stock and their transfer from one pen to another, thereby facilitating the cleansing operation.

The detail of design of animal walkways and races is important if animals are to move easily through the lairage. The positioning of a drainage gully in the middle of a walkway frequently causes animals to baulk, as do harsh shadows, puddles of water or shafts of light. It is well established that, owing to their natural curiosity, animals move more readily along curved rather than straight passageways and that sharp corners slow movement considerably. A bend in a raceway of 45° slowed the progress of pigs by about 10%; a bend of 90° or 120° slowed progress by 19%; and a 180° bend slowed their progress by 44% (Warriss *et al.*, 1992a).

Pigs rest more contentedly if they can lie against a solid wall rather than rails, and there is less fighting if they are confined to long narrow pens rather than square ones. Either rails or walls are satisfactory for cattle and sheep. With walls, it is possible to wash out a pen without causing stress, by splash and noise, to animals in neighbouring pens. However, animals are much easier to inspect in railed pens, unless an overhead catwalk is provided. Vertical supports should be cylindrical and tubular to reduce the possibility of injury, and the tops capped to allow effective cleansing and disinfection to be carried out. Horizontal rails should also be cylindrical and tubular, as they are easier to clean effectively with a pressure washer than rails of tubular box cross section.

The introduction of *automatic systems* to move pigs through the lairage in groups in larger slaughter establishments has improved both the welfare of the animals and the efficiency with which the facility operates. The push gates move the pigs in groups of 15 along the passageways at a steady pace from the loading to a holding position. Pigs rest within 20 minutes, contrasted with an hour under normal lairage conditions; and aggression is much reduced.

Facilities should be checked to ensure there are no defects which could cause bruising or even death. Projections and sharp corners are taboo, and if rails are being used for pen partitions, it is essential that there is no possibility of animals getting their heads between rails and being strangled; rail gaps must be of the proper width.

In some countries, cattle are sprayed with jets of water and walked through footbaths before entering the slaughterhouse area. This practice is of benefit in warmer climates where the hair is short and the skin of cattle is fine, but where hair is long in housed stock and there is a build-up of manure and dirt on the hair, spraying would only serve to make matters worse. A light spraying of pigs is widely considered of value in preventing pigs fighting and also reduces the build-up of contamination in the scald tank. However, research work has failed to demonstrate that sprays actually reduce fighting, and it has been suggested the improvement in meat quality in sprayed pigs is due to a cooling effect, rather than a reduction in stress.

Facilities in the lairage which are required for the carrying out of ante-mortem inspection effectively include:

1 A race, with a crush gate for cattle, where the animal can be identified.
2 An adequate number of well-lit pens, with a system for identification or numbering of pens; for inspection purposes, a light intensity of 220 lux is necessary.
3 An isolation pen, with facilities for examination of individual animals.
4 Competent lairage staff to assist with the identification, movement and examination of animals.
5 An office for the use of the veterinarian is useful for the completion of records.

Animal husbandry in the lairage

Moving animals within the lairage

The avoidance of stress in the animal in the period immediately prior to slaughter is important for economic reasons of meat quality as well as for animal welfare reasons. Animals must therefore be handled with consideration at all times with minimal use of force of any type. Electrical goads have been banned by management from many pig lairages as it has been demonstrated they result in an increased heart rate and an increased level of carcase damage (Guise and Penny 1989) and replaced with gentler driving aids such as solid push boards. The use of flags to move bovine animals through the lairage has been shown to be very effective with range or feedlot cattle in Brazil. The flags are typically 50–75 cm² or consist of plastic stips or streamers on the end of poles.

The attitude of lairage attendants can be all-important to the calm and efficient operation of the facility. Persons experienced in animal husbandry know instinctively where to stand when moving stock and can carry out their task using only encouraging noises and the occasional tap or wave of a stick. Inexperienced operatives frequently excite, confuse and antagonise the animals, making handling at best difficult and at worst dangerous and impossible. The good stockman will automatically recognise the individual characteristics of an animal and will adapt his or her technique to get the work completed in the least stressful way for both animal and handler.

Good abattoir management committed to high operating standards is essential if animal welfare in the lairage is to be maintained at an acceptable level.

A useful concept which can assist in training lairage staff is that of 'flight zones'. Each animal can be considered to be surrounded by an imaginary zone or personal space which it will endeavour to maintain. In a semi-wild unhandled animal, such as a range steer, this area will be very large (e.g. >30 m), while in a dairy cow, it will be small. When the handler enters the 'flight zone', the animal will move away to try to re-establish the space between itself and the handler. The direction in which the animal moves depends on where, in relation to the animal, the handler enters the zone; for example, if he enters the zone at a point in front of the animal's shoulder, the animal will move backwards, and if behind the shoulder, it will walk forwards (www.grandin. com//behaviour/principles/flight.zone.html) (Fig. 6.4).

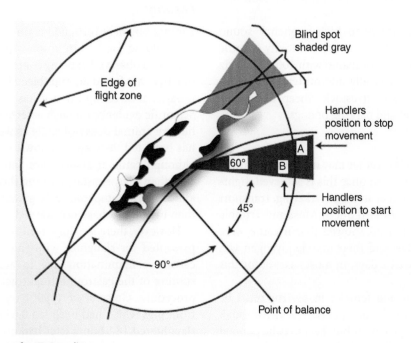

Figure 6.4 Flight zones – after T. Grandin.

The movement of sheep through a lairage may be facilitated by the use of a decoy or 'Judas' sheep. This procedure utilises the innate tendency of sheep to follow one another by 'training' one particular sheep, or allowing it to become accustomed, to pass through the lairage leading the others. Use can be made of a mirror, strategically placed, to assist the movement of sheep out of a pen (Franklin and Hutson, 1982). It is particularly important when driving sheep to exercise patience and give them time to move at their own pace. Attempts to rush will result in those at the rear climbing over or riding on those in front, resulting in bruising.

Pigs can be particularly awkward to drive. They move only as a loose group, optimum group size 5 or 6, preferring to move along beside rather than behind their comrades. The maximum number of pigs which should be moved as a group is 15. This is also considered to be the ideal group size per pen at a stocking density of 0.55–0.67 m²/100 kg. Lewis and McGlone (2007) demonstrated that it took the same time to load 170 pigs in groups of 5 or 6 compared with a group size of 10 but the latter had elevated heart rates.

Excessive or strident *noise* can be very stressful to livestock, especially pigs. Measurements indicate that noise levels average 75 dB in lairage pens, rising to 100 dB in the pre-stunning pen. This may arise from human voices, the use of whips, noisy machinery, barking dogs, compressed-air brakes on vehicles, alarm bells, thunder, etc. The manufacturers of meat plant equipment have a duty to ensure that equipment operates as quietly as possible, especially in the stunning area and its immediate surroundings. The provision of rubber baffles on doors and gates is essential.

Cattle are more sensitive to high-frequency sound than are human beings. The auditory sensitivity of cattle is at its greatest at 8000 Hz compared with 1000–3000 Hz in man. Unusual and especially intermittent sounds are upsetting to all classes of livestock. Sheep are visibly frightened by the sight and barking of dogs.

Social stress

Mixing strange animals together may make them fight to establish a new social order; once this is achieved, fighting ceases. This may occur during marketing, transport or in the lairage. Work carried out by Moss and Trimble (1988) in Northern Ireland showed that if cattle were mixed and were active, and their muscle glycogen was depleted, it took at least 2 days, in most cases 3, for this to be replaced.

Aggressive animals and females in oestrus must be isolated, as must horned from polled stock. Although young bulls reared in groups as bull beef may be penned together, breeding bulls and boars should always be penned separately. Larger animals will usually be aggressive to smaller ones. It is important to recognise, however, that both are stressed. This can be seen especially in young bulls which, if mixed in the lairage, can rapidly become exhausted through constant mounting. Mixing of young bulls is therefore contraindicated, and they should be slaughtered as soon as possible after arrival in the lairage. It has been noted that if these animals remain in the lairage for only 2–3 hours, they may produce dark-cutting meat.

Watering

The drinking water supply to pens should be designed to allow all animals access to clean water at all times. This simple principle can be obstructed if pens are overstocked so making it physically impossible for some animals to access the drinkers. Ample drinking water during their retention in the lairage also serves to lower the bacterial load in the intestine and facilitates removal of the hide or pelt during dressing of the carcass. Stunning of animals by electrical means is rendered more efficacious if they have received unlimited water during their detention prior to slaughter. The positioning and design of water troughs or drinkers is of particular importance in order that faecal contamination of the water is avoided. Self-filling bowls are generally more satisfactory than large concrete troughs for cattle, and drinkers recessed into the walls of the pens are preferred for pigs. Water nipples are not always readily used by pigs, and some protrude from the pen wall at a height which renders them a welfare hazard.

Fasting

Among butchers throughout the world, the practice of withholding food from animals prior to slaughter has long been observed, it being contended in support of this practice that fasted animals bleed better, that the carcase is easier to dress and that it has a brighter appearance. Scientific evidence for such assertions is lacking and the hungry animal does not settle as well as the animal that has been fed. It is also a known physiological fact that although cattle and sheep are better able to withstand cold than pigs, resistance to the shock of a severe fall in atmospheric temperature is greater in the fed animal than in one that has been starved.

However, there is a duty to ensure that animals are not presented for slaughter with full stomachs to prevent carcase contamination due to accidental incision or rupture of the gastrointestinal tract during the dressing procedure. Guise *et al.* (1995) reported that stomachs from pigs which had been fed 0.64 kg of dry matter and slaughtered 18.5 hours later had on average a wet stomach content of 0.87 kg (0.24–1.33). In recognition of these arguments, EU Regulation 1099/2009 requires animals which have not been slaughtered within 12 hours of arrival at the slaughterhouse to be fed and subsequently to be given moderate amounts of food at appropriate intervals.

Resting of animals prior to slaughter

The actual duration of the resting period necessary to ensure normal physiological changes in the muscle after slaughter depends on many factors. These include the species, age, sex, class and condition, time of year, length of journey, method of transportation, etc. Where different species are handled within the one lairage, it is important to ensure that proper arrangements are made for movement forwards for slaughter after an adequate resting period for the particular animals involved. Cows in good condition in temperate countries should not be held for long periods during winter because of the possibility of hypomagnesaemic tetany. Spring lambs require a relatively shorter period of rest than adult sheep and tend to lose weight with prolonged holding.

However, the quality of the rest encountered in the lairage has been brought into question. Cockram (1991) argues persuasively that the novel environment of the lairage, with people moving around, may not provide optimal conditions for cattle to rest, as measured by lying behaviour. Although conditions may improve overnight, with cattle lying down and resting, he suggests that the evidence is unclear as to whether the meat quality from cattle held overnight in the lairage shows a significant improvement.

It has been determined in Australia that the ultimate pH in steer carcases was lower in animals that had been rested and fed for 4 days than in animals rested for only 2 days after a 320 km (200 mile) journey. In the same country, the ultimate pH values in the carcases of rams were higher, and the meat colour was darker in animals rested for 120 hours after a journey by road of 1110 km (690 miles). In Bulgaria, blood and muscle values in calves transported by road for up to 450 km were back to normal in 24 hours.

McNally and Warriss (1996) demonstrated that as the time cattle were held in the lairage increased, the amount of bruising increased significantly.

In New Zealand, Purchas (1992) investigated the effect of decreasing the holding time in the lairage from 28 to 4 hours, after 2 hours' transport. Overall, the dressing-out percentage based on full live weights was significantly lower for the 28 hour group, so that for the mean live weight of 483 kg, the extra 24 hours of holding time led to 4.5 kg less carcase weight, with the rate of loss being slightly greater for the heifers. Perhaps surprisingly, if the lairage is to be considered as a place of rest, the mean ultimate muscle pH was significantly higher for the 28 hour group (0.34 pH units), but this effect was much more apparent for bulls (0.60 pH units) than for steers (0.27 pH units) or heifers (no change), presumably owing to the greater activity that characterises the behaviour of bulls. On the basis of this work, it may be suggested that in order to maximise carcase yield and meat quality, holding of cattle in the lairage should be restricted to 4 hours. The number of variables between lairages, however, means that such a recommendation should be treated with caution.

Warriss et al. (1992b) demonstrated that in pigs, blood cortisol and beta-endorphin levels return to normal values after 2–3 hours in the lairage. These blood constituents measure mainly psychological stress and support the observation that the majority of pigs, whether in single or mixed producer lots, cease to fight after the first hour in the lairage and settle down to rest (Moss, 1977). A period of rest of 2–3 hours for pigs has therefore been recommended. It allows sufficient time to recover from previous stresses without significantly increasing the problems of long food deprivation, muscle glycogen depletion and skin blemish seen after longer periods, particularly after holding overnight.

Excessively long periods of retention only serve to make the task of lairage cleaning – one of the most difficult tasks in the meat plant – even more difficult, as well as increasing the possibility of cross infection. *It has been found, for example, that the longer pigs and calves are held prior to slaughter, the greater is the build-up of infection, particularly of Salmonella organisms, and the greater the risk of cross infection.* In one experiment with calves awaiting slaughter, it was shown that after a few hours' detention, only 0.6% of the animals harboured salmonellae, whereas after 2–5 days, 55.6% had *Salmonella* in their intestine. Other authorities have recorded *Salmonella* in 7% of farm pigs, 25% of pigs in the lairage pen and 50% of pigs at slaughter; 75% of lairage drinking water was also infected. It is recommended, therefore, that young calves be slaughtered as soon as possible after arrival at an abattoir because of the risk of cross-contamination and because it is difficult to induce calves to eat. Small pens with solid bases to the partitions, given regular cleansing and disinfection, will considerably lower the risk of cross infection with *Salmonella* organisms.

Pre-slaughter handling and meat quality

Stress and the animal

During the process of loading at the farm, the journey to the abattoir or market, the holding at the market, the offloading, the detention in the abattoir lairage and the subsequent handling up to the point of slaughter, the animal is subjected to a wide variety of stressors, many of which have an adverse effect with subsequent deleterious changes in the carcase. Even death may occur.

Stressors may include physical trauma and fear and environmental excesses of noise, heat, cold, light, wind chill or humidity. These may make excessive demands on the animal and may result in handling problems which may be reflected in abnormal bodily changes at slaughter.

A husbandry system can be said to be stressful if it makes abnormal demands on the animals. An individual factor may be called a *stressor* if it contributes to the stressful nature of a system of husbandry.

Seyle (1974) defined stress as a *non-specific response* in an animal attempting to resist or adapt to maintain homeostasis, that is, the tendency for the internal environment of the body to be maintained constant and in equilibrium. This suggests that, whatever the trigger for the stress, the physiological response is identical.

There are two main reactions of an animal to stress: the *alarm or emergency reaction* and the *general adaptive syndrome* (together termed the *fight-or-flight syndrome*). The alarm reaction is the result of a sudden adverse stimulus and takes place immediately. It is reflected in an increased activity of the sympathetic nervous system which supplies the involuntary muscles, the secretory glands and the heart. The result is an outpouring into the bloodstream of the catecholamines, noradrenaline and adrenaline by the medulla of the adrenal gland, leading to increased heart rate and force of cardiac contraction, constriction of peripheral blood vessels, elevated blood pressure, dilation of bronchi, cessation of digestion and mobilisation of liver glycogen with increases in blood sugar. Glucagon, a peptide produced by the alpha cells of the islets of Langerhans in the pancreas, is more powerful than adrenaline in the production of blood glucose by the mobilisation of liver glycogen.

While the alarm reaction is immediate, the general adaptive syndrome is the essential stress reaction and is longer lasting. Adrenocorticotrophic hormone (ACTH) is produced by the anterior pituitary gland and brings about the production of corticosteroids such as cortisone and hydrocortisone (cortisol), which regulate the general metabolism of carbohydrates, proteins and fats on a long-term basis. There is a decrease in carbohydrate metabolism, and an increase in protein metabolism, the amino acids being converted to glycogen in the liver. Fat is metabolised from the fat deposits and is metabolised in the liver, producing ketone bodies. *The overall result is an increase in the level of blood glucose and ketones.* Other changes in the general adaptation syndrome include hypertrophy of the adrenal gland with reduction in its ascorbic acid and cholesterol stores, eosinophilia (reduc-

tion in the number of eosinophils), lymphopenia (reduction in the number of lymphocytes), polynucleosis (an increase in polymorpho-nuclear leukocytes) and an increased susceptibility to disease. Sustained adaptation syndrome leads to reduced growth rate in young animals and loss of weight in adult animals.

This non-specific response of the body, irrespective of the origin of the stress, has been questioned and adapted by Moberg (1987) and others. They suggest that corticosteroids may not be produced as a response to all stressful stimuli, that different species may react differently to the same stressor and that in some cases other endocrine pathways may be involved. It may be wrong to assume, therefore, that a lack of adrenal response indicates that there is no stress. There appears to be an important role played by the brain, including the limbic system, the pituitary and the hypothalamus, especially in the mechanism by which animals cope with stress. *When an animal puts substantial effort and resources into coping with a stressful situation, it can be considered to be suffering distress.*

Stress and meat quality

The physiological changes described previously which occur when an animal is stressed can have a very significant effect on the quality of the meat if the stress occurs in the period prior to slaughter. In order to understand these changes, it is necessary to have some knowledge of the biochemical events which occur in muscle in the period immediately after the animal's death.

After slaughter, the supply of oxygen to the muscle ceases with the cessation of blood circulation. Normal aerobic respiration in the muscle therefore stops, to be replaced by anaerobic reactions. Anaerobic glycolysis, the breakdown of hexose sugars, results in the production and accumulation of lactic acid in muscle and a characteristic fall in the pH from 7.0–7.2 to around 5.5. This fall normally takes 4–8 hours in pigs, 12–24 hours in sheep and 24–48 hours in cattle.

Anaerobic glycolysis results in the production of much less energy, stored as adenosine triphosphate (ATP), than its aerobic alternative. After death, the levels of ATP therefore fall. Energy is required to keep muscle in its relaxed state. When the levels of ATP fall to a critically low level after death, the relaxed state can no longer be maintained. The muscle's component molecules, actin and myosin, combine irreversibly to form actomyosin, and the muscle contracts slightly in what is known as *rigor mortis* – the carcase 'setting'.

The rate of onset of rigor is therefore dependent on the supply of ATP in the muscle at death. Any external factor which depletes this supply of ATP will hasten the onset of rigor mortis. This fact is demonstrated in exhausted bulls, the carcases of which set rapidly after slaughter owing to low levels of glycogen, and therefore of ATP, in the muscle at the time of death. These animals will, in addition, have a high muscle pH since little lactic acid will have been produced. It is important to recognise that rigor mortis depends only on the availability of ATP, not on the pH of the meat.

Pre-slaughter stress, therefore, affects both the rate of onset of rigor mortis and the rate and the extent of the fall in muscle pH. Alterations in these parameters affect the appearance and eating quality of the meat, the most common manifestations being pale, soft, exudative (PSE) pork and DFD beef. These economically significant conditions are described in detail in Chapter 2.

Pre-slaughter feeding of sugars

In order to ensure adequate pre-slaughter levels of glycogen in the muscle, which will result in sufficient lactic acid being produced to cause the required fall in pH, it is necessary either to minimise stress, fear, excitement, fatigue or excessive exertion on the animal or to allow for an adequate period of rest prior to slaughter in order for muscle glycogen levels to replenish. Another approach is to feed easily digestible carbohydrates, such as sugar, while the animals are in the lairage. As far back as 1937, experiments in pre-slaughter feeding of molasses to pigs showed a restoration of muscle glycogen and subsequent low tissue pH. Later work emphasised this; the psoas muscle, fillet, had a post-mortem pH of 6.0 when pigs were starved overnight, compared with 5.43 when 1.4 kg sucrose was fed 22 and 6 hours before slaughter. The cuts from carcases of sucrose-fed pigs also gained more weight during curing, the bacon and ham underwent less shrink while maturing, and a further advantage was a significant increase in liver weight. Better keeping qualities of bacon and ham were also reported.

Sugar solutions have been used to overcome some of the storage, handling and feeding problems of solid sugar. A study at the bacon factory of Cavaghan and Gray in Carlisle showed that carcase yields were increased by 2.8% and liver weights by 27%, and muscle pH was reduced by 0.2–0.3 units, when pigs fed a glucose syrup solution and water and held overnight were compared with those receiving water only. When compared with pigs slaughtered on arrival, the differences were 1.3%, 13% and 0.2–0.3 units, respectively.

In cattle detained for 2 days in the lairage, a 25% loss in liver weight may occur. In one plant in Chicago, the effects of stress in cattle are reduced by incorporating molasses in the drinking water. It has also been shown that the feeding of sugar rapidly restores the energy-yielding carbohydrate reserve (glycogen) of the muscles and liver, allowing the development of normal acidity in the former and preventing loss of weight in the latter. The feeding of up to 1.3 kg of sugar for 3 or more days before slaughter of cattle or pigs has increased daily weights. Some workers have found that loss in live weight can be prevented by feeding sugar.

Under present-day abattoir conditions, it is doubtful whether pre-slaughter feeding is always a practical or economic proposition.

Traumatic injury

Bruising is defined as traumatic injury without penetration of the skin where blood vessels are damaged to such an extent that there is extravasation into the surrounding tissues. Several studies of cattle bruising have shown that approximately 31% of bruises occur in the loin and hip area, 36% on the shoulder, 13% on the ribs and 20% on other parts of the body. In sheep, many of the bruises are due to rough handling, resulting either from animals being lifted by the wool or grabbed by the legs during sorting, weighing and loading on the farm, during unloading or while being handled prior to being stunned.

Fasting has been shown to increase bruising and there is some evidence that chronic stress makes animals more susceptible to it.

Time of bruising

Although the presence of bruises at slaughter is apparent to the eye, knowledge of the exact time of infliction is necessary if steps are to be taken to prevent bruising. At slaughter, a bruise may be dated approximately by the physical criteria listed in Table 6.4.

Although its use is largely historic, a more specific method of dating is based on a test which utilises the formation of *bilirubin* from haemoglobin in the area of the bruise. A sample of bruised meat is soaked in Fouchet's reagent (trichloracetic acid and ferric chloride); bruises up to 50 hours old give no reaction; those 60–72 hours old turn the solution light blue; those 4–5 days old give a dark-green reaction. The bilirubin test has been used to show, for example, that 90% of poultry bruises are inflicted 0–13 hours before slaughter.

It has also been suggested that the age of a bruise can also be estimated by measuring the *electrical conductivity*

Table 6.4 Approximate ageing of bruises by physical appearance

0–10 hours old	Red and haemorrhagic
Approximately 24 hours old	Dark coloured
24–38 hours old	Watery consistency
Over 3 days	Rusty orange colour (bilirubin) and soapy to the touch

of the tissue, which increases up to a maximum at 40 hours. *Histological methods* have been developed which claim to be able to differentiate between bruises occurring at various times between 48 hours' pre-slaughter and stunning (McCausland and Dougherty, 1978)

Rough handling

Observations in over 100 packing stations in the United States have shown that rough handling and the abusive use of clubs, whips and electric goads are responsible for the majority of injuries. If animals become stubborn or fractious, and refuse to enter or emerge from a vehicle, they are all too often beaten and shouted at until they fall, or in the case of pigs are dragged by the ears, sustaining injuries, even fractures and bruises. This senseless form of animal handling is not confined to the United States – it occurs the world over. McNally and Warriss (1996), in a survey carried out in the United Kingdom, report that over 35% of cattle bruising was due to stick marks. Giving animals time and space to move is a prerequisite not adopted by all handlers. Some knowledge of animal behaviour, with attention to detail in the design of animal handling/loading/unloading facilities, can remove the stress and danger for both handler and animal.

Three categories of sheep were examined for evidence of bruising: sheep transported direct from farms and those transported from local and distant markets in Scotland (Jarvis, Cockram and McGilp, 1996). In sheep coming directly from farms, 93% had no bruises compared with 86% from local markets and 74% from distant markets.

Blood biochemistry showed significantly higher levels of serum creatine kinase and plasma osmolality in the sheep from distant markets than in the other two groups, suggesting greater muscle damage and dehydration, respectively. However, there were no substantial differences between the three groups in terms of packed cell volume, total plasma protein and beta-hydroxybutyrate.

A survey of 4473 cattle delivered to one slaughter plant from 21 live auction markets in England revealed an overall prevalence of bruising of 8.1% and of stick marking of 2.2%. Differences existed between the prevalences of both bruising in carcase from steers, heifers and bulls. Overall, steers had the greatest amount of carcase damage and young bulls the lowest amount. Variations also occurred in the frequency of bruising (range 2.4–17.9%) and of stick marking (range 0–9.6%) from different markets. There was no evidence that longer journeys (distances ranged from 80 to 464 km) were associated with greater carcase damage. There was a relationship between a high degree of bruising and stick marking at one particular market (McNally and Warriss, 1997).

Presence of horns

An important factor in the frequency of bruising is whether the animal is hornless or horned. The Australian Meat Board has shown that approximately half the bruising in horned cattle is due to the horns and that the incidence of bruising in horned cattle is twice as high as in hornless breeds. The tipping of horns, by the removal of 10–15 cm, has been recommended but was not found to make any significant difference to the incidence of bruising. The only answer is to have all cattle polled, either by dehorning young calves or by breeding naturally polled stock.

Temperament

The temperament of cattle obviously has an effect on the incidence of bruising and, as every cattle farmer knows, temperament varies between breeds and individuals. It is considered that the bruising of cattle in a confined space, for example, a cattle wagon or lairage pen, is due to the natural 'milling about' of a mob of cattle rather than to malicious aggression. Practical farmers, however, are unanimous in the assertion that a bad-tempered animal can create havoc in a mob of cattle, especially under confined conditions, and personnel in every abattoir have noticed how an old cow may persistently harass its fellows. The same occurs with pigs, where one animal in a group can persistently bully its mates.

Over-crowding undoubtedly increases aggressiveness and may be responsible for a high incidence of bruises in animals awaiting slaughter. Among the food animals, fat pigs are the most likely to be affected during transport as their heat-eliminating powers are very limited and they soon succumb to overexertion.

Stunning box design

Bruising can be produced in an animal both before and after stunning, but not once the animal has been bled when the blood pressure drops to zero. The design of the stunning box can, therefore, be of importance in the problem of bruising. In Australia, it has been shown that over 60% of cattle fall from the stunning box so heavily that they are bruised, the extent of the bruise depending on the severity of the fall and the time between stunning and bleeding.

In Australia, bruising in cattle causes an estimated annual loss of up to $26 million (1976), and horn damage plus stunning box bruising accounts for 48% of this loss. The incidence of stunning box bruising can be reduced by a proper design which ensures that the animal slides out of the box. In some abattoirs, the animal is ejected onto a thick rubber mat.

Mixing of animals

Bruising and bite marks on the surface of the skin of pigs cause depreciation in market value. The incidence of this type of damage, severe enough to result in downgrading, has been recorded as 7.3% (MLC, 1985) with a difference between boars and non-boars of 10 and 5.4%, respectively (Warriss, 1984). Most bruises occur during transport, a minor proportion during loading and unloading. Pigs from different farms loaded on the same lorry behave comparatively quietly once the lorry is in motion but start fighting as soon as the lorry stops. Reducing the stopping periods by 50% reduces the incidence of bite marks by 25%. Pre-mixing of socially unfamiliar groups of pigs in a holding pen for a couple of days prior to transport also considerably reduces injuries from fighting. In the lairage, it is important to avoid mixing pigs from different sources, different social groups and different ages if at all possible. Spraying pigs with water on arrival has been used to decrease the incidence of PSE pork by cooling the pigs, but care must be taken in cold weather not to induce hypothermia by leaving the sprays on for extended periods.

Breed

Some breeds of cattle, for example, the Brahman and Afrikaner, are notoriously excitable. Certain breeds of pigs are so susceptible to the effects of stress, for example, the Piétrain and Poland China, that steps are being taken to identify the 'stress gene' and remove it from the population by breeding strategy and genetic engineering.

Incentives and education

An effective tool in the education of animal handlers about the damage careless handling can do to stock is to allow them to see the results on the carcase. Bruises on cattle, stick marks on pigs and wool pulls on sheep all leave their obvious, permanent and costly marks on the dressed meat. When producers are made aware that they are losing money through the loss of carcase weight due to the trimming of these defects, the pressure to improve handling facilities and stockmanship to prevent bruising is increased.

References

Abbott, T.A., Guise, H.J., Hunter, E.J. *et al* (1995) *Animal Welfare*, 4, 29–40.

Allen, W.M. and Smith, L.P. (1974) Proceedings of the 20th European Meeting of Meat Research Workers, Dublin, p. 45.

Biss, M.E. and Hathaway, S.C. (1996) *Veterinary Record*, 138, 82–86.

Bradshaw, R.H., Hall, S.J.G. and Broom, D.M. (1996) *Veterinary Record*, 138, 233–234.

Broom, D.M. (1986) *British Veterinary Journal*, 142, 524–526.

Cockram, M.S. (1991) *British Veterinary Journal*, 147, 109.

Dexter, D.R., Cowman, G.L., Morgan, J.B. *et al* (1994) *Journal of Animal Science*, 4, 824–827.

Findlay, C.R. (1972) *Veterinary Record*, 91, 233–235.

Franklin, J.R. and Hutson, G.D. (1982) *Applied Animal Ethology*, 8, 457–478.

Grigor, P.N., Goddard, P.J., MacDonald, A.J. *et al.* (1997) *Veterinary Record*, 140, 8–12.

Guise, H.J. and Penny, R.H.C. (1989) *Animal Production*, 49, 517–521.

Guise, H.J., Penny, R.H.C., Baynes, P.J. *et al* (1995) *British Veterinary Journal*, 151 (6), 659–670.

Ingram, J.M. (1972) *Agriculture (Northern Ireland)*, 47 (8), 279.

Jarvis, A.M., Cockram, M.S. and McGilp, I.M. (1996) *British Veterinary Journal*, 152, 719.

Jones, P.W. (1980) *Veterinary Record*, 106, 4–7.

Kephart, K.B., Harper, M.T. and Raines, C.R. (2010) *Journal of Animal Science*, 88, 2199–2203.

Knowles, T.G., Warriss, P.D., Brown, S.N. and Kestin, S.C. (1993) *Applied Animal Behaviour Science*, 38, 75–84.

Lambooij, E., Broom, D.M., von Mickwilz, G. and Schutte, A. (1999) in *Vet Aspects of Meat Production, Processing and Inspection* (ed F.J.M. Smulders), ECCAMST, pp. 113–128.

Lambrooij, E. (2007) in *Livestock Handling and Transport* (ed T. Grandin), CABI Publishing, Wallingford, pp. 228–244.

Lapworth, J.W. (1990) *Applied Animal Behaviour Science*, 28, 203–211.

Lewis, C.R.G. and McGlone, J.J. (2007) *Livestock Science*, 107, 86–90.

McCausland, I.P. and Dougherty, R. (1978) *Australian Veterinary Journal*, 54, 525.

McNally, P.W. and Warriss, P. (1996) *Veterinary Record*, 138, 126–128.

McNally, P.W. and Warriss, P.D. (1997) *Veterinary Record*, 147, 231–232.

MLC (1985) Technical Notes, No. 4, 14–16.

Moberg, G.P. (1987) *Journal of Animal Science*, 65, 1228–1235.

Moss, B.W. (1977) *Applied Animal Ethology*, 4, 4323–4339.

Moss, B.W. and Trimble, D. (1988) *Record of Agricultural Research*, vol. 36, Department of Agriculture for Northern Ireland, Great Britain.

Northern Ireland Department of Agriculture (1984) Code of practice for the pre-slaughter handling of pigs, www.dardni.uk/pigs_code_of_practice_-2.pdf (accessed 29 April 2014).

Philips, P.A., Thompson, B.K. and Fraser, D. (1988) *Canadian Journal of Animal Science*, 68, 41–48.

Purchas, R.W. (1992) *27th Meat Industry Research Conference Hamilton, New Zealand*, Meat Industry Research Institute, New Zealand.

Rankin, J.D. and Taylor, R.J. (1969) *Veterinary Record*, 85, 575–581.

Ridell, J. and Korkeala, H. (1993) *Meat Science*, 35, 223–228.

Seyle, H. (1974) *Biochemistry and Experimental Biology*, 11, 190.

Shepherd, M.W., Jr, Liang, P., Doyle, M.P. and Erickson, M.C. (2007) *Journal of Food Protection*, 70, 2708–2716.

Smith, L.P. and Allen, W.M. (1976) *Agricultural Meteorology*, 16, 115.

Stosic, P.J. (1996) *Hide Improvement Project. Dung Contamination of Cattle Hides*, The Leather Technology Centre, Northampton.

Thompson, J.M., Halloran, W.J., McNeill, D.M.J. *et al* (1987) *Meat Science*, 20, 293–309.

Warriss, P.D. (1984) *Principles of Pig Science*, Nottingham University Press, Nottingham, pp. 425–432.

Warriss, P.D. (1995) *Meat Focus International*, 1, 491–494.

Warriss, P.D. and Bevis, E.A. (1986) *British Veterinary Journal*, 142, 124–130.

Warriss, P.D. and Brown, S.N. (1994) *Veterinary Record*, 134, 513–515.

Warriss, P.D., Bevis, E.A. and Young, C.S. (1990) *Veterinary Record*, 127, 5–8.

Warriss, P.D., Bevis, E.A., Edwards, J.E. *et al* (1991) *Veterinary Record*, 128, 419–421.

Warriss, P.D., Brown, S.N., Knowles, T.G. and Edwards, J.E. (1992a) *Veterinary Record*, 130, 202–204.

Warriss, P.D., Brown, S.N., Edwards, J.E. *et al* (1992b) *Veterinary Record*, 131, 194–196.

Further reading

Food Safety Implications of Land-spreading Agricultural. Municipal and Industrial Organic Materials on Agricultural Land used for Food Production in Ireland, Food Safety Authority of Ireland (2008) www.fsai.ie (accessed 10 April 2014).

Scientific Opinion Concerning the Welfare of Animals during Transport, adopted by the European Food Safety Authority (EFSA) in December 2010. *EFSA Journal* (2011), 9(1):1966

7

Humane slaughter

'A righteous man regardeth the life of his beast'.

Proverbs 12:10.

The moral and ethical answers to the questions raised when humans kill animals for food can only be answered for each individual according to their own religious, political or economic circumstances. All can agree, however, that if it is to be done, the act of killing must be carried out in such a way as to cause minimum of stress, or distress, to the animal. There are no 'nice' ways of killing animals: only the acceptable and the unacceptable. It is the duty of the veterinarian in the meat plant to have the knowledge and authority to ensure that only acceptable methods are applied.

Thorpe (1965) states that 'there are two opposite pitfalls which beset those who, like ourselves, attempt to decide on the limits of physical injury and restraint which are not permissible for a civilised people to exceed in their treatment of domestic animals. First is the error of supposing that domestic animals in their feelings and anxieties are essentially like human beings; second is the equally serious error of assuming they are mere insentient automata. To avoid these two pitfalls is relatively easy. To know what path to choose between them is extremely difficult'.

In conventional slaughtering methods in most developed countries, it is normal practice to render the animal insensible by stunning, except by the Jewish and Muslim methods, and then to kill it by bleeding. Stunning has two purposes: to induce an immediate state of insensibility and to produce sufficient immobility to facilitate the sticking process to initiate bleeding. In this two-stage system of slaughter, it is vital that insensibility lasts until anoxia resulting from exsanguination makes the loss of consciousness irreversible. This depends on the length of the interval between stunning and sticking, *which must be as short as possible*, and the efficiency of the sticking itself. It is a matter for great concern that faults occur all too often in both areas owing to lack of training, care or supervision and, not least, to the usual high speed of operations in the modern high throughput slaughter establishment.

The discovery that satisfactory bleeding can occur where *cardiac arrest* has been induced introduces the possibility of stunning to kill rather than merely rendering the animal insensible. This obviates all risk of cruelty and should be the ideal for the future for all the food animals.

The European Union Treaty of Amsterdam, in force since May 1999, explicitly acknowledges that farm animals are sentient beings rather than agricultural products or commodities. Through the 'Protocol on the Protection and Welfare of Animals' (1997), it obliges the European Union institutions to pay full regard to animal welfare requirements when formulating and implementing EU legislation.

The responsibility for the welfare of animals from the time they arrive at the slaughterhouse until they are dead lies with the operator of the establishment. European Union Council Regulation 1099/2009 recognises this by requiring the operator to produce a 'Standard Operating Procedure' describing how animals will 'be spared any avoidable pain, distress or suffering during their killing and related operations' and specifically what measures will be taken to ensure that animals

1 are provided with physical comfort and protection, in particular by being kept clean in adequate thermal conditions and prevented from falling or slipping;
2 are protected from injury;
3 are handled and housed taking into consideration their normal behaviour;

Gracey's Meat Hygiene, Eleventh Edition. Edited by David S. Collins and Robert J. Huey.
© 2015 John Wiley & Sons, Ltd. Published 2015 by John Wiley & Sons, Ltd.

4 do not show signs of avoidable pain or fear or exhibit abnormal behaviour;

5 do not suffer from prolonged withdrawal of feed or water; and

6 are prevented from avoidable interaction with other animals that could harm their welfare.

In addition to the above requirements, establishments slaughtering more than 1000 livestock units/year, that is, more than 1 000 cattle, or 150 000 poultry, or equivalent, are required to designate an 'animal welfare officer' (AWO) to assist in ensuring that animal welfare standards are met. The AWO will be directly responsible to the operator of the establishment for animal welfare matters and must hold a certificate of competence in all the operations he/she oversees, having received training from the competent authority in the learning objectives laid out in EC 1099/2009 and having passed an examination. An important provision of the regulation is that the AWO shall be in a position to require that slaughterhouse personnel carry out any remedial actions necessary to ensure compliance with the regulation.

However, while it is correct that the responsibility for welfare of the animals lies with the operator of an establishment, the Official Veterinarian maintains his/her role of verification, audit and enforcement of the required animal welfare standards.

No legislation is of any value unless it clearly incorporates the ethic that the quest for production must never take precedence over the far more important issues of hygiene, meat safety and animal welfare.

Pre-slaughter handling/restraint

It is generally regarded as undesirable that an animal awaiting slaughter should view the slaughtering process. While the higher animals undoubtedly share some sensations with human beings, it is questionable whether any trepidation is felt specifically by an animal at the sight and smell of blood. Nevertheless, fear is undoubtedly engendered by strange noises, movements, surroundings and smells, and this fear is accentuated by the separation of the animal from its fellows and the consequent disappearance of the feeling of protection that a gregarious animal enjoys in the presence of its comrades. Group stunning, for example, for sheep utilising low-voltage head-only electrical tongs, can reduce the isolation factor; however, it must not be allowed to compromise the stun-to-stick interval.

The design of the *handling facility in the lairage* which delivers the animals to the point of slaughter should utilise knowledge of animal behaviour to reduce the fear or apprehension felt by the animal to a minimum. The tendency for one sheep to follow its comrade up a single file race, the preference most animals have to walk up rather than down a slope and the movement of pigs in optimum-sized groups of about 15 individuals are all examples of good practices. The theory of moving animals within the lairage is dealt with in detail in Chapter 6.

Cattle movement and restraint

Cattle are usually moved from the pens in the lairage to the *stunning box* via a solid-walled race. Cattle have been shown to move more readily along a race with *curved walls*. A *raised walkway* along one side assists the handlers in their effort to keep the animals moving. The animal should spend the minimum possible time in the actual stunning box where they are finally isolated from their cohorts. They should not be moved into the box until the operative responsible for the stunning procedure signals that they are ready to stun the animal.

Cattle head restraint

There have been a number of types of *head restraint* for cattle used to present the head of the animal in a position to assist accurate stunning, but a simple *shelf* which extends to the floor of the stunning box, preventing the animal dropping its head, seems to be the most successful. However, with all head restraints, smaller than average animals present problems by having sufficient space within the stunning box to position themselves in such a way as to avoid the restraint system. This can be overcome by the provision of a hydraulically operated *tail pusher* in the back of the box. Personal observations of these mechanisms have shown that, if incorrectly used to force cattle into this head restraint, the animal's spine can be fractured by the pressures applied. Pneumatic head restraints and tail pushers can also be problematic as the noise of escaping air can frighten the animal.

The positioning of *lights* above the animal's head to attract its attention is reported as being a useful addition in maintaining the head in a raised position.

Ewbank, Parker and Mason (1992) reported on the use of active head restraints at slaughter and concluded that 'while the introduction of head restraint devices into cattle stunning pens had a positive effect in terms of improving the stunning accuracy, behaviour and cortisol results suggest that enforced usage of this type of head restrainer could be a cause of distress to the cattle involved'. The fixed shelf-restraint was found to improve the accuracy of stunning without increasing the length of time the animal spent in the stunning box and without causing the animal increased stress.

A head restrainer, which prevents lateral and vertical movement, is a necessity if a pneumatic captive bolt is used to stun cattle in order to ensure accuracy of application.

Pig movement and restraint

One of the greatest problems in delivering animals to the point of slaughter is presented by the necessity for pigs to be stunned by high-voltage electric current to arrive at the point of stunning continuously at a rate of several hundred/hour, in single file, and to become confined in a 'V'-shaped restrainer. With their feet off the floor, animals are less likely to attempt to struggle and be injured. Restrainers which support the animal on the chest have been shown to be less stressful for pigs than 'V'-shaped restrainers. Pigs prefer to move as a group, with their comrades on either side. They resent being forced into single file. The answer, to some extent, has been to utilise a *curved double race* where the pig can see his comrades moving along beside him, but there still comes a point in most cases where the double race must feed into one single restrainer. The single-file chute should be at least 6 m long to achieve continuous flow, but no more than 10.5 m long, to keep the pigs moving without excessive goading.

A common alternative for high line speeds is to use a *gas stunning system* which allows several pigs to be stunned simultaneously. The pigs may be allowed to move along a passageway with the group size gradually decreasing as pigs progress at different speeds, until the required number is attained. This group, usually of about five or six pigs, is moved into a small pen which descends into the gaseous environment where stunning occurs. Line speeds of 800 pigs/hour can be accommodated by this system.

The effect on pigs of immediate pre-slaughter stress, as measured by post-mortem blood biochemistry and meat quality, has been studied by Warriss, Brown and Adams (1994). They concluded that these subjective assessments of the stress suffered by pigs correlated well with objective measures, specifically the sound level immediately before stunning, and that as expected higher stress levels were associated with poorer meat quality. They confirmed that the confinement and restraint associated with race-restrainers were stressful to the animals, and that the use of *electric goads* to coerce pigs to move along these systems, particularly at high line speeds, increased the levels of stress.

The slaughtering process

In the past, all too often, the task of stunning was given to untrained individuals. It cannot be emphasised too strongly that, *in addition to the important matter of animal welfare, proper stunning/killing plays a significant part in preventing injuries to staff engaged in the subsequent shackling and bleeding processes.* EU Council Regulation 1099/2009 requires those involved in the killing of animals and 'related operations' to be trained and receive certificates of competence relevant for the categories of animals concerned and the operations that they carry out. Related operations are defined as handling, restraining, stunning, assessment of effective stunning, shackling or hoisting of live animals and bleeding live animals.

Farm animals may be stunned utilising the following:

1 Percussive blow to the head
2 Penetrative captive bolt
3 Non-penetrative captive bolt
4 Electrical stunning
5 Exposure to gas mixtures

They may be killed using the following:

1 Firearm with free projectile
2 Electrocution
3 Exposure to gas mixtures

Assessment of unconsciousness at slaughter

The nervous system, composed of the brain and spinal cord (central nervous system), and the peripheral nerves, is the important control and communication system of the body. The brain, consisting of two cerebral hemispheres, cerebellum and medulla oblongata, is responsible for coordinating all the activities necessary for the maintenance of life. Situated in the bony cranial cavity, to which it closely conforms, it contains all the vital centres controlling the body's many activities.

The *waking state*, or *state of consciousness*, has been described as 'a dynamic equilibrium between the activation of cerebral neuronal networks maintained by the incessant impact of innumerable ascendant and associative impulses and the cumulative functional depression resulting from the very continuity of this state of excitation' (Bremner, 1954). Consciousness involves an awareness of the environment and the ability to appreciate pain.

In the act of slaughter, it is essential that a state of *unconsciousness* or *insensibility* be *instantaneously* produced to ensure total freedom from pain, this being further ensured by immediate exsanguination. Where *cardiac arrest* has been created, there is an almost immediate insensibility which is *permanent*. The discovery that adequate bleeding ensues despite cardiac dysfunction in this method makes this a most important development in the slaughter of animals. It had been always thought that a beating heart was necessary for proper bleeding, but this has been discounted, provided sticking is performed within 3 minutes of cardiac arrest.

The *time taken to reach insensibility* due to exsanguination depends upon the technique utilised in sticking, the species, the age of the animal, whether the carcase is suspended or recumbent and the method of pre-stunning used. Based on electroencephalographic data, sheep have been shown to achieve 'brain death' in 2–7 seconds, pigs in

12–30 seconds (average 18 seconds) and cattle in 20–102 seconds (average 55 seconds). The species differences are due to differences in the arteries which supply the blood to the brain via the Circle of Willis. In all cases, in the interests of the animal, it should be assumed that the upper limit applies.

Electroencephalograms (EEGs) and electrocorticograms (EcoGs) are widely used to record brain electrical activity in order to determine the state of consciousness. Efficient stunning methods disrupt the neurons or neurotransmitter regulatory mechanisms in the brain. EEG brain wave patterns show changes from the normal which are incompatible with consciousness, such as grand mal epilepsy or prolonged periods of quiescence. In addition, external stimuli fail to evoke electrical activity in the brain (somatosensory evoked potentials) indicating the brain's incapacity to receive and process external stimuli.

Within the abattoir however, observation of clinical signs is the only method available to assess an effective stun. The *typical signs of effective stunning by electricity* are immediate collapse of the animal with flexion, followed by rigid extension of the limbs, opisthotonus (extreme arching back of the neck and spine), downward rolling of the eyeballs with tonic (continuous) muscular spasm changing into clonic (repeated) violent spasms and eventual muscle flaccidity. The term *electroplectic fit* has been used to describe these signs of an *effective stun*. The tonic spasms last for some 10–25 seconds, and the clonic phase 15–45 seconds, in both pigs and sheep.

The *typical signs of an effective stun using concussive methods* in cattle are immediate collapse of the animal followed by tonic spasm lasting about 10–15 seconds, then slow clonic movements of the hind legs and eventually vigorous hind leg movements. In pigs, the tonic phase lasts 3–5 seconds, followed immediately by violent, clonic muscle spasms which make bleeding the animal difficult and often dangerous. In an effective stun, normal rhythmic breathing must cease immediately, and the eyeball should face outwards with a fixed gaze and not be rotated inwards.

In *carbon dioxide anaesthesia in pigs*, the effects are those of a chemical anaesthetic, with the eventual onset of insensibility. A period of increased respiratory rate is followed by slow respiratory movements and final dyspnoea (difficult breathing). Corneal and palpebral reflexes are absent, and extreme muscle flaccidity supervenes. The limbs and jaw are consequently relaxed.

The use of palpebral, corneal or pupillary reflexes to ascertain the effectiveness of stunning is inappropriate for most methods of stunning. Palpebral and corneal reflexes are not under cortical control and may therefore be present in an animal or bird which has been rendered insensible. Conversely, the palpebral reflex may be absent in an animal which has been ineffectively electrically stunned. Although complete pupillary dilatation is a reliable sign of total insensibility of an animal nearing the point of death, it is of little practical use since, for example, it has been demonstrated that while sensibility as measured by electrical activity occurs 8 seconds after the decapitation of a sheep's head, complete pupillary dilatation does not occur until 87 seconds.

The most reliable objective sign of loss of sensibility is the *absence of respiratory activity*. The return of regular respiratory movements after stunning, but not irregular respiratory gasps, should always be a cause of concern. 'Gagging' respiratory movements, agonal breathing, are generally a sign of imminent brain death. In general, vocalisation in animals during the induction of unconsciousness with any stunning method is indicative of pain or suffering. Absence of vocalisation does not however guarantee absence of pain or suffering.

Methods of stunning

The choice of a particular method of stunning depends on many different factors – species, breed and age of animal, intended line speed, humane aspects, capital and maintenance costs, efficiency of equipment, ease of operation, safety of personnel and effects on carcase and brain, along with religious and legal requirements.

The number of variable factors involved in modern stunning systems, especially electrical and gaseous methods, makes a system of approval prior to operation desirable. The parameters under which a particular system operates should be recorded; for example, the required line speed, class of animal, current as measured in average amps, waveform and frequency. Methods by which the system's operation is measured, calibration of the monitoring equipment, records to be completed and audited should also be agreed with the competent authority.

Percussive stunning

Many different types of percussive stunning pistol are in use throughout the world, having been introduced at the end of the nineteenth century. They are generally operated by means of a blank cartridge, although some are pneumatic in design. With the most common type, the *captive bolt pistol*, a bolt is propelled forward on discharge of the blank cartridge and automatically recoils into the barrel. The tip of the bolt is concave and has a relatively sharp rim. Ideally, the bolt, which varies in length from 70 to 121 mm and in diameter from 12 to 14 mm, should be recessed into the body of the pistol so that when the muzzle is held firmly against the animal's head, the bolt can gain velocity before penetration of the skull occurs.

It is important when using captive bolt pistol to ensure that the correct strength of cartridge is used for the different species. With *Cash* instruments, these range in strength from 1 grain for small animals such as milk

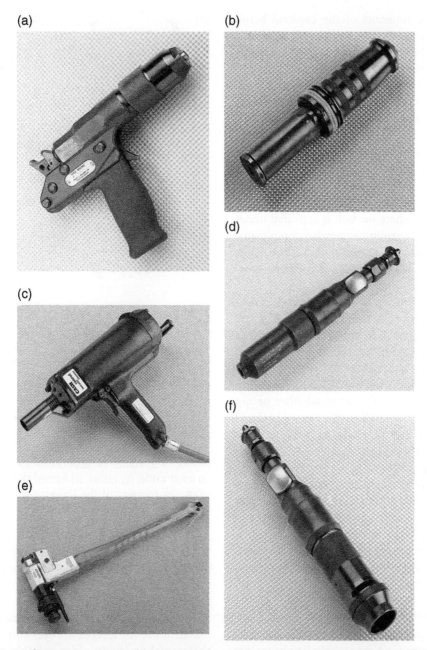

Figure 7.1 Various types of percussive stunners. (a) Penetrative percussion stunner; incorporates special 'no fire' system with low noise level. (b) Contact firing penetrative concussive stunner available for large and small animals. (c) Air-powered penetrative stunner for sheep and goats; contact and 'no-fire' systems incorporated. (d) Penetrative concussive stunner 0.22 calibre; palm- or finger-activated trigger; firing pin pull to cock instrument. (e) Contact and failsafe non-penetrative concussive stunner for use in deep stunning pens; suitable for ritual slaughter. (f) Non-penetrative concussive stunner incorporating 'no-fire' system; suitable for ritual slaughter (by kind permission of Messrs Accles and Shelvoke, Witton, www.acclesandshlevoke.co.uk).

lambs, up to 3 and 4 grains for large cattle and mature bulls (1 grain = 0.065 g).

Properly used, captive bolt equipment is very effective in finished cattle, sheep and calves, but less so in bulls and pigs, especially sows and boars, in which the frontal bone structure is very thick and restraint to allow accurate application is difficult (Fig. 7.1).

The important force in producing unconsciousness with the captive bolt pistol is the impact energy of the bolt, which is heavily dependent on the speed at which it strikes the brain, rather than the penetration of the brain *per se*. A velocity of about 55 m/s is recommended for steers, heifers and cows, and between 65 and 70 m/s for young bulls. The strength of the cartridge must be matched with the robustness of the gun to prevent metal fatigue and breaks in washers, buffers, etc.

Percussive stunners achieve their effect as a result of the energy imparted to the brain generating turbulent rotatory and other movements of the cerebral hemispheres, increasing the chance of a tissue-deforming collision or impact between the cortex and the skull. This in turn causes diffuse depolarisation and synchronised discharge of cortical neurons (Shaw, 2002). In addition to these changes, penetrative percussive stunners cause direct damage and trauma to the cerebral hemispheres and brainstem.

The captive bolt pistol is a very useful instrument, but it cannot be used for slaughter at rates of over 240–250/hour owing to difficulties in reloading. In these cases, an automatically resetting stunner can be used.

Pneumatic stunners, where the bolt is activated under a pressure of 80–120 psi, require somewhat complicated actions to fire them, and there may be occasions when air pressure is inadequate. With proper pressure, however, a high bolt velocity can be achieved.

Non-penetrative concussion stunners using a mushroom-shaped head were sometimes used in calves and lambs. However, EU Council Regulation 1099/2009 has banned the use of non-penetrative captive bolt devices in ruminants above 10 kg bodyweight. Properly used, this method is capable of producing immediate insensibility. Much depends on the operative as to whether or not blood splashing results, especially in the case of lambs. If the animals are handled properly and the interval between stunning and bleeding is short, blood splashing in muscle will be minimal.

If the first blow using a non-penetrative concussive stunner fails to produce an effective stun, subsequent shots are unlikely to be effective due to the swelling of the skin and subcutaneous tissue caused by the first shot. An alternative backup system, such as penetrative percussion or electrical stunning, should therefore always be immediately available for use.

Head sites for percussive stunning

With both types of percussive stunners, care must be taken to hold the instrument reasonably firmly against the animal's head at the proper point and direction. In *adult cattle*, the correct point is in the middle of the forehead where two lines taken from the medial canthus of each eye to the base of the opposite horn or horn prominence cross. The stunner is placed at right angles to the forehead and after discharge is lifted away from the falling animal. In *calves*, the pistol should be placed slightly lower on the head than for adult cattle, while for *bulls* and *old cows*, the muzzle is placed 1.5 cm to the side of the ridge running down the centre of the forehead. Cattle should never be stunned in the poll position.

In *hornless sheep and goats*, the stunner is placed on the top of the head and aimed towards the gullet, while

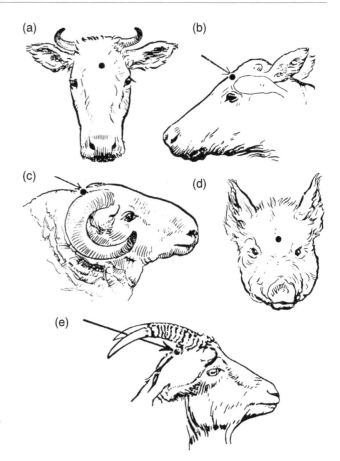

Figure 7.2 Points of application for concussive stunning: (a) adult cattle; (b) calves; (c) horned sheep; (d) pigs; (e) horned goats (by courtesy of the Universities Federation for Animal Welfare).

for *horned sheep and goats*, the muzzle is placed behind the ridge which runs between the horns, the direction of aim being the same.

For *bacon weight pigs*, the stunner is placed about 2.5 cm above the level of the eyes and fired upwards into the cranial cavity. In older animals, captive bolt stunning is less reliable owing to the massive nature of the skulls and the large frontal sinuses of older pigs. The muzzle should be placed about 5 cm above the level of the eyes to the side of the ridge which is in the mid-line of the skull, and at right angles to the frontal surface (Fig. 7.2).

The *contact-firing types* of *captive bolt stunner* are much more satisfactory than the trigger-operated ones, only a light tap on the animal's head being necessary to fire them. With cattle restrained in a stunning box, they are easier to operate than trigger-operated pistols. However, if they are dropped on the floor or struck against the stunning box wall, the whole gun can become a dangerous missile (Fig. 7.3).

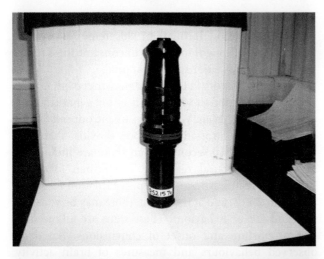

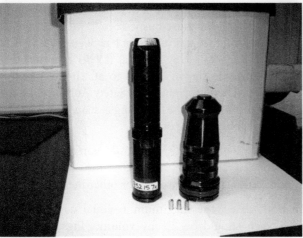

Figure 7.3 Contact firing penetrative concussive stunner for cattle.

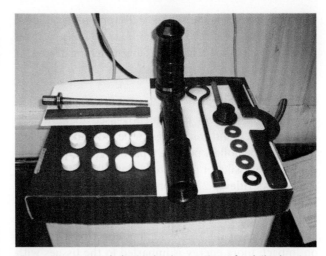

Figure 7.4 Captive bolt pistol, taken to pieces for daily cleaning.

A defect of percussive stunning and the use of the free bullet is noise. Most of the really serious defects, however, arise from misuse or from instruments in poor state of repair, as is the case with all forms of stunning. The Official Veterinarian must be satisfied that the instruments used for stunning, and for restraint, are in a good state of repair.

If equipment is to function correctly, the importance of *regular maintenance* cannot be overemphasised. The velocity of the bolt may be significantly reduced by a build-up of carbon or corrosion on the piston, which drives the bolt forward, or by excessive wear in any of the moving parts. While some manufacturers recommend cleaning every 70 shots, *daily dismantling and thorough cleaning must be carried out*. A record of cleaning and maintenance should be kept by the operator and audited by the Official Veterinarian as part of a regular check of the equipment (Fig. 7.4).

A common indication that a stunner requires cleaning is the tip of the bolt protruding from the muzzle more than the usual distance when the bolt returns to the barrel.

All forms of mechanical stunning devices should be fitted with safety levers to minimise the chances of accidents.

A backup stunner should always be on hand in case of emergency.

Bolt velocity check

A device is now available for checking the bolt velocity of all Cash penetrative stunners. The stunner is placed upright in the device and fired, stunning performance of the various cartridges being recorded as FAST, OK or SLOW by means of indicator lights on a separate recorder. Accurate monitoring of stunner performance means more effective stunning, fewer second shots, greater operator efficiency and safety, and a high standard of animal welfare.

Neural tissue embolism in cattle

With the realisation that Transmissible Spongiform Encephalopathies (TSEs) were zoonotic, considerable interest focused on the possibility that percussive stunning could result in emboli of brain tissue entering edible tissues. Garland, Bauer and Bailey (1996) in the United States reported the condition in 2.5–5% of cattle stunned by a pneumatic-actuated penetrative captive bolt pistol, the diaphragmatic lobe of the lung being the area most commonly affected. Pneumatic stunners, which inject compressed air through the captive bolt into the cranium, disintegrate the brain and are most likely to result in emboli. Pneumatic powered stunners that do not inject air present a reduced risk but greater than that of cartridge-driven stunners. However, penetrating captive bolt stunning has been demonstrated to result in central nervous system (CNS) embolism in jugular blood in a large percentage of both cattle and sheep. In non-penetrative captive bolt stunning, CNS material was detected in jugular blood of 2% of animals, Coore *et al.* (2005).

Pithing, described later, has been demonstrated to increase the risk of neural emboli.

Free bullet pistol

The free bullet pistol is frequently used to humanely destroy horses, and sometimes cattle, humanely. Bullets may be of the hollow pointed type, frangible iron plastic composite missiles or powdered iron bullets fired from a small-bore rifle (0.22 calibre), 9 mm or 0.38 calibre handgun, or a small instrument held against the forehead. The benefit of hollow point projectiles is a greater enhancement of the mushrooming effect or expansion on impact; more energy is imparted to the tissues with increased tissue destruction, and there is less likelihood of the missile exiting the head.

The points of application are in general the same as those for the captive bolt pistol, in the case of horses this being high up in the forehead immediately below the roots of the forelock where two lines from the medial canthus of each eye to the base of the opposite ear cross. The direction of aim in horses is slightly below the right-angle plane to the forehead.

Great care must be taken to avoid accidents when using free projectiles, and each instrument should be fitted with a safety device. In future, the use of the free bullet is likely to be increasingly discouraged for reasons of safety.

Water jet stunning

This experimental form of percussive stunning, described by Lambooij (1996), utilises a fine jet of water to penetrate the skull and mechanically destroy the brain by the induction of laceration, crushing and/or shock-waves to such an extent that immediate unconsciousness is induced. The 0.5 mm jet, applied at pressures of 3500–4000 bar at a similar site as for the captive bolt, drills through the skin and skull in 0.2–0.4 seconds.

Destruction of the brain results in convulsions, which can be controlled using an immobilising current of 400 mA applied using 40 V. Initial work has indicated that it may be possible to produce meat of superior quality, compared to either electrical or CO_2 stunning, using this method.

Carbon dioxide and other gas mixtures

Carbon dioxide was first used to induce pre-slaughter anaesthesia in animals in 1904 but was not used successfully on a commercial scale until 1950. Since then the method has been modified in several different ways and is now widely used throughout the world, although not as extensively as it could be, probably because of the high

cost of installation and operation. The technique was banned for a period during the 1980s in the Netherlands because it was thought to lead to unconsciousness under very stressful conditions for the animal.

Raj and Gregory (1995) demonstrated that pigs showed no aversion to 30% CO_2 in air but a marked aversion to 90% CO_2 in air. When pigs are introduced to 80% or higher concentrations of carbon dioxide, there is a period of about 10 seconds when there are little or no signs of behavioural reaction. There then follows a period of breathlessness and hyperventilation for a further 10 seconds, and at this point, there may be vocalisation and escape behaviour. These signs are followed by loss of posture and onset of convulsions. Based on observed behaviours and measures of brain activity, there is a considerable period of time, up to 15 seconds, before the pig loses consciousness.

The use of other gas mixtures has been investigated. Raj and Gregory (1995) and Raj (1999) reported that no aversion was shown by pigs to an environment of 90% *argon*. The European Food Safety Authority report (2004) recommended the following gaseous atmospheres for the stunning/killing of pigs:

- A mixture of 30% CO_2 and 60% argon or nitrogen in air, or
- with 90% argon or nitrogen (or other inert gas) in air.

In both cases, the maximum residual concentration of oxygen should be 2% by volume. Pigs should be immersed into these recommended gas concentrations within 10 seconds from leaving the atmospheric air, and they should be exposed to gas mixtures for a minimum of 3 minutes. These regimes will, however, only give an effective stun for less than 50 seconds so bleeding must commence within 25 seconds. An exposure time of 7 minutes to these recommended atmospheres will result in a stun/kill, but this is too long a period to be commercially viable in practice.

Currently, however, carbon dioxide is the only gas widely used for stunning animals commercially. It is usually stored in cylinders or bulk tanks as a liquid under pressure. It is also available in solid form for which a converter is necessary. The gas is non-flammable and has a higher specific gravity than air, sinking to the bottom of any container, a fact which has to be borne in mind when it is being used for anaesthesia or euthanasia purposes. It presents no hazard to the operator.

Inhalation of carbon dioxide induces respiratory and metabolic acidosis and, hence, reduces the pH of the cerebrospinal fluid (CSF) and neurons thereby exerting its neuronal inhibitory and anaesthetic effects. These are measured as quiescent EEG recordings and abolition of somatosensory evoked potentials in the brain. A concentration of 80–95% CO_2 in air should be utilised with sufficient exposure time to kill the majority of the pigs and render others unconscious until death occurs by exsanguination. If the concentration is too low, the pigs will not be properly stunned; if it is too high, pigs may become stiff, show reflex muscular activity and bleed poorly. If the exposure period is too long, superficial congestion of the skin occurs and when pigs are scalded the skin is bluish in colour.

The type of *apparatus* employed to administer the gas depends mainly upon the required rate of slaughter.

1 The *oval tunnel* is now largely historic but was used for killing rates of up to 600 pigs/hour. As the name suggests the gas tunnel is in the form of an oval through which a slot conveyor carries the pigs, the actual tunnel sloping downwards at an angle of 30° to the anaesthetising chamber. On exit, the pigs are shackled, hoisted to an overhead rail and bled. The actual conveyor in the tunnel is divided into 10 compartments, one pig being accommodated in each compartment. Pigs up to 113 kg can be handled in this equipment, which is not suitable for other species.

2 The *dip lift* is suitable for any size of pig, as well as calves and sheep. It consists of a cage 200 cm long, 70 cm high and 50 cm wide which, when the animal enters it, descends vertically to the CO_2 pit where it remains for the pre-set time and then automatically returns to ground level, ejecting the unconscious animal for shackling and bleeding. The greatest advantage of the system is that it allows several pigs to be stunned simultaneously, assisting immediate pre-slaughter handling. This is suitable for low throughput establishments.

3 The Compact CO_2 stunner, was the second system to be developed and consists of a horizontally revolving apparatus divided into four to eight compartments each holding one animal. It operates in such a way that, when one section is uppermost for loading, the others are rotating to submerge in the gas chamber. Once the pig is loaded, the floor flips down and the pig is suspended in the cage, supported on each side, to minimise escape behaviour. The unit usually has a capacity of up to 600 pigs/hour. In a commonly used design, the pigs are exposed to 10% CO_2 at the first position, 30% for 10 seconds at the second, 60% for 10 seconds at the third and over 90% for 20 seconds at the fourth and fifth, after which the pigs are discharged from the unit.

4 The 'Compact stunner' was developed into the 'Combi-compact stunner' which is similar to the 'Compact' but permits three or four pigs per compartment allowing group loading and is consequently less stressful to the pigs. The group loading system can be partially automated using panels fitted with sensor which gently ease group of pigs into the system (Fig. 7.5).

With all systems, the chamber must be fitted with a *device for measuring the gas concentration* at the point of maximum exposure and for giving a clearly visible and audible warning if the concentration of the gas concentration falls below the required level. All systems should allow efficient evacuation of the pigs in the event of mechanical failure.

The *advantages* claimed for carbon dioxide stunning/killing include relaxed carcases, allowing easier dehairing and dressing, less noise and reduced labour requirements. It has also been contended that the yield of blood from pigs stunned by this method is 0.75% better because carbon dioxide stimulates respiration and thus favours blood circulation and consequently bleeding. Muscular

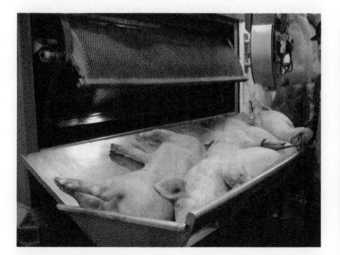
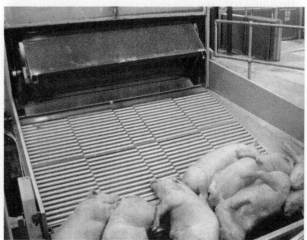

Figure 7.5 CO_2 anaesthesia. Combi-compact system showing convenient shackling position after stunning (Reproduced with permission from David Armstrong).

haemorrhages are said to be avoided, the number of bone fractures is reduced to zero and the amount of pale soft exudative (PSE) may be reduced.

Electrical stunning

There are many different types of electrical stunning systems in use, most being manually operated while some are automatic in operation, especially for pigs and poultry.

This method consists of passing an alternating current (AC) through the brain and, with some techniques, also the heart of the animal, the instrument most commonly employed being one which resembles a pair of *tongs*. The current causes massive depolarisation of neurons in the brain, resulting in EEG patterns similar to that recorded in humans with a generalised epileptic seizure and the associated tonic–clonic muscle contractions. This epileptiform activity is analogous to a loss of consciousness and appears to be associated with loss of sensory awareness.

The epileptiform activity in the brain is induced by a release of neurotransmitters, glutamate and aspartate, into the extracellular space. This is a reversible process with the animal starting to regain consciousness about 40 seconds after the stun.

The conditions necessary to produce an effective electrical stun are as follows:

1 The strength of the electric current should be sufficient to ensure that the animal is killed outright by cardiac arrest or remains insensible until death occurs by exsanguination.
2 Provided sufficient current is applied, a genuine *electroplectic shock* will be induced. The mains voltage may fluctuate considerably and at times fall to a dangerously low level in the stunning apparatus, and it is therefore required that every electrical stunning apparatus is fitted with indicators visible to the operator that provide a warning if the current or voltage drops, or the time of application falls short of 7 seconds for low-voltage systems and below 3 seconds for high-voltage equipment. Many systems apply a minimal test current immediately before the stun current is applied to gauge the resistance. If the resistance is too high for an effective stun, the stun current will not be applied.
3 The electrodes should be correctly positioned so that the current will pass through the thalamus and cortex, the chief sensory centres in the forebrain. This relates to the space between the eyes and the base of the ears on most species. The electrical resistance of contact with the hair and skin may be lowered by ensuring that the electrodes are kept moist by immersion in brine and the skin of the head is kept clean but dry. The presence of wool on the sheep's head can increase electrical resistance significantly. The practice of wetting the pig's head should be discouraged since it may result in current tracking over the surface of the pig's skin rather than through the brain.

There is little doubt that the failure of operators to observe these criteria has been the cause of much of the criticism of electrical stunning methods, firstly on the grounds that the method was not always humane and secondly because *haemorrhages* were often observed in the muscular tissue of animals stunned by electrical means.

It is necessary for an adequate amount of electrical current to pass through the brain in a sufficiently short period of time. This depends on the voltage applied and the resistance, or more correctly impedance, present. If too high a voltage is employed, carcase quality may be compromised by the production of *muscle haemorrhages and broken bones*; if too low a voltage is used, the animal may be paralysed but still conscious of pain. Operator safety also plays a part in determining voltage levels; levels under 150 V are not generally effective, especially allowing for fluctuations in mains voltage.

Whatever type of electrical stunning is used, a *backup stunner*, in the form of a portable captive bolt device should be available for use, not only on incorrectly stunned animals, but also for casualty animals in their transport vehicle or in the lairage. It may be advisable to have an additional set of stunning tongs for use in several electrical sockets positioned throughout the lairage and casualty accommodation. This is particularly useful if sows and boars, which are difficult to stun effectively with a captive bolt, are to be slaughtered.

Since the brains of animals are relatively small, it is important that electrodes are accurately and firmly placed high up on the sides of the head. The irregular anatomy of the head makes this difficult, especially if the animal is moving. The electrodes are easier to position if the tongs are relatively heavy and if the operator is able to apply them to the animal downwards rather than upwards or horizontally. Placement of tongs is also achieved with less effort in efficient restrainer-conveyor systems. *Head-to-body* equipment should be correctly counterbalanced. The electrodes must be in good repair and not be corroded or coated with carbon. It is essential that the equipment is earthed properly for operator safety (Fig. 7.6).

The passage of electric current through the brain results in a rapid rise of blood pressure due to vasoconstriction and increased heart rate, hence the need for immediate bleeding in order to avoid blood splashing.

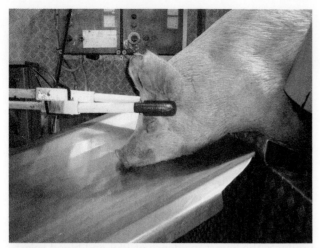

Figure 7.6 Electrical stunning tongs in use (Reproduced with permission from John Hood).

Low-voltage electrical stunning

Low-voltage electrical stunning, defined as using less than 150 V is no longer recommended by many authorities, including the Humane Slaughter Association. It consists of a control panel, on which voltage can be adjusted, meters capable of measuring the current and voltage as it is applied, and a pair of tongs with terminal electrodes for application to the sides of the animal's head. In order to create a better contact, the electrodes are immersed in a saline solution before use or possess in-built water jets. Many tongs systems are now capable of delivering in excess of 250 V safely.

For *head-only* electrical stunning systems, a minimum electric current of 400 mA for pigs, and 250 mA for sheep and lambs, has been recommended to produce an effective stun when the tongs are placed in the ideal position. However, most experts set their recommendations considerably higher at 1.0 A for sheep, 0.6 A for lambs, 1.3 A for pigs and 1.5 A for cattle, having made the assumption that tong placement on the head would frequently be far from ideal.

High-voltage electrical stunning

Investigations into electrical stunning have shown that high-voltage systems using 300 V or above are more effective than low-voltage systems provided they are used with automatic restrainers and with due regard to operator safety. The application time must be at least 3 seconds. Fractures (vertebrae and scapula) may occur in pigs stunned on the floor.

High-voltage electrical systems for pigs are available in a fully automatic form which incorporates two V-shaped restrainer-conveyors. These are placed in series and move at different speeds so that the animals are separated sufficiently to present their heads for stunning to a set of specially shaped electrodes suspended on

hinged metal plates which hang down inside the second conveyer and contact the animal's head as it passes through. The stunning voltage is of the order 600–1000 V. Ninety percent of the pigs are killed; the remaining 10% are only stunned. Difficulties may be encountered with this system in maintaining a consistently correct positioning of the electrodes across the brain of the pig. It is particularly important that a backup stunner is always present to deal with any animal which suffers poor positioning of the electrodes, resulting in only partial stunning. Automated electrical stunning systems using chest belt conveyers have an improved accuracy due to the use of photo sensors to aid accurate placement of the electrodes and accurate positioning of the animal's head.

Head-to-brisket stunning of cattle

The high-voltage *head-to-brisket* system was first developed in New Zealand for religious slaughter of cattle. Electrodes are applied to the animal in a purpose-built stunning pen following capture in a neck yoke. On capture, a chin lift operates from which a nose contact plate is applied. A current to a maximum of 3.5 A (at 550 V, 50 Hz) is applied between the nose and neck yoke for 3 seconds to stun the animal, with an additional current applied between the neck and brisket via a pneumatically positioned electrode between the animal's forelegs, to produce cardiac arrest.

Studies carried out by Wotton *et al.* (2000) demonstrated that an effective stun could be achieved in cattle utilising the head electrodes only with currents as low as 0.46 A when applied for 3 seconds or 1.15 A for 1 second. In the cardiac arrest cycle, the maximum current survived by an animal was 1.51A from which it can be deduced that if the current is sufficient to cause cardiac arrest there must always be sufficient to cause an effective stun. Evidence suggests that successful induction of unconsciousness and cardiac fibrillation is associated with gasping and/or rhythmic breathing movements in the majority of animals and rotation of the eyeball in some, and resumption of corneal and palpebral reflexes in a few. However, these responses are subsequently lost and brain death occurs without the resumption of consciousness. It has been suggested that these brainstem reflexes observed particularly after short duration cardiac arrest stuns do not indicate recovery and can therefore be ignored under these specific circumstances as long as ventricular fibrillation has been achieved.

Head to back/leg stunning of pigs and sheep

High-voltage electrical stunning in addition to being used for head-only application, may incorporate special electrodes through which current is applied simultaneously to the head and back/leg. In this system, the brain is anaesthetised and the heart put into arrest, thus cutting off the blood supply to the brain, which suffers death before anaesthesia ends. Research work has shown that brain function ceased 23 seconds after this system of stunning, whereas this time was extended to some 50 seconds with head-only stunning. The animal is, in fact, killed, thus improving animal welfare and making the stun-to-stick interval less important. Provided sticking is performed intrathoracically within 3 minutes, bleeding is satisfactory. A minimum current of 1.3 A applied with a minimum of 250 V is recommended for pigs and 1.0 A at 375 V for sheep.

In order to be fully effective, head-to-back/leg stunning must be combined with automatic restraining systems which prevent adverse reflex muscular movements and the possibility of fractures as well as making the task of shackling and bleeding easier for operatives. 'Pelt-burn' in sheep occasionally occurs on the back with this method.

Effect of stunning on meat quality

Most of the problems associated with penetrative percussive stunning (captive bolt) appear to result from an unduly long interval between stunning and sticking and/or inadequate penetration of the bolt, resulting in *blood splashing in muscles*, particularly of the diaphragm, the abdominal wall, the intercostal muscles and the heart.

The all-too-frequent, and illegal, habit of group stunning a number of animals before shackling/bleeding – especially in sheep – is a practice that leads to this result, the animals first 'stunned' being the ones affected. This lesion tends to occur where there is a marked rise in arterial blood pressure, the highest rates taking place in head-only electrical stunning, where the incidence can be markedly reduced by the adoption of a short stun-to-stick interval.

Head-to-back/leg electrical stunning produces a very low incidence of blood splashing, but petechiae may on occasions occur in connective tissues and fat. High-voltage head-only stunning in pigs sometimes results in petechial haemorrhages throughout the loin. High-voltage electrical stunning may also result in the *fracture of bones* with associated haemorrhage into surrounding tissue. The fracture is thought to be due to the force of the tonic convulsion induced during and immediately after stunning and to be reduced by increasing the frequency of the sinusoidal AC from 50 Hz, the norm, upwards towards 1500 Hz. However, increasing the frequency of the current has the disadvantage of reducing the fibrillating effect on the heart. Fractures occur in the scapula, pelvis, the neck of the femur and around the fifth or sixth thoracic vertebrae and are much more common in pigs, which have greater muscle mass than sheep.

It has also been demonstrated that the use of tongs with 300 V in a restrainer-conveyor resulted in superior pig meat quality compared with automatic stunning with 680 V, the incidence of PSE being much less in the former method which also showed superior values in relation to pH, temperature, rigor mortis, bacteriological status, etc. It is likely that these differences were due to variations in the amperage and in the number of interruptions in the flow of the current during stunning (Van der Wal, 1983).

Since carbon dioxide–anaesthetised pigs do not exhibit clonic convulsions post-stunning, they are safer to handle for the operators even when blood is being collected for human use. It is generally accepted that carbon dioxide produces the lowest incidence of PSE and blood splash, and that overall the quality of meat produced is superior.

Slaughter of minor species

For further detailed information, the European Food Safety Authority (EFSA) report on the welfare aspects of the main systems of stunning and killing applied to commercially farmed deer, goats, rabbits, ostriches, ducks, geese and quail is recommended.

Slaughter of deer

The family Cervidae includes red deer, fallow deer, muntjaks, moose, caribou and roe deer. They are often characterised as being either 'farmed' or 'wild', but for the purposes of considering their welfare at time of slaughter or killing, it is more appropriate to categorise them as domesticated, semi-domesticated or wild.

Domesticated deer may be transported in specially adapted vehicles to abattoirs which have handling facilities adapted to deal with their welfare needs. The most common method of slaughter is percussive penetrating captive bolt, but head-only low-voltage electrical stunning and free bullet are also used.

The bolt velocity and hence the size of charge and type of pistol will vary with different types of deer in addition to their age and sex.

Head-only low-voltage electrical stunning requires a minimum current of 1.0 A for fallow deer and a minimum current of 1.3 A for red deer, applied across the brain using tongs. While fallow deer show similar tonic–clonic reactions as other domestic livestock, red deer either exhibit a very short tonic phase or none at all. Clonic activity characterised by violent kicking lasts approximately 30–45 seconds in red deer and approximately 20 seconds in fallow.

The use of a free bullet to kill deer in the slaughterhouse has been used, but more frequently, it is the method of choice for semi-domesticated or wild deer shot in the field so avoiding the stress of transport. A .22 calibre rifle has been recommended for use at short range or a .32 calibre 'humane killer', but not placed directly against the head. The recommended sites include the following:

1 Frontally, using the intersection point of the lines from the base of each ear to the opposite eye and firing horizontally into the forehead
2 Firing through the skull just behind the base of the antlers in the direction of the animals muzzle
3 For reindeer with large antlers in a lateral position (temporal region) under the base of the antlers, between the outer canthus of the eye and the base of the ear

Slaughter of ostriches

Ostriches are slaughtered at 9 or 10 months of age for meat and at approximately 14 months of age to obtain optimal leather quality. The most common methods of slaughter are percussive penetrative captive bolt and low-voltage electrical stunning.

While the penetrative captive bolt stuns ostriches effectively, it is not known whether this is produced by physical destruction of the neural tissue, bleeding of the brain or concussion. Parts of the skull overlying the hemispheres were found to be very thin (especially in Emus), and it is not known whether sufficient energy to produce concussion could be generated. The recommended sites are as follows:

1 The intersection point of two lines drawn between the base of the ears and the contralateral eyes
2 Placing the penetrative captive bolt on the crown with the bolt pointing in the direction of the throat

With both sites, the head has to be restrained to allow for accurate operation of the pistol. Following an effective stun, the bird collapses and enters a tonic followed by a violent clonic phase which may compromise operator safety and make it difficult to bleed the ostrich quickly.

Electrical stunning of ostriches is carried out using scissor-like tongs with spiked electrodes, applied between the eye and ear for 3–6 seconds delivering on average 500 mA (500 V). Due to the duration of the stunned state (25 seconds), it has been recommended that a short stun-to-stick interval be used or that birds should be killed by a current of long duration, for instance, over 6 seconds. A damp hood placed over the ostrich's head in the lairage has been found to greatly assist in the handling of the bird and accurate placement of the electrodes.

Slaughter of rabbits

Traditionally, rabbits were slaughtered by a percussive blow to the head using a wooden baton or a metal pipe. In commercial abattoirs, the main method used is

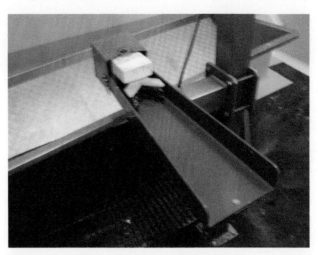

Figure 7.7 Device for electrical stunning of rabbits.

electrical stunning although penetrative captive bolts have been used.

Electrical stunning is carried out using a handheld or wall-mounted V-shaped spiked electrode. The rabbit is supported by the operative in one hand while the other guides the rabbits head into the V-shaped electrode so that contact is made between the outer corners of the eye and the base of the ears thus spanning the brain. The impedance across rabbits' heads due to their fur is considerable, between 300 and 1500 Ohms, so it is difficult to recommend minimum voltages to deliver the current required for an effective stun. However, extrapolation from other species suggests that 400 mA should be used. Operator safety must be considered as the rabbits are held throughout stunning (Fig. 7.7).

For percussive penetrative captive bolt stunning, the rabbit is restrained in sternal recumbency to allow accurate positioning of the pistol at right angles to the skull with the muzzle positioned slightly paramedial on the animal's head between or as close to its ears as possible.

Gaseous stunning of rabbits would remove the inevitable stress which occurs when they are handled pre-stunning in the abattoir environment. However, it has not been scientifically investigated whether the induction phase might cause the animal pain or distress or, indeed, the correct exposure time/concentrations required to give a reliable stun.

Other methods of slaughter

In Spain, parts of Italy, Mexico and some South American countries, *cattle* were traditionally slaughtered by the *neck-stab* or *evernazione* method, in which a short double-edged knife (*puntilla*) is plunged into the occipito-atlantal space at the nape of the neck, severing the medulla oblongata. This effectively immobilises the animal without inducing insensibility. The technique has been criticised since animals slaughtered in this way show a photomotor reflex considered by some experts to be indicative of a state of sensibility (Lumb and Jones, 1973).

In the Arctic, *reindeer* are killed by a curved single-edged knife which after being inserted into the occipito-atlantal space, is directed forwards to destroy the brain.

In India and in the Far East, practically all animals are slaughtered while conscious. In India, the majority of sheep and goats are killed by a method in which the throat is cut transversely as in the Jewish method of slaughter. The Sikh or Jakta method is also practised, the sheep or goat being decapitated by one stroke of a special sword.

Slaughter of poultry (see also Ch. 10)

With poultry, the speed of operations, which may be typically 6000 birds/hour, complicates the stunning procedure, as it does all other procedures. Indeed *the requirement for speed is a major factor in reducing the standard of all operations in modern slaughter and processing plants for all species of animals.*

With all stunning methods used for poultry, it is important that both common carotid arteries are severed by the bleeding system, whether automated or manual, in order to ensure that birds to not regain consciousness. Gregory and Wilkins (1989a) demonstrated that cutting all the major blood vessels in the necks of electrically stunned chickens resulted in loss of blood amounting to 2% of body weight in less than 25 seconds after neck cutting.

Electrical stunning of poultry

Several types of electrical stunning device are utilised for poultry depending on the processing speed.

Handheld head-only stunning devices must be of a design suitable for the species of bird to be stunned. Electrodes vary in size, in the surface area in contact with the head of the bird, in the impedance of the electrode and in the pressure which can be applied to the bird's head. In addition the nature of the current, whether pulsed direct current (DC) or sine wave AC, the frequency of the current and its waveform significantly alter the time/voltage combination required to deliver the current which will result in an effective stun. As an example of this, the voltage necessary to deliver a fixed amount of current at a given resistance seems to be higher with a pulsed DC than sine wave AC and it also increases with increasing frequency (Fig. 7.8).

Given these difficulties, it has been recommended that a minimum average current of 240 and 400 mA should be applied for a minimum of 7 seconds to chickens and

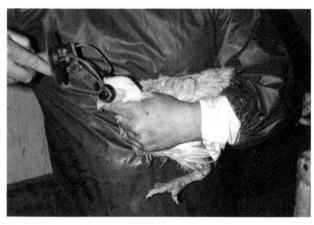

Figure 7.8 Handheld electrical stunning of poultry.

turkeys, respectively, when using a handheld head-only constant voltage stunner (110 V) supplied with a frequency of 50 Hz AC. Neck cutting should be carried out, incising both carotids, within 15 seconds from the end of the stun. If a variable-voltage, constant-current stunner delivering sine wave AC, with low impedance electrodes is used, minimum average currents of 100 mA/50 Hz, 150 mA/400 Hz or 200 mA/1500 Hz are recommended and applied for a minimum of 1 second.

For ducks, a constant current of not less than 600 mA/50 Hz, applied for 4 seconds, is recommended.

Manually operated stunning devices are only suitable for low rates of kill – up to 300 birds/hour. Assessment of the effectiveness of stunning with handheld electrodes can be difficult. This is particularly the case with ducks and geese where the birds may be confined in cones. An initial period of wing flapping and leg flexion on induction is followed by a distinct tonic seizure with stiffening and arching of the neck, rigidly extended legs, wings folded tightly around the breast and constant body movements. It is important to emphasise that correctly stunned birds can maintain a nictitating membrane and other eye reflexes.

Electric water baths can be used for both stunning and killing poultry. The method requires the hanging of birds upside down, their legs having been placed in a metal shackle specifically designed for the particular species and type of bird. The shackling procedure causes birds significant distress; wing flapping is normal and, under commercial line speeds of 6 000–10 000/hour, dislocations and fractures do occur. Birds are transferred in the inverted position to the water bath. Their heads pass through the electrified water, and the current passes through the whole body towards the shackle, stunning or killing the bird. It is imperative that birds cease flapping prior to the water bath or they may receive pre-stun electrical shocks which are thought to be extremely painful and distressing for them. This is a particular problem with turkeys where, due to their wingspan, the wings tend to hang below the level of the head. Pre-stun shocks can be reduced by providing an insulated entry ramp to the bath, avoiding overflow of water at the entrance and by providing a moving belt to support the breast of the bird so that the turkey is presented to the stunner at an angle which raises the wings above the level of the head.

In an attempt to calm the birds, 'hanging on' is usually carried out in either dim (<5 lux) or blue lighting, a breast comforting strip which rubs along and supports each birds ventral surface as it passes is provided (compulsory in the EU from 2013) and a minimum time interval between shackling and stunning of 12 seconds for poultry, 20 seconds for turkeys, is allowed during which the birds may calm down. Given these parameters, the shackling to stunning period should be kept as short as possible, 1 minute for chickens and 2 minutes for turkeys.

The height of the water bath in relation to the shackles, and the level of water in the bath, should be adjusted to the size of bird to be stunned or killed so that there is at least complete immersion of the birds' heads in the water or preferably immersion up to the base of the wings. Food grade salt may be added to improve the conductivity of the water and sufficient voltage provided to deliver the recommended average currents given in Table 7.1. However, overflow from the water bath and the addition of water to maintain levels means that the salt concentration can drop quickly, so the initial addition of salt should not be relied upon to compensate for deficient water bath current. It may be necessary to add more salt or increase the voltage when the conductivity of the water drops (Perez-Palacios and Wotton, 2006).

The poor bird welfare inherent with the need to hang birds in an inverted position on shackles has been addressed in a prototype system which restrains the birds on a moving conveyer and applies an electrical stun through dry electrodes first to the head only and then head to body to induce cardiac arrest. A constant current of 150 mA/50 Hz is applied for at least 1 second across the head followed by at least 1 second across the heart. This system may have particular benefits for heavy turkeys.

Table 7.1 Minimum recommended average current (mA) delivered to birds in water bath stunning systems EFSA (2004, 2006)

Frequency (Hz)	Chickens	Turkeys	Ducks and geese
Up to 200	100	250	130
200–400	150	400	
400–1500	200	400	

Assessment of unconsciousness in electrical water bath stunned poultry

The most reliable indicator that a bird is properly stunned by a low-voltage method is the electroplectic fit. The characteristics of this condition are the neck arched with the head directly vertical, open eyes, absence of corneal reflex, wings arched, rigidly extended legs and constant rapid body tremors.

When cardiac arrest is induced, these signs are shorter lasting and they are followed by a completely limp carcase, no breathing (absence of abdominal movements in the vent area), loss of nictating membrane reflex and dilated pupils. The comb reflex can also determine whether sensibility has resumed after stunning or neck cutting. It should be borne in mind that the absence of rhythmic breathing is not a valid sign of unconsciousness in birds that have had their neck broken or severed, for example, during neck cutting.

Although cardiac arrest is preferable from a welfare standpoint, the use of high stunning currents is thought to be associated with quality issues such as wing haemorrhage, red skin conditions including red wing tips and pyrostyles, poor plucking, broken bones (in particular the furculum) and ruptured blood vessels causing blood splashing in the breast muscle.

Stunning/killing poultry with controlled atmospheres

The use of *gaseous mixtures* for the stunning of poultry in their transport crates prior to shackling has obvious benefits for welfare. Various concentrations of CO_2 and argon in air have been studied experimentally. It has been concluded that poultry do not find concentrations of CO_2 up to 30% by volume aversive. The EFSA report of 2006 recommends the following gas mixtures for use in chickens:

1 Minimum of 1 minute exposure to 40% CO_2, 30% oxygen and 30% nitrogen, the *induction phase*, followed by a minimum exposure to 80% CO_2 in air, the *finishing phase* or

2 Minimum of 2 minute exposure to any mixture of argon, nitrogen or other inert gases with atmospheric air and CO_2, provided that the CO_2 concentration does not exceed 30% by volume and the residual oxygen does not exceed 2% by volume or

3 Minimum of 2 minute exposure to argon, nitrogen, other inert gases or any mixture of these gases in atmospheric air with a maximum of 2% residual oxygen by volume.

Birds stunned with argon alone take twice as long to lose sensibility as those stunned using other mixtures, but the birds show none of the behavioural signs, such as gasping and head shaking, associated with the irritant properties of CO_2 (Raj and Gregory, 1993, 1994). It is recommended that birds should be exposed to the gaseous environment for a minimum of 2 minutes and that hanging and neck cutting in broilers should be carried out within 3 minutes of gas stunning if carcase defects such as red wing tips, wing vein engorgement/haemorrhage, shoulder haemorrhage and red feather tracts are to be minimised. However, gas stunning does result in fewer broken bones than electrical stunning, especially the broken wing bones which can enter the breast muscle, the so-called chokers; and breast muscle haemorrhages are eliminated.

It has been discovered that stunning with argon-induced anoxia accelerates the fall in muscle pH during the early post-mortem stage without inducing a PSE-like condition. Used in conjunction with air chilling at 1°C, filleting can be performed at 2 hours post-mortem. The eating quality of this meat was rated in tests as superior to that of control fillets.

Percussive stunning of poultry

Percussion stunning using both penetrative and non-penetrative captive bolt results in severe skull fractures and structural damage to the brain of poultry. A commercially available captive bolt device fitted with a non-penetrating percussive head is used to kill poultry on farm and as a backup method in commercial poultry slaughter establishments. When penetrative captive bolts are used, the bolt diameter, velocity and penetration depth are critical to achieving a humane stun/kill. The captive bolt should be fired perpendicular to the frontal bone surface with the bird restrained, usually in a cone, and the head supported by the operative's hand. The bolt diameter should be a minimum of 6 mm. Signs of an effective stun include uncontrolled and severe wing flapping, immediate loss of breathing, loss of neck tension, leg flexion and extension.

Other methods of slaughter

Traditionally *cervical dislocation* has been widely used on farm and as a backup method for slaughter in commercial poultry slaughter establishment. It is not permitted by current EU legislation to be used in slaughterhouses except as a backup method and on farm only in birds weighing less than 5 kg. It is widely considered not to cause immediate loss of consciousness but to result in death from asphyxiation or ischemia. There is also the possibility that the tissue damage inflicted by the technique may be perceived by the bird as painful.

Similarly, *decapitation* does not result in instantaneous loss of brain responsiveness. Although a flat Electrocorticogram (EcoG) is elicited within a few seconds, corneal reflexes remain in completely isolated heads for periods up to 30 seconds. In his commentary article, Bates (2010) concluded that

1 Severing the spinal cord and the tissues immediately surrounding is likely to be painful.
2 Decapitation is a painful procedure and that conscious awareness may persist for up to 29 seconds in the disembodied heads.

Effects of stunning on poultry meat quality

As with the larger farm animals, deleterious changes sometimes occur in poultry carcases after slaughter which are attributed to defects in the slaughter methods. These frequently result in downgrading and even condemnation. However, conclusions about the effects of stunning are often contradictory and at least some of the changes encountered may be occasioned by the stress of handling and transport in part, if not in whole.

A disadvantage of using 50 Hz AC water bath stunners is that, at current levels greater than 105 mA per chicken and 150 mA per turkey, there are significant increases in the incidence of haemorrhaging in the breast and leg muscles, broken bones in the carcase and the appearance of other conditions which result in carcase downgrading (Gregory and Wilkins, 1989a, 1989b).

Pithing

After *cattle* are stunned, they were sometimes pithed before bleeding by the insertion of a long thin rod or closely coiled wire into the hole made by the penetrating bolt of the pistol. The insertion of this rod destroys the motor centres of the brain so that reflex muscular action does not occur at sticking, thus avoiding injury to operatives and speeding carcase dressing. There is little evidence that this operation interferes with the bleeding of the carcase to any appreciable degree, but the pithing rod or cane should not be any longer than 0.6 m; if it is too long, the spinal cord roots of the greater splanchnic nerve, which is the main vasoconstrictor of the abdominal cavity, are destroyed. The resultant dilatation of the splanchnic blood vessels causes congestion of the liver, kidneys and intestines and, in addition, congestion and enlargement of the spleen, producing the '*slaughter spleen*'.

Pithing was used with the bed system of carcase dressing. *Under modern conditions, where cattle carcases are suspended for dressing, it is completely unnecessary provided efficient stunning and shackling are carried out, besides being very unhygienic and time-consuming.* Pithing is also contraindicated in those countries where BSE is known to exist because of the risk of contamination of meat through an increased risk of neural emboli and the potential for infection of operatives. In addition, the complete removal of a damaged spinal cord is rendered impossible. Consequently, as a result of European Commission Decision 2000/418, pithing is no longer permitted for animals slaughtered for human consumption within the EU.

There is some evidence that bacteria can be introduced into the carcase on the pithing cane and subsequently dispersed throughout the carcase before the heart stops beating. It is therefore imperative that if pithing is carried out, the cane is sterilised between use on each animal.

Bleeding

Bleeding following stunning must always be carried out without delay since even when stun-to-kill methods are deployed, they may not always be effective.

The circulating blood volume in animals is estimated to be 8% of body weight. Specific volumes for each species are given in the following text. Approximately 40–60% of the total blood is lost at bleeding.

Cattle

There are two main methods of bleeding *cattle*:

1 *Bilateral severance of the carotid arteries and jugular veins* by an incision across the throat region caudal to the larynx as in ritual slaughter
2 Incision in the jugular furrow at the base of the neck, the knife being directed towards the entrance of the chest to sever the *brachiocephalic trunk* and *anterior vena cava*

Care must be taken not to pass the knife too far towards the chest for, if the pleura is punctured, blood may be aspirated into the thoracic cavity and adhere to the parietal pleura, particularly along the posterior edges of the ribs. This contamination is known as *back bleeding or over sticking* and, may necessitate stripping of the pleura. In cattle, the blood cannot infiltrate between the pleura and contiguous chest wall; this may occasionally occur in pigs but over a small area immediately posterior to the first rib.

Current abattoir practice is to stun cattle and then hoist them, by the shackling of a hind leg, over a bleeding gully. The advantage of a bleeding rail is that it permits centralised collection of blood and also accelerates the throughput of animals, allowing them to be stunned and removed in quick succession through the same stunning pen. Observations have shown that bleeding was 40% more effective in cattle bled on the rail than in those bled in a horizontal position (Fig. 7.9).

If unilateral sticking at the base of the neck is performed, it is of value to make other small bilateral incisions at the angle of the jaw, severing the jugulars at

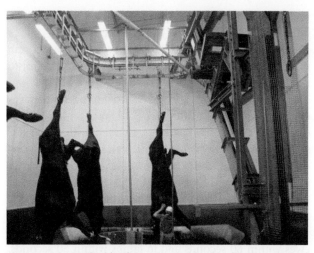

Figure 7.9 Cattle bleeding over a blood collection channel (Reproduced with permission from Sarah Jackson).

their division into *internal and external maxillary veins*; this permits easier skinning of heads and also reduces the quantity of blood in the lingual artery. The vertical head-down position of the suspended carcase otherwise causes blood to be retained in the head.

The ordinary bleeding knife severs blood vessels more rapidly if the blade is held at right angles to the direction of the vessels and longitudinal axis of the body.

Whichever method is employed, bleeding should continue for 6 minutes. The average *yield of blood* obtained in *cattle* slaughter is 13.6 kg. *Cows* yield more blood than bulls or bullocks of the same weight, in some cases up to 22.6 kg in old cows. About 57.3% of the blood is yielded in the first 30 seconds after sticking, 76.6% after 60 seconds and 90% after 120 seconds.

In *calves*, the incision was at one time at the side of the neck with the severing of the jugular vein. The purpose of this was to produce slow bleeding after the carcase was hung up prior to dressing, for slow bleeding ensure the desirable white colour of veal. Calves are now bled rapidly at the level of the first rib, and yield 2.7 kg of blood.

Sheep

In the slaughter of sheep, bleeding is usually carried out by an incision in the jugular furrows close to the head, severing both *carotid arteries* and *jugular veins*. However, *thoracic inlet bleeding* is superior as it reduces the risk of contamination of the cut surfaces with ruminal content from the severed oesophagus which frequently occurs with the former method. However, accidental cutting of the oesophagus may still occur with this method. At one time, when cradle dressing was carried out, it was customary to jerk the head back sharply in order to rupture the spinal cord where it enters the skull, the purpose being, as in the pithing of cattle, to minimise reflex muscular action before dressing of the carcase. Like pithing, it is an unnecessary procedure.

The most satisfactory type of knife for the lateral stab method, where the bleeding knife is inserted posterior to the trachea and oesophagus, is one with a blade about 23 cm long and 4 cm wide with a straight back unsharpened except at the tip, and a tapered point on the cutting edge of about 8 cm. The knife is fitted with a circular safety guard between blade and handle. The unsharpened edge is placed in contact with the oesophagus, but it may puncture this organ if the knife is withdrawn at the wrong angle. Even when great care is taken with this technique, both carotid arteries may not be severed.

Approximately 75% of the available blood is lost from ewes within 60 seconds and in lambs within 50 seconds. Electrically stunned lambs bleed more rapidly than those stunned with the captive bolt. There was no significant difference in the rates of bleeding between sheep that are not stunned and those stunned with the captive bolt pistol.

Bilateral severance is the easiest technique to perform and produces satisfactory bleeding. This is the best method for bleeding sheep in lateral recumbency. When both carotid arteries are severed, the sheep loses brain response in less than 14 seconds; if only one carotid artery is severed, insensibility can take more than 70 seconds to occur.

In contrast with cattle, which bleed more fully in the head-down position, trials with sheep at the UK Meat Research Institute have shown that sheep bled in the horizontal position lose approximately 10% more blood than those suspended vertically.

Bleeding of the sheep carcase should last for 5 minutes, the amount of blood obtained from a slaughtered sheep being 1–2.5 kg, lambs having the lower weights.

Pigs

In pigs, the knife is inserted in the midline of the neck at the depression in front of the sternum, and is then pushed towards the heart to sever the *anterior vena cava* brachiocephalic trunk at the entrance of the chest; sometimes the carotid artery is also pierced. Care should be taken not to insert the knife too far as it may penetrate into the shoulder, allowing blood and water from the scalding tank to run back into the shoulder 'pocket' beneath the scapula giving its wall a cooked appearance. The carcase should not be placed immediately in the scalding tank; too large a sticking wound and contaminated scalding water facilitate the entry of microorganisms into the carcase tissues by way of the jugular vein and may lead to spoilage. In some abattoirs, pigs are stunned, then hoisted and bled while suspended (Fig. 7.10).

Urination occurring, after electric stunning, while the pig is bleeding renders the blood unmarketable, but this

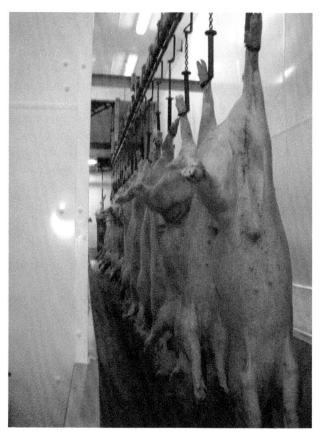

Figure 7.10 Pigs bleeding over a blood collection channel (Reproduced with permission from David Armstrong).

may be overcome by using the hollow knife. Pigs should be allowed to bleed for 6 minutes, as during this period the muscles relax and the hair is more readily removed during scalding.

Pork pigs yield 2.2 kg of blood, bacon pigs 3 kg, while boars and sows yield 3.6 kg.

In many abattoirs, *prone sticking* of pigs has been adopted. After being rendered unconscious, the animal is discharged on to a conveyor belt and is stuck while lying prone in the tonic phase, the blood draining into a trough running parallel to the conveyor.

Immediately after sticking, the animals may come under a holding-down belt which continues the full length of the conveyor and restrains the involuntary struggling that occurs during the clonic phase. The advantages of prone sticking of electrically stunned pigs are the more efficient recovery of blood and the elimination of ruptured joints and joint capsules, which are a troublesome condition in pigs bled while suspended and are the cause of the so-called *internal ham bruising*. In addition, a study in Austria found that the incidence of PSE meat was reduced from 62–63% in vertically bled pigs, to 22–27% in those bled in the horizontal position.

For *sterile collection* of quantities of blood, the necessary equipment (stainless steel hollow knifes, vacuum pump, sterilisation facilities, anticoagulant injection, containers, etc.) must be available. The incision at the base of the neck provides a larger flow of blood evenly and more hygienically than procedures not so geared. Sterile blood collection must be efficient and rapid; otherwise the rate of kill will be considerably reduced.

Efficiency of bleeding

It was once thought that the efficiency of bleeding had a most important bearing on the subsequent keeping quality of the carcase. Studies have been unable to demonstrate any correlation between the amount of blood lost at the time of slaughter and subsequent pH values, water content, bacterial counts, flavour and tenderness of beef or lamb. The extra blood retained by the poorly bled animal is retained mainly in the viscera and skin.

The stunning of an animal by any means produces a rise in the blood pressure of the arterial, capillary and venous systems, and in sheep, the normal arterial blood pressure of 120–145 mm Hg may rise to 260 mm Hg or over when the animal is stunned prior to bleeding. This is accompanied by a transitory increase in the heart rate. Both of these factors will facilitate immediate bleeding. The importance of *immediate bleeding* is obvious when it is realised that the rate of flow of blood from a cut vessel is 5–10 times more rapid than blood flow in the intact vessel, and not until 20% of the blood has been lost does the pressure begin to fall. If an undue interval is allowed to elapse between stunning and bleeding, the carcase may be imperfectly bled and may exhibit blood splashing.

Slaughter without pre-stunning

The Farm Animal Welfare Council (2003) concluded that slaughter without pre-stunning was unacceptable since, even under ideal conditions, the basic principles that pre-slaughter handling facilities should minimise stress and that unconsciousness should be induced without distress were not satisfactorily observed. However, it remains a fact that this same accusation could be laid at the door of many of the other accepted slaughter techniques previously described in this chapter. There is room for considerable argument as to the pain caused by the cut itself. It is unlikely that the slaughter process will be sufficiently stressful to induce the physiological flight response which would result in endogenous opioid analgesia, and it can be argued that the restraint prevents normal escape reactions. The cut across the throat severing the trachea will prevent the normal vocalisation associated with injury. Attempts to assess the distress

that may be inherent in cutting the tissues, by measuring the reaction of blood hormone levels, are likely to be unreliable since the cut prevents ACTH from the adrenal cortex reaching the adrenal glands.

A study by Gibson *et al.* (2009), measuring EcoG effects in calves, demonstrated that the act of slaughter by ventral neck incision is associated with substantial noxious stimulation that would be expected to be perceived as painful in the period between incision and loss of consciousness.

There have been calls, particularly from animal welfare organisations, that meat produced from animals slaughtered without pre-stunning should be labelled as such. This is in recognition of the fact that the significant quantities of meat slaughtered without stunning are placed on the market for general sale.

Shechita – Jewish religious slaughter

The Jewish method of slaughter is controlled in Britain by the Jewish Board of Shechita, and Jewish slaughter men have to undergo several years of training before being licensed by the Rabbinical Commission. They are also subject to annual examination of skills by the Commission.

In order for meat to be *kosher*, that is, right, fulfilling the requirements of Jewish law, animals must be slaughtered and dressed according to ritual methods specified in the Talmud, the body of Jewish law and legend based on the Torah which is the substance of God's revelation to man in the Old Testament (Pentateuch, first five books). The reference to Shechita is said to be found in Deuteronomy 12:21 – 'thou shalt kill of thy herd and of thy flock, which the Lord hath given thee, as I have commanded thee'.

At slaughter, the animal must be healthy and have suffered no injury. Pre-stunning of the animal is therefore forbidden. Animals that do not conform to these ideals and any defects at slaughter in the form of faults in *shechita* (act of killing for food) or disease lesions discovered in the carcase render the meat *terefa*, that is, unfit for consumption by Jews. Likewise, animals that lie quietly and cannot be made to rise must not be slaughtered according to Jewish ritual. This early recognition of the inadmissibility of ill or moribund animals for human food is worthy of note.

Shechita is performed by a *shochet*, or cutter, who slaughters the fully conscious animal with a single, deliberate, swift action of a razor-sharp knife, the *chalaf*. It is roughly twice the width of the animal's neck and is devoid of any notch or flaw, and has been examined before the slaughter of each animal. All the soft structures anterior to the cervical spine are severed, including the carotid arteries and jugular veins. It is essential that the neck be fully extended in order to keep the edges of the wound open and thereby, it is said, prevent any pain.

The *five rules of Jewish ritual slaughter*, in their traditional order, are that the neck incision shall be completed without pause, pressure, stabbing, slanting or tearing. If the knife receives any nick, however small, during the act of shechita, the slaughter is not correctly performed and the use of the meat is not permitted for Jewish food.

The shochet ('cutter') is normally assisted by a sealer (*shomer*) who is responsible for putting the kosher mark on the brisket and on edible offal. In some instances, for example, large kosher slaughter plants, several shochets may work together in the task of slaughter and tagging meat.

Besides performing the act of slaughter, the shochet offers prayers and carries out a 'postmortem examination' by making an incision posterior to the xiphoid process and inserting the arm to detect any adhesions in the thoracic cavity ('searching'). Full meat inspection may be performed by a shochet or by the government inspector. Should the carcase be held in the chill room for more than 24 hours, it must be washed in order to remove blood; further washing and curing, *mehila*, or broiling is carried out in the home.

Carcases found fit for consumption must have the meat porged by removing the large blood vessels in the forequarter prior to retail sale. Only forequarters are normally used, since the hindquarters, which are said to contain over 50 blood vessels, can only be porged by highly skilled kosher butchers and are therefore rarely eaten. 'Only be sure that thou eat not the blood; for the blood is the life; and thou mayest not eat the life with the flesh' (*Deuteronomy* 12:23).

Kosher slaughter restraining systems (also used for Halal slaughter) were developed to overcome the pain and distress associated with the practice of 'shackling and hoisting' conscious cattle. The shackling and hoisting of conscious cattle is forbidden in most western societies, but kosher slaughter is exempt from this requirement. The Weinberg restraint pen permits a bovine animal to be rotated through 180° causing significant distress to the animal. Its use has consequently been banned in some countries. A version of the Weinberg, the Facomia pen, is considered by some observers to induce less stress in the cattle. Turning cattle to a position between upright and lateral recumbency (45° or 90°) has the potential to decrease stress. This has been recognised by the Netherlands where it is mandatory for all cattle slaughtered without stunning to be placed on their side (Fig. 7.11).

The ASPCA (American Society for the Prevention of Cruelty to Animals) restrainer pen, first invented by Peter Hoad of Canada Packers, Toronto, Canada, was further developed and modified by the Cincinnati Butchers' Supply Company and by Temple Grandin (1980). It takes the form of a metal pen fitted with a belly plate, a rear pusher on a guillotine door and a front neck yoke and chin lift. Hydraulic controls are used to operate the equipment and position the animal for kosher and halal slaughter. The rear pusher and chin lift should be equipped with

<table>
<tr><td>(a)</td><td>(b)</td></tr>
<tr><td>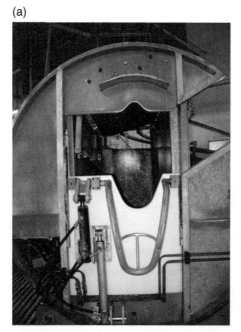</td><td>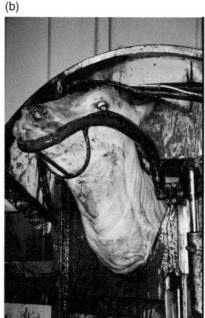</td></tr>
</table>

Figure 7.11 (a) Rotating restraint pen of the Facomia type; (b) close-up of the head restraint (Reproduced with permission from Karen von Holleben).

pressure-limiting devices. While the cut is being made, the hind leg is shackled to withdraw the animal from the pen. There is no doubt that the Cincinnati-Boss (CB) pen is much less stressful on the animal than the Weinberg pen, but it is by no means perfect. One defect is the manner of withdrawal of the animal from the pen, which in some types of CB pen pulls the hind leg in an unnatural manner which must result in hip joint damage. Some stress inevitably occurs due to restraint and raising of the head. Dunn (1990) compared a rotating Weinberg pen and the ASPCA pen for slaughter of cattle in the upright position. He found that the mean time for which the animal was restrained in the Weinberg pen, from the rear gate was secure until the throat was cut was 103.8 seconds, of which the animal spent on average 70% (73 seconds) in the inverted position. By contrast, the animal spent on average 11.1 seconds in the ASPCA pen before its throat was severed. In addition, the animal struggled more, especially during inversion and vocalised more, with the Weinberg than with the ASPCA pen (Fig. 7.12).

A problem with all types of casting pen is that the cattle tend to aspirate blood. This does not occur when the animal is held in the upright position. It has been reported that the presence of blood on the equipment does not appear to upset the cattle and that in fact some animals have been observed to lick the blood.

Restrainer systems have been manufactured to deal with *small farm animals* – calves and sheep. In one of these US items of equipment, which is used for both conventional and religious slaughter, the animal is conveyed straddlewise along a double rail above which is a head cage which positions the head upwards for the neck cut. Many sheep are slaughtered without pre-stunning by manually restraining them on the floor with their head lifted or by placing them on their side on a cradle.

It is claimed that the Jewish method of slaughter does not involve any act of cruelty because the knife is particularly sharp, the cut is made dextrously by a trained person and the severance of the carotid vessels is followed by a very rapid fall in blood pressure within the cephalic arteries. It is therefore suggested that the anoxia from the diminished blood supply to the brain tissues, causing loss of brain structure, brings about almost immediate unconsciousness. Others contend that it is not anoxia which results in the collapse of the animal but rather cerebral shock due to the sudden fall in pressure of the CSF. Gibson *et al.* (2009) carried out histological examination of the brains from animals slaughtered by ventral neck incision and found no evidence to support these hypotheses.

Opponents of the Jewish method of slaughter have also contended that additional blood, via the *vertebral artery*, and therefore independent of the carotid supply, may still reach the brain of cattle and prolong the period of consciousness. (The vertebral artery, being enclosed in the vertebral column, is not severed in the Jewish or Muslim method of slaughter.) Anatomical differences in the blood supply to the brain occur in the various species of animals. In the sheep and goat, the complete brain is supplied with blood from the common carotid arteries; the vertebral arteries supply only the anterior spinal cord and the posterior medulla oblongata. However, it has been shown experimentally in calves that the vertebral arteries can carry enough blood to maintain consciousness when both common carotid arteries are occluded. Very little blood is required to maintain consciousness, especially in the head-down position and in young animals which have a greater resistance to anoxia. It has been estimated that without stunning, the time between cutting through the major blood vessels and insensibility, as deduced from behavioural and brain responses, is up to 20 seconds in sheep, up to 25 seconds in pigs and up to 2 minutes in cattle. Some estimates have suggested that calves can take up to 5 minutes to become insensible. However, Rosen (2004) in his defence of shechita argues that the experimental evidence demonstrates that on severing the carotids, the flow of blood through the vertebral artery of calves is reversed, away from the brain, taking the route of least resistance.

A factor of considerable importance is that after the carotid arteries of cattle are severed transversely, they tend, by virtue of their elasticity and as a physiological response to the fall in blood pressure, to retract rapidly within their own external connective tissue coat, thus narrowing the arteries and slowing bleeding. As the blood pressure in the anterior aorta will then be maintained by the heart action, the blood pressure in the vertebral artery may likewise be maintained at a substantial level, and unconsciousness may therefore be delayed. Such sealing can and does occur, in some cases very rapidly, and provides an explanation why some cattle, the throats of which have been cut by the Jewish method, have been known to regain their feet and walk a considerable distance before they have eventually succumbed some minutes later. It is imperative that the slaughterman does not interfere with the neck in an attempt to ensure a good blood flow in the period immediately following the cut as this is likely to cause unnecessary distress and is unlikely to achieve its objective.

The assertion by supporters of Jewish slaughter that bleeding of the animal is more complete than in other methods of slaughter has been challenged by some authorities who contend that the paler colour of the flesh of Jewish slaughtered animals is due to the violent respiratory efforts which accompany ritual slaughter, these having the effect of increasing the proportion of oxyhaemoglobin in the

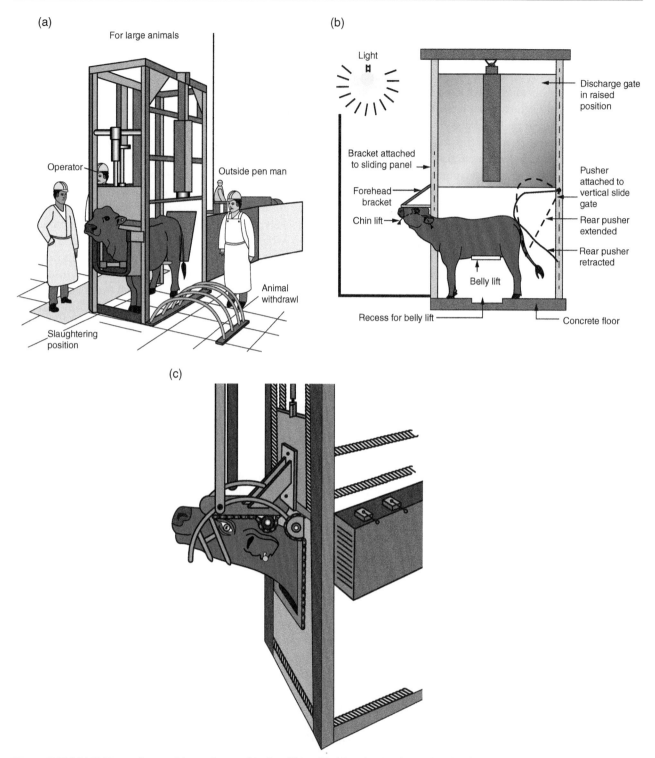

Figure 7.12 (a) ASPCA restraint pen; (b) restraint pen side view; (c) head-hold mechanism (Reproduced with permission from Karen von Holleben).

blood, thus rendering the residual blood in the carcase paler than normal and giving the flesh a well-bled appearance.

The important issue is whether or not the animal is suffering pain during the period of consciousness following cutting of the carotids and jugulars. The evidence presented by the studies of Gibson *et al.*

(2009) would suggest that, in cattle, the answer is that they are.

Muslim methods of slaughter

Many of the practices relating to the slaughter of animals and the consumption of meat by members of the Jewish faith also apply to Muslims. The welfare of the animal is a major consideration in both cases, and the eating of dead animals, blood and swine is forbidden.

The actual method of slaughter is virtually the same for both religions. The Quran describes the procedure of carotid and jugular section as the 'cutting and draining of blood'. The act of slaughter (*Al-Dhabh*) is allowed in the name of God; therefore, pronouncing the name of Allah is the usual practice. This is to remind the slaughterer that he is taking the life of a living creature.

Animals must not be slaughtered in the sight of other beasts, and those to be killed are to be fed and watered beforehand. The act of cutting the skin with a sharp knife is regarded as painless, or almost so, and the rapid loss of blood is said to produce instantaneous insensibility. Just as defective methods may be used in stunning by mechanical means so also can throat cutting be imperfectly performed with the result that not all four blood vessels are severed. Islamic law demands that the animal is alive at the time of slaughter and that it is slaughtered in a humane manner. The Prophet Mohammed is reported as saying that 'God who is blessed and exalted has declared that everything should be done in a good way; so when you kill, use a good method, and when you cut an animal's throat, you should use a good method; for each of you should sharpen his knife and give the animal as little pain as possible'.

Unlike Shechita, the Muslim method of slaughter is not controlled by a central board but is overseen by the local Islamic authority who decides whether or not particular acts and thoughts conform to the tenets of Islamic Law (*Shariah*). So in some instances, prior stunning with electricity or captive bolt pistol is allowed. (In New Zealand, a head-only stun of 0.5–0.9 A for 3 seconds is performed for sheep and 2.5 A for cattle, the major blood vessels being severed within 10 seconds of the stun.) Immediate post-cutting electrical stunning is increasingly used a practice which is to be encouraged. It is also understood that non-penetrative concussive, stunning has been permitted in some quarters. Provided it can be shown that the heart is still beating after stunning, prior anaesthesia is approved, at least in some instances.

Slaughter of poultry without stunning

For slaughter without stunning, poultry are usually manually restrained or confined to cones of appropriate size before neck cutting.

Most chickens lose consciousness in 12–15 seconds, but signs of consciousness are possible up to 26 seconds after the cut (Barnett, Cronin and Scott, 2007). This is similar to the mean time reported for loss of posture, 13.9 seconds.

The efficiency of the process depends on the cutting of both carotid arteries and both jugular veins. In contrast with cattle, the vertebral artery is not involved in the blood supply to the brain. The cutting of all four blood vessels can be difficult to achieve in practice due to the carotid arteries being close to the spine and the need not to touch the spine with the knife which could render the carcase unfit for kosher requirements.

This slaughter method can be considered to have the advantage over conventional water bath electrical stunning in that in this low throughput method the birds are not shackled until they are dead.

References

Barnett, J.L., Cronin, G.M. and Scott, P.C. (2007) *Veterinary Record*, **160**, 45–49.

Bates, G. (2010) *Journal of the American Veterinary Medical Association*, **237** (9), 1024–1026.

Bremner, F. (1954) *Brain Mechanisms and Consciousness* (ed. J.F. Delafresnaye), Oxford University Press, London.

Coore, R.R., Love, S., McKinstry, J.L. *et al.* (2005) *Journal of Food Protection*, **68** (4), 882–884.

Dunn, C.S. (1990) *Veterinary Record*, **26**, 522–525.

Ewbank, R., Parker M.J. and Mason C. (1992) *Animal Welfare*, **1**, 55–64.

Farm Animal Welfare Council (2003) *Report on the Welfare of Farmed Animals at Slaughter or Killing – Part 1, Red Meat animals*, DEFRA Publications, London.

Garland, T.D., Bauer, N. and Bailey, M. (1996) *The Lancet*, **348**, 610.

Gibson, T.J., Johnson, C.B., Mellor, D.J. and Stafford, K.J. (2009) *New Zealand Veterinary Journal*, **57**, 77–95.

Grandin, T. (1980) *International Journal of the Study of Animal Problems*, **1** (6), 375.

Gregory, N.G. and Wilkins, L.J. (1989a) *Journal of Science of Food and Agriculture*, **47**, 13–20.

Gregory, N.G. and Wilkins, L.J. (1989b) *Veterinary Record*, **124**, 530–532.

Lambooij, D.L.O. (1996) *Meat Focus International* (April), pp. 124–125.

Lumb, W.V. and Jones, E.W. (1973) *Veterinary Anaesthesia*. Lea & Febiger, Philadelphia, pp. 338–340.

Perez-Palacios, S. and Wotton, S.B. (2006) *Veterinary record*, **158**, 654–657.

Raj, A.B.M. (1999) *Veterinary Record*, **144**, 165–168.

Raj, A.B.M. and Gregory, N.G. (1993) *Veterinary Record*, **133**, 317.

Raj, A.B.M. and Gregory, N.G. (1994) *Veterinary Record*, **135**, 222–223.

Raj, A.B.M. and Gregory, N.G. (1995) *Animal Welfare*, **4**, 273–280.

Rosen, S.D. (2004) *Veterinary Record*, **154**, 759–765.

Shaw, N.A. (2002) *Progress in Neurobiology*, **67**, 281–344.

Thorpe, W.H. (1965) The assessment of pain and stress in animals. Appendix III. Report of Technical Committee to enquire into the welfare of animals kept under intensive livestock husbandry systems. Cmnd 2836. HMSO, London.

Van der Wal, P.G. (1983) in *Stunning Animals for Slaughter* (ed G. Eikelenboom), Martinus Nijhof, The Hague.

Warriss, P.D., Brown, S.N. and Adams, S.J.M. (1994) *Meat Science*, **38**, 329–340.

Wotton, S.B., Gregory, N.G., Whittington, P.E. and Parkman, I.D. (2000) *Veterinary Record*, **147**, 681–684.

Further reading

European Union (2002) Scientific Steering Committee report, Scientific Opinion on Stunning Methods and BSE Risks.

European Food Safety Authority (2004) EFSA – AHAW/04-027 Welfare Aspects of Animal Stunning and Killing Methods. Scientific Report of the Scientific Panel for Animal Health and Welfare on a request from the Commission relating to welfare aspects of animal stunning and killing methods, http://www.efsa.europa.eu/cs/BlobServer/ScientificOpinion/opinion ahaw 02 ei45 stunnina report v2 en1.pdf?ssbinarv=true (accessed on 16 April 2014).

EFSA (2006) EFSA report on the welfare aspects of the main systems of stunning and killing applied to commercially farmed deer, goats, rabbits, ostriches, ducks, geese and quail. *Annex to the EFSA Journal*, **326**, 1–18.

Humane Slaughter Association (1993) Guidance Notes 2: Captive Bolt Stunning of Livestock, www.hsa.org.uk/publications/publications (accessed 29 April 2014).

Humane Slaughter Association (1994) Guidance Notes 1: Electrical Stunning of Sheep, Goats and Pigs, 2nd edn, www.hsa.org.uk/publications/publications (accessed 29 April 2014).Humane Slaughter Association (1995) Practical Slaughter of Poultry: A Guide for the Small Producer, 2nd edn, www.hsa.org.uk/publications/publications (accessed 29 April 2014).

8

Meat hygiene practice

Meat and animal by-products

Hygienic production

Slaughterhouse operators are responsible for developing and implementing effective food safety management procedures to eliminate or minimise the impact, as far as possible, of all the hazards encountered during dressing. Good manufacturing practice (GMP) and good hygiene practice (GHP) are the cornerstones of hazard control systems. These must be supported by robust prerequisites, also known as sanitary performance standards, and be enhanced and consolidated by applied hazard analysis and critical control point (HACCP)-based procedures – see also Chapter 9.

One of the most important roles of the meat hygiene team within the abattoir is the independent verification of the food safety management system in place. This involves the inspectors allowing the operator the autonomy to operate their own system of monitoring, verification and corrective action, while evaluating the outcome of these controls to ensure they deliver hygienically prepared meat and raw material for edible co-products as well as controlling waste and rejected materials. The inspectorate must be prepared to take effective action when the operators system is flawed or not implemented as intended and the operator fails to identify or correct the problem.

Sources of contamination (See also Chapter 6)

The classic work of Empey and Scott (1939) in Australia dealt with the sources of contamination of meat. They showed that the main sources of contamination were hides and hair, soil, contents of the stomach and gut, water, airborne pollution, utensils and equipment.

The chief source of bacteriological contamination was found to be the hide and hair of the slaughtered animals, deriving mainly from the microflora of the pasture soil, but with a higher incidence of yeasts. Then, as today, the transfer of microorganisms from the hide to the underlying tissues was found to begin during the first stage of removal of the pelt by means of knives used for skinning. Further transfer occurs via the hands, arms, legs and clothing of operatives.

A similar study carried out in 1996 by Bell and Hathaway in New Zealand demonstrated that there has been little improvement in the general hygienic status of dressed carcases over the intervening years.

Outer integument – hide, hair, fleece or skin

One of the main sources of carcase contamination is the outer surface of the live animal itself, particularly in winter months when the animals are housed. A survey of 600 cattle hides in Northern Ireland during the 1960s showed that the average weight of manure, soil and other dirt adhering to them was 4 kg, with a range of 0.9–15.8 kg; weights of 36 kg have been recorded in England (Gracey, unpublished data). The prevalence of zoonotic bacteria, on both hide and fleece, has been confirmed by a number of studies, the conclusions of which are summarised in Table 8.1.

Current observations would suggest that although husbandry practices have changed since the 1960s, the filthy state of many cattle entering the abattoir as a raw material for food has not. It is essential, as discussed in previous chapters, that livestock be presented for slaughter in as clean and dry a condition as possible, this being achieved by hygienic practices on the farm, in transport lorries and in market and in the slaughter establishment's lairage pens.

Gracey's Meat Hygiene, Eleventh Edition. Edited by David S. Collins and Robert J. Huey.
© 2015 John Wiley & Sons, Ltd. Published 2015 by John Wiley & Sons, Ltd.

Table 8.1 Prevalence of zoonotic agents on cattle hides (various studies)

Zoonotic agent	Prevalence on cattle hides (%)
E. coli O157	1.0–27.8
Salmonella	5.5–10
Campylobacter	0–33

In Finland, the problem of excessively dirty cattle being presented for slaughter was greatly reduced by the application of a series of rules agreed by meat inspection veterinarians, farmers, the meat industry, the leather industry and the state veterinary department. Under this agreement, excessively dirty animals are detained to be slaughtered separately after the clean animals, the extra cost incurred being billed to the owners involved. This has resulted in a decrease in the numbers of excessively dirty cattle by 85% (Ridell and Korkeala, 1993).

In the United Kingdom, a clean livestock policy was introduced during 1997. It was very successful in ensuring that cleaner cattle and sheep were slaughtered for human consumption. Until the advent of the revised European food hygiene legislation in 2006, those considered by the official veterinarian to be in an unacceptable state at ante-mortem inspection had to be cleaned up in the lairage before being re-presented for ante-mortem inspection. Animals unable to be adequately or effectively cleaned for welfare or health and safety reasons were consigned to by-product or, in rare cases, allowed to return home. Since 2006 in Europe, the slaughterhouse operator has assumed the responsibility for determining the condition of cleanliness that their production process can effectively deal with. These procedures must be built into the food safety management controls to be monitored and verified by their own system and meeting the process hygiene criteria set in European microbiological criteria regulation. The slaughterhouse operator's system is subject to the independent verification of the official veterinarian and inspection team.

Gastrointestinal tract

Accidental puncture of the stomach and intestines is a source of contamination on occasions, as is spillage from the rectum and oesophagus. It has been estimated that the mixed bacterial flora of the gastrointestinal tract may reach 10^{10} colony-forming units (cfu) per gram of contents.

Rupture of the stomach or intestines is more likely where there is an underlying pathology, for example, navel abscess in lambs, traumatic reticulitis in cattle and peritonitis in pigs.

Transport of cattle or sheep to the slaughterhouse may increase the number of salmonella organisms shed into livestock waste and the percentage of animals shedding, but this is not the case for all food poisoning bacteria, for example, E. coli O157. The longer the animals remain in the lairage, the greater the potential for cross-contamination. This is particularly the case for pigs if pens are not properly cleaned between batches and if they are held overnight.

Stunning and sticking

Work carried out by Daly et al. (2002) and Buncic et al. (2002) suggests that bacterial contamination introduced into the carcase during penetrative captive bolt stunning may become widely dispersed across the slaughter line environment and within carcases, their surfaces and edible offals. During the act of sticking, bacteria can enter the jugular vein or anterior vena cava and travel in the bloodstream to the muscles, lungs and bone marrow. Many have questioned whether bacterial contamination by this route is of great importance (Troeger, 1994). However, since it has been demonstrated that marker bacteria can enter the circulation by this route (Daly et al., 2002), it is imperative that hygienic two-knife technique, initial spear cut through the skin followed by severing of the blood vessels using a second, is a routine part of GHP.

Physical contact with structures

The design of the line must allow for a full range of sizes of stock so that legs do not touch stands or supports and necks or heads do not drag along the floor, walkways or tables. A common weak point occurs at the point on the line where the bovine gastrointestinal tract is dropped on to the gut table, chute or conveyor. Gross cleaning, with squeegee and shovel, etc., must be ongoing throughout the working day to prevent the build-up of blood and debris. As part of GMP/GHP, every opportunity must be taken during breaks in production when the slaughter floor is free of carcases and offal to rinse down the line.

Care must also be taken to ensure that the position and height of offal rails is such as to prevent contact with the floor or structures. Swinging viscera, particularly at corners, may come into contact with supporting structures, while poor positioning of the line frequently leads to operatives dragging viscera across the floor, platforms or the line structure for hanging.

Operatives

All persons working in the slaughter hall are an important, and extremely mobile, source of contamination and means of cross-contamination for the meat. Movement of all personnel about the plant must be strictly controlled, and in the ideal situation, movement would occur only from clean to dirtier parts of the plant. In practice, this is impossible. To minimise the risk of contamination, upgrade stations must be provided where washing, disinfection and, if necessary, a change of outer clothes can take place. Although the movement about the plant of general operatives making social visits can generally be controlled, practical experience has shown that managers, quality control staff, but most of all engineers and fitters, can be the greatest problem in this respect.

There is a commonly held misconception among operatives that protective clothing is to protect them from getting dirty, rather than to protect the meat from them. This underlines a basic widespread lack of knowledge of hygiene matters among workers in the food industry. Current European legislation requires that all personnel involved in food manufacture receive an appropriate level of training and supervision.

The operator of the slaughterhouse must establish a staff training programme enabling workers to understand and follow the procedures required to implement the GMP/GHP, prerequisites or sanitary performance standards and critical control point monitoring, verification and corrective action where appropriate. Training must be commensurate with the role of the operative; thus supervisors and managers will get different training to a operative eviscerating or the cleaners although there will always be some common topics. The official veterinarian responsible for the establishment will evaluate the training policy and procedures during the course of verification.

Equipment and utensils

The equipment used within the slaughter hall is a potential source of contamination. This includes knives, saws and hock cutters which come into direct contact with the meat and so must be regularly cleaned and sterilised. However, it also involves indirect sources of dirt and debris such as the moving overhead line itself, from which oil or grease may drop on to the meat, and the hide-puller from which faeces may flick on to the exposed carcase and adjacent carcases.

The slaughter hall environment

Ventilation in the workroom must be sufficient to evacuate steam and to prevent condensation forming on the ceiling or inner surface of the roof and overhead structures. A common source of steam emanates from sterilisers which are allowed to operate in excess of 82°C and in which no system is incorporated to discharge the steam. Steam may act as a vector for bacteria and can in addition condense on the carcases, adding to surface moisture and assisting bacterial growth. Condensation

dripping on to the carcase from above brings with it dirt, bacteria and moulds. The traditional reliance on hot water sterilisers could be significantly reduced with the advent of effective alternative sanitising systems with the equivalent or possibly even greater effect.

Water is also a problem if allowed to pool on the floor owing to blocked drains or uneven surfaces. Gullies around the splitting saw frequently become blocked with debris and, if water accumulates, the carcase may be splashed with water from the floor. Ineffective or incomplete ducting of waste water from sinks or scald water rinse stations can also lead to excessive dirty water on the floor.

Another source of water splash can be poorly positioned hand wash stations or *apron washes*. This problem is exaggerated if the water supply does not cut off immediately the operative steps out of the apron wash cabinet.

Pressure differences between the workroom and the outside frequently result in draughts which enter if doors are left open. The temptation to leave exterior doors open in temperate climates during the summer is understandable but must be resisted since flies, dust and dirt gain easy access. This is frequently the case when the doors are adjacent to the waste skips, hide stores and green offal rooms.

Poorly maintained structure may result in contamination of the meat from, for example, rust or paint flakes dropping on to the meat or into trays intended for meat. Excessive lubrication of overhead moving chains or cogs is another potential contamination hazard.

Vermin and pests

All measures necessary to exclude vermin and pests from the food-producing factory must be taken. Physical exclusion begins with a fence around the entire premises to keep out cats and dogs, and also includes self-closing external doors and fly-screening on windows. Vermin and pests which manage to gain entrance must be systematically destroyed. The operator's arrangements for detection and elimination must be documented and effectively implemented by the operator themselves. The procedures in place should include the nature of any poison bait, the bait points and the frequency of the inspections. A regular check should be made of all insectocutor trays and a record kept of the dead fly count. A large fly count indicates that the insectocutor is working, but more importantly, that the exclusion practices are not. The official veterinarian must scrutinise these arrangements at audit.

Plant surrounds must be kept clean and tidy so that vermin such as rodents, cats and dogs are not attracted to the site. All external waste bins must be covered; otherwise gulls, starlings and other scavenging birds will be attracted. Food containers must never be stored outside even when the intention is to wash them before reuse. They provide attraction and harbourage for vermin and pests and could inadvertently be brought into use before effective sanitation had occurred.

Chemical contamination

Cleaning chemicals may contaminate the meat if they have not been used in accordance with the manufactures' instructions. Only chemicals suitable for use in the food industry should be used for sanitising the slaughterhouse. Most cleaning agents need to be rinsed off the structures correctly. It is not uncommon to find a residue of chemical on sanitised stands and equipment after they have dried. Some sanitising agents are designed to be left on surfaces and do evaporate to leave a residue-free surface. All rail grease and lubricating oils should be food grade. Chemicals used in the food factory cannot be stored in rooms where food is handled. Ideally they should be stored in a specifically designated store away not only from food but any materials that might come into contact with food, for example, wrapping or packaging materials. The operator must be able to provide evidence of the suitability of the chemicals used and information on their correct use.

The hazard of intrinsic chemical residues in the meat is dealt with in Chapter 13.

Methods of reducing contamination

Dealing with the dirty animal

It is almost inevitable that, despite all efforts to prevent it, dirty animals will be presented for slaughter, especially in the winter months in the British Isles. The operator must have a procedure for screening and subsequently handing and hygienically dressing the varying degrees and nature of dirty animal presented taking account of animal disease control restrictions and animal welfare considerations.

The first option to be considered should always be to reject without slaughtering, but disease restrictions or animal welfare considerations may make this impossible. It is widely agreed that in most cases it is easier to hygienically dress dirty, dry cattle and sheep than dirty, wet ones. Slaughter should then be delayed until the animals are dry by resting them in straw yards or, in the case of sheep or lambs, on expanded metal floors. A technique recommended by one experienced veterinarian to assess when dirty wet lambs are sufficiently dry to allow hygienic dressing is that lambs should be detained until their underside can be rubbed without dirtying the hand. It should be recognised, however, that in warm climates, and where lambs have been fattened on root crops, dry-

ing the animals may result in release of dust which adheres to the hot carcase while the fleece is being removed. *In all cases, the welfare aspects of the husbandry practices which have resulted in the dirty animals should be borne in mind, and farm inspections by the appropriate agency instituted where necessary.*

In New Zealand, it has been common practice for many years to wash lambs through plunge dips prior to slaughter. A study of this practice by Biss and Hathaway (1996) indicated that, although the carcases of washed lambs showed evidence of less visible contamination than those of unwashed lambs, washing had a detrimental effect on the microbiological load as measured by *E. coli* and aerobic plate counts. The same study showed that the levels of visible and microbiological contamination were lower on carcases derived from clipped when compared with 'woolly' lambs. In the United Kingdom, many slaughter establishments routinely clip the incision lines and 'crutch' of dirty lambs in the lairage and charge the producer for the service.

Washing heavily cladded cattle in the lairage is futile from a hygiene perspective, and may be highly detrimental to animal welfare. It is impossible to wash the legs, hooves and ventral aspect of cattle effectively. Commercial application of an apparatus to wash bovine carcases post-bleeding and pre-evisceration has been trialled. The treatment involved spraying the carcase for 10 seconds with a 1.5% solution of sodium hydroxide at a temperature of 65°C followed by a rinse with a solution of sodium hypochlorite containing 1 ppm free chlorine. The treatment had little effect on the total number of aerobic bacteria or enterobacteria on the surface of the dressed carcase but resulted in a significant reduction in the prevalence of *E. coli* O157:H7.

A process for *chemically de-hairing* cattle between stunning and sticking has been patented in the United States. It involves repeated applications of 10% sodium sulphide solution and rinses with 3% hydrogen peroxide within a closed cabinet and results in the complete removal of dirt, faeces and hair. However, a study of the process by Schnell *et al.* (1995) demonstrated that, although there was less visible contamination on the treated carcases than on conventionally slaughtered controls, total bacterial counts, measured as aerobic plate counts and total coliform counts, showed no decrease in the overall bacterial load. A further study of this process, Nou *et al.* (2003), however concluded that there may be value in the process.

Bosilevac *et al.* (2004) applied a detergent surfactant, cetylpyridinium chloride (CPC 1% w/v), to the hides of cattle in the lairage immediately before stunning in order to determine its effectiveness as an intervention for carcase contamination from the hide. The treatment was found to reduce *E. coli* O157 prevalence on hides from 56 to 34% and on carcases from 23 to 3%. Although concerns remain relating to the chemical contamination of the carcase with the detergent, commercial application is possible.

Once the operator has applied his pre-slaughter controls, the animals go forward for ante-mortem inspection. The official veterinarian can authorise slaughter provided he is satisfied that the condition of the animals is such that controls further down the dressing line, for example, appropriate line speed, use of spacing etc. are likely to be effective. At any stage, where the official veterinarian feels that carcase hygiene may be compromised, he can impose addition controls over and above those proposed by the operator. Where additional controls have to be imposed, the operator should review and adjust his own controls for future processing. When the animals are judged ready for slaughter, the quality control team must monitor the operation closely and control the *speed of the line* accordingly. As important as line speed, which gives the operatives sufficient time to carry out the extra washing of hands, arms, aprons and sterilising equipment which will be necessary, is the spacing of the animals. On a moving line, the placing of carcases on every other overhead hanger decreases the possibility of carcases touching each other and also gives the slaughtermen more room to work hygienically. Each slaughterman must be trained to remove contamination by trimming as soon as it occurs. The supervisor or quality control operative must verify that this process is effective and where contamination is occurring investigate and address the problems that are causing it. A useful technique that can be used as part of the verification process is to mark the location of contamination with an X on a carcase template the very time it is detected. Over the course of a day, this builds up a picture of where on the carcase most contamination is occurring and allows trace back in the dressing process to where corrective action needs to be taken, for example, operative retraining, more space, clips or waxed paper sheets to protect. The inspection team must verify that the operator's controls, both monitoring and verification, are effective and insist on modification to the process or stop operations if contamination is occurring and not being effectively addressed.

It goes without saying, however, that the real answer to dirty animals lies primarily with livestock producers on the farm and to a lesser extent with hauliers. Slaughterhouse operators have to deal with what is delivered to them. However, it may be necessary to provide an attractive bonus payment for suppliers of clean animals or a significant penalty for the others to bring about real change in the supply chain.

Clipping cattle on line

Clipping after slaughter on the dressing line, as an alternative to clipping cattle in the lairage, has the advantage of removing all animal welfare and handler health and safety concerns. McCleery *et al.* (2008) demonstrated that both interventions effectively reduced carcase surface contamination under commercial slaughter conditions in Northern Ireland. On-line clipping, when compared with clipping in the lairage, resulted in a small but significance difference in ultimate carcase pH, mean 5.59 rather than 5.66. However, the on-line clipping facility must be so designed as to eliminate all risk to the exposed carcase from dust created during the clipping process. This can be achieved by physical separation of the clipping from the exposed carcase by, for example, a two-level slaughterhouse, clipping after the bleeding channel but before the carcase is elevated to the floor above for dressing, making use of air curtains or by other physical barriers. The amount of dust in the immediate area can be reduced by using vacuum incorporated into the clipper mechanism (Fig. 8.1).

Protecting the meat from the worker
Clothing

Under European law, each food business operator must determine what clothing is suitable to protect the food they produce from contamination from the work force. The key stipulation is that whatever clothing is worn, it must be clean. Slaughterhouse operators would be wise to look to some of the more prescriptive requirements of the previous meat hygiene legislation as a guide to what might be suitable. This stipulated that

'Staff handling exposed or wrapped fresh meat or working in rooms and areas in which such meat is handled, packaged or transported must in particular wear clean and

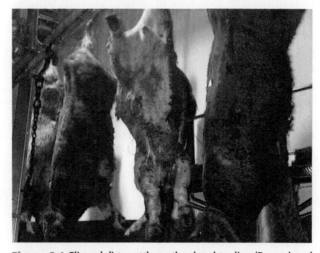

Figure 8.1 Clipped dirty cattle on the slaughter line (Reproduced with permission from John Hood).

easily cleanable headgear, footwear and light-coloured working clothes and, where necessary, clean neck shields or other protective clothing. Staff engaged in slaughtering animals or working on or handling meat must wear clean working clothes at the commencement of each working day and must renew such clothing during the day as necessary'.

Laundry arrangements must be under the control of the operator, either on-site or contracted out. The laundering standards must be verified by the supervisors or quality control team. The outdated practice of operatives laundering their own protective clothing at home should be resisted, as the monitoring and verification of standards is made impossible.

Headgear should be easily cleanable and kept clean, and should cover the crown of the head, with all hair retained within a hairnet and beards within a net or snood. For both hygiene and health and safety reasons, white bump caps are to be recommended for all staff. Easily cleaned footwear means, in effect, that it must be waterproof so that boot washers can be used to remove adherent fat and soils.

Hands

All operatives in the slaughter hall must have facilities readily available to wash their hands during the working day. The water supply must be premixed to a suitable temperature – too cold and it will not remove the dirt and the operative will not use it; too hot and it will produce steam and the operative will not use it – and must be supplied through taps designed to prevent the spread of contamination. In practice, this means a non-hand- or arm-operated outlet. Arm-operated outlets may be suitable in processing areas other than the slaughter hall where there is less risk of the operatives' arm having gross contamination. Outlets in the slaughter hall may be controlled by foot, knee or 'magic eye'. Soap, suitable for use in the food production environment, must be available. Bactericidal soap is marginally more effective than plain soap and should be non-perfumed to avoid the potential to taint the product. Disposable paper towels should also be provided and bins should be provided to hold the towel waste.

Bell and Hathaway (1996) reported that a 44°C water hand rinse removed 90% of the microbial contamination from workers' hands, but rinsed hands, particularly those contacting the fleece, still carried a microbial population exceeding 10^4 cfu/cm.

Gloves

The wearing of rubber and chain mail gloves presents a dichotomy between hygiene and health and safety. In the slaughter hall, it is likely that with many of the tasks,

gloves will become grossly contaminated from the hide with faeces and other soils. With rubber gloves of the 'washing-up' type in common usage, it is almost impossible to wash the entire length of the glove. There is frequently, therefore, a rim of gross contamination around the top of the glove which is readily transferred to the meat. Attempts to seal the glove to the arm with tape are rarely successful. Chain mail gloves also become contaminated and can only be effectively cleaned after removal. Although this allows the chain to be cleaned, the fastening tapes frequently remain in a filthy state. The best compromise is probably to cover the chain mail glove, which is usually worn only on the free hand, with a skin-tight rubber latex type glove.

Cut-resistant polyester yarn gloves are manufactured by several companies for use instead of chain mail. Some claim that an antibacterial agent has been built into the yarn from which the glove is made which has an activity against Gram-positive and Gram-negative bacteria, including salmonellae. The gloves can be laundered through a washing machine and reused many times.

Control of hazards from medical conditions

The requirement for certification by a medical practitioner that operatives were fit to work with meat has very sensibly been dropped from European legislation. Instead the food business operator determines how he will ensure that the operatives who pose a risk to food are prevented from handling food or entering food handling areas. Key elements of the operators' controls include the following:

1 Pre-employment screening by health questionnaire with reference to the medical profession only when necessary
2 Induction training that covers all medical conditions that must be reported to the employer and in particular those that mean the operative should refrain from work
3 Return to work screening following illness or travel to particular countries, again with reference to the medical profession as necessary
4 Periodic refresher training regarding significant symptoms and the action to take
5 Observation of operatives by supervisors to spot any sign that there may be an unreported condition

It is important that workers who are suffering or who have recently suffered from bouts of gastroenteritis are excluded from duties where they are handling exposed meat. Workers with septic lesions must cover such sores with appropriate waterproof dressings.

An example of a staff self-declaration form which may be used as a pre-employment questionnaire for prospective employees in the food industry is shown in

Table 8.2 Fitness to work questionnaire

Pre-employment questionnaire

	Yes	No

1. Have you now, or have you over the last 7 days, suffered from diarrhoea and/or vomiting
2. At present, are you suffering from:
   (i) skin trouble affecting hands, arms or face?
   (ii) boils, styes or septic fingers?
   (iii) discharge from eye, ear or gums/mouth?
3. Do you suffer from:
   (i) recurring skin or ear trouble?
   (ii) a recurring bowel disorder?
4. Have you ever had, or are you known to be, a carrier of typhoid or paratyphoid?
5. In the last 21 days, have you been in contact with anyone, at home or abroad, who may have been suffering from typhoid or paratyphoid?
   If the answer to any question is 'yes', the individual should not be employed as a food handler until medical advice has been obtained.

Table 8.2. The effectiveness of this one-off certificate in preventing persons carrying readily transferable infections is dubious. Some companies require regular faecal samples to attempt to identify salmonella carriers, but since excretion of pathogens is frequently intermittent, this is unlikely to be very effective.

The World Health Organisation (Health Surveillance and Management Procedures for Food-Handling Personnel Technical Report Series 785, 1989) concluded that 'the pre-employment and subsequent routine medical examination of food handlers are ineffective and thus unnecessary. Examination may, however, be appropriate in the case of food handlers reporting sick or in the investigation of outbreaks of food-borne disease'. Reference was also made to the policy in the state of Florida in the United States where similar conclusions were reached.

These conclusions were based on a study of the following: physical examination, medical history, throat swabs, blood tests, X-rays and skin tests for TB and other lung infections, and the examination of faeces for pathogens and parasites.

A study of countries where pre-employment and routine periodic medical examinations are mandatory disclosed high costs of medical and laboratory examinations aggravated by the high labour turnover, seasonal employment and the use of part-time staff in the food industry. Many of these countries no longer adopt routine medical examinations.

The most cost-effective measures were considered to be education and training involving both managers and food handlers.

Good hygiene practice
Hygienic use of knives

Regulation (EC) No 852/2004, the general regulation on the hygienic production of all foodstuffs, at Annex II, Chapter V, requires that 'all articles, fittings and equipment with which food comes into contact are to be effectively cleaned and, where necessary, disinfected. Cleaning and disinfection are to take place at a frequency sufficient to avoid any risk of contamination'.

The most common method of sterilising implements is in a cabinet containing water at 82°C, the knife, saw or whatever piece of equipment is to be sterilised being left *in situ* for at least 2 minutes. It is essential that the level of the water covers the handle/blade junction and that the knife or implement is visibly clean before being placed in the steriliser. If it is not washed first, the blood and debris will merely harden on to the blade, which should not be considered sanitised. A 44°C rinse followed by a dip into a steriliser at 82°C will reduce the contamination on a knife to less than 10^3 cfu/cm (Bell and Hathaway, 1996). Sterilising equipment without a flow-through of water is not to be recommended as it can quickly become filthy. This is particularly the case for splitting saws where, if a plunge bath is used, the water rapidly takes on the colour and consistency of a thick soup. For this type of equipment, a cabinet into which the blade of the implement is placed and sprayed with a foot-operated stream of water is preferred. The water from the cabinet can be positively ducted, reducing steam and splash.

Current legislation in many countries, including the EU, permits the use of alternative methods, to water at 82°C, for sterilisation of knives and equipment, as long as they are proven to be effective. Food Science Australia (FSA) investigated the origin of 82°C water as the standard accepted method and found it to be based on a study carried out in the United States into methods of sterilising splitting saws in the 1950s. They identified the following benefits of using lower water temperatures for sterilisation of equipment:

- Reducing risk of operator injury (scalds)
- Reducing hot water consumption, particularly by knife sterilisers
- Less water, particularly hot water, going to effluent ponds
- Saving on energy costs for heating
- Reducing fogging and condensation
- Potential reduction in maintenance requirements

Table 8.3 Minimum water temperatures for knife sanitation, according to the minimum observed immersion time of knives during routine operation

Observed minimum immersion time (seconds)	Immersion temperature without pre-rinsing (°C)	Immersion temperature following a pre-rinse in 40°C running water (°C)
1	82	75
5	80	70
10	70	70
20 or more	65	60

A study by Goulter, Dykes and Small (2008) established the importance of pre-rinsing of knives prior to immersion in the steriliser. They also established that at a range of temperatures, increasing the immersion time from 1 to 5 seconds gave a significant increase in bacterial reduction. FSA suggested combination of temperature and time for effective knife sterilisation, with and without rinsing as given in Table 8.3.

In order that knives in particular spend sufficient time in the water at 82°C, or alternative temperatures, it is necessary for each operative to have several knives. This modus operandi is known rather grandly as the *multiple knife technique*. When the operative arrives at the workstation to commence work, he or she places a number of clean knives in the steriliser. Each time a knife becomes contaminated, it is washed and placed in the steriliser and another knife is selected. The knives are used serially so that each has spent the maximum possible period in the steriliser.

This technique is suitable for knives. However, for larger equipment like hock cutters, it may be necessary on some lines for equipment to be doubled up so that each item can spend sufficient time being decontaminated.

Operator's wishing to use alternative systems of sterilisation to water at 82°C must be able to demonstrate that the alternative systems are indeed equivalent or better. In addition to efficacy, alternative systems must not introduce any new hazard to the process. Suggested alternatives include chemical-based systems and use of ultraviolet light. Given the amount of gross contamination that any system on the slaughter line will have to deal with, there has been considerable scepticism about viable alternatives. Any trial to demonstrate equivalence must do so under commercial conditions and as such be tailored to each individual slaughter line. The trials must be run in parallel with use of water at 82°C so that the resultant meat has been produced in accordance with European law. Results from chemical trials conducted to date remain commercial in confidence due to the

financial investment in demonstrating equivalence. However, it is claimed that chemical sterilisation systems can be more cost-effective in the long term mainly on account of the reduction in energy costs. A somewhat unforeseen advantage to the chemical alternative is that knife blades are not dulled by the hot water of the steriliser, remain sharp for longer and so require less steeling to keep their edge.

Hygienic use of the scabbard

Scabbards of the closed type can usually be considered to be unhygienic and a source of contamination to a sterilised knife. The newer open stainless steel scabbard is a considerable improvement.

A scabbard is necessary, for health and safety reasons, for the transportation of knives to the workstation. Once at the workstation, all knives should be unloaded into the steriliser from which they are used for the rest of the working day. The only major exception to this rule on the slaughter line is the operative who removes the head from the bovine. On most slaughter lines, he must carry the head from the point of removal to the washing cabinet, where the head is hung, trimmed and washed inside and out with a high-pressure spray. It would be unsafe for him or her to do so with the head in one hand and the knife in the other.

Hygienic use of the steel

The steel, which is used to keep the knife sharp, is a source of contamination frequently overlooked in daily operations. A traditional bar steel which is hanging from the user's belt, dangling either inside or against the outside of a wellington boot, cannot be considered as a suitably hygienic surface against which to rub a knife which has just been removed from a steriliser. The cleanliness of the steel, and its storage when not in use, are therefore very important. On arrival at the workstation, the steel should be removed from the belt or scabbard and sterilised. It is unreasonable to expect the steel to be stored throughout the day in the steriliser, since most operatives believe that this practice destroys the effectiveness of the steel. It should therefore be stored hanging freely from a hook at the workstation where it will remain effectively sterile, provided only sterilised knives are used on it. The steel should not be stored in the wash-hand basin, where it will be contaminated from waste water during washing and which may contain stagnant water, on ledges, behind pipework or in most of the other ingenious places in which it is often found in the workplace.

The widespread introduction of the 'flip flap' type steel has made it possible for this steel to be fixed, either temporarily or permanently to the structure of the slaughter line close to the wash, to the steriliser facility.

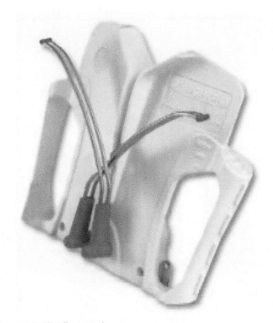

Figure 8.2 Flip/flap steel.

Again, if only washed and sterilised knives are sharpened, most opportunities for cross-contamination should be eliminated (Fig. 8.2).

Layout and flow lines

The layout of the slaughter hall and the flow lines for the entry and exit of carcases, operatives, bins and other equipment is particularly important and must be properly designed at the planning stage. Adequate space is a fundamental requirement for subsequent hygienic operation. There should be a clear demarcation and, as far as possible, physical separation between clean and dirty parts of the abattoir. Operatives must be able to reach their workstation without risking contamination of themselves or the meat by walking through or under carcases on the lines or passing through 'less fit' parts of the abattoir such as green offal rooms, rendering plants or waste storage areas. During breaks, procedures must be in place to ensure that work clothes and equipment remain clean. Insufficient thought in this area frequently leads to workers from different parts of the abattoir using the same facilities during breaks, with the potential for cross-contamination. It is not unknown for food factory operatives to be seen playing football in the factory surrounds still wearing their protective clothing and footwear during their breaks from the line.

It is obvious that waste bins and the hide conveyor should never cross the slaughter line because of the risk of contamination, but poor design, especially in the older factories with twisted lines, sometimes makes this impossible to avoid. It is not only the bin of, for example pet food, but also the operative who propels it. He or she will by necessity be passing back and forth from clean workroom to the waste skip area.

At the initial design stage or any subsequent modification to the slaughter hall and associated areas, the slaughterhouse operator should consider the following:

How will the carcase get to and then progress down the line?
How will each operative get to his/her workstation?
What is to be harvested?
Where will that harvesting occur?
How and where will all parts requiring inspection be presented for official inspection?
Is a batching system required?
How will correlation be maintained?
How will inspected material get to the chills?
What equipment or containers will be required?
Where will they come from?
How will that equipment/container be cleaned before reuse?
What waste will be generated?
Where will it be generated?
How can the waste be contained and removed?

The use of chutes removing waste without the need for personnel movements is clearly advantageous. As part of the audit and review of approval, the official veterinarian should always consider whether the slaughterhouse operator has done the best he can in terms of the design and layout of the premises as a whole as well as within individual workrooms. Where layout or flow lines are less than optimal, the official veterinarian must consider whether the operator is managing the inherent food safety risks that result.

Another important consideration is the layout of the individual workstation. It is important that the washing and sanitising equipment is sited so that it is simple and convenient to use. To put it bluntly, if the equipment is not positioned so that it is easier for the operative to use it than not, it is inevitable that in the hurly-burly of the workplace and the repetitive nature of the tasks, shortcuts will be taken. An apron wash with the steriliser positioned on its outer wall is one such example, where the operative steps into the apron wash, washes the knife as he enters and places it in the steriliser, washes his apron, hands and arms in the apron wash, and collects a clean knife on his way out.

Dressing techniques – Removal of hide/fleece/hair

The contamination of the carcase by dirt, debris and hair from the outer integument of the animal must be prevented as far as possible by good dressing technique. In many cases, complete prevention is almost impossible, for example, with deer which have been allowed to wallow, are caked with mud and in addition shed their hair profusely. Details of some recommended techniques are outlined in

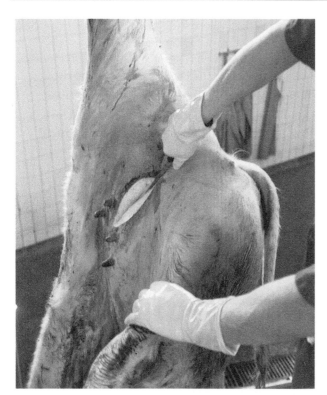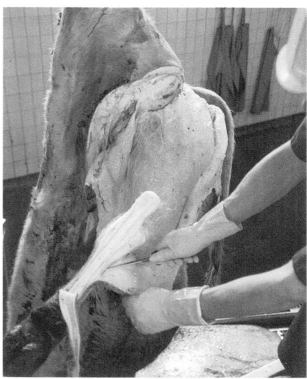

Figure 8.3 The initial incision, which will be extended using the spear cut technique. Effective out-rolling of hide is shown at right (by courtesy of R. H. S. Moore BA, MVE, MRCVS).

the following text. These are, however, only suggestions and not all will be appropriate under every circumstance. The skill of the professionally trained veterinarian is to understand the general principles so that they can assess the efficacy of the slaughterhouse operator's procedures in achieving the desired outcome and when required can advise the operator how to adapt procedures to address a particular practical situation or problem encountered.

Cattle

Dry, clean cattle, having been stunned, are allowed to slide or tumble from the stunning box. The use of raised slats or metal grid in this area – the dry landing area – is essential in order to keep the animals as clean and dry as possible. Small *et al.* (2002) concluded that the stunning box area was a potential source of cross-contamination of zoonotic bacteria as animals with clean hides fall out onto the same area of floor following stunning as contaminated ones. The cattle are then hoisted by the leading hindleg on to the line and bled before the removal of the hide commences.

An incision through the skin, the knife moving as it must through the dirty exterior towards and into the clean interior, is always fraught with the hygienic risk of pushing dirt or hair on to the carcase. These initial cuts must, therefore, be carried out with great care and kept as short as possible. Once through the skin, the knife must be washed and sterilised, and/or exchanged for a clean

knife. All incisions from this initial one should then be made using a *spear cut technique*, where the blade of the knife is reversed so that its back is against the carcase and the cut is made from the inside of the skin towards the outside, or to put it another way, from clean towards dirty. This results in reduced contamination (Fig. 8.3).

To illustrate the point, consider a common procedure for freeing the hide from the rear quarters during on-line dressing of cattle. An initial short incision is made along the ventral midline between the hindlegs of the suspended animal. The knife used is washed and placed in the steriliser, hands, arms and apron washed and a clean sterilised knife is collected from the steriliser. The initial incision is extended downwards towards the umbilicus, and upwards along the free hind limb towards the hock, using the spear technique. Skinning then proceeds from these incisions.

During skinning, the carcase frequently becomes contaminated from in-rolling at the edges of the hide. Small alterations to the positioning of the skinning incisions is often sufficient to alter the way in which the hide hangs and so eradicate the problem. The use of pairs of crocodile clips joined by an elastic cord has been found to be a useful tool in the prevention of in-rolling, especially when used at the hide-puller.

A particular problem with hide-pullers, especially those which pull upwards, is dirt flicking from the hide on to the exposed carcase as the hide finally detaches

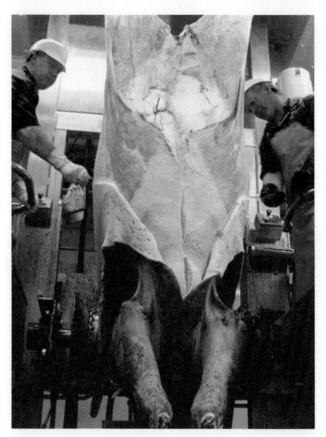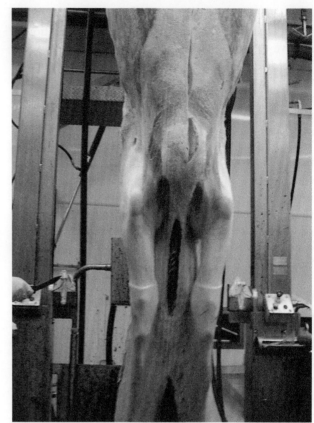

Figure 8.4 Downward hide-puller; more hygienic than upward puller and can also skin head, previously prepared.

from the carcase and head. These flecks must be removed immediately by trimming. Work by Madden, Murray and Gilmour (2004) in Northern Ireland indicated that hide-pulling was the major point of bacterial contamination of beef carcases and hence an important potential intervention stage for controlling the final microbiological quality of the carcases (Fig. 8.4).

A particularly important initial cut through the skin is the one which exposes the major vessels in the neck for sticking. As previously described, the knife contaminated while incising the skin must be washed and sterilised, and a clean knife used to sever the blood vessels.

Sheep

Most of the techniques described for cattle are also applicable to sheep. Adequate spacing on the line is particularly important when dressing sheep. Many of the problems occur with the ventral incision and with in-rolling of the fleece. Again the elasticised crocodile clips are useful. Judicious use of glossy paper sheets placed on the sternum and inguinal regions can be very successful. It is imperative that the right sort of paper, which will remain in place but not adhere permanently to the carcase, is used.

A particular problem may be encountered where dry, dirty sheep release dust while the fleece is being mechanically removed. This dust can be virtually impossible to remove from the carcase surface. Pelting machines which allow the pelt to flap about and recoil excessively when it is released from the carcase are most likely to result in the exposed meat surface being showered with loose hairs and other debris from the fleece.

In the *traditional sheep dressing system*, the lamb was suspended initially by the hindlegs. The pelt was freed manually from the hind-quarters and removed to the level of the shoulders by a combination of 'punching out' and pulling downwards from tail to head. The forelegs were then lifted and hung on a rail running parallel to that suspending the hind-feet, and the fore-quarter was skinned using knife work and a horizontal pull. This technique has been replaced in many sheep slaughter lines by a more hygienic system, known as *inverted dressing*. The lamb is suspended initially by the forelegs, and the pelt is loosened from around the shoulders. Some knife work is utilised to partially free the pelt from the hindquarters, before it is removed by a mechanical pelter pulling from head to tail. Gill *et al.* (2000) studied the microbiological difference between carcases dressed conventionally and by the inverted method and found the latter to be 1.5 log units less coliforms or *E. coli*.

It is common practice, particularly in New Zealand, to wash the carcases after pelting and before evisceration to remove visible contamination such as wool, blood and faeces. It is likely that, although this practice improves the appearance of the carcase, it actually assists in spreading contamination to otherwise clean parts of the carcase and adds water to the warm exposed meat surface to assist bacterial metabolism.

Bell and Hathaway (1996) found that the areas of highest contamination were the forequarter region with inverted dressing and the hindquarter with conventional dressing. In both cases, these regions are the sites where cuts are made through the skin. With both systems, contamination around these cuts was entirely consistent with direct fleece contact resulting from 'rollback'.

In Italy, mechanical subcutaneous inflation has been used to assist in skinning lightweight lambs. Producers claim that the resultant carcase has a better appearance and that there are fewer cuts in the subcutaneous fat and muscle. The technique has been shown to produce carcases of comparable microbiological standard to those produced by conventional dressing. Sheridan (1998) suggested that washing the carcase after the hide or fleece has been removed and before evisceration reduced the pathogen load on carcases at the end of the dressing process.

Pigs

Most pigs in the British Isles are scalded, de-haired, singed and scraped as a preparation for bacon production rather than being skinned. The scalding water may contain many different types of bacteria originating from the pigs' skin and gastrointestinal tract, including *Salmonella* spp. The temperature of the water in the drag-through scalding tank, at 60°C, is generally sufficient to reduce vegetative growth and can result in as much as a 4 log reduction in bacterial numbers on the surface of the carcase. If, however, the temperature of the scald water is not properly maintained, contamination of the water with enteric bacteria may reach 2 log units/ml. The skins of scalded pigs were found to have low numbers of both enteric pathogens and spoilage bacteria (Sorqvist and Danielsson-Tham, 1986; Troeger, 1994), but the subsequent de-hairing process re-contaminates the skin.

Vertical scalding of pigs on the line with humidified air reduces the opportunity for contamination of the carcase via the stick wound. Humidified air is blown under pressure through nozzles to reach all parts of the carcases. Scalding at a temperature of 61°C continues for about 7 minutes. Water consumption is about 15% of the normal method. There is no cross-contamination,

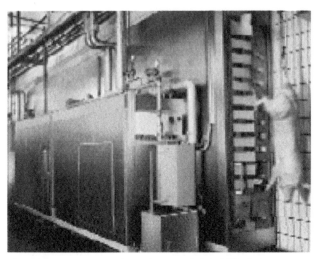

Figure 8.5 Vertical scalding of pigs with humidified air.

no water in lungs, no infection of thorax through the stick wound and no recirculation of dirty water (Fig. 8.5).

Following singeing, the bacterial load on the carcase surface is of the order of tens of bacteria/cm², but the scraping and polishing procedures which follow recontaminate the surface to the order of 10^3 bacteria/cm². The majority of these are spoilage bacteria, predominantly acinetobacteria, moraxellae and pseudomonads, with enteric organism such as *E. coli* and *Campylobacter* at single figures per cm².

An apparatus, described by Gill *et al.* (1995), has been developed and trialled commercially on a pig line operating at 800 pigs/hour, and is capable of reducing the contamination on the surface of uneviscerated pigs by a factor of 10^2. The machine washes the pigs with sheets of water heated to 85°C for a treatment time of 15 seconds. Water is recirculated from a tank beneath the line through screens to header tanks which feed the nozzles.

One common problem, or perceived problem, is the failure of the automatic equipment to remove all of the pig's *toe nails* all of the time. Although they look dirty, personal investigation would suggest that toe nails carry no greater a bacterial load than the rest of the carcase.

Preventing contamination from the gastrointestinal tract

After the outer integument, the gastrointestinal tract is the next most important potential source of contamination. However, if the rectum and oesophagus can be sealed, and the tract removed intact, the contamination can be effectively controlled.

Cattle

The technique used for sealing the rectum is known as *bunging*. The system depends to some extent on skinning technique and on the type of hide-puller being utilised. If an upwards hide-puller is in use, the skin is pulled away from the perineal region with the rest of the hide leaving the perineal region hygienically exposed. The technique which is recommended involves the operative placing a plastic bag over his left hand with a strong elastic band around his wrist. The exposed end of the rectum is grasped with this hand and a circular incision made around the rectum, freeing it from adherent tissues within the pelvis. The plastic bag is then unfurled over the rectum with the elastic band. The protected rectum can now be allowed to pass or be pushed down into the abdominal cavity. If a downward hide-puller is utilised, the rectum must be freed prior to removal of the hide. This is a more difficult task to complete hygienically since the circular cut around the rectum to free it has to be made through the contaminated hide.

Automation of this process has transformed the task of bung removal, reducing faecal contamination significantly, improving carcase dressing technique and minimising operative fatigue and risk of knife damage (to operative and carcase meat).

A machine developed in Australia known as the Beef Bung Bagging Machine automatically grasps the rectum, leaving the operative to clear the rectum from its attachments with a circular incision. A plastic bag and rubber ring are applied to make a secure seal on the rectum, and all operations are carried out without hand contact with the carcase.

A less sophisticated hydraulically operated elastrator can also be used for sealing a plastic bag with a rubber ring (Fig. 8.6).

The oesophagus (weasand) in cattle is usually sealed by an elastrator ring applied at the oesophageal–ruminal junction in a procedure known as *rodding*. The procedure involves the separation out of the oesophagus and, using a stainless steel instrument, forcing a rubber ring up the length of the oesophagus, through the thoracic cavity, to deposit it using a trigger device at the oesophageal–ruminal junction. Rodding is best carried out immediately bleeding is completed to prevent the escape of ruminal fluid, which would contaminate the tissues of the head and neck (Fig. 8.7).

Sheep

In sheep, after the pelt is removed, the rectum is freed from the attachments within the pelvis and a length of 30 cm, or more, is exteriorised. Although several alternative practices exist, it is acceptable to 'milk' the

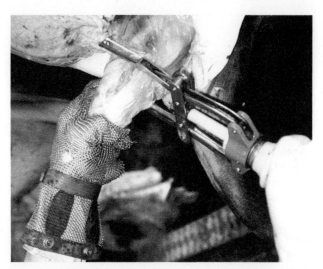

Figure 8.6 Elastrators with expanded rubber ring ready for placing over plastic bag or rectum (by courtesy of R. H. S. Moore MRCVS).

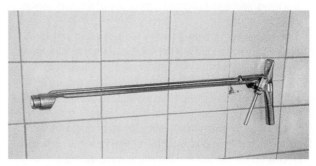

Figure 8.7 Stainless steel rodder.

solid faeces back up the rectum, cut off the posterior few centimetres and allow the cut end to drop into the abdominal cavity.

The oesophagus in sheep may be sealed using a smaller version of the bovine rodding equipment, but more frequently clips are used.

Pigs

In pigs, the abdominal cavity is opened, and the pubic synthesis of the pelvis is split prior to the freeing of the rectum. The anal sphincter is removed intact and, since the pelvis is split, the rectum can be detached and removed from the abdominal cavity with the entire gastrointestinal tract in one movement. Commonly, the only attempt made to seal the rectum to prevent faecal spillage is a simple knot tied in the posterior rectum. The most common reason for contamination of the carcase is accidental incision of the wall of the rectum while the operative is cutting round to free it. The procedure leaves little margin for error since the operative does not want to cut into the hams, one of the most expensive cuts.

Smokies

Within the United Kingdom, there is a market, especially among recent immigrants from West Africa and parts of Asia, for smoked skin-on sheep meat, known colloquially as 'smokies'.

The production process involves the slaughtering of sheep that have been recently shorn, to a wool length of about 5 mm. Following shackling and bleeding, the carcase is singed and then pressure washed to remove the burnt wool and expose the golden brown, smoked sheep skin. Following evisceration and removal of the head and, if necessary, the spinal cord as specified risk material (SRM), the carcase is inspected before undergoing a final 'toasting' to dry the carcase surface and produce an even golden brown colour.

A microbiological study of the surface of the carcase indicated that the 'smokies' had lower total aerobic microbiological counts than conventionally dressed sheep carcases. As the presence of the skin might hinder visual inspection of the surface of the carcase for the presence of abscesses, additional palpation, especially of the neck region, might be appropriate.

Investigations into the potential for residues of veterinary medicinal products, particularly subcutaneously administered vaccines, anthelmintics and topically applied sheep scab treatments, confirmed that existing controls on the use of authorised veterinary medicines would in all likelihood provide adequate consumer protection. Similarly, concerns that residues of potentially genotoxic and/or carcinogenic polycyclic hydrocarbons might be present from the smoking process on the carcase at harmful levels proved to be unfounded.

As in cattle, bunging of pigs can be improved by automation. A device with a tubular blade is positioned by a central pin which is placed up the rectum. The blade cuts down around the rectum, loosening it.

No attempt is usually made to seal the porcine oesophagus.

Post-slaughter decontamination

The emergence of *E. coli* O157: H7, especially in Canada, the United States and Scotland, as a significant food poisoning pathogen of animal origin has initiated a search for methods by which the consumer can be given even greater assurances as to the safety of the meat to be consumed. The deaths of children and the elderly during the 1990s who had consumed beef burgers or meat products contaminated with low numbers of the O157: H7 organisms have caused understandable anxiety especially as it followed upon increased public concern about other food poisoning organisms such as

Salmonella and *Listeria*. To answer these concerns and in an attempt to improve meat safety, the United States Department for Agriculture (USDA) Food Safety Inspection Service (FSIS) suggests that all carcases must receive at least one antimicrobial treatment before chilling. These treatments may include hot water, organic acid sprays, antimicrobials, hydrogen peroxide, trisodium phosphate (TSP) and chlorinated water. European food law permits potable water and approved substances only.

Water

Historically it was not uncommon to wash the carcases of both cattle and sheep with large volumes of hot or cold water to remove any visible contamination which had found its way on to the carcase during processing. The general movement in Europe has been away from this practice towards the use of the minimal amount of water necessary to remove bone dust from the spinal column, with faecal and other contamination being removed by trimming. This approach was supported by a great deal of scientific research and comment, such as that of Ellerbroek, Wegener and Arndt (1993), who demonstrated that spray washing did not reduce or increase bacterial contamination of the ventral area of sheep carcases, the portion of the carcase most likely to be contaminated by slaughter personnel, but led to bacterial contamination of the clean dorsal surface of the carcase. The conclusion was therefore drawn that spray washing with water at 12°C, 6 bar pressure for 20 seconds did not improve the microbial status of sheep carcases and that the additional water remaining on the carcase enhanced the multiplication of bacteria in the long run.

Having reviewed the available evidence, Gill (2009) concluded that when carcases or sides are relatively heavily contaminated during skinning or subsequent operations, washing for relatively long times will substantially reduce the numbers of bacteria on the meat, probably by removing bacteria that are associated with particles that are flushed from the carcases or sides. However, if the contamination of carcases is well controlled throughout the dressing process, washing will have little or no beneficial effect on the microbiological condition of the meat.

Studies suggest that to have any beneficial effect, large volumes of water are required to flush contaminants from the surface of the carcase or the temperature of the water must be high enough, and the contact time long enough, to cause heating of the surface of the meat sufficient to kill the specific bacteria being measured.

The Food Safety and Inspection Service of the USDA has approved two novel methods of cleansing beef

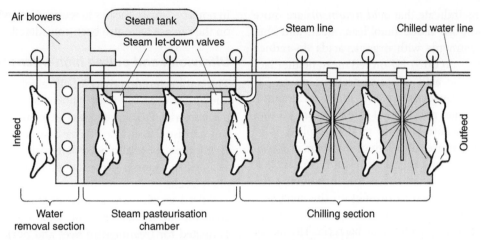

Figure 8.8 Steam pasteurisation chamber – water removal, pasteurisation and chill sections.

carcases. The first is a *steam vacuum sterilisation process* which uses water at 88°C, vacuum and steam at 45 psi to remove contamination and sterilise the meat surface through means of a nozzle similar to a vacuum carpet cleaner (Dorsa, 1996). The second is a system of *steam sterilisation* in which, after removal of surface water, the split carcases are passed through a sealed chamber where they are exposed to low-pressure steam at over 85°C for 8 seconds and then cooled with a chilled water spray (Phebus, 1996). Available data indicate that the system of carcase 'pasteurisation' can reduce the numbers of aerobes and *E. coli* by at least 1–2 log units. However, the temperatures utilised can result in gross discolouration of the treated surfaces rendering them unacceptable within some markets (Fig. 8.8).

A study by Gill *et al.* (1995) considered that treatment of pig carcases prior to evisceration with water at 85°C for 20 seconds gave maximum destruction of the surface bacteria present.

Trimming

Prasai *et al.* (1995) demonstrated that removing visible contamination by trimming and then washing was the most practical and effective method for reducing microbial contamination of the beef carcase. They emphasised that frequent sterilisation of knives and other tools used in the trimming process was essential to reduce or minimise bacterial contamination, and that individual operative technique was the most important factor in the efficiency of trimming.

Gill (2009) reported that trimming of visible contamination from carcases had little effect on the microbiological status of the carcase as he found that there was not necessarily any correlation between visible and microbiological contamination.

Chemical treatments

The following *chemicals* have been used to reduce the bacterial load on meat after slaughter:

1 Chlorine
2 Organic acids: for example, acetic acid, lactic acid, citric acid and fumaric acid
3 Hydrogen peroxide
4 Antimicrobials: for example, nisin, bactericin and lactoferrin
5 Phosphates: trisodium phosphate

The effectiveness of chemical treatments in reducing the numbers of pathogenic organisms is far from being definitely established. Methods demonstrated to be effective in the laboratory have frequently been found to be less effective under commercial application. Efficacy may vary with the particular chemical used, the concentration of the chemical which may be effected by excessive dilution on wet carcases, the contact time, the tissue type, the length of time which has elapsed between contamination and treatment, the organism, the temperature of the solution and the method of delivery.

A study utilising *chlorine* at 20 ppm in a beef carcase wash at 16°C for 10 and 60 seconds demonstrated that treatments with chlorine at this concentration and temperature were no more effective than water alone for reducing faecal contamination on meat (Cutter and Dorsa, 1995). However, higher concentrations of chlorine up to and above 350 ppm have been utilised and reported to be effective, although such high concentrations of chlorine are neither advisable nor acceptable. Chlorine is readily inactivated by organic matter and combines with amino nitrogen to form the less active chloramines.

Investigations indicate that *acid treatments* are more effective on adipose tissue than lean meat, and that while spray treatments with organic acids do reduce populations of *E. coli* O157:H7 on red meat, neither lactic, citric or acetic acid at concentrations up to 5% reduced the pathogen levels to zero (Cutter and Siragusa, 1994). Brackett, Hao and Doyle (1994) confirmed that these acids at concentrations up to 1.5% applied at 20 and 55°C did not appreciably reduce numbers of *E. coli* O157:H7 on beef. In general, it would appear that although organic acids are successful in reducing the numbers of spoilage bacteria present on the meat surface, they are of much less use when expected to render meat safer by removing pathogenic bacteria. The use of lactic acid is permitted within the EU applied as a 2–5% solution by spraying or misting, up to a temperature of 55°C. Its use must be within the context of a HACCP system to visibly clean beef carcasses, half carcases or quarters.

Trisodium phosphate has been used to reduce the total viable counts on poultry carcasses by 50% and the incidence of salmonella-contaminated carcasses from 9.5% to 0%. Phosphates are, however, potential environmental pollutants.

The abuse of post-processing treatment to mask poor hygiene practice during dressing and an ineffective inspection processes must be rigorously opposed. The FSIS in the United States recognises this and states categorically that 'antimicrobial treatments will not be permitted to substitute for strict compliance with sanitary slaughter and carcase dressing procedures, e.g. no visible faecal contamination will be permitted on the carcase before the treatment is applied'. Suitably controlled, and as part of an integrated approach to the reduction in the total numbers of pathogenic and spoilage bacteria present on the carcase before it enters the chillers, these treatments may have an important role to play. Public demand for meat which is naturally produced and residue-free, however, may make the concept of treating meat with antimicrobials, acids or high levels of chlorine difficult to establish.

Bacteriophages

Bacteriophages (phages) are viruses that attack and kill specific strains of bacteria. They were first discovered in the early twentieth century and have been utilised to treat infectious disease, but in 2006, bacteriophages were approved in the United States as a 'food additive' that could be sprayed on ready-to-eat meat and deli products to reduce the presence of Listeria monocytogenes. This was followed in 2007 by a bacteriophage product designed to be sprayed, misted or washed onto cattle hides to reduce the presence of *E. coli*. Phage products to include

in poultry carcase washes to reduce Campylobacter jejuni on the carcase have also been considered.

Ultraviolet and pulsed high-intensity light

The antibacterial activity of ultraviolet light has been known for over 100 years. Short wavelengths acts upon the bacterial DNA preventing it from multiplying and can sanitise the surface of a carcase at exposure times of 10 minutes. It has also been demonstrated to be effective as a post-packing treatment applied to modified atmosphere packs.

Pulsed visible light at wavelengths between 170 and 2600 nm and intensities of up to 50 joules/cm^2 has been evaluated for treatment of beef and pork for exposures ranging from one millionth up to one tenth of a second. At longer exposure intervals and higher intensities, the surface temperature of the meat heats quickly causing inactivation of bacteria and, in some cases, cooking at the meat surface.

A commercial system which has a combination of pulsed light and ultraviolet is available and is reported to reduce total numbers of aerobes significantly.

Outputs of the slaughterhouse

Essentially there are two categories of material arising from the slaughter process – that which goes for human consumption and that which does not. The former group is made up of a mixture of that which progresses into the food chain with minimal processing – the obviously edible meat – and that which needs significant further processing before it is suitable for ingestion – the edible co-product. Of the material that does not go for human consumption, the animal by-product, some goes as waste, some to pet food production and some for technical or pharmaceutical uses.

The principle has already been established that the live animal, farmed for human consumption, is food. Obviously the live animal requires a degree of processing for it to actually be eaten, but virtually all parts of the healthy animal, with appropriate processing, can be used for human consumption. Biologically, most non-carcase material is edible, with appropriate cleaning, handling or processing, but variable use is made throughout the world owing to custom, religion, palatability and reputation of the product. After the carcase, the most commonly used organs and parts for human consumption are liver, heart, tongue, kidney, tripe and intestines as sausage casings, except for the bovine intestine in areas with Specified Risk Material (SRM) controls. Some cultures will use other parts of the animal – cattle, pig and poultry feet, pigs' ears, etc.

The edible output from the animal can be subdivided into those parts where minimal processing is required prior to consumption and those parts and material where more significant processing is required, commonly referred to as edible co-product, as follows:

Edible output – minimal processing: carcase meat, mechanically separated meat (MSM), blood and red offal, for example, liver and kidney

Edible co-product: treated stomachs, bladders and intestines, collagen and gelatine from hides and bones, rendered fats, etc.

The non-edible output of the slaughterhouse is the animal by-products. However, animal by-products are not simply those parts which cannot be eaten, like the SRM, content of the gastrointestinal tract and material declared unfit for human consumption. Animal by-product includes that material which could be used for human consumption but which for commercial reasons the food business operator has decided will not be sold for human consumption. In other words, **animal by-products are all those parts that are not intended for human consumption.** It should be noted that once the decision has been taken that the material which could have been used for human consumption is an animal by-product, it cannot later return to the human food chain.

It is essential that controls are in place to ensure that, in particular, products categorised as animal by-products cannot be later be reintroduced to the human food chain. The practice of diverting animal by-product to the food chain has led to serious incidences of fraud and public health concern in the past with not only unfit meat being upgraded from animal by-product to meat or edible product but also animal by-products destined for pet food such as chicken feet, pig stomachs and tripe.

The yield from meat animals during the slaughter process of non-edible outputs ranges from 20 to 30% of the live weight for beef, pork and lamb and from 5 to 6% of the live weight of chickens.

The non-muscle parts of animals, owing to their higher glycogen content and lesser fat covering, are more perishable than the carcase meat, and they must be chilled quickly to lower temperatures than the muscle to control the microbiological load. They should be kept at a temperature of not more than 3°C. Freezing does not significantly decrease the bacterial numbers in edible products or co-products, but a temperature of −12°C will arrest all microbial growth. Vacuum packaging will also increase the shelf life, which in some cases can be doubled using this technique. Some of these products can also be cured, smoked, pickled and/or canned. All material intended for human consumption must come from animals which have passed both ante-mortem and post-mortem inspection and have been harvested and handled hygienically and stored appropriately.

Table 8.4 Average breakdown of 450 kg steer and 21 kg lamb

	Steer %	Lamb %
Carcase and other edible output	62–64	62–64
Edible fat	3–4	5–6
Blood	3–4	3.5–4
Animal by-product	8–10	6–7
Stomach and intestine contents	8	5.5
Hide (skin and fleece in lamb)	7	15

The *pet food industry* utilises materials which are not acceptable for human consumption, that is, those which, although edible, are not in demand from the consumer and so have a low monetary value, such as cow's liver. Material that is considered unfit for human consumption but which does not present a risk to animal or human health can be used for pet food, for example, parasitic livers. The handling and storage should be hygienic, but chilling is not essential for 24 hours if the material is to be processed. However, there must be complete separation from material for human consumption as some of the pet food products will not have been presented for veterinary post-mortem inspection, for example, chickens' feet.

The use of specialised glands for *pharmaceutical* purposes, although still carried out, has decreased owing to the biotechnical manufacture of medicines, which allows for a more consistent product (Table 8.4).

Treatment of edible co-products

Fats

With the exception of the hide, the most valuable output of the abattoir is the fat trimmed from the intestines (except mesentery which is SRM), kidney area, channel and other internal organs of cattle. Fats are graded as follows: 1 refers to edible fat and 2–6 inedible fat. The grades are dependent on free fatty acid (FFA) content and colour. Caul (omentum and its contained fat droplets) and kidney fat are rendered to produce premier jus, which is separated into oleo oil and oleo stearin (suet). Dripping is made from caul, kidney and body fat. Grades 2–6 are used in animal feeds, soaps (mainly 2–4) and the chemical industry (predominately 6). The latter uses them in such diverse products as toothpaste, lubricating oils (where they can be used in two-stroke marine biodegradable fuel), plastic, cotton and liquid washing detergents. More traditionally they have been used in the dressing of leather, and production of commercial glycerine, which itself is used in medicinal preparations, nitroglycerine, gunpowder, cordite and dynamite.

Table 8.5 Standards of rendered animal fat, depending on type

	Ruminants			Porcine animals			Other animal fat	
	Edible tallow		Tallow for refining	Edible fat		Lard and other fat for refining	Edible	For refining
	Premier jus[a]	Other		Lard[b]	Other			
FFA (m/m% oleic acid) maximum	0.75	1.25	3.0	0.75	1.25	2.0	1.25	3.0
Peroxide maximum	4 meq/kg	4 meq/kg	4 meq/kg	4 meq/kg	4 meq/kg	4 meq/kg	4 meq/kg	4 meq/kg
Total insoluble impurities		Maximum 0.15%				Maximum 0.5%		
Odour, taste, colour	Normal							

[a] Rendered animal fat obtained by low-temperature rendering of fresh fat from the heart, caul, kidneys and the mesentery of bovine animals, and fat from cutting rooms.
[b] Rendered animal fat from the adipose tissues of porcine animals.

Fat occurs in many area of the *pig carcase*, the best quality fat being obtained from the peritoneal lining (leaf fat) and the next best from the back fat, mesentery and omentum. The surplus fat of pigs is worked up into various qualities of lard. A pig of 90 kg live weight yields about 6.3 kg of lard.

Sheep fat is rendered in the same way as beef fat or lard and, though it is not converted into oleo oil or oleo stearin because of its flavour, it may be used as dripping when blended with other fats. Mutton fat is firmer and contains more stearin than ox or pig fat, and historically was used as a preservative layer on the top of glass jars of meat paste (Table 8.5).

Edible fat rendering

High-quality fats have low FFA values and are usually stable. Efficient rendering processes ensure that the FFA content remains low by means of initial cold storage of the raw material where it is not immediately used, followed by keeping the processing temperatures as low as possible and the cooking times minimised. There are three main methods of processing edible fat: wet rendering, dry rendering and continuous low-temperature rendering.

The *wet rendering* method involves the use of pressure batch cookers in which the pre-cut raw material is injected with live steam to a temperature of 140°C under pressure, for 3–4 hours. After this time, the pressure is slowly released and the fat is run into a receiver and further purified by gravity or centrifugation to settle out the water and fines. The proteinaceous solids or greaves are emptied from the cooker, and the fat is removed by pressure. Historically, solvent extraction methods were also used. Greaves are then ground and dried if intended for human consumption or used in the pet food industry.

The *dry rendering* process uses heat in the form of steam and water over a period of $1\frac{1}{2}$ hours at atmospheric pressure to drive off water indirectly from the fat in the cooker. The rest of the process is the same as for the wet rendering method.

The *continuous low-temperature wet rendering* system uses heating, separation and cooling on a continuous basis, and is usually regarded as the ideal process. The process involves mincing of the raw material, melting by live steam injection at 90°C, continuous separation of solids from the liquid fat in a decanter centrifuge, further heating, centrifugation to remove the fines and cooling in a plate heat exchanger to below solidification point.

An important principle in the rendering of fat is the prevention of the breakdown of fat into fatty acids and glycerides by the action of the enzyme lipase, which is active at temperatures of 40–60°C. Above 60°C, lipase is inactivated. The continuous low-temperature system utilises this action and at the same time minimises undesirable chemical activity, burning, oxidation and off-flavours.

Stomach and intestines

The contents of the rumen, reticulum, omasum and abomasum are generally emptied in the gut room and the intestines are separated from the stomachs. In the United Kingdom, the bovine intestines and mesentery are collected, along with the other SRM, as animal by-product Category 1, and stained and rendered accordingly.

Tripe is most commonly produced from the first stomach (rumen or paunch) and second stomach (reticulum) of the ruminant and occasionally from the third stomach (omasum). It can also be derived from the stomach of the pig. The stomachs are first emptied and washed, and the fat is trimmed off. The pillars of the rumen (mountain chain) may be removed, trimmed, packaged and frozen for human consumption, Japan being the traditional consumer, but also in other countries. The remaining material is cleaned in one stainless steel drum which operates rather like a cylindrical washing machine and then transferred to a second similar machine but on this occasion with a roughened interior which removes the external fat. The stomachs are then scalded in water containing washing soda, scraped and placed in cold water to clean them, and finally cooked for 3–3½ hours at a temperature of 49–60°C. The reticulum is the source of 'honeycomb' tripe. In some countries, the omasum is made into 'bible' tripe; in others, it is considered uneconomical because of the difficulty of removing the mucous membrane.

Rennet is manufactured from the abomasum of the calf.

Intestines – casing preparation

The first operation in handling intestines is 'running', that is, the separating the intestines from the mesentery. This is carried out either manually or by machine. The next step is to run the intestine through a 'manure stripper' comprising large rollers (which resemble a laundry wringer), to squeeze out the contents of the intestines. This step requires the use of a great quantity of potable water to wash the casings and the correct arrangement and alignment of equipment to ensure control and removal of dirty water from the process without back flow, to ensure progressive cleaning of the intestines. The casing should then be soaked in water for approximately 30 minutes at 38–42°C. In some areas of the world, casings then go through a fermentation cycle, but in other countries (e.g. the United Kingdom and the United States), casings processed by fermentation are no longer acceptable. Intestines which have not been fermented are run through a crushing machine and soaking tank. This breaks the intermucosal membrane and separates it from the rest of the intestine. Next, the intestine goes through a mucosa stripper, which looks and acts essentially like the manure stripper used for the initial emptying. Potable water at 42°C is again used to wash away the waste material. Any remaining string-like material and mucosa are removed by rolling. After cleaning, the casings are placed in a cold salt solution and held overnight. The next day they are graded, salted with fine salt until they have absorbed 40% salt and packed into barrels.

Blood for human consumption

Approximately 4.5% of the live weight of an animal is collectable blood, which represents around 10% of the protein available in an animal. Dried blood is high in protein (80–90%) and rich in lysine.

Blood for human consumption is collected via a hollow knife inserted into the blood vessels where sticking is performed. Normally, an anticoagulant such as sodium citrate (0.2% w/v) is supplied to the knifepoint through a hollow pipe in the knife handle. It should be collected in a primary tank and held there until the animal from which the blood originated has passed meat inspection. Should the animal not pass post-mortem inspection, only the small holding tank of blood need be condemned.

In a typical blood meal plant separation of the plasma and cell fractions is accomplished in the high-speed centrifuge or separator. After separation, the plasma is frozen or spray-dried at low temperature in order to maintain its solubility and binding properties. The red cells can be used for black sausages or blood puddings or dried into blood meal.

It is important to prevent haemolysis or rupture of the red cell membranes during processing. Haemolysis will occur if the red cells come into contact with solutions of lower osmotic pressure, causing the absorption of water and bursting of the corpuscles, and the presence of fat, which will dissolve cell membranes, bringing about haemolysis. The same problem can be caused by sudden variations of temperature, freezing and damage through rough handling.

Bones

Bones attached to the musculature are handled and sold as fresh meat. However, today, because of the increasing production of boneless meat, there is an increasing amount of bone available for processing. Once separated from the musculature, bone must be processed without undue delay, with attention to temperature control and of course hygiene. The end products of bone processing are fat, bone meal and gelatine, with meat-and-bone meal being produced when there is meat in the original raw material.

Gelatine is produced from bones, tendons and sinews subsequent to the extraction of fat and under carefully controlled pressure. Current EU legislation requires that ruminant bone material from animals born, reared or slaughtered in countries or regions classified as having a low incidence of bovine spongiform encephalopathy (BSE) is subjected to a process which ensures that all bone material is finely crushed and degreased with hot water and treated with dilute hydrochloric acid (at minimum concentration of 4% and pH <12.5) for a period of at least 20 days with a sterilisation step of 138–140°C for 4 seconds or by any approved equivalent process. Gelatine is used in making brawn, pies, ice cream and capsules for medicines, in photography, as a culture medium for bacteria and in the production of smokeless gunpowder. Some of the gelatine used for these purposes comes from veal and a smaller amount from beef. Nowadays pig skin supplies a large quantity of gelatine.

Hides and skins

Edible products manufactured from hides and skins include gelatine and collagen. In addition, pig skins are used to manufacture a rind emulsion for sausage production. In order to reduce the risk to human health, hides and skins must derive from animals that have passed ante-mortem and post-mortem inspection. A system must therefore be implemented to ensure hides/skins from carcases that have been classified as unfit or detained for further investigation can be identified and segregated. The raw material and processing must be carried out in a manner which removes any physical, chemical or bacteriological hazard.

Gelatine is manufactured from the hides and skins of farmed ruminants, pigs, poultry and wild game. In this case, raw material is subjected to a treatment with acid or alkali, followed by one or more rinses. The pH must be adjusted subsequently. Gelatine must be extracted by heating one or several times in succession, followed by purification by means of filtration and sterilisation.

Collagen is manufactured from hides and skins of ruminant farm animals and wild game, pig and poultry skins and bones and tendons. Collagen must be produced by a process that ensures that the raw material is subjected to a treatment involving washing, pH adjustment followed by one or more rinses, filtration, extrusion or by an approved equivalent process. The collagen may then be dried.

Animal by-products

Animal by-products are any animal carcase, part of an animal carcase or any material of animal origin not intended for human consumption. Material becomes animal by-product when either they are unfit and/or unsafe, or the food business operator decides that they will not be used for human consumption.

Animal by-product collection, identification processing and storage in Europe is regulated under Regulation (EC) No 1069/2009 and the food hygiene and transmissible spongiform encephalopathy (TSE) regulations. Under Regulation (EC) No 1069/2009, they are categorised as follows:

Category 1

a. Entire bodies and all body parts, including hides and skins, of the following animals:
  i Animals suspected of being infected by a TSE in accordance with Regulation (EC) No 999/2001 or in which the presence of a TSE has been officially confirmed
  ii Animals killed in the context of TSE eradication measures
  iii Animals other than farmed and wild animals, including in particular pet animals, zoo animals and circus animals
  iv Animals used for experiments as defined by Article 2(d) of Directive 86/609/EEC without prejudice to Article 3(2) of Regulation (EC) No 1831/2003
  v Wild animals, when suspected of being infected with diseases communicable to humans or animals
b. The following material:
  i SRM; see Table 8.6
  ii Entire bodies or parts of dead animals containing SRM at the time of disposal
c. Animal by-products derived from animals which have been submitted to illegal treatment as defined in Article 1(2)(d) of Directive 96/22/EC or Article 2(b) of Directive 96/23/EC

Table 8.6 Specified Risk Material (SRM)

Age	Parts classified as SRM
Cattle – within the EU	
All ages	Tonsils
	Intestine from the duodenum to the rectum
	Mesentery
Over 12 months	The skull excluding the mandible and including the brain and eyes
	Spinal cord
Over 30 months	Vertebral column including the dorsal root ganglia, but excluding vertebrae of the tail, the spinous and transverse process of the cervical, thoracic and lumbar vertebrae, median sacral crest and wings of the sacrum
Sheep and goats – within the EU	
All ages	The spleen and ileum (To ensure that all is removed, approximately 60 cm of the terminal small intestine should be removed and disposed of as SRM from the ileo-caecal junction, upwards and away from the caecum.)
Over 12 months, or with one permanent incisor erupted	Skull including the brain and eyes, tonsils and spinal cord (Skull does not include horns.)

This table may be subject to change as per requirements of the EU and national legislation.

d. Animal by-products containing residues of other substances and environmental contaminants listed in Group B(3) of Annex I to Directive 96/23/EC, if such residues exceed the permitted level laid down by Community legislation or, in the absence thereof, by national legislation
e. Animal by-products collected during the treatment of waste water required by implementing rules adopted under point (c) of the first paragraph of Article 27:
    i From establishments or plants processing Category 1 material
    ii From other establishments or plants where SRM is being removed
f. Catering waste from means of transport operating internationally
g. Mixtures of Category 1 material with either Category 2 material or Category 3 material or both

Examples of Category 1

- Whole bodies of cattle, sheep, goats, water buffalo and bison either rejected at ante-mortem inspection, or found dead on arrival, or found dead in the lairage (unless SRM has been removed at the point of disposal)
- Carcases, blood and all parts (including hide/skin) from animals which do not prove negative for a TSE following testing
- All parts (including hides, skins and blood) of TSE-sampled carcases disposed of prior to test results being obtained
- Products suspected of containing EC-prohibited non-medicinal treatments or illegal substances, for example, elevated dioxin or heavy metal contaminants (but does NOT include products containing residues of permitted veterinary medicinal products)
- Bodies of wild game animals affected by disease communicable to humans or animals

Category 2

Category 2 material shall comprise the following animal by-products:

a. Manure, non-mineralised guano and digestive tract content
b. Animal by-products collected during the treatment of waste water required by implementing rules adopted under point (c) of the first paragraph of Article 27:
    i From establishments or plants processing Category 2 material
    ii From slaughterhouses other than those covered by Article 8(e)
c. Animal by-products containing residues of authorised substances or contaminants exceeding the permitted levels as referred to in Article 15(3) of Directive 96/23/EC
d. Products of animal origin which have been declared unfit for human consumption due to the presence of foreign bodies in those products
e. Products of animal origin, other than Category 1 material, that are
    i Imported or introduced from a third country and fail to comply with Community veterinary legislation for their import or introduction into the Community except where Community legislation allows their import or introduction subject to specific restrictions or their return to the third country
    ii Dispatched to another Member State and fail to comply with requirements laid down or authorised by Community legislation except where they are returned with the authorisation of the competent authority of the Member State of origin
f. Animals and parts of animals, other than those referred to in Article 8 or Article 10,
    i That died other than by being slaughtered or killed for human consumption, including animals killed for disease control purposes
    ii Foetuses
    iii Oocytes, embryos and semen which are not destined for breeding purposes
    iv Dead-in-shell poultry
g. Mixtures of Category 2 material with Category 3 material
h. Animal by-products other than Category 1 material or Category 3 material

Examples of Category 2

- Any carcase, part of a carcase or offal which comes from an animal or bird which was not presented for full ante-mortem inspection, or not presented with food chain information
- Any carcases, parts of carcases or offal which comes from an animal or bird and was not presented for post-mortem inspection, at whatever stage it was rejected, for example, unskinned lambs heads, tails, udders and the penis; post-mortem rejects containing pathological lesions indicating disease communicable to man or animal, for example, septicaemic carcases, pneumonic lungs, cysticercus bovis lesions, pericarditis, muscle abscesses, septic arthritic joints, tuberculous lesions, etc.
- Whole bodies of pigs or poultry either rejected at ante-mortem inspection, found dead on arrival or found dead in the lairage
- Meat found to contain pathological lesions during cutting, for example, abscesses

- Any meat or offal not handled or stored in accordance with the EU Fresh Meat Hygiene Regulations, which results in the meat becoming spoiled and a risk to either human or animal health
- Any meat that is unfit for human consumption or is spoiled in any way as to present a risk to human or animal health
- Mouldy or decomposing meat or offal including discoloured contents of blown vacuum packs
- Any meat found to have residues of substances which may pose a risk to animal or public health

Category 3 (can be used for pet food)

Category 3 material shall comprise the following animal by-products:

a. Carcases and parts of animals slaughtered or, in the case of game, bodies or parts of animals killed, and which are fit for human consumption in accordance with Community legislation, but are not intended for human consumption for commercial reasons
b. Carcases and the following parts originating either from animals that have been slaughtered in a slaughterhouse and were considered fit for slaughter for human consumption following an ante-mortem inspection or bodies and the following parts of animals from game killed for human consumption in accordance with Community legislation:
  i Carcases or bodies and parts of animals which are rejected as unfit for human consumption in accordance with Community legislation, but which did not show any signs of disease communicable to humans or animals
  ii Heads of poultry
  iii Hides and skins, including trimmings and splitting thereof, and horns and feet, including the phalanges and the carpus and metacarpus bones, and tarsus and metatarsus bones of the following:
    - Animals, other than ruminants requiring TSE testing
    - Ruminants which have been tested with a negative result in accordance with Article 6(1) of Regulation (EC) No 999/2001
  iv Pig bristles
  v Feathers
c. Animal by-products from poultry and lagomorphs slaughtered on the farm as referred to in Article 1(3) (d) of Regulation (EC) No 853/2004, which did not show any signs of disease communicable to humans or animals
d. Blood of animals which did not show any signs of disease communicable through blood to humans or animals obtained from the following animals that

have been slaughtered in a slaughterhouse after having been considered fit for slaughter for human consumption following an ante-mortem inspection in accordance with Community legislation:
  i Animals other than ruminants requiring TSE testing
  ii Ruminants which have been tested with a negative result in accordance with Article 6(1) of Regulation (EC) No 999/2001
e. Animal by-products arising from the production of products intended for human consumption, including degreased bones, greaves and centrifuge or separator sludge from milk processing
f. Products of animal origin, or foodstuffs containing products of animal origin, which are no longer intended for human consumption for commercial reasons or due to problems of manufacturing or packaging defects or other defects from which no risk to public or animal health arise
g. Pet food and feedingstuffs of animal origin, or feedingstuffs containing animal by-products or derived products, which are no longer intended for feeding for commercial reasons or due to problems of manufacturing or packaging defects or other defects from which no risk to public or animal health arises
h. Blood, placenta, wool, feathers, hair, horns, hoof cuts and raw milk originating from live animals that did not show any signs of disease communicable through that product to humans or animals
i. Aquatic animals, and parts of such animals, except sea mammals, which did not show any signs of disease communicable to humans or animals
j. Animal by-products from aquatic animals originating from establishments or plants manufacturing products for human consumption
k. The following material originating from animals which did not show any signs of disease communicable through that material to humans or animals:
  i Shells from shellfish with soft tissue or flesh
  ii The following originating from terrestrial animals:
    - Hatchery by-products
    - Eggs
    - Egg by-products, including egg shells
  iii Day-old chicks killed for commercial reasons
l. Aquatic and terrestrial invertebrates other than species pathogenic to humans or animals
m. Animals and parts thereof of the zoological orders of Rodentia and Lagomorpha, except Category 1 material as referred to in Article 8(a)(iii), (iv) and (v) and Category 2 material as referred to in Article 9(a) to (g)
n. Hides and skins, hooves, feathers, wool, horns, hair and fur originating from dead animals that did not show any signs of disease communicable through that

product to humans or animals, other than those referred to in point (b) of this Article

o. Adipose tissue from animals which did not show any signs of disease communicable through that material to humans or animals, which were slaughtered in a slaughterhouse and which were considered fit for slaughter for human consumption following an ante-mortem inspection in accordance with Community legislation

p. Catering waste other than as referred to in Article 8(f)

Examples of Category 3

- Whole carcases or parts of carcases which have passed ante-mortem and post-mortem inspection, but for commercial or other reasons are not intended for human consumption, for example, unincised pig offal, pig spleens, stomachs and pig feet, intestines from mammals or ratites empty of digestive material (except bovine/ovine/caprine SRM), poultry necks, poultry intestines, testicles, pig rind and bones from a cutting establishment
- Parts of a carcase or offal that are not permitted by the EU Food Hygiene Regulations to be used for human consumption but which are nevertheless no risk to human or animal health, for example, livers with fluke lesions, milk spot lesions, muelerius lung lesions and melanosis
- Any carcase, part of a carcase or offal certified as not being produced, stored or transported in accordance with the EU Food Hygiene Regulations which consequently cannot be sold for human consumption, for example, meat stored or found over temperature
- Meat which falls on the floor which is not visibly soiled to create a risk to human or animal health
- Trimmed fat or waste carcase meat not intended for human consumption
- Meat rejected by the producer because it no longer meets specification
- Poultry offal harvested after delayed evisceration

Transport

Category 1 animal by-products pose the highest risk to human and animal health and Category 3 the lowest. If the categories of waste are mixed, the entire consignment is considered as the higher of the categories involved (Table 8.6).

Animal by-products must be collected and transported in suitable leakproof containers or vehicles. The containers or vehicles used for transport must be adequately covered and all must be maintained in a clean condition. These containers must be labelled according to the category of by-product to be transported as follows:

- 'Category 1 for disposal only'
- 'Category 2 not for animal consumption' (other than manure and digestive tract contents)
- 'Category 2 for feeding to [specified species of animal]' when a permitted derogation to feed to certain animals is used
- 'Category 3 not for human consumption'
- 'Manure' in the case of manure and digestive tract content

Staining

Animal by-product must be stained in accordance with animal by-product and SRM legislation. SRM must be stained with Patent Blue V(E131, 1971 Colour Index No 42051) prepared to give a 0.5% weight/volume solution, immediately after removal from the carcase and in such a way as to avoids any risk of contamination of fresh meat. Category 1 material, which does not contain SRM, and Category 2 material, with the exception of blood, gut contents and green offal, must be stained with Brilliant Black BN (E151, Colour Index 197 No 28440). Stain is applied to every surface of the material at a sufficient strength to provide a dark covering. The surface of pieces of material weighing more than 25 kgs must be opened by multiple deep incisions. Entire poultry carcases consigned as animal by-products must be opened by multiple and deep incisions, whether they have been de-feathered or eviscerated or not. Animal by-products which are removed immediately through a sealed and leakproof pipe which connects the meat processing establishment or animal by-products establishment to an approved rendering or incineration establishment need not be stained. Category 3 material does not require staining, unless it is mixed with higher category material.

Materials for technical uses
Intestines

Animal small intestines can be utilised for a variety of non-food purposes such as surgical sutures, collagen sheets (used for burn dressing burns), strings for musical instruments and sports equipment, pet food, animal feed, tallow or fertiliser.

Blood for pet food

Blood for inclusion as pet food, Category 3, must come from pigs or poultry which have passed ante-mortem inspection or ruminants that have passed both ante-mortem and post-mortem inspection.

For purposes other than human consumption, blood can be collected very easily by placing troughs below the carcases. They should be designed so that they are easily dry-cleaned with rubber squeegees. It is essential that water does not come in contact with the blood for two reasons: (i) water will cause haemolysis of the red blood cells and prevent the adequate separation of plasma and red blood cells and (ii) should blood get into the plant effluent system, it will greatly increase the biological oxygen demands (BODs) by around ten times and the suspended solids by three times.

Before being allowed to enter the collecting tank, inedible blood should be strained to exclude foreign matter.

Drying of blood meal by removing the water is carried out in three main ways as follows:

1 *Direct batch drying* carried out in batch dryers similar to rendering batch coolers. The raw blood is dried to 2–10% moisture by simply boiling off the water.
2 *Batch coagulation followed by batch drying*. The raw blood is initially coagulated by injecting direct steam into an open tank containing the raw blood. The coagulum, which is around 25% total solids (TS) is then separated by draining or hand pressing and dried in a batch dryer.
3 *Continuous coagulation before drying*. This is the most common method of processing blood. Strained blood from a blood holding tank is pumped into an intermediate pre-heating tank equipped with a low-speed agitator and the blood is pre-heated to 60°C by steam. The blood then passes to the coagulator and as a result of steam injection nozzles, positioned at several points in the coagulator, at the exit, the blood is at an optimum temperature of 90°C. A decanter then separates the solids, which are dried, and the liquid.

Bone in pet food

Some, mainly pig bone and chicken necks, are emulsified and used in pet food.

Calcined bone, obtained by roasting in air, is used in the manufacture of high-class pottery and china, in the refining of silver and in copper smelting. Bone charcoal is utilised in bleaching, sugar refining and case-hardening of compounds in the manufacture of steel. Special bone powders are employed for the removal of fluorine from drinking water.

Hides and skins for leather production

Hides and skins constitute the most valuable material removed from the animal carcase. *Skins* come from smaller animals, for example, sheep, calves and goats, while larger skins such as those from cattle, horses, elephants are called *hides*. Leather from cattle hides is used to produce shoes, garment leather, upholstery leather and accessory leather. *Pig skin*, the second most common leather-making raw material worldwide, is thinner than cattle hides and is primarily manufactured into garment leather. The largest producer of pig skins is the People's Republic of China.

The quality of leather to a large degree depends on the techniques used for hide removal (flaying) and the processing that follows.

Bovine hides can be removed manually, which requires great skill to avoid damage, but nowadays in commercial meat plants, hides are removed mechanically by hide-pulling machines following initial knife work.

Pig skins are scalded and de-haired, and this generally makes them unsuitable for further processing. Pigs can be skinned with a knife, but considerable skill is required owing to the softness of the fat. Mechanical pulling of the hides is gaining popularity because of energy and labour savings when compared to scalding. However, it results in a 6–8% loss in carcase weight, and it is generally slower (150–300 per hour) than scalding (150–850 per hour).

Goat skins are more valuable than sheep skins because they are larger and produce a better-lasting leather. *Sheep skins* require a longer time (up to several hours) to cool after slaughter than other hides owing to the insulating properties of the wool and the presence of grease.

As well as for leather, hides and skins are used for non-food purposes such as cosmetic ingredients and medicinal prosthetics such as skin grafts and sutures.

After flaying, hides and skins should be chilled or cured quickly to arrest bacterial and enzymatic decomposition or spoilage. In areas with low relative humidity, they may be air-dried for preservation, but salt is mainly used as the curing ingredient. Salt-pack curing involves a flesh-side up stack of hides, usually 90–130 cm high, with an equal weight of salt to hide spread evenly over the flesh-side of each hide in the stack. This draws moisture out of the hides. Preservatives are often used with salt-pack curing. Curing takes 20–30 days for cattle.

Hide curing

Ox hides arrive at the tannery either fresh from the abattoir, chilled or more usually salted and dried to prevent putrefaction. Tanning is defined as the hardening of hides, using vegetable tanning agents, chromium salts or other substances such as aluminium salts, ferric salts, silicic salts, aldehydes and quinones, or other synthetic hardening agents (EC 853/2004, Annex III, Section XIV, 2).

After soaking in water to cleanse and soften the hides, they are placed in tanks filled with milk of lime for 1–4 weeks to loosen the hair and open up the fibre. The hair on the outside, and flesh and meat on the inside, are then scraped off and, after removal of lime by washing in weak acid, the hides are tanned. Tanning may be done by a vegetable process using the barks of trees, or by a chemical process known as 'chrome tanning'. The tannery process, from raw hide to finished leather, takes about 3 months. The hide from bullocks and heifers, when tanned, is used as sole leather or for belting. Sole leather is obtained from the butt, the area of the hide lying on either side of the backbone.

Hygiene requirements for animal by-product processing establishments

The premises of the processing plant must be adequately separated from other processing establishments such as meat plants. Premises for the processing of high-risk material must not be on the same site as meat plants, unless in a completely separate part of a building. Only authorised personnel should be allowed access.

The establishment should have a clean and an unclean section, which must be clearly separated. The unclean section must have a covered area to receive the animal waste and must be constructed so that it is easy to clean and disinfect. Floors must be laid to facilitate the draining of liquids. The plant must have adequate lavatories, changing rooms and washbasins for staff. In the unclean section, where required, there must be adequate facilities for de-skinning or de-hairing of animals and a storage room for hides.

The establishment should be of sufficient size and have enough hot water and steam to process hygienically the waste received. The unclean section must, if appropriate, contain equipment to reduce the size of animal waste and equipment for loading the crushed animal waste into the processing unit. A closed processing installation is required in which to process the waste, and where heat treatment is required, this installation must be equipped with measuring equipment to check temperature and, if necessary, pressure at critical points, recording devices to record continuously the results of measurements and an adequate safety system to prevent insufficient heating.

To ensure that there is no cross-contamination of finished processed material by incoming raw material, there must be clear separation between the area of the plant where the incoming raw material is unloaded and processed and the areas set aside for further processing of the heated material and the storage of the finished processed product.

There must be adequate facilities for cleaning and disinfecting the containers in which animal by-product is received and the vehicles in which it is transported. The wheels of the vehicles carrying high-risk material must be disinfected before departure or before leaving the unclean section of the processing plant.

There must be a waste water disposal system which hygienically removes waste water and a laboratory to carry out the required testing or of the services of an outside agency.

Containers, equipment and vehicles used for the transport of animal by-product must be cleaned, washed and disinfected after use.

Personnel wWorking in the unclean section must not enter the clean section without changing their clothes and footwear. Equipment and utensils must not be taken from the unclean to the clean area.

Waste water originating in the unclean section must be treated to ensure no pathogens remain.

There must be a systematic method to prevent the ingress of birds, rodents, insects or other vermin.

Rendering processes

While some meat plants have rendering departments for the treatment of condemned and other inedible material, it is better, from a public health standpoint as well as the efficiency of processing, that the premises should be located away from food outlets and be large enough to handle material from a large area.

The best and most economical method of processing unfit meat and offal is by heat treatment in a jacketed cylinder, which gives complete sterilisation and maximum return from the rendered material. A number of different methods are available for handling inedible material, all of which are concerned with the separation of the three main constituents, fat, water and fat-free substance, and the production of sterilised technical fat and meat-and-bone meal.

There are four categories of rendering systems which are as follows:

1 Conventional batch dry rendering with mechanical defatting
2 Continuous dry rendering with screw press defatting
3 Semi-continuous wet rendering with centrifugal defatting

The batch systems are more labour intensive but less expensive to install than continuous systems.

In these three systems, the raw material is cooked to sterilise the components (water, fat and meal) for separation, the fat being finally purified. There are major differences in the type and order of the various operations.

In the *continuous dry rendering process* (which resembles batch dry rendering except that the operation is continuous), the system operates at atmospheric pressure. After cooking, the material is pre-strained and discharged to a screw press for defatting. The length of the cooking process depends on the method of filling and the cooker size.

4 Continuous wet pressing and centrifugal defatting
Various models of this process have been developed, but the main principle consists of mincing of the raw material, melting to liberate the fat, wet pressing and drying/sterilising. Water, fat and fine solids are separated by centrifugation. A disadvantage of this process is that, similar to continuous dry rendering with screw press defatting, it does not fulfil existing sterilising regulations in some countries, necessitating a further sterilisation of the meal.

References

Bell, R.G. and Hathaway, S.C. (1996) *Journal of Applied Bacteriology*, **81**, 225–234.

Biss, M.E. and Hathaway, S.C. (1996) *Veterinary Record*, **138**, 82–86.

Bosilevac, J.M., Authir, T.M., Wheeler, T.L. *et al.* (2004) *Journal of Food Protection*, **67**, 646–650.

Brackett, R.E., Hao, Y.Y. and Doyle, M.P. (1994) *Journal of Food Protection*, **57** (3), 198–203.

Buncic, S., McKinstry, J., Reid, C.A. *et al.* (2002) *Food Control*, **13**, 425–430.

Cutter, C.N. and Dorsa, W.J. (1995) *Journal of Food Protection*, **58** (2), 1294–1296.

Cutter, C.N. and Siragusa, G.R. (1994) *Journal of Food Protection*, **57** (2), 97–103.

Daly, D.J., Prendergast, D.M., Sheridan, J.J. *et al.* (2002) *Applied and Environmental Microbiology*, **68**, 791–798.

Dorsa, W. (1996) *Proceedings of the 49th Reciprocal Meat Conference, June 1996, Provo, Utah*, pp. 114–120.

Ellerbroek, L.I., Wegener, J.F. and Arndt, G. (1993) *Journal of Food Protection*, **56** (5), 432–436.

Empey, W.A. and Scott, W.J. (1939) Council of Scientific and Industrial Research, Bulletin No. **126**.

Gill, C.O. (2009) *J. Food Protection*, **72** (8), 1790–1801.

Gill, C.O., Bryant, J. and Brereton, D.A. (2000) *Journal of Food Protection*, **63**, 1291–1294.

Gill, C.O., McGinnis, D.S., Bryant, J. and Chabot, B. (1995) *Food Microbiology*, **12**, 143–149.

Goulter, R.M., Dykes, G.A. and Small, A. (2008) *Journal of Food Protection*, **71** (7), 1338–1342.

Madden, R.H., Murray, K.A. and Gilmour, A. (2004) *Journal of Food Protection*, **67**, 1494–1496.

McCleery, D.R., Stirling, J.M.E., McIvor, K. and Patterson, M.F. (2008) *Journal of Applied Microbiology*, **104** (5), 1471–1479.

Meat & Livestock Australia (2003). Water at less than 82°C for sanitization knives in abattoirs: a guide to gaining regulatory approval, www.mla.com.au/off-farm/Project-outcomes/Food-Safety/Water-at-less-than-82-degrees-for-sanitising-knives-in-abattoirs (accessed on 30 April 2014).

Nou, X.W., Rivera-Batoncourt, M., Bosilevac, J.M. *et al.* (2003) *Journal of Food Protection*, **66**, 2005–2009.

Phebus, R. (1996) Proceedings of the 49th Reciprocal Meat Conference, *June 1996*, Provo, Utah, pp. 121–124.

Prasai, R.K., Phebus, R.K., Garcia Zepeda, C.A. *et al.* (1995) *Journal of Food Protection*, **58** (10), 1114–1117.

Ridell, J. and Korkeala, H. (1993) *Meat Science*, **35**, 223–228.

Schnell, T.D., Sofos, J.N., Littlefield, V.G. *et al.* (1995) *Journal of Food Protection*, **58** (12), 1297–1302.

Sheridan, J.J. (1998) *Journal of Food Safety*, **18**, 321–339.

Small, A., Reid, C.A., Avery, S. *et al.* (2002) *Journal of Food Protection*, **65**, 931–936.

Sorqvist, S. and Danielsson-Tham, M.L. (1986) *Fleischwirtschaft*, **66**, 1745–1748.

Troeger, K. (1994) *Fleischwirtschaft*, **74** (6), 624–626.

9

Meat inspection protocols

Ever since mankind has realised that food could make him sick, there has been meat inspection protocols. The books of *Leviticus* (Chapter 11) and *Deuteronomy* (Chapter 14), common to Judaism, Christianity and Islam, list animals that are clean, that is, fit to eat: the ox, the sheep, the goat, the buck, the gazelle, the roebuck, the wild goat, the deer and the antelopes and all clean birds. In the thirteenth and fourteenth centuries in Europe, beginning in Italy, the butchers' guilds were established which set and enforced sanitary standards, encompassing butchery skills and 'tidiness' (Fig. 9.1).

During the second half of the nineteenth century, the traditional slaughter of animals throughout the growing industrialised cities led to an increasing sanitary problem. The 'city fathers' acted, bringing in rules which had the result of centralising slaughter into municipal slaughterhouses permitting for the first time rules of meat inspection based upon the growing understanding of zoonotic parasites and infectious disease, particularly tuberculosis (TB), to be implemented. These emerging rules were brought together and published in Berlin in 1890 by Robert von Ostertag, translated into English in 1906.

In the United States, the first Federal Meat Inspection Act was introduced in the 1890s with the objective of maintaining exports of meat into Europe. However, the legislation did little to improve overall standards, and in 1906, a novel by Upton Sinclair, *The Jungle*, which described the unsanitary conditions in US slaughterhouses, galvanised public opinion for change. Despite opposition from the slaughter industry, a government investigation followed, the Neill–Reynolds report, which led to a new Meat Inspection Act making ante-mortem, post-mortem inspection and hygienic processing mandatory.

The case for change

It is beyond dispute that the inspection procedures which have served the meat industry since they were first introduced in the late nineteenth century are in need of a radical overhaul. The necessity for change has been championed by recognised authorities in meat hygiene worldwide over the last 35 years: Blackmore (1983), Hathaway *et al.* (1987), Hathaway *et al* (1989), Berends *et al.* (1993), Johnston (1994) and many others. It is widely agreed that, even when carried out conscientiously, traditional post-mortem inspection techniques are ineffective even in detecting the macroscopic lesions they are designed to identify. McCool (1979) and Heath *et al.* (1985) reported that <20% of *Cysticercus bovis* and only 41% of *Cysticercus ovis*, respectively, were detected by online inspection. A Dutch research project 'Integrated quality control approach', carried out over 20 years ago, showed that only 50% of the abnormalities present were detected either by 'traditional post-mortem meat inspection or by visual inspection and palpation only' (Berends *et al.* 1993). Hathaway *et al.* (1987) and Blackmore (1983) suggested that *incision of the lymph nodes*, especially the mesenterics, may result in the cross-contamination of other carcases and organs with *Salmonella* or *Campylobacter* via the inspector's knife. An assessment carried out on the routine examination of some of the regional lymph nodes of the viscera in lambs in New Zealand (Hathaway and Pullen, 1990) indicated that examination of these nodes added nothing to inspection of the primary organs.

Using a quantitative risk assessment approach, Mousing *et al.* (1997) determined the consequences of a change from traditional meat inspection procedures (which included manual handling, palpation and

Gracey's Meat Hygiene, Eleventh Edition. Edited by David S. Collins and Robert J. Huey.
© 2015 John Wiley & Sons, Ltd. Published 2015 by John Wiley & Sons, Ltd.

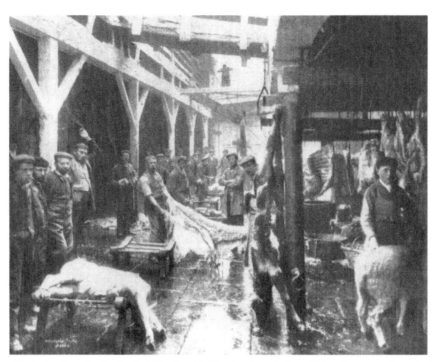

Figure 9.1 Early centralised slaughter facility in the UK – Provided by the Association of Meat Inspector from their archive.

incision) to an entirely visual form of inspection in 183 000 Danish slaughter pigs. Out of 58 lesion codes, 26 (45%) were assessed as merely aesthetic or as the healed stage of an earlier lesion; 9 (15%) were active but local lesions, occurring only in non-edible tissue; 5 lesion codes (9%) were assessed as active, non-septic lesions occurring in edible tissue caused by swine-specific pathogens; and 10 (17%) were abscessal or pyaemic lesions occurring in edible tissue. Seven lesion codes (12%) may be associated with consumer health hazards (two frequently and five rarely). One lesion code was associated with an occupational health hazard.

It was estimated that per 1000 pig carcases, an additional 2.5 with abscessal or pyaemic lesions in edible tissue containing *Staphylococcus aureus*, 0.2 with arthritis due to *Erysipelothrix rhusiopathiae*, 0.2 with caseous lymphadenitis (*M. avium-intracellulare*), 0.7 faecally contaminated with *Salmonella* species and 3.4 faecally contaminated with *Yersinia enterocolitica* would remain undetected as a result from changing from the traditional to the visual inspection procedure.

These authors concluded that the visual system would result in about 4 additional pigs per 1000 carcases being passed which might cross-contaminate other carcases with *Salmonella/Y. enterocolitica* and that the main direct benefit of the visual system (without manual handling, palpation and incision) would probably be a lower level of cross-contamination with hazardous bacteria, especially from the pharyngeal region and the plucks. In addition, the visual system allows for less labour, with

the release of control resources for hygienic surveillance programmes and wider risk assessment strategies.

The European Food Safety Authority (EFSA) opinion on 'the public health hazards to be covered by the inspection of meat (swine) 2011' concluded that 'palpation/incision used in traditional post-mortem inspection should be omitted in pigs subject to routine slaughter, because the risk of micro-biological cross-contamination is higher than the risk associated with potentially reduced detection of conditions targeted by these techniques'. The opinion identified *Salmonella* spp., *Y. enterocolitica*, *Toxoplasma gondii* and *Trichinella* spp. by qualitative risk assessment as the only significant hazards. The (bovine) opinion 2013 again identified *Salmonella* spp. as a significant hazard along with verotoxigenic *Escherichia coli*, with the risk from *T. gondii* and extended-spectrum and/or AmpC β-lactamases being undeterminable due to lack of data. In this case, the EFSA panel considered that 'palpation/incision, as used in current post-mortem inspection, should be omitted in the case of bovine animals subjected to routine slaughter, because these procedures do not add to the identification and control of the high priority bovine meat-borne hazards and **may** increase their spreading and cross contamination'. The use of 'may' is explained as a need for further research into the extent to which manual manipulation during post-mortem inspection contributes to increasing spread and cross contamination. This opinion also highlights the important role played by post-mortem inspection in surveillance for animal health pathogens particularly bovine TB and liver fluke.

However, any alterations to the existing systems must be based on sound scientific principles of food hygiene and not unduly influenced by political pressures from interested parties either from within the meat industry seeking short-term financial savings or from the 'inspection industry' seeking to defend their positions and the status quo. Food safety is of paramount importance.

The holistic approach

These opinions emphasise that meat inspection is not just about food safety although this is an important aspect of its purpose. Following upon the bovine spongiform encephalopathy (BSE) crisis in 1996, the increase in incidence of food poisoning and deaths due to verotoxigenic *E. coli* associated with beef, particularly minced/ground beef, and the resultant loss in consumer confidence in the safety of foods of animal origin, many countries saw fit to transfer responsibility for meat inspection from agricultural to health departments. This inevitably resulted in a change in the focus of priorities from the other purposes of meat inspection, that is, meat quality, animal health, animal welfare and protection of the environment, to concentrate on the appropriateness of the current controls for food safety. While the focus of government altered, it is significant that the general public and consumer organisations did not perceive a need for change but rather for current controls to be carried out better and augmented.

Integrated Food Safety Assurance

Farm to fork

The realisation that food safety was the responsibility of everyone in the food chain, from farm to consumer, and not just the processor, grew from a number of food safety incidents where investigations highlighted that the contamination incident occurred beyond the controls present within the processing establishment. The importance of the role of the primary producer, the farmer, in the safety and quality of all foods of animal origin has come to the fore. Feed contamination incidents in Europe, such as with dioxin or arsenic, emphasise the important role that the integrity of feed plays in food safety, particularly when unusual raw materials are used in an effort to produce least cost rations. Globalisation presents its own unique challenges for food safety with raw materials being sourced worldwide, remote from the user and the possibility of personal audit of the material's integrity at point of origin. Globalisation also results in the rapid dispersal of completed food products to widely distributed markets with technology permitting improved 'shelf life' for fresh or frozen product.

EFSA has identified the role of the farm in safe food production in all of their opinions on the 'public health hazards to be covered by the inspection of meat' and emphasised the importance of information from the farm being transmitted to the decision-makers at the slaughterhouse through *food chain information*.

Food chain information

Within current EU legislation, food chain information is the mechanism by which information is communicated from the farm to the slaughterhouse. Prior to 2006, information on poultry production was transferred via production reports which performed a similar task. The responsibility for securing this information lies with the food business operator of the establishment, while the official veterinarian uses it to inform ante-mortem and post-mortem decisions.

Unfortunately, to date, the good intentions of the regulation have largely not been achieved except for the vertically integrated poultry producers and in pigs in a few countries, for example, Denmark. The integrated high-intensity pig and poultry farming systems often employ their own on-farm veterinary team and can provide detailed information about husbandry; veterinary medicine use; the results of production sampling schemes and testing, for example, for *Salmonella*; morbidity and mortality figures; production figures per group of livestock, for example, daily live weight gain; etc. When linked to information relating to previous ante-mortem and post-mortem findings, a meaningful picture of the disease status, animal welfare and veterinary medicine use of the production unit can be established. This information forms the foundation on which a risk-based inspection protocol can be built.

With less intensive or integrated pig and poultry production and for cattle sheep and goats, food chain information is received by the operator but is often so lacking in detail or integrity as to be meaningless. It is obviously in the short-term interests of the producer to conceal problems on farm rather than to declare them to the operator of the slaughterhouse who may reject the animal or consignment. If there is no verification through any form of farm audit in place, little real information is available to inform ante-mortem decisions. Farm audit or checks could be achieved through farm quality assurance schemes, with third-party checks or through 'herd health' programmes with involvement of the producer's private veterinary practitioner both in the provision of advice to inform the programme and in the interpretation of the significance of the ante-mortem and post-mortem information provided by the official veterinarian at the slaughterhouse.

Ante-mortem inspection

The purpose of ante-mortem inspection is to ensure that only clean, healthy residue and stress-free animals are presented for slaughter. As illustrated in Figure 9.2, the effective preselection of animals on farm into high and low risk is key to an 'Integrated Food Safety Assurance'. To allow farms to be categorised into groups with animals presenting equivalent risk to public health, EFSA has suggested the use of harmonised epidemiological indicators (HEIs) for potential hazards (EFSA, 2011, 2012).

As examples, the EFSA opinions propose HEIs for *Trichinella*, *T. gondii*, *Salmonella* and *Y. enterocolitica* in pigs; *Salmonella*, *Campylobacter* and extended-spectrum/AmpC β-lactamase producing *E. coli* in poultry; and *Salmonella*

> An *epidemiological indicator* is defined as the prevalence or incidence of the hazard at a certain stage of the food chain or an indirect measure of the hazard that correlates to human health risk caused by the hazard.

and verotoxigenic *E. coli* in cattle. The application of these requires actions on farm, for example, controlled housing for pigs or 'clean hide' interventions for cattle. The standards for these interventions must be harmonised if the HEIs are to have any meaning.

The concept is applicable to the consideration of risk from 'farm to fork' and could be used to standardise risk not just between production units but also between slaughter establishments.

As discussed, the inspection of individual animals, or groups of animals in the slaughterhouse lairage without reliable information from the farm, akin to a veterinary examination without a history, is limited. Selection of animals into groups of greater or lesser risk based, at this point, on incomplete data, for example, on age alone, is impossible to justify.

Consequently, any suggestion that a less rigorous online post-mortem inspection regimes should be introduced before a reliable system of food chain information on which public health risk can be assessed is in place would be foolhardy.

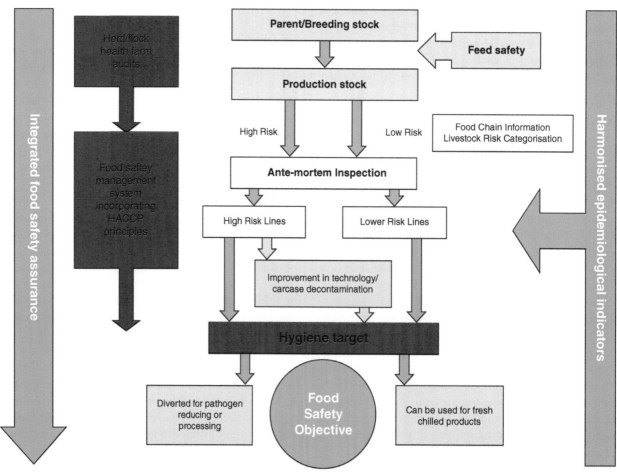

Figure 9.2 Integrated food safety assurance.

Ante-mortem inspection procedure in the slaughter establishment

Animals must undergo veterinary ante-mortem inspection on the day of their arrival at the slaughterhouse or before the beginning of daily slaughtering. The inspection must be repeated immediately before slaughter if the animal has been in the lairage overnight. The operator of the slaughterhouse must facilitate operations for performing ante-mortem health inspections and in particular any handling which is considered necessary.

In summary, the inspection must determine:

1 Whether the animals are suffering from a disease which is communicable to man and to animals or whether they show symptoms or are in a general condition such as to indicate that such a disease may occur.
2 Whether they show symptoms of disease or of a disorder of their general condition which is likely to make their meat unfit for human consumption; attention must also be paid to any signs that the animals have had any substances with pharmacological effects administered to them or have consumed any other substances which may make their meat harmful to human health.
3 Whether they are tired, agitated or injured.
4 Whether they are sufficiently clean to enter the normal slaughter protocol.

Where the post-mortem inspection is necessary in order to make a diagnosis, the official veterinarian shall request that the animals in question are slaughtered separately or at the end of normal slaughtering.

A system of communication of ante-mortem findings to those carrying out the post-mortem findings is essential in order to ensure that post-mortem inspection is supplemented by additional detailed inspection, palpation or incisions, or if the veterinarian considers it necessary for confirmation, by an appropriate bacteriological examination and a search for residues of substances with a pharmacological effect which may be presumed to have been administered to treat the pathological state observed.

For *public health* purposes, the veterinarian must separate normal animals from those which may be suffering from a potentially zoonotic disease or present a hygiene risk to the slaughterhall environment owing to the soiled condition of their hide/fleece. Animals which may contain residues of pharmaceutical product must be detained for testing post-mortem.

It is also very important that the workers within the abattoir are alerted to the presence of any *zoonotic condition*, such as orf or ringworm, or where brucellosis or TB reactor cattle are being slaughtered, so that appropriate health and safety measures can be taken. In the United Kingdom, the action to be taken in the event of each condition being identified should be assessed and written down under the 'Control of Substances Hazardous to Health Regulations 2002' which are a series of statutory regulations made under the framework of the Health and Safety at Work Act 1974.

The *animal health* aspect requires the veterinarian to identify *notifiable disease*. It is recognised within the state veterinary service that it is likely that a serious epizootic, such as foot-and-mouth disease or swine fever, will first be recognised at an abattoir, as was the case in the UK 2001 foot and mouth outbreak.

The ante-mortem procedure allows the veterinarian to assess the *welfare* implications of the structures and procedures within the lairage. In the ideal situation, this would involve *inspections on the farm of origin*, during transport, as well as in the lairage prior to death.

Following inspection, the veterinarian may make one of the following five decisions:

1 Animals may progress for normal slaughter.
2 Animals should not enter the plant or should be condemned ante-mortem. In this group, they will be dead, moribund, emaciated or excessively dirty animals and those showing evidence of a septicaemia or other conditions which would result in the meat being unfit for human consumption.
3 Animals should be slaughtered but may need a special detailed post-mortem examination, or may need to be slaughtered in a special area or at a different time from other animals, owing perhaps to a localised infection or suspicion of a more generalised condition. Animals suspected of being treated with illegal drugs for the purposes of growth promotion, or of having residues of therapeutic substances, may be included in this group. Emergency on-farm slaughtered cases will require particular attention.
4 Stock should be segregated for slaughter under special conditions, for example, dirty stock at a slow line speed.
5 Slaughter may be delayed, for example, for excessively fatigued or excited animals or those requiring treatment.

For reasons of animal health, animals should only be allowed to leave the lairage, for example, to return home, under the most exceptional circumstances and under animal health restrictions. An alternative is to consign them to another abattoir, with the capacity and approvals to slaughter them. This is the only option permitted under EU law – Regulation 854/2004, Annex I, Section II, Chapter III (8).

(a)

(b)

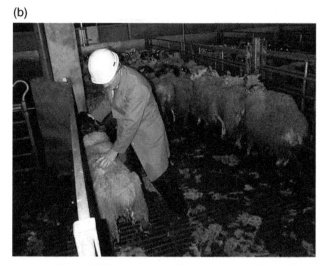

Figure 9.3 Ante-mortem inspection. (a) Taking the temperature of a suspect heifer and (b) examination of a suspect lamb (Reproduced with permission from Harold Moore).

Practical ante-mortem procedure

Livestock in the lairage should be inspected at rest and while in motion. Both sides of the animal should be observed. In practice, this is simple to carry out while the animals are being unloaded, but their excited state during this procedure may mask some conditions such as mild lamenesses, making a second check necessary. In the case of sick or suspect diseased animals and those in poor condition, the species, class, age, condition, colour or markings and identification number are recorded. The general behaviour of the animals, whether fatigued or excited, their level of nutrition, cleanliness, obvious signs of disease and any abnormalities should be observed and recorded. In addition to the segregation of diseased and suspect stock, females in oestrus, aggressive animals and horned stock should be isolated. If *unacceptably dirty animals*, that is, ones which, in the opinion of the veterinarian, cannot be dressed at normal line speed without an unacceptable risk of carcase contamination, have been allowed by factory management to enter the lairage, they must be segregated and detained until their condition becomes more acceptable, or they can be dressed at a line speed which decreases the risk of contamination.

Animals showing evidence of localised conditions such as injuries, fractures, abscesses and benign tumours (e.g. papillomata) or conditions which will show up lesions on post-mortem inspection need to be segregated and given a detailed clinical examination. Such animals may pass forward with the normal kill if the condition proves to be a minor one, slaughtered at the end of the day's kill or slaughtered separately and given a thorough post-mortem examination.

In the case of *sick animals*, the temperature should be taken; a rise in temperature may be the first indication of a communicable disease, although in moribund animals the temperature may frequently be subnormal. In sheep, body temperature may be a somewhat misleading guide as, of all the food animals, its temperature is subject to the greatest daily fluctuation; variations between 39 and 40°C are common, and in heavily woolled sheep in summer, the temperature can vary between 38.2 and 40.1°C in healthy animals. Pigs that show a temperature of 41°C or over and cattle and sheep that show a temperature of 40.5°C or higher should be isolated until the temperature falls for, if they are slaughtered while suffering from this degree of fever, the carcase will be congested and will invariably require condemnation (Fig. 9.3).

Animals showing signs of systemic disturbance and an elevated temperature should not be slaughtered for human consumption but slaughtered either in the lairage or at the end of the day and disposed of as animal byproduct. Only on very exceptional occasions should the animal be treated in isolation in the lairage.

It is absolutely essential that good contemporaneous *records* are kept of the ante-mortem findings. These records must be available to the inspectors at the time of post-mortem inspection so that the findings can be acted upon at that stage. A system which correlates the ante-mortem and post-mortem findings should be kept as simple and transparent as possible. In addition, there must be a simple method, usually *pen cards*, which allows the lairage staff to easily identify which animals have received ante-mortem inspection and what the outcome has been (Fig. 9.4).

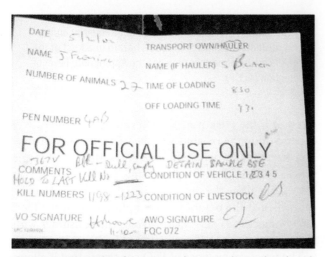

Figure 9.4 Example of a pen card system (Reproduced with permission from Harold Moore).

Emergency slaughter animals

An exception to the general rule that only live animals be accepted into the slaughterhouse for human consumption permits the emergency slaughter of livestock elsewhere. This has gained importance thanks to the improvements made to tighten up the rules on the welfare during transport of animals within the EU which has virtually eliminated what was once common practice – the transportation of acutely lame or recumbent animals to the meat plant. Historically, this was particularly a problem with post-parturient dairy cows, cull sows and pork pigs with vertebral abscess as a result of tail biting. Data from the United States, 2005–2007, show that under the USDA/FSIS system (White and Moore, 2009), 0.8% of cows sent for slaughter were condemned during ante-mortem inspection and 3.04% at post-mortem (Table 9.1).

These figures demonstrate the extent of the problem of transporting end-of-use cull dairy cows.

As a guide to frequency of occurrence of emergency slaughter, Northern Ireland, with a cattle population of 1.7 million, had during the years 2010 and 2011 approximately 500 carcases presented as having had on-farm emergency slaughter carried out.

Under current rules, meat from a red meat animal that has undergone *emergency* slaughter outside the slaughterhouse may only be used for human consumption if it is from 'an otherwise *healthy* animal that has suffered an *accident* that prevented its transport to the slaughterhouse for welfare reasons'. Animals cannot be transported for welfare reasons if, under one definition, it cannot walk unaided or under alternative it cannot bear weight on all four limbs.

Emergency implies that slaughter takes place as a result of an event requiring immediate attention.

Table 9.1 USDA/FSIS data on carcase condemnation of dairy cows 2005–2007

Ante-mortem failure 0.8% of total		Post-mortem failure 3.04% of total	
Dead	62.5%	Malignant lymphoma	26.9%
Non-ambulatory or moribund	35.0%	Pneumonia	13.1%
Epithelioma	0.8%	Septicaemia	10.2%
Pneumonia	0.5%	Peritonitis	8.9%
Pyrexia	0.3%	Pericarditis	6.8%

An *accident* is defined as 'a specific, identifiable, unexpected, unusual and unintended external action which occurs in a particular time and place, without apparent or deliberate cause but with marked effects or alternatively as an unforeseen or unexpected event especially one causing loss or damage'. Examples of accidents may include fractured limbs; road traffic accidents; serious lacerations or injuries from, for example, feed shear grabs; 'bulling injuries' and 'doing the splits'; serious haemorrhage; obturator paralysis assessed immediately post calving; or clearly identifiable spinal injury from an accident.

Emergency slaughter: The decision on farm

If a farmer considers that an animal which has had an accident may still be suitable for food, he should seek the advice of his private veterinary practitioner. It is the responsibility of the veterinary practitioner to confirm whether or not the animal is suitable for food, taking into consideration its clinical history, clinical signs and history of veterinary medicines administered and the required withdrawal periods.

The veterinarian may decide on one of the three options:

1 The animal is fit to be transported alive to the slaughterhouse for human consumption accompanied by complete food chain information.

2 The animal may be slaughtered on farm, or elsewhere outside the slaughterhouse, and the carcase transported to the slaughterhouse, accompanied by complete food chain information supplemented by a veterinary declaration.

3 The animal may be slaughtered and disposed of as animal by-product, remembering that currently within the EU, bovines over 48 moths must be sampled and tested for BSE.

Having confirmed that the animal is fit for food, is healthy, is not emaciated, is clean enough to be sent to a

---

Veterinary Declaration

Should confirm:
The favourable outcome of the ante-mortem inspection
The reason for emergency slaughter, including details of the
    accident that required emergency slaughter of the animal
Any treatment administered to the animal
The date and time of slaughter
The requirement for the declaration to include the time and
    date of slaughter dictates that the veterinarian signing the
    declaration must be present at the time of slaughter.

A Food Safety Objective is the maximum frequency and/or
concentration of a (microbiological) hazard in a food at the
time of consumption that provides the Appropriate Level of
Protection (ALOP).

---

food factory and does not potentially contain residues
of veterinary medicines, the practitioner may confirm
the findings on the 'food chain information' document.
The British Cattle Veterinary Association and the Pig
Veterinary Society in the United Kingdom have both
produced useful notes for guidance for the veterinary
practitioner. If he or she is in any doubt, they may find it
useful to discuss the details of the case with the official
veterinarian in the slaughter establishment to which the
carcase is to be conveyed.

The farmer should confirm with the food business
operator for the slaughter establishment that they will
accept the carcase for dressing. The slaughterhouse must
be less than 2 hours' transport time from the farm of origin. Since the carcase is likely to fall outside the specification of many of the abattoir's customers, they may only
accept it on the understanding that it returns to the
farmer presenting it for his/her own consumption.

In all cases, the private practitioner must ensure that
the welfare of the animal takes precedence over all other
considerations. The slaughter and bleeding of the animal
must be carried out efficiently by the veterinarian or by
an appropriately trained and experienced slaughterman.

Emergency slaughter: The decision at the slaughter establishment

On arrival at the slaughter establishment, the food chain
information and veterinary declaration are conveyed via
the operator to the official veterinarian. The official veterinarian must confirm that the carcase can proceed to
be dressed for food before hygienic dressing and processing commences. A detailed post-mortem should be
carried out to confirm the on-farm diagnosis, and in all
cases, samples should be collected to confirm freedom
particularly from residues of antimicrobial substances.

Post-mortem inspection

Within the framework of Integrated Food Safety
Assurance (Fig. 9.2), ante-mortem should differentiate
the animals for slaughter into high and low risk. As

discussed, the effectiveness of this risk assessment will
depend upon the reliability of the information available.
The key to improving the current system is that the
actions taken during processing and post-mortem
inspection allow the meat to emerge which meets a target, which at the point of consumption can meet a food
safety objective (FSO) that provides the consumer with
an appropriate level of protection (ALOP).

The practical purpose of FSO concept is that it allows
flexibility of regulatory control and operation of the
process in that it does not prescribe how compliance is
achieved but rather defines the goal. There are however
significant challenges to agreeing an ALOP, that is, the
acceptable level of cases permissible at the level of a population through risk assessment. Despite this difficulty,
setting an FSO for specific hazards does assist risk management in the Integrated Food Safety Assurance by
setting an ultimate target at consumer level that can
be translated into milestones, the HEIs at various steps
along the road from farm to fork.

This concept is also applicable to the control of hygiene
described later in this chapter but is an important concept to consider when dealing with those hazards best
controlled through the setting of HEI for the post-mortem inspection process.

Facilities for post-mortem inspection

In addition to the usual structural and mechanical
facilities which provide for good working conditions and
enable carcases and their parts to be delivered for inspection in a satisfactory manner, each inspection point on
the slaughter line should have well-distributed lighting
of at least 540 lux in intensity which does not distort
colours. There must also be sufficient sanitising units
for equipment, hands and aprons, with disinfectant soap
and disposable paper towels available. A system for the
effective sterilisation of knives, cleavers and saws must
be available, be this a wash facility adjacent to a water
bath operating at 82°C which will encompass the blade–
handle junction or an equivalent method.

These requirements extend to the routine inspection
points on the slaughter line and to the 'detained' area
where further detailed examination is performed. It is
essential that there should be coordination and communication between inspection points and that the inspectors on the inspection line can confidently identify
correlated carcases and viscera. For most domestic farm

animals, there are normally three main inspection points: head, viscera and carcase. Ideally, the inspection station for the viscera should be slightly before the carcase inspection point so that significant findings can be communicated to the carcase inspector. Synchronisation of conveyorised lines carrying carcases and offal is absolutely fundamental for accurate identification of carcases and their related organs. A fail-safe method must be put in place to ensure that, when a carcase is condemned, all carcase parts including the head, viscera, blood and hide can also be retrieved for condemnation. Increasingly, other carcase parts such as the feet, trachea, aorta and bladder are used for human consumption, so these must also be condemned. There must also be a mechanism by which, when a carcase is detained, the viscera and other body parts are also sent to the detained room. In many cases, it is almost impossible for the veterinarian to make a proper informed judgement on a carcase without the evidence which the viscera can provide (Fig. 9.5).

Systems of recording disease data vary according to the particular operation and the type and rate of slaughter. For low slaughter rates, a manual system of recording findings on a washable 'Nobo' board may be satisfactory, but for fast lines, computerised systems with automatic recording of the 'kill number' from a transponder on the hook or gambrel, with a touch- or voice-operated information recorder, must be considered. When a *universal microchip* for *the electronic identification of cattle* is accepted within Europe, this 'number' could be read automatically throughout the animal's life and through to the end of the slaughter line (Fig. 9.6).

Every inspection station should have a line stop button within easy reach. The inspectors/official auxiliaries must have the authority to stop production immediately in the event of a contamination incident or if correlation between the inspection points is lost.

Carcase identification and traceability

It is essential that *live animal identification* be retained on the carcase until it passes over the weighbridge. For the day's kill, or batches within this, a *slaughter programme* will have been compiled giving details of stock, their class, identification, name and address of owner, lot, pen and slaughter sequence numbers, etc., copies of which are made available to appropriate persons including the meat inspection staff. If live animal tags are not actually retained on the carcase because of hygiene concerns, it is important to have a reliable system of substituting 'dead' for 'live' identifications so that accurate details of producer (or wholesaler, retailer), ownership, carcase weight, grade, classification and disease information are maintained.

Practically, all the current forms of *meat identification* have drawbacks, from the standpoint of hygiene, legibility or practicality. For example, the commonly used labels with plastic or metal clips must be carefully removed before the carcase meat enters the cutting room. Leaving the bovine ear complete with its ear tag on the animal as it travels up the slaughter line has obvious advantages and equally obvious disadvantages from a hygiene perspective. The use of *transponders* implanted in the ear which can be read at the inspection and grading/weighing points as long as the ear remains with the carcase adds added benefit to this practice. A compromise is to remove the ear during skinning and place it hygienically in a plastic bag which is clipped to the first side of the carcase with a reusable stainless steel hook. Metal and polypropylene stamps with *marking dyes* are in common use for carcase identification, and *roller strips* are used for indicating grades especially on pigs. *Pigs* are generally identified

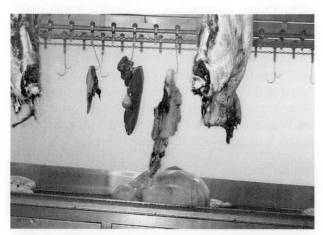

Figure 9.5 Visual correlation of carcase with offals (Reproduced with permission from Harold Moore).

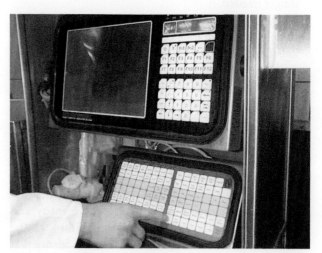

Figure 9.6 DARD Northern Ireland system for online recording of post-mortem findings (Reproduced with permission from Harold Moore).

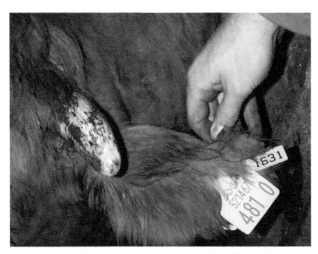

Figure 9.7 Bovine ear tag, correlated with kill number ante-mortem (Reproduced with permission from Harold Moore).

by a tattoo, or slap mark, applied ante-mortem but legible only after scalding and scraping. Grades on pigs are frequently identified by writing on the exposed dermis with a special wax pencil (Fig. 9.7).

Any good system of carcase meat identification must be clearly legible, easily applied, cheap, non-toxic, non-corrosive and suitable for use with modern data retrieval systems. The UK Meat and Livestock Commission issued a guide on the labelling of carcase meat and prime cuts some years ago. It concluded:

1 Do not label, write or stamp unless essential.
2 Fix labels in a consistent position to aid checking and removal.
3 Do not apply labels to parts of the carcase likely to be used for manufacturing, such as flank or brisket.
4 Remove all labels and clips as soon as they are no longer needed.
5 On bone-in cuts, apply the label close to the bone and to only one cut in each customer's batch.
6 Label pork carcases high on the front of the hock, away from the ham.
7 Label lamb carcases on the front of the shank.
8 Label beef carcases on the rib cage or chine bone or vertebral column and veal carcases on the leg.

Meat detained for re-inspection must also be identified in a place and by a means acceptable to both the abattoir food business operator and the official veterinarian. A system developed post-BSE ensured that the inspection team were aware of the exact identity and category of every carcase and offal passing through the abattoir. This involved a system which could ensure that correlation was maintained in order that specified bovine offal was properly removed and that meat and offal from officially BSE-free holdings are separated from those of 'lower' status.

Traditional post-mortem inspection

This post-mortem inspection system described by von Ostertag at the end of the nineteenth century was a paradigm shift in public health control and was designed to control the hazards known at that time. These were primarily bovine TB and parasites. Its significance is illustrated by the fact that it became established as the standard to be followed worldwide and maintained acceptance for 100 years. The basics of the observations required, the palpations and incisions, are outlined in the following paragraphs. The principal purpose of this inspection protocol is to determine if the carcase and offal are 'normal' and to separate the normal from the abnormal. The lymph nodes are considered in this system to be the sentinels for infection of the body systems, so emphasis is put on their size, colour and structure on incision.

Traditional post-mortem inspection of cattle

The traditional EU requirements for post-mortem inspection of carcases intended for human consumption are specified in Regulation (EC) 854/2004, Annex I. Inspection of a carcase and its organs should proceed in the following order although this may be enhanced if justified by specific hazards being suspected (Fig. 9.8).

Head

An examination of the outer surfaces and eyes is followed by an inspection of the gums, lips and tongue for foot-and-mouth disease, necrosis and other forms of stomatitis, actinomycosis and actinobacillosis, the tongue being palpated from the dorsum to the tip for the latter disease. Incisions of the internal and external masseters for *C. bovis* should be made parallel with the lower jaw. After the tongue is dropped, routine incisions of the retropharyngeal, submaxillary and parotid lymph nodes should be made for tuberculous lesions, abscesses and actinobacillosis. The tonsils of cattle and pigs frequently harbour pathogens such as tubercle bacilli, *Salmonella* and *Yersinia*. Consequently, regulations may specify that they should be removed and should not be used as ingredients of meat products. As part of the BSE controls, the tonsils must be classified as specified risk material (SRM) and must be removed and disposed of as such.

Lymph nodes

The detailed examination of lymph nodes, often recommended in different meat inspection codes, is mainly for the detection of TB and is fully justified where this disease is a problem.

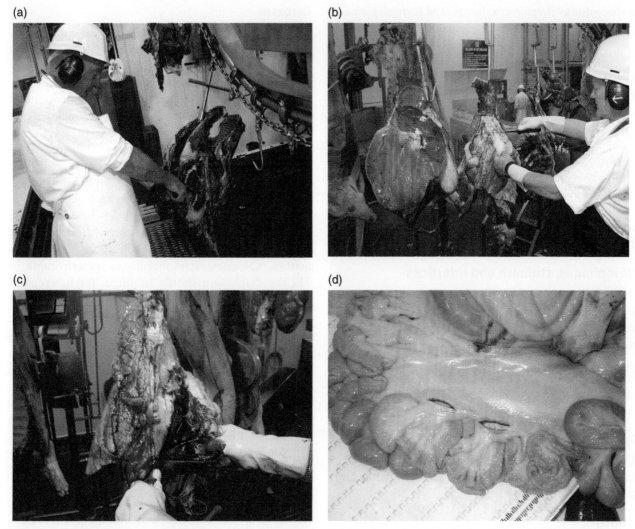

Figure 9.8 Traditional post-mortem inspection of (a) the bovine head, (b) bovine red offal, (c) bovine heart and (d) bovine mesenteric lymph nodes (Reproduced with permission from Harold Moore).

The situation with regard to the *gastric* and *mesenteric lymph nodes* in *cattle* is more problematic. Historically, examination of TB reactors (1978 in Northern Ireland) showed that 1.9% of the cattle had lesions in the mesenteric lymph nodes only, *Mycobacterium bovis* being recovered from these lesions. In spite of this finding, however, it is likely that the saving in time and costs of inspection outweigh any slight animal health benefits accruing (Goodhand, 1983).

Lungs

Visual examination, which should be followed by palpation, should be carried out for evidence of pleurisy, pneumonia, TB, fascioliasis, hydatid cysts, etc. The bronchial and mediastinal lymph nodes should be incised. The lung substance should be exposed by a long, deep incision from the base to the apex of each lung, and the trachea

and main branches of the bronchi opened lengthways, only when they are to be used for human consumption.

Heart

The pericardium should be examined for evidence of pericarditis, haemorrhages, etc. The ventricles are then incised, and the outer and inner surfaces are observed, particular attention being paid to the presence of petechial haemorrhages on the epicardium or endocardium and to cysticerci, hydatid cysts and occasionally linguatulae in the myocardium. Alternatively, the heart may be everted after cutting through the interventricular septum with four lengthways incisions into the septum and the ventricular wall – this latter procedure reduces the heart's value. A flabby condition of the myocardium is often associated with septic conditions in the cow, while vegetative endocarditis occurs in chronic swine erysipelas and in sheep due to *Streptococcus faecalis* and *E. rhusiopathiae*, the causal organisms of swine erysipelas.

Liver

A visual examination with palpation should be made for fatty change, actinobacillosis, abscesses, telangiectasis and parasitic infections such as hydatid cysts, *C. bovis*, fascioliasis or linguatulae. The larval stage of *Oesophagostomum radiatum* may occasionally be found in the ox liver. Observe and, if necessary, palpate the gall bladder. An incision should be made on the gastric surface of the liver and, in bovines, an incision at the base of the caudate lobe to examine the bile ducts. Where necessary for a diagnosis, incise as necessary into the bile ducts and liver substance.

Oesophagus, stomach and intestines

Observe and, if necessary, palpate these organs. The serous surface may show evidence of TB or actinobacillosis, while the anterior aspect of the reticulum may show evidence of a foreign body.

Kidney

Enucleation of the kidney to allow visual inspection and, if necessary, incision of the kidney and renal lymph nodes.

Spleen

The surface and substance should be examined for TB, haematomata and the presence of infarcts with observation, palpation and, if necessary, incision.

Uterus

The uterus should be viewed, palpated and, if necessary, incised, care being taken to prevent contamination of the carcase. Evidence of pregnancy or of recent parturition in the well-bled and well-set carcase is not significant.

Udders

The potential for the presence of food-poisoning microorganisms in the udder is such that it is questionable if they should ever be considered as fit for human consumption. If they are, they should be palpated, and each half of the udder opened by a long, deep incision, preferably multiple and about 5 cm apart, and the lymph nodes incised. Abscesses or septic mastitis may be present, and the supramammary lymph nodes, even in a dry cow, should be incised for evidence of abscesses or TB. In brucellosis reactors, the udder is removed intact without incision and without handling.

Testes

If destined for human consumption, the testes should be viewed and palpated.

Carcase

The cut surfaces of bone and muscle, carcase exterior, pleura, peritoneum and diaphragm should be observed, attention being given to condition, efficiency of bleeding, colour, cleanliness, odours and evidence of bruising and other abnormalities. If necessary, palpation and incision of parts may be indicated, for example, triceps brachii muscle for *C. bovis*. The superficial inguinal, external and internal iliac, prepectoral and renal lymph nodes should be observed and, if necessary, palpated and incised. Where a systemic or generalised disease is suspected, in tuberculin reactors and where tuberculous lesions have been detected in the viscera, the main carcase lymph nodes must be examined. The thoracic and abdominal cavities should be inspected for inflammation, abscesses, actinobacillosis, mesothelioma or TB; the diaphragm should be lifted, for tuberculous lesions may be hidden between the diaphragm and the thoracic wall.

Traditional post-mortem inspection of calves

The routine post-mortem of calves is virtually the same as for adult bovines, with special attention to particular sites. A visual examination of the mouth and tongue should be made for foot-and-mouth disease and calf diphtheria. Attention should also be paid to the abomasum for evidence of peptic ulcers, the small intestine for white scour or dysentery and the liver, portal lymph nodes and posterior mediastinal lymph nodes for congenital TB. The lungs, kidneys and spinal cord should be examined for melanotic deposits and the umbilicus and joints for septic omphalophlebitis. The consistency of the synovial fluid of the hock can be readily determined by puncturing the protrusion on the inner aspect of the joint with the point of a knife. The appearance and consistency of the renal fat should be carefully noted.

Traditional post-mortem inspection of sheep and goats

Sheep and goats require a less detailed inspection than cattle, calves and pigs, the routine inspection requiring no incisions. The carcase should be visually examined for satisfactory bleeding and setting, the lungs for parasitic infections, especially hydatid cysts and nematodes, and the liver for fascioliasis. In Australia and New Zealand, it is routine procedure to palpate the carcase for evidence of arthritis, caseous lymphadenitis, inoculation abscesses and lesions due to grass seed awns (Fig. 9.9).

Traditional post-mortem inspection of pigs

Post-mortem examination of pigs follows the same overall routine as for cattle.

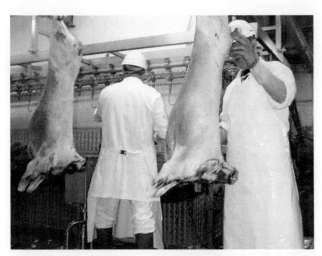

Figure 9.9 Traditional post-mortem inspection of lamb carcases (Reproduced with permission from Harold Moore).

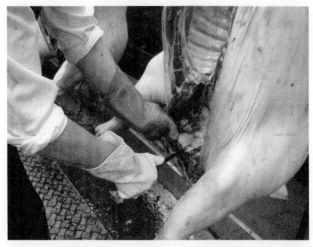

Figure 9.10 Traditional post-mortem inspection of the porcine head and submaxillary lymph nodes (Reproduced with permission from Harold Moore).

Skin lesions are an important diagnostic feature of swine erysipelas, swine fever and urticaria. The skin should also be examined for 'shotty eruption', the tail for necrosis, the feet for abscess formation and the udder for actinomycosis.

The viscera require inspection in the manner detailed for cattle, with particular attention to pneumonia and the secondary complications that develop in virus pneumonia, mainly pleurisy, pericarditis and, to a lesser extent, peritonitis.

The submaxillary lymph nodes are routinely examined for TB. Abscesses in the submaxillary lymph node may be caused by the passage of sharp foreign bodies through the wall of the pharynx or, in some countries, a beta-haemolytic *streptococcus* which also often causes tongue abscesses. Small yellow, necrotic foci resembling TB but caused by *Corynebacterium equi* are sometimes found in these nodes. The presence of metal spicules in the dorsum of the tongue has been identified as a problem in the United Kingdom by the manufacturers of pressed tongue. Some of these fragments have been identified as hypodermic needles, but others are pieces of wire and would appear to have originated from car tyres given to the pigs as 'toys'. The liver need not be incised except when it appears cirrhotic. The kidney surface should be examined for cysts and systemic changes (Fig. 9.10).

Where *Cysticercus cellulosae* is prevalent, the investigation must include examination of the directly visible muscular surfaces, in particular the thigh muscles, the pillars of the diaphragm, the intercostal muscles, the heart, the tongue and the larynx and, if necessary, the abdominal wall and the psoas muscles freed from fatty tissue. Where trichinosis is known or suspected, appropriate examination and muscle sampling must be carried out.

Current post-mortem inspection in the pig requires that only the submaxillary lymph nodes and the supramammary lymph nodes in sows are routinely incised. Within the EU, the mesenteric lymph nodes of pigs are no longer incised because of the frequent contamination of knives with *Salmonella* organisms which may be present in the nodes.

Traditional post-mortem inspection of equines

Post-mortem inspection of equidae follows the same general pattern for cattle and all other livestock. Although equidae generally possess fewer lesions than other animals, particular attention should be paid to the lungs and liver for evidence of echinococcal cysts and to the muscles and lymph nodes for melanosis. The main carcase lymph nodes should be examined when systemic or generalised disease is suspected, when TB lesions are detected and when the live animal has shown a reaction to the mallein test. The possibility of glanders requires that the mucous membranes, trachea, larynx, nasal cavities, sinuses and their ramifications are carefully examined, after splitting the head in the median plane and excision of the nasal septum.

Traditional post-mortem inspection of poultry

Facilities should be available for whole-carcase inspection after defeathering and washing. Cases with obvious disease, fractures, injuries, blood blisters, etc. can be detected and detained at this stage.

Second-stage inspection takes place on the partially eviscerated carcase where it is possible to relate carcase and viscera. The viscera, hock joints and tibias are observed and the latter palpated. The body cavity and internal organs are viewed. In some cases, one inspector examines the carcase, while another examines the viscera – of value in turkeys but not in broilers. In the United States, it is recommended that the spleen of adult birds be crushed. The trimmer is instructed to trim, remove viscera, condemn, etc. as necessary.

It is essential that the inspector in charge arranges for a line speed consistent with the number and competence of his inspectors, type of poultry, presentation methods, incidence of disease, efficiency of evisceration procedures, etc. Line speeds should be reduced in any unfavourable situation and brought back to normal only when conditions are satisfactory. If necessary, operations should cease until the situation is satisfactory. It is recommended that the line start and stop control be within reach of the inspector in charge.

Decisions at post-mortem examination

The *final judgement* as to the action to be taken with a carcase or parts of a carcase *is based on the total evidence produced by observation, palpation, incision, smell, ante-mortem signs and the results of any laboratory test*. It is essential, therefore, that the results of ante-mortem and supporting laboratory tests are available to the veterinarian when he is making the final decision.

For some conditions, legislation, such as that based on EC Regulation 854/2004, Annex 1, Section II, Chapter V, declares unfit all meat, offal or blood which has originated from animals found on inspection to exhibit signs of the disease. This includes:

a. Derives from animals that have not undergone ante-mortem inspection, except for hunted wild game
b. Derives from animals the offal of which has not undergone post-mortem inspection unless otherwise provided for under Regulation (EC) 854/2004 or 853/2004
c. Derives from animals which are dead before slaughter, stillborn, unborn or slaughtered under the age of 7 days
d. Results from the trimming of sticking points
e. Derives from animals affected by an OIE List A or, where appropriate, OIE List B disease, unless otherwise provided for in Section IV
f. Derives from animals affected by generalised disease such as generalised septicaemia, pyaemia, toxaemia or viraemia
g. Is not in conformity with microbiological criteria laid down under Community legislation to determine whether food may be placed on the market
h. Exhibits parasitic infestation, unless otherwise provided for in Section IV

i. Contains residues or contaminants in excess of the levels laid down in Community legislation. Any overshooting of the relevant level should lead to additional analyses whenever appropriate
j. Without prejudice to more specific Community legislation, derives from animals or carcasses containing residues of forbidden substances or from animals treated with forbidden substances
k. Consists of the liver and kidneys of animals more than 2 years old from regions where implementation of plans approved in accordance with Article 5 of Directive 96/23/EC has revealed the generalised presence of heavy metals in the environment
l. Has been treated illegally with decontaminating substances
m. Has been treated illegally with ionising or UV rays
n. Contains foreign bodies (except, in the case of wild game, material used to hunt the animal)
o. Exceeds the maximum permitted radioactivity levels laid down under Community legislation
p. Indicates pathophysiological changes, anomalies in consistency, insufficient bleeding (except for wild game) or organoleptic anomalies, in particular a pronounced sexual odour
q. Derives from emaciated animals
r. Contains specific risk material, except as provided for under Community legislation
s. Shows soiling, faecal or other contamination
t. Consists of blood that may constitute a risk to public health owing to the health status of any animal from which it derives or contamination arising during the slaughter process
u. In the opinion of the official veterinarian, after examination of all the relevant information, it may constitute a risk to public and animal health or is for any other reason not suitable for human consumption

The regulation also identifies (Annex I, Section IV, Chapter IX) six specific conditions for which specific directions are given. These are as follows:

1 **Transmissible Spongiform Encephalopathies (BSE and Scrapie)**
Controls have varied over the years as the risk to public health has varied.

A short history of BSE
There have been few conditions that have had such a major impact on meat inspection theory, thinking and controls as BSE. As a direct result of the disease, the EFSA was established. Ministers across Europe were forced to resign, thousands of cattle were destroyed and/or removed from the food chain and completely new testing and inspection regimes were

1979	Changes to rendering treatment parameters
1985	First suspect cases of BSE
1986	BSE identified as a new disease entity
1988	BSE made a notifiable disease
1988	Ban on use of milk from BSE suspects other than for feeding to the cow's own calf
1989	Meat and bone meal in animal feed identified as source of infectivity and banned from ruminant feed
1990	Specified material (certain tissues likely to contain most infectivity) controlled and removed from food chain
1995	First cases of variant Creutzfeldt–Jakob disease (vCJD) identified in Great Britain
1996	Link between vCJD and BSE established – March 1996
	EU ban on trade of beef from the United Kingdom
	Ban on use of meat from cattle more than 30 months of age at slaughter. The Over Thirty Month Scheme (OTMS) set up to dispose of cattle aged over 30 months at slaughter. Specified material extended to other cattle tissues and to sheep.
	Approval of XAP scheme which allowed beef processors to bring beef from outside the United Kingdom, process it under supervision and export it to other member states
1997	Bone in beef prohibited for retail sale due to risk identified in experimental work. Ban was short lived due to apparent public demand for T-bone steaks
1998	The Export Certified Herd Scheme was agreed only for Northern Ireland to allow beef from animals from certain herds slaughtered and processed under certain conditions to be exported to other member states. The scheme collapsed due to the slaughter of ineligible animals
1999	The Date-Based Export Scheme agreed for United Kingdom allowing beef from animals born after 1 August 1996 meeting additional criteria and slaughtered and processed under controlled conditions to be exported to other member states
2000	Introduction of transmissible spongiform encephalopathy (TSE) testing of brainstem samples collected from animals at slaughter and OTMS animals at the rendering plant
2001	EU legislation introducing controls in all member states to control and eradicate BSE and scrapie in sheep, specified tissue and animal feed controls. BSE testing fully implemented
2005	Beef from over-thirty-month (OTM) animals returns to the food chain. Testing of all OTM animals required as part of disease surveillance. Animals born before 1 August 1996 cannot be used for human consumption
2006	UK export ban lifted
	The OTM Scheme ends and the Old Cow Disposal Scheme (OCDS) begins as an outlet for animals born before 1 August 1996
2009	End of the OCDS
	TSE testing of animals at slaughter moved from over 30 to over 48 months. All surviving pre-1996 animals banned from the food chain permanently
2011	TSE testing of animals at slaughter moved from over 48 to over 72 months
2012	No recorded deaths or new suspect vCJD cases in United Kingdom since first cases were recorded in 1995
	Total of 176 vCJD deaths since 1995
	Routine TSE testing of animals at slaughter stopped with testing of a small number of 'high-risk' animals only

put in place. The following is a brief chronology of the disease and its control from its first diagnosis as a clinical disease to the dismantling of the additional controls put in place to control it and to provide reassurance to consumers.

We do not know what the future will bring, and it is difficult to define success, given that 177 people died from vCJD in the UK, but it is fair to say that the disease has been controlled. Given that the incubation period (time from infection to clinical signs) for BSE is estimated to be 5 years and that the causal agent has not been identified, it is reassuring that the control procedures put in place have controlled this new disease within five incubation periods.

2 **Cysticercosis**

Taenia solium – *C. cellulosae* – human pork tapeworms. The adult tapeworm is 3–5 cm long. They can survive in humans for many years. Eggs are passed out in the faeces, and after ingestion by a susceptible pig, the ova hatch in the intestine and the resultant oncospheres travel via the blood to muscles but can also go to the lungs and liver, kidney and brain. Humans become infected by ingesting raw or inadequately cooked pork containing viable cysticerci. The human final host may also act as an intermediate host and become infected with cysticerci, most likely from the accidental ingestion of *T. solium* eggs via unwashed hands or contaminated food. It is most prevalent

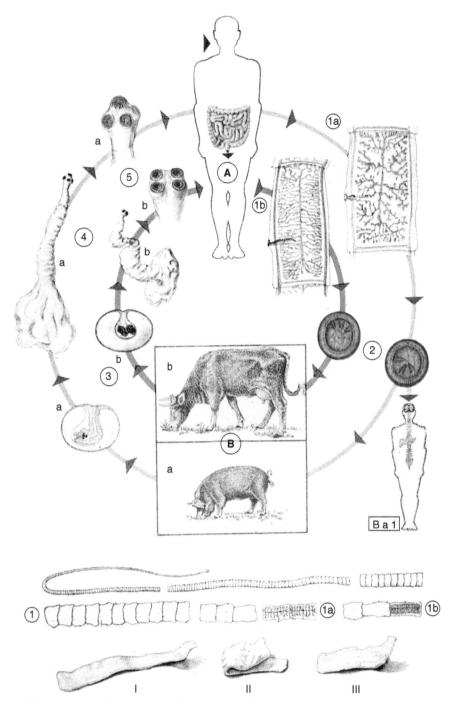

Figure 9.11 Life cycle of *T. saginata/T. solium* (Courtesy of Prof. A.J. Trees).

in South and Central America, India, Africa and parts of the Far East, apart from areas where there are religious sanctions on the eating of pork. The condition is now very uncommon in most developed countries (Fig. 9.11).

Taenia saginata, C. bovis – beef tapeworm, 'beef measles'. The condition is present worldwide, particularly important in Africa and South America. Prevalence studies within the EU vary from 0.01% in

Italy, 0.02% in Germany and 0.22% in Belgium (EFSA, 2010). The adult tapeworm is found only in humans and is 5–15 cm in length. An infected human can pass million of eggs daily.

After ingestion, the ova hatch to form oncospheres which travel via the blood to striated muscles. It is first grossly visible about 2 weeks later as a pale, semi-transparent spot about 1.0 mm in diameter, but it is not infective to man until about 12 weeks later when it has reached its full size of 1.0 cm and is greyish white, oval and enclosed by the host in a thin fibrous capsule. The scolex is usually clearly visible. The cysts last from weeks to years. When they die, they are usually replaced by a caseous, crumbly mass which may become calcified. Both living and dead cysts are frequently present in the same carcase. Humans become infected by ingesting raw or inadequately cooked meat. Development to patency takes 2–3 months.

Although *C. bovis* may occur anywhere in the striated muscles, the predilection sites are the heart, the tongue and the masseter and intercostal muscles.

There are two quite distinct epidemiological patterns found in developing countries and developed countries.

In many parts of Africa, Asia and Latin America, cattle are reared on an extensive scale, and human sanitation is poor. Human infection can be over 20% and cattle infection 30–60% on routine carcase infection although the prevalence is thought to be much higher. In areas such as Europe, North America, Australia and New Zealand, standards of sanitation are high, and meat is carefully inspected and generally thoroughly cooked before consumption. In these countries, the prevalence of cysticercosis is low, but this may vary with the diligence of inspection, although one has to weigh the requirements of detection of cysticercus against the damage to the carcase and consequent lower value.

Occasionally, a cysticercosis 'storm' can occur when a high proportion of cattle are infected. This is associated with the improper use of human sewage as a fertiliser or the use of a farm slurry tanker to empty a human septic tank.

T. saginata eggs may survive for more than 200 days in sludge. In agricultural practice, the use of human sludge as a fertiliser should be confined to elevated fields or to those on which cattle will not be grazed for 2 years.

Other causes of sudden high incidence on a farm may be due to a tapeworm infection in a stockman either as a random event or as a result of migrant labour from a country with a high incidence of infection.

The cause of the low but persistent infection in cattle is thought to be due to the access of cattle to water contaminated with sewage effluents, to the carriage and dispersal of *T. saginata* eggs by birds which frequent sewage works or feed on effluent discharge into rivers or sea and, transport the eggs to pasture and occasional fouling of pasture by itinerant infected individuals. In contrast to the developing countries, cattle of any age are susceptible. When cattle are first infected as adults, the longevity of the cysticerci is limited, most being dead within 9 months.

Meat infected with *C. bovis* is considered to be unfit for human if generalised, that is, more than one area or part affected. If the infestation is localised, the parts not infected may be considered fit following upon cold treatment – at less than −7°C for at least 3 weeks or −10°C for at least 2 weeks. Table 9.2 may be used to assist judgements.

3 Trichinellosis

Trichinella spiralis is a roundworm found in pig, rat, man and most mammals. The life cycle is indirect. Adult parasites and infective larvae are unusual in being present within a single host.

The developing adults (Fig. 9.13) live between the villi of the small intestine. After fertilisation, the males die, while females bury deeper into the intestinal mucosa.

After a week, they produce L1 larvae which enter the bloodstream and make their way to the skeletal muscles. The larvae penetrate striated muscle cells where they grow rapidly and begin to coil within the cell. This takes 3–6 weeks after which the larvae are infective. Development is resumed when the muscle is ingested by another host. Infection in man is acquired by eating inadequately cooked pork or its by-products such as sausages, ham and salami. Smoking, drying or curing meat does not necessarily kill the larvae. Horse meat has increasingly been implicated in the transmission to man (Fig. 9.12).

Table 9.2 Guide to judgements on *C. bovis* findings

Post-mortem finding				Judgement
Number	Location	Status	Cyst	
More than one	Generalised	Viable	1	Reject the carcase and the offal
One or more	Localised	Viable	1 (v)	Reject affected organ or carcase part.
		Caseous or calcified	1 or more (nv)	Require cold treatment of remainder
More than one	Generalised	Caseous or calcified	1 (nv)	Reject the affected organs or carcase parts Require cold treatment of remainder

nv, non-viable; degeneration has occurred; v, viable.

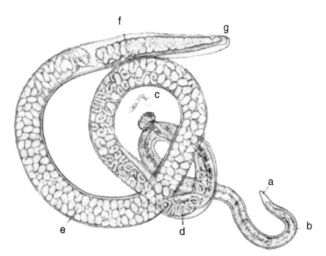

Figure 9.12 Adult female *T. spiralis*: (a) oral opening; (b) oesophagus; (c) newborn larva, just expelled from vulva; (d) larvae in interior portion of uterus; (e) fertilised and developing ova; (f) ovary; and (g) rectum, ×100 (By courtesy of Dr. S.E. Gould).

Table 9.3 Summary of time/temperature combinations for treatment of domestic pig meat for *Trichinella*

Cold treatment	Maximum thickness of pieces of pork (cm)	Maximum temperature of the chill (°C)	Minimum consecutive time for cold treatment (days)
1	Up to 15	−15	20
	Up to 15	−23	10
	Up to 15	−29	6
2	15–50	−15	30
	15–50	−25	20
	15–50	−29	12
3	Up to 25	−25	10
	25–50	−25	20

Trichinella testing of potentially infected swine and equines is an official control within the EU, with the specific technical detail of the testing regime laid down in legislation, Regulation 2075/2005 and its successors. Except for those few countries considered to be free from *Trichinella*, both in livestock and wildlife, samples must be collected from breeding domestic pigs, that is, sows and boars, wild boar, solipeds and pigs reared and fattened outdoors, not in controlled housing. Examination is either by direct observation of flattened striated muscle samples through a stereoscopic microscope, a trichinoscope, or through a bulk digest method, in which compounded samples are treated with hydrochloric acid and pepsin prior to microscopic examination.

Cold treatment of meat may be used as an alternative to *Trichinella* testing for domestic pig meat. The time/

Table 9.4 Time/temperature combination for treatment of domestic pig meat where core temperatures can be measured

Maximum core temp of pig meat (°C)	Minimum consecutive time period for the cold treatment
−18	106 hours
−21	82 hours
−23.5	63 hours
26	48 hours
29	35 hours
32	22 hours
35	8 hours
37	30 minutes

temperature combination for cold treatment is dependent on the thickness of the pieces of meat (see Table 9.3 for a summary). However, if it is possible to monitor the core temperature of the pig meat, alternate time/temperature combinations are allowed (Table 9.4).

4 **Glanders**

Where appropriate, solipeds are to be examined for glanders. This requires careful inspection of the mucous membranes from the trachea, larynx, nasal cavities and sinuses and their ramifications. This requires the head to be split lengthways.

Meat from horses found to have glanders is unfit for human consumption.

5 **Tuberculosis**

Human infection with bovine TB from the consumption of meat from infected cattle has never been recorded. However, EU regulations require that animals that have reacted positively to an intradermal tuberculin test are slaughtered separately and that precautions are taken to avoid cross-contamination. Where inspection reveals localised tuberculous lesions in more than one organ or area of the carcase, the whole carcase and its offals and blood should be declared unfit for human consumption. If tuberculous lesions are found only in a single organ or part of a carcase, the affected organ or carcase area need only be removed.

The EFSA opinion on the public health hazards to be covered by inspection of meat (bovine animals) (2013) recognised that while there was no evidence that *M. bovis*, bovine TB, could infect humans through meat in the EU, traditional inspection through lymph node incision provided important surveillance information, particularly in low-incidence or officially tuberculosis-free (OTF) member states or zones (Fig. 9.13).

6 **Brucellosis**

The carcase and offal from an animal with lesions suggestive of acute brucellosis must be considered unfit for human consumption.

(a)

(b)

(c)

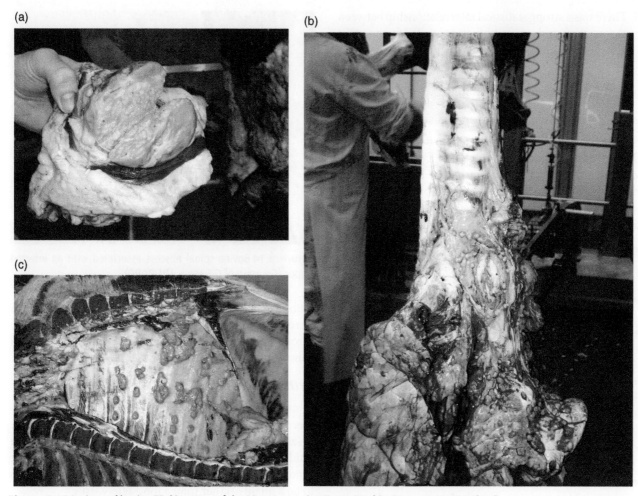

Figure 9.13 Lesions of bovine TB (Courtesy of the Meat Inspection Team, Dunbia, Dungannon, N. Ireland).

Common post-mortem findings

Inspectors often disagree about how best to interprete common post-mortem findings. Decisions require the detailed examination of suspect animals including all parts of the carcase and viscera, even organs and parts whose position is remote from what is considered to be the primary lesion. This will determine whether the lesions are *localised* or *generalised* and consequently the extent of condemnation necessary.

Similarly, the nature of the specific lesion, along with the entire carcase and viscera, must be considered to decide whether the condition is *acute* or *chronic*.

As a general rule, the *acute* and *generalised* condition will require the *total condemnation* of the carcase and the viscera, while the *chronic* and *localised* may require only *local condemnation* or in some cases *no condemnation* at all. This emphasises the importance of correlation of inspection procedures and the importance of ensuring that viscera follow the carcase on to the detained rail since there may be significant lesions in both. If we consider some specific lesions, some general guidance can be suggested.

Abscesses

Abscesses are one of the most common lesions routinely encountered in pigs. A study carried out to map the position of abscesses in 75 130 pigs produced the following findings (Huey, 1996):

1 2.87% of pigs examined had an abscess at one site.
2 The dominant bacterium isolated from all abscesses was *Actinomyces pyogenes*. It has been argued (Berends *et al.*, 1993) that since this bacterium poses little threat to the consumer's physical health, only local condemnation is ever justified. However, any indication of a bacteraemia or pyaemia can do little for the quality of the meat and nothing to reassure the public as to the safety of their food. As Norval stated in 1966, 'there can be nothing more disgusting to the butcher or housewife than to slice through an abscess when preparing meat'.
3 0.26% of pigs slaughtered possessed abscesses at more than one site.
4 Of these, 80% had the tail as one of the sites, indicating the importance of tail biting in the aetiology.

5 There was a strong statistical interrelationship between abscesses found in combination at tail/lungs, tail/vertebrae, tail/legs, tail/ribs and tail/peritoneum.

As stated earlier, the following are the two most important questions to be answered.

Is the lesion localised or generalised?

A study of the literature indicates that it is most likely that infection spreads from the tail of a pig to the pelvis via the local lymphatic system, from the tail to the lungs, ribs and legs via the bloodstream and from the tail to the spinal vertebrae via the cerebrospinal fluid. This would indicate the following in terms of condemnation:

- *Abscesses at a single site*: Condemnation of the part is usually sufficient, after careful examination of the rest of the carcase and the viscera.
- *Abscess in the tail and one or more in the spinal vertebrae*: Remove the tail and the spinal column only.
- *Abscess in the tail and one or more in the lungs, ribs, peritoneum or forelegs*: Condemnation of the carcase is justified.
- *Abscess in the tail and hindleg*: Local condemnation may be sufficient.
- There is no apparent interrelationship between abscesses in the head or the neck and those elsewhere, for example, the tail or lungs, so only local condemnation is indicated.
- A statistically significant interrelationship was demonstrated between abscesses in fore- and hindlegs. In each case, the aetiology must be considered before a judgement can be made. If, for example, the cause is thought to be rough floors and there is no evidence of haematogenous spread, local condemnation may suffice.

Is the lesion acute or chronic?

If an abscess is in the acute stage of development, in that there is poor or no capsule formation, accompanied by systemic changes, it will usually be necessary to totally condemn the carcase and viscera (Fig. 9.14).

Omphalophlebitis

Omphalophlebitis or navel ill is a relatively common post-mortem finding in countries where very young calves, 4–8 days old, are slaughtered. A study in New Zealand (Biss *et al.*, 1994) suggested that there was histopathological evidence that a low-grade bacteraemia was present in approximately 25% of these calves and that routine condemnation of the carcase was justified in *extended* or *systemic*, but not in *localised* cases. *Localised* was defined where lesions were restricted to the umbilicus, *extended* where lesions were also evident in the

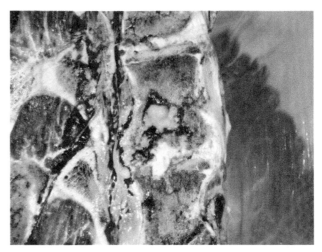

Figure 9.14 Bovine spinal abscess associated with an infected carpus (Courtesy of G Rankin, OV, DARD).

umbilical vessels and *systemic* navel ill where lesions were present in the liver and/or other viscera and the carcase as well as the umbilical tissues. Localised navel ill constituted about 75% of all navel ill cases.

Arthritis

A small quantity of blood-tinged fluid in a joint is neither unusual nor significant. In all but the most acute cases, the causative agent cannot be cultured from the fluid found in the joint; it can only be isolated from the synovial membrane. Most authorities consider arthritis to be a quality rather than a food safety issue.

However, on either safety or aesthetic grounds, the following can be used as a basis for judgement:

- If there is purulent material present, the limb should be condemned to the joint above the one affected.
- The limb should be condemned if there is iliac, prescapular or prepectoral lymph node involvement.
- If three or more limbs show lymphatic involvement, the carcase warrants rejection.
- If the popliteal lymph node is enlarged but the iliacs are normal, it may be sufficient to reject only the lower limb.
- If there are systemic changes in the viscera indicating that the arthritis is generalised or acute, the carcase and viscera should be condemned.

Oedema

In the healthy animal, there is osmotic equilibrium between intracellular and extracellular parts. Disturbances of water and sodium homeostasis (sodium retention), hydrostatic pressure or decreased plasma pressure, hypoproteinaemia, heart or kidney failure, lymphatic obstruction, etc. lead to the accumulation of fluid in the intercellular spaces and cavities of the body.

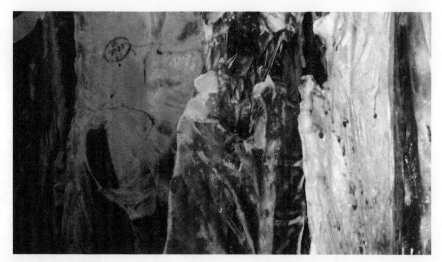

Figure 9.15 Oedema on bovine shoulder.

Oedema fluid, with its low protein content, is termed a *transudate* as opposed to an *exudate* of inflammation, which is rich in protein, leukocytes and fibrin.

When this fluid collects in the peritoneal cavity, it is called *ascites*; in the pleural cavity, *hydrothorax*; in the pericardial sac, *hydropericardium*; in the brain, *hydrocephalus*; and in the subcutaneous and connective tissue spaces, *anasarca*. The term *effusion* is also used to denote an escape of fluid into a part, for example, pericardial effusion.

Oedema may be *localised*, as in acute inflammation, photosensitisation and cerebral and pulmonary oedema; *generalised* as in severe malnutrition, parasitic gastroenteritis, fascioliasis and *brisket disease* of cattle. It may be *inflammatory* or *non-inflammatory* in origin.

In cases of malnutrition and starvation where there is severe protein deficiency, oedema is evident in a generalised form – *nutritional oedema*.

Oedema may also be produced by an *increased permeability* of capillary walls as a result of damage by toxins or to an increased filtrability of the blood. Such changes are evident in allergic conditions like urticaria and purpura haemorrhagica and in bacterial diseases like bowel oedema, malignant oedema, anthrax and mulberry heart disease.

Obstruction to the lymphatic flow from a part, for example, by tumours or granulomas, may result in oedema.

In oedema, the affected area is swollen (often several centimetres in depth and mostly well defined), firm, painless and pits on pressure. Section incision reveals a pale yellowish fluid or gelatinous mass from drips which fluid, which has a tendency to clot.

Localised, minor forms of oedema and ascites and hydrothorax are of less serious import than anasarca and

---

Test for oedema

A test for oedema involves the estimation of water content of bone marrow. This consists of floating pea-sized pieces of fat from a long bone in alcohol of strengths 32, 47 and 52%. Marrow containing less than 25% of water will float in each solution of alcohol, in which case the carcase may be released provided there are no other abnormalities; if the water content of the marrow is 50% or more, the marrow sinks in two or three of the solutions and the carcase is judged unfit for food.

---

much easier to judge. Oedema combined with poorness is probably one of the most difficult decisions to make in meat inspection. Detention of the carcase for 12 hours is indicated in all generalised cases while tests are being undertaken (Fig. 9.15).

If the serous cavities have dried out well and the carcase has set properly with reasonable or good condition, the carcase may be passed for food. However, in *anasarca* (oedema) involving the subcutaneous and connective tissues or any form of oedema accompanied by emaciation and non-setting, the carcase should be condemned. (In healthy cattle, the bone marrow contains not more than 25% of water, but in anasarca, it holds more than 50%.)

Pneumonia and pleurisy

Carcases must be condemned if there are any signs of systemic change in the viscera, especially the liver, kidney and carcase lymph nodes. If there is no such evidence, condemnation of the carcase cannot be justified, and stripping of the pleura or removal of the rib cage may suffice. In almost all cases where it is necessary

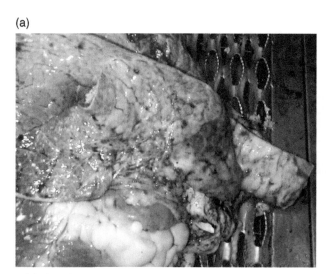

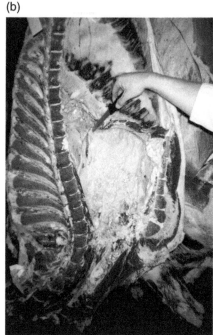

Figure 9.16 (a) Chronic pneumonia in apical and part cardiac lobes. (b) Bovine suppurative pneumonia.

to strip the pleura, the diaphragm should be removed (Fig. 9.16).

The possibility of *antimicrobial residues* being present must be considered.

Endocarditis

Endocarditis (inflammation of the endothelial lining of the heart) is bacterial, parasitic or mycotic in origin, most often affecting the valves. The most common lesion is *verrucose* or *vegetative endocarditis* of pigs, a valuable diagnostic lesion of chronic swine erysipelas. The mitral valve is the main part involved, varying degrees of rough yellowish or greyish yellow adhering to the valve, sometimes large enough to occlude the atrioventricular orifice. The chordae tendineae may also show vegetations. Streptococci, especially *Str. suis* type 2, are common causes of acute endocarditis in pigs.

An extensive analysis of the results of bacteriological investigations and judgements of samples obtained from 117 pigs and cattle diagnosed at post-mortem with endocarditis, between 1977 and 1989 in Hungary, was carried out by Szazados (1991). In pigs, *Erysipelothrix rhusiopathiae*, a beta-haemolytic streptococci, streptococci belonging to the viridans group, *Arcanobacterium pyogenes* (formally Corynebacterium pyogenes) and *Staphylococcus aureus*, were isolated in decreasing order of frequency. In cattle, *A. pyogenes* was isolated most frequently.

Ulcerative valvular endocarditis due to streptococci or *Corynebacterium (A.) pyogenes* is occasionally met with in the bovine, appearing as rough valvular plaques.

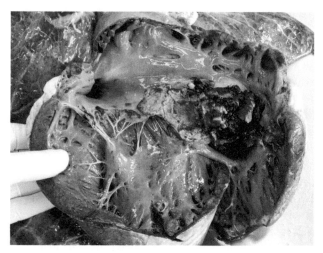

Figure 9.17 Endocarditis – classic vegetative lesion right side of heart (Courtesy of Hal Thompson).

In sheep, verrucose endocarditis, when caused by *Streptoccus faecalis*, is usually seen on the bicuspid valve.

Bacteria were present in the spleen, liver and kidney of over 60% of the samples examined, and muscle and lymph nodes were positive in over 30% of samples.

Of the 117 cases, 79 cases (67.5%) were condemned for septicaemia. Without this type of detailed bacteriological examination, however, given these statistics, condemnation of the carcase is justified in all cases of endocarditis (Fig. 9.17).

Pericarditis

Pericarditis (inflammation of the pericardium) may be serous (early stages), fibrinous or septic. Early stages show hyperaemia with a thin, clear exudate.

Fibrinous pericarditis: In later stages, greyish-white fibrin strands are formed, sometimes flecked with blood, and the exudate is reduced in amount. In chronic fibrinous pericarditis, the fibrinous exudate appears as villous strands when the epicardium and pericardium are separated – 'bread-and-butter' pericarditis.

Septic or purulent pericarditis: The presence of pyogenic bacteria is indicated by the appearance of pus which varies in consistency and colour according to the types of organisms involved – thin, whitish pus or thick creamy, yellowish, yellowish-green or greenish pus. Putrefactive bacteria produce a foul smelling pus (Fig. 9.18).

(a)

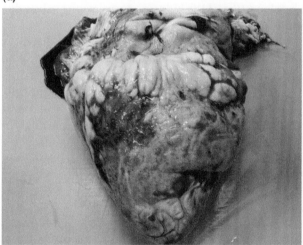

(b)

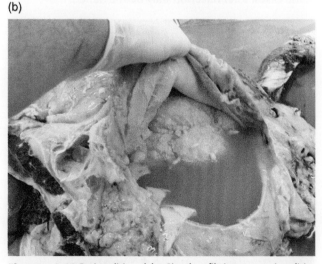

Figure 9.18 Pericarditis. (a) Simple fibrinous pericarditis. (b) Suppurative pericarditis with fibrino-purulent exudate (Courtesy of Hal Thompson).

Septic pericarditis is the form occurring in *traumatic reticulopericarditis* in cattle. (Traumatic pericarditis can also occur in the horse and sheep.) Early forms show the aforementioned septic changes, but more chronic cases reveal varying deposits of fibrin which fuse the epicardium and pericardium together. The pericardial sac itself is thickened, and there is usually a fistulous cord-like fibrous tract (which may contain some pus) connecting the reticulum and pericardium. *A. (formally C.) pyogenes* is the most common organism in a mixed flora which may contain anaerobic gas-forming bacteria. A local chronic peritonitis is frequently associated with the fistulous tract and may give rise to adhesions between the diaphragm, pericardial sac and anterior aspect of the reticulum. Pleural and pneumonic changes are frequent associates. Bacteria may pass from the infected pericardial sac into the bloodstream, producing septicaemia, but more commonly the infective material remains encapsulated with toxins being released to cause cachexia.

Traumatic reticulopericarditis occurs most often in cows over 4 years of age, often shortly after parturition. Its frequency is related to the bovine habit of licking and swallowing various foreign bodies and the close relationship of the reticulum and the heart. These organs are about 5 cm apart during expiration and 2.5 cm during inspiration. The regular movement of the diaphragm during respiration facilitates the forward movement of sharp objects through the anteroventral border of the reticulum and the diaphragm to penetrate the pericardial sac at the apex of the heart. Occasionally, sharp objects may penetrate the myocardium, lung, pleura, liver or spleen.

Pyelonephritis

Pyelonephritis is a fairly common disease in cows, generally occurring as a sequel to parturition, but it also affects sows (mainly the acute form). It is rare in calves, horses, sheep and goats. It attacks the kidney pelvis and parenchyma and results from ascending infection. As with other kidney infections, it may be acute, chronic, septic or non-septic.

The condition is probably a mixed bacterial one, but a prominent organism appears to be *Actinobaculum suis*.

Pyelonephritis may be unilateral or bilateral and is manifested by catarrh and dilatation of the renal pelvis which is filled with a slimy detritus which may contain fibrinous clot or pus and possesses a strong ammoniacal odour. The acute form begins with inflammation and necrosis of the renal crest (projection of the renal medulla into the pelvis containing the openings of the tubules). At this stage, the parenchyma is swollen, dark red and firm. Haemorrhages may also be present in the acute stage. If infection extends along the uriniferous tubules, it may give rise to abscesses in the cortex and irregular grey areas on the kidney surface. Occasionally, the infection causes complete obliteration of the kidney parenchyma, making the organ a purulent sac.

As the disease progresses in more typical situations, chronic tubulointerstitial nephritis supervenes with progressive fibrosis. Scarring with contraction of the fibrous tissue and loss of kidney tissue produce marked contraction and distortion of the organ even to virtual obliteration of some lobes. In very severe cases, the kidney assumes a greyish, nodular appearance, becoming very small in size.

Bruising

It is now broadly accepted that:
Muscle tissue is generally sterile until it is exposed to extraneous contamination.
Extraneous contaminants grow no faster on bruised than unbruised tissue.
There is no difference in the microbiological condition of meat from bled and unbled lamb carcases.

The trimming of bruised tissue is therefore purely aesthetic.

Pigmentation

Pigments may emanate from outside the body (*exogenous* pigments) or from within the body (*endogenous* pigments).

Exogenous pigments are normally associated with the grazing of livestock in proximity to certain industries and with urban pollution. The most common is *carbon* or *coal dust* which causes pneumoconiosis in coal miners and various dusts. Carbon appears as black particles in the lung tissue and associated lymph nodes.

Carotenoid pigments derived from carotene A and B (precursors of vitamin A) and *xanthophyll* are of plant origin. These *lipochrome pigments* are normal constituents of many different body tissues – adrenal gland, Kupffer cells of the liver, corpus luteum, testes and the adipose tissue of Jersey and Guernsey cattle as well as the yolk of eggs and butter fat. They are also found in the so-called subcutaneous xanthomas of poultry. These are not true tumours but collections of connective tissue cells and cholesterol-containing phagocytes.

Endogenous pigments in animals include melanin, haematin, haemosiderin, bile pigments, porphyrin, lipofuscin and cloisonné kidney pigment in sheep and goats.

Melanin

All healthy pigmented skin contains a brownish-black protein colouring substance, *melanin*, produced in melanocytes by the oxidation of the amino acid tyrosine. It is especially evident on the surface of the bovine palate, tongue and cheeks and in the hair, horns and eyes of dark-skinned cattle, black and grey horses and black and red pigs. The deposits are black or brown in colour and usually of irregular shape and size, most being about a centimetre in diameter.

Abnormal deposits of melanin (*melanosis*) are encountered chiefly in the bovine and less commonly in sheep and pigs. In the *ox*, melanosis is commonly found in the lungs, liver and meninges, where it usually involves the pia mater and more rarely the dura mater and is termed *black pith*. The pigmentation may also be found on the pleura and peritoneum, in cartilages and bone and between muscles. The black colouration of the kidneys of adult cattle, especially the Red Danish breed, may be due to melanin or *lipofuscin*, an endogenous pigment closely allied to melanin. In calves, the liver and the cortex of the kidney are frequently affected, but this must be distinguished from the blackish colouration of the kidneys of very young calves due to bile pigments.

In *sheep*, melanosis is most common in the liver, but some black hepatic pigmentation is due to lipofuscin, especially in Australia (Fig. 9.19).

In the *pig*, the condition is most often seen in the belly fat or in the udder of females, often being revealed as radiating lines or patches distributed along the ducts of the mammary glands.

Melanomas are malignant tumours which arise from melanin-forming cells (melanocytes).

Melanin in itself is not harmful, but affected organs should be condemned. Where the condition is generalised, total condemnation is warranted. The presence of a melanoma justifies a very detailed examination; in metastatic cases, total rejection may be warranted.

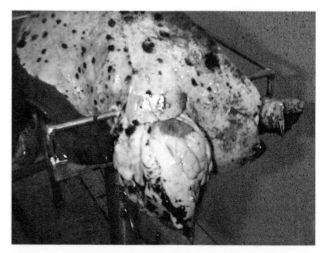

Figure 9.19 Melanosis in a bovine lung.

Haematogenous pigments

Haemoglobin (Hb) is a compound protein in red blood cells (RBCs) which consists of the iron-containing porphyrin pigment *haem* combined with the protein globin.

Certain pigments derived from Hb metabolism are encountered in some abnormal conditions.

Haematin is a pigment formed by the oxidation of haem from the ferrous to the ferric state. It occurs as a dark-brown, black or yellow granular pigment in the parasitised RBCs and reticuloendothelial cells in the spleen, liver, lymph nodes and bone marrow in diseases like babesiosis in which there is widespread destruction of RBCs. Several trematodes, for example, *Fascioloides magna*, and some schistosomes also produce haematins locally in the tissues.

Haemosiderin, an iron-containing pigment and store of iron (the other important iron storage pool is *ferritin*), occurs normally in hepatic cells, bone marrow and spleen (in macrophages). It appears in excess as yellowish granules in severe cases of RBC haemolysis as with haematin, in cases of extensive haemorrhage and chronic passive congestion. Haemosiderin combined with ferritin is occasionally observed in Angora goats in which a brownish or blackish pigmentation in kidneys has the appearance of enamelled jewellery – *cloisonné kidney*.

Bile pigments

Biliverdin is a green bile pigment formed from porphyrin by the breakdown of RBCs in the liver and bone marrow. It is rapidly reduced, mainly in the spleen, to *bilirubin*, an orange-yellow pigment, and then, bound with albumin, transported to the liver via the reticuloendothelial system. Most of the bilirubin passes from the liver to the gall bladder and eventually to the small intestine where it is reduced to meso-bilirubinogen and urobilinogen by bacteria. The latter, in association with stercobilin, colours the faeces brown.

Icterus

Icterus (*jaundice, hyperbilirubinaemia*), arising from haemolytic, obstructive hepatic or toxic causes, occurs when the balance between bilirubin production and clearance is disturbed. Bile pigments, mainly bilirubin, accumulate in the tissues, which are tinged yellow. The condition is caused by the reabsorption of bile pigment into the circulatory system and displays three main types (Fig. 9.20).

Obstructive jaundice may be due to mechanical obstruction to the flow of bile by gallstones; parasites such as liver flukes (especially *Dicrocoelium dendriti-*

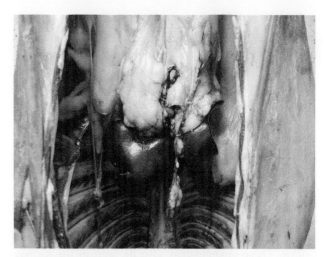

Figure 9.20 Icterus/jaundice in a lamb carcase.

cum), ascarids or tapeworms like *Thysanosoma actinoides* in the bile ducts; biliary cirrhosis (especially in the pig but rarely in cattle or sheep); cholangitis (inflammation of the gall bladder); and pressure from tumours, abscesses or granulomas. In pigs, the most common parasite in temperate regions to invade the bile ducts from the intestine is *Ascaris suum*.

Haemolytic jaundice denotes the excessive destruction of RBCs by infective organisms, for example, in babesiosis, eperythrozoonosis, anaplasmosis, equine infectious anaemia and leptospirosis in pigs. The yellow colouration is less marked in this form than in the obstructive and toxic types.

Toxic jaundice is brought about by the action of toxic substances on liver cells resulting in fatty change, necrosis and the liberation of plasma bilirubin. *Poisonous plants* incriminated are members of the *Senecio* species (ragwort and groundsel) such as *S. jacobaea* (ragwort, benweed), *S. vulgaris* (groundsel), *S. burchelli* and *S. cunninghamii* in North America and the latter with *S. quadridentatus and S. lautus* in Australia. These contain pyrrolizidine alkaloids which are potent hepatic toxins also found in certain *Crotalaria*, *Gossypium* (cotton plant) and *Allium* (garlic, onion) species. The mycotoxins associated with some *Lupin* spp. also cause hepatocyte injury and icterus. Some *inorganic poisons*, especially copper and selenium, and *organic compounds* such as phenothiazine can also cause severe jaundice. Excess copper in the diet of calves may cause icterus due to toxic hepatitis, cirrhosis and fatty change resulting in carcase condemnations.

A form of hyperbilirubinaemia which is not obstructive, haemolytic or toxic occurs in horses on starvation rations or from anorexia secondary to other diseases, for example, colic. Most cases are subclinical but some progress to frank disease.

In many cases, diagnosis of icterus can present a problem. In both live animals and carcases (especially of cattle and horses), yellow colouration occurs even when serum bile acids/bilirubin levels are normal. Conversely, hyperbilirubinaemia can occur where jaundice is not very evident, perhaps owing to masking by erythema of the mucous membranes. In cases of doubt, therefore, it is necessary to resort to *tests for plasma bilirubin*.

There is marked yellowish colouration of the superficial fatty tissues, the fat deposits within the visceral cavities and the serous membranes. Closer inspection may reveal an abnormal colour in connective tissue which varies from lemon to orange yellow or greenish yellow. These changes may also be seen in the kidney cortex, calyces and renal pelvis. Yellow pigmentation is often evident in large nerve trunks and in the endothelium of medium-sized arteries such as the internal and external iliacs and brachial and femoral arteries, which are coloured even in slightly icteric carcases. Icteric colouration may also be seen in the lungs, sclera of the eye, tendons and cartilaginous extremities of long bones.

In doubtful cases, for example, the presence of slight icterus in a well-nourished carcase, it should be detained for 24 hours and then re-examined since the action of normal muscle enzymes may remove the yellow colour. If the pigmentation is only slightly evident after the 24-hour detention, the carcase may be safely released for food. This is especially so in mild cases of obstructive jaundice, icterus associated with fractures, torsion of the spleen, etc.

Icterus in the pig associated with hepatic cirrhosis may also be accompanied by an abnormal odour and taste; overnight cooling tends to deepen the yellow colour, and the skin then appears freckled. Icteric pig carcases should therefore be detained for a similar period and then subjected to a *bile acids* and/or *boiling test*, the latter to detect abnormal odours. In the absence of these changes, the carcase may be passed as fit.

In all animals, a marked degree of icterus present after a 24 hour detention of the carcase warrants total condemnation. This is the situation in haemolytic, toxic and the more severe cases of obstructive jaundice. Icteric carcases should preferably be examined in daylight since artificial light may distort colours. If, under natural light, carcases show any degree of icterus along with parenchymatous degeneration of organs (the result of bacterial infection) or show an intense yellow or greenish discolouration without evidence of infection, they should be totally condemned.

Jaundice must be distinguished from the yellow colour of fat commonly seen in old bovines and certain dairy breeds like Jerseys and Guernseys in which it is

---

> **Laboratory tests for icterus**
>
> Icterus index (depth of colour of serum compared with standard solution) and serum bile acid assay are used.
>
> A useful test is to boil 2 g of fat from the suspect carcase in 5 ml of a 5% solution of NaOH for 1 minute in a boiling tube. Cool under the tap and carefully add 3–5 ml of ether. Shake and allow to stand. Layers will separate.
>
> A greenish-yellow colour in the *upper* layer indicates presence of carotenoid pigments; if colour is in the *lower* layer, bile pigments are indicated.

confined to the adipose tissues as the pigment carotene. This yellow colouration is also occasionally met with in pigs and sheep.

Porphyrin

Porphyrins are a group of reddish constituents of haem, the red iron-containing pigment of Hb in animals, of green photosynthetic chlorophylls of higher plants, of cytochrome (a red enzyme found in most cells) and of catalase, an enzyme responsible for the breakdown of hydrogen peroxide in mammalian tissues.

The porphyrias are a group of disorders in which there is excessive production of porphyrins or their precursors in the tissues due to enzymic deficiencies in haem biosynthesis. Symptoms include skin fragility and blistering, abdominal pain, paralysis, anaemia, reddish-brown teeth and bones with death in acute attacks.

In man and animals (cattle, sheep, horses, goats and pigs), the presence of photodynamic porphyrins and other substances in the blood (ingested, injected or present as a result of liver damage) causes them to be hypersensitive to sunlight, resulting in dermatitis and oedema – *photosensitisation*.

A rare *congenital* form (pink tooth, congenital porphyria) occurs in cattle, pigs, cats and man in which urine, bones and teeth are discoloured pink or reddish brown owing to excess porphyrin along with typical skin lesions on exposure to sunlight in cattle but not in pigs and cats. The lesions also occur in the lungs, kidneys, liver and lymph nodes.

The cattle type (*bovine congenital erythropoietic protoporphyria* (BCEP)) affects herds in which inbreeding and close linebreeding are practised – particularly Limousins. Cattle show signs of agitation, head shaking and ear twitching. Scaliness, oozing small scabs and flaking debris affected the pinnae of the ears, which were very sensitive to the touch.

Various plants contain photosensitising substances, such as hypericin in *Hypericum perforatum* (St. John's wort), fagopyrin in *Fagopyrum esculentum* and

Fagopyrum sagittatum (buckwheat), furocoumarin in *Ammi majus* (bishop's weed), *Cymopterus* spp. (spring parsley, wild carrot, various clovers, alfalfa and brassicas) and perloline in *Lolium perenne* (perennial ryegrass). Ingestion of these plants in active growth can cause primary photosensitisation.

Secondary or *hepatogenous photosensitisation* occurs when liver cells are damaged, for example, in hepatitis or biliary duct obstruction. *Phylloerythrin*, an end product of chlorophyll metabolism normally excreted in the bile, is then liberated into the bloodstream and accumulates in the tissues to cause photosensitisation. *Plants* responsible for hepatotoxic damage and secondary photosensitisation include bog asphodel (*Narthecium ossifragum*), *Lupin* spp. (*Lupinus*), *Lantana* spp. (*Lantana*) and panic grass spp. (*Panicum*). Various fungi can be responsible, for example, *Pithomyces chartarum*, which contains sporidesmin, is found in perennial ryegrass (*L. perenne*) and is the cause of *facial eczema* in New Zealand sheep (*big head* or *geeldikop* in South Africa). Certain *chemicals* such as phenothiazine, carbon tetrachloride and corticosteroids may also induce photosensitisation.

The *lesions* of photosensitisation are confined to the white, unpigmented, less hairy and woolly areas of the skin which become reddened and oedematous. Commonly affected parts are the face and ears, but teats, vulva and perineum may also be involved. Skin necrosis and gangrene often ensue. General signs of weakness, fever, anaemia, posterior paralysis and nervous symptoms with death are not uncommon.

The condition must be distinguished from 'big head' in sheep caused by *Cl. oedematiens* (*Cl. novyi*).

When bony structures are affected with pigmentation, consideration should be given to boning-out with release of the unaffected muscular tissue for food. In local affections, the affected part only need be rejected.

Lipofuscin ('wear-and-tear pigment', pigment of brown atrophy, lipochrome, haemofuscin)

A yellowish-brown granular pigment which accumulates in the cytoplasm of cells, especially of the heart, liver, adrenal gland and brain, and is associated with ageing, apoptosis and chronic wasting diseases. It occurs in Devon cattle, Nubian goats and Hampshire Down sheep, being sometimes described as *ceroid lipofuscinosis*, which is also seen in man. Affected animals show hindlimb ataxia and blindness, post-mortem findings including cerebral and retinal atrophy, neuronal and macrophage granulation and storage of ceroid lipofuscin in nervous tissue especially the brain.

Lipofuscins are derived from the oxidation of tissue lipids and/or lipoproteins. Granules of the pigment can be seen in stained sections (Sudan Black and Fontana Silver) as clumps near cell nuclei. They are resistant to fat solvents, acid-fast in reaction and negative to iron stains.

Xanthosis (xanthomatosis, osteohaematochromatosis, brown atrophy)

Xanthosis affects the heart most often but also involves the diaphragm, masseters, tongue, muscles of the forelimb and organs such as the adrenal gland, liver, kidney, thyroid, parathyroids, ovary and testis. The actual cause of pigment (lipofuscin) deposition is unknown, and there is doubt as to its significance.

Xanthosis is encountered especially in old animals but is not confined to them, being seen in otherwise healthy animals. It is being recorded fairly frequently in Ayrshire cattle and their crosses indicating a possible recessive gene.

Examination of affected carcases shows that the *heart* is affected in all cases and the *adrenal cortex* to be commonly involved. Of the skeletal muscles, the *masseters* are most severely pigmented but generally less than the heart, the *diaphragm* being the next in order of importance.

Yellow fat disease. Yellowish or brownish fat is sometimes seen in pigs fed on fish diets. The staining is due to the deposition of *ceroid*, a waxy substance similar to *lipofuscin*. Ceroid is resistant to fat solvents, is acid-fast and is stainable with fat stains.

Ochronosis (alkaptonuria) is a rare hereditary disease of cattle, pigs, horses and man in which *homogentisic acid* accumulates in tissues and is excreted in the urine due to a deficiency of its acid oxidase.

Homogentisic acid polymerises to form a brownish-black melanin-like pigment which is deposited mainly in the fibrous tissue (tendon sheaths, ligaments, cartilage), kidneys, endocrine gland and lungs. (Homogentisic acid is an intermediate product in the breakdown of the amino acids, phenylalanine and tyrosine.)

Tumours

A *tumour* or *neoplasm* is an abnormal growth of new cells which have become insensitive to normal growth control mechanisms and which (i) usually resemble the cells from which they have derived; (ii) proliferate in an unrestrained and disorderly manner; (iii) possess no organised structural arrangement; (iv) persist after cessation of the causal stimuli; (v) serve no useful purpose, especially in malignancy; and (vi) result from one or more mutations of the cellular DNA, especially malignant forms. (In some cases, tumours need not proliferate progressively and may even regress spontaneously.)

The word *tumour* means a swelling, which is an indication of the general gross appearance, although this is not always the case. For example, some malignant carcinomas are relatively small yet capable of causing early death, and some mesotheliomas are flattened in appearance. Much depends on the invasive properties (which vary in degree) and location, type of tissue involved, type of tumour, etc.

Structure. All forms of tumours (benign and malignant) consist of a parenchyma of neoplastic cells and a supporting stroma or matrix of connective tissue, blood vessels and sometimes lymphatics. The parenchyma is responsible for the functioning of the tumour and determines its classification.

Classes of tumours

Benign tumours usually grow slowly by expansion and by compressing or displacing adjacent tissues. They remain localised (although several may appear in an area) and are often spherical in shape with a fibrous capsule. They are thus capable of excision. There is a tendency for benign tumours to resemble the original cells more than malignant tumours.

Malignant tumours (cancers) in contrast grow more rapidly by invasion and destruction of the tissues they invade. Although the resemblance to original cells is usual, some types differ in cell structure. Pleomorphism (wide variety in cell morphology and staining) is more common with malignant tumours which contain more abnormal products of mitosis (cell division) such as broken chromosomes, huge, dark staining nucleoli and various protein and polypeptide products. They have a great tendency to metastasise, reaching distant sites in the body via the bloodstream, lymphatics and across tissue spaces.

Benign and malignant tumours occurring in endocrine glands may elaborate hormones, for example, insulin in the pancreas and corticosteroids in the adrenal gland.

Causes of tumours

Although the exact cause of many neoplasms is unknown, several specific factors, environmental and genetic, are involved:

1 *Physical carcinogens*, for example, ionising and ultra-violet radiation, chronic irritation, etc., cause DNA damage.
2 *Chemical carcinogens* such as benzene, vinyl chloride, arsenic, chromium, β-naphthylamine, etc. also lead to DNA damage.
3 *Viruses.* Tumour-inducing (oncogenic) viruses which cause tumours in animals include the DNA viruses of the adenovirus, herpesvirus, papovavirus and poxvirus groups and the RNA retroviruses.
4 *Hormones.* Disordered hormone metabolism (pituitary, ovary, thyroid, adrenal gland, parathyroid, pancreas) may produce neoplasia (adenomas and carcinomas), especially in man.
5 *Heredity.* Some strains of animals are prone to develop tumours, being inherited in the germ line.
6 *Parasites*, for example, *Gongylonema neoplasticum*, can produce gastric carcinoma in the rat and *Cysticercus fasciolaris* (cystic stage of *Taenia taeniaeformis*) sarcoma in rat livers.
7 *Ageing.* Tumours occur more commonly in older animals. Some, however, like malignant lymphoma, tend to affect young animals more often. Since most food animals are slaughtered at a young age, tumour formation is encountered relatively infrequently in them. The increased incidence with age may be a reflection of the longer period of exposure to carcinogens or to innate changes in metabolism or both.

Gene mutation (genetic damage) is the basic characteristic in all cases of neoplasia and is associated with the activity of proto-oncogenes and oncogenes, the former non-transforming genes being converted into transforming cellular oncogenes under special circumstances to initiate the neoplastic events. Fundamental to all tumour formation is the total lack of response to normal growth controls.

Effect on host

Malignant tumours are more life threatening than benign tumours. The latter can occur in animals without any untoward effects, for example, papillomata. In both types, much depends on their location and proximity to vital structures: obstruction of blood vessels, intestine, trachea, oesophagus, bile ducts, etc. may result in addition to ulceration of natural surfaces with haemorrhage and secondary infection. Tumours themselves, being well vascularised, can bleed profusely, even causing anaemia.

Hormone production can result in excess insulin from the pancreas with hypoglycaemia and overproduction of corticosteroids from the adrenal gland to cause sodium retention and hypertension.

The usual accompaniment of *malignant tumours* with their metastatic effect is severe loss of condition with anaemia, anorexia, weakness and prostration. In some cases, however, for example, lymphosarcoma, malignancy does not appear to cause undue loss of weight.

Nomenclature of neoplasms

In general, the parenchyma (the essential cellular elements) of the neoplasm determines its behaviour and its name. However, there are serious inconsistencies in the nomenclature of tumours.

Benign tumours usually have the suffix -*oma* attached to the cell type from which they originate, for example, fibroma from fibrous tissue, osteoma from bone, adenoma (Greek, *aden*, gland) from glandular tissue, chondroma from cartilage, leiomyoma from smooth muscle and so on. *Polyp* is a benign adenoma arising as a projection from a mucous surface. However, the suffix *-oma* can be deceptive since *lymphomas* and *sarcomas* are malignant collections of lymphocytes and melanomas, mesotheliomas and seminomas are also malignant. Some gliomas (tumours of CNS astrocytes and oligodendrocytes), myelomas (plasma cell collections) and teratomas (tumours containing different cell types found in the ovary and testis) are benign and some malignant.

Malignant tumours arising from *mesenchymal* tissues (connective tissue, muscle, cartilage, bone, blood and blood vessels, lymphoid tissues, kidneys and gonads) are termed *sarcomas*, for example, fibrosarcoma, chondrosarcoma and adenosarcoma. Those arising from *epithelial* tissues are called *carcinomas*. The carcinomas can be further differentiated, for example, squamous cell carcinoma which is a cancer with cells resembling stratified squamous (scaly or plate-like) epithelium.

Leukaemias are malignancies in which the normal white blood cells (WBC) are replaced by large numbers of lymphocytes, monocytes or myelocytes.

Judgement of neoplasia

Careful examination of the lesions as to shape, size, colour, consistency, location, number, distribution, etc., along with general carcase signs, may give some idea as to identification, whether benign or malignant, to provide a basis for provisional judgement.

However, it is difficult visually to distinguish many tumours, for example, between fibromas and equine sarcoids, between fibropapillomas and fibrosarcomas and between the latter and myxosarcomas and undifferentiated carcinomas. Judgement is usually simpler in poultry, in which poor condition is a common accompaniment.

An accurate diagnosis can only be made by detailed histopathological examination of samples of suspect lesions, a procedure which should always be resorted to when suspect neoplastic lesions are encountered.

Enzootic bovine leukosis is a *notifiable disease* in the United Kingdom, and all suspect cases, including those in meat plants, must be notified to the state veterinary service.

A single or a few localised benign tumours require *condemnation of the affected part or organ*, provided there are no other adverse signs. Numerous benign tumours in different organs and multiple malignant growths warrant *total condemnation*. While poor carcase condition, oedema, etc. may exist to assist in this judgement, it should be remembered that this support is not always present.

Poor condition/emaciation

The difference between *leanness* and *emaciation* is one of degree, but both may possess the same basic causes.

Thinness may be an expression of physiological normality, but the more serious emaciation is usually associated with other signs of disease.

Both conditions may involve *aphagia* (decreased food intake) in the form of inappetence (reduced appetite), *anorexia* (complete absence of appetite), *pica* (depraved appetite) or complete starvation.

Decreased food intake (*aphagia*) has a variety of different causes; many, however, are unknown. They include all the febrile diseases, stomatitis, pharyngitis, metabolic toxaemia, gastrointestinal parasitism and cobalt deficiency in ruminants, nutritional deficiencies (thiamin in pigs, protein, energy, copper, phosphorus, salt, iron, zinc, manganese, iodine, etc.), thirst, severe pain, stress and inadequate level of feeding.

Pica or *depraved appetite* (*allotriophagia*) involves eating, licking or drinking of foreign materials. The materials consumed on occasions are hair, wool, wood, faeces, litter (by all species including poultry), soil, bark, bones, cloth, poisons such as lead and foreign bodies (especially by cattle) and cannibalism (foetuses, tails and ears of pigs, etc.). The drinking of urine occasionally observed in dairy cattle is a form of pica but can also be seen in cows deprived of adequate drinking facilities.

Malnutrition (*inanition*) is the state in which the diet contains all the essential nutrients but in reduced amounts – a stage on the way to complete starvation. It is more common than starvation and is associated with some loss of body weight, ketosis, reduced metabolic respiratory and heart rates, hypothermia and sexual activity. Malnutrition commonly occurs during inclement weather in horses, cattle and sheep, in particular where supplementary feeding is absent.

Starvation involves complete cessation of food intake (proteins, carbohydrates, fats, vitamins, minerals and trace elements) and quickly leads to a great loss of weight with exhaustion of glycogen stores, breakdown of muscle protein to amino acids and increase in urinary urea, increased fat catabolism with release of fatty acids and formation of ketones and hypoglycaemia and decrease in insulin production. Starvation does not commonly occur today in developed countries, only being observed in cruelty cases.

In pica, malnutrition and starvation, there is an increased susceptibility to infection with higher morbidity and mortality rates.

Emaciation is a wasted condition of the animal body that may be pathological, occurring during the course of a disease such as TB and Johne's disease in cattle and parasitic gastroenteritis, chronic fascioliasis and caseous lymphadenitis in sheep. In old ewes, the teeth may be lost and the animal unable to eat. Erysipelas, swine fever and paratyphoid in pigs can produce great loss of condition in pigs. It may also be the result of prolonged starvation.

The *live animal*, especially equines and ruminants, shows a great loss of skin turgor and an increase in skin extensibility owing to the huge loss of subcutaneous fat. The skin *tenting test* (picking up of a fold of skin and noting the time for the fold to disappear) in an emaciated animal usually takes some 45 seconds or more. The eyes are sunken in their orbits because of the reduction of orbital fat, giving the eyes a gaunt, sunken appearance. All the bony prominences – spinous processes of vertebrae, hip bones, ischial tubers, stifle, elbow, shoulder joint, etc. – are conspicuous, while the ribs stand out clearly. Weakness is very evident, the heart rate is reduced, the pulse is full and blood pressure is raised. Body weight loss may be as great as 50–60%. Recumbency eventually ensues with death due to circulatory failure.

The blood chemistry changes follow those of starvation. There is abnormal regression of body condition with diminution in size of the organs, especially the muscles, liver and spleen. The outstanding feature, however, is the *loss of body fat* and an alteration in its consistency. The locations that normally carry adipose tissue – mesentery, omentum, perirenal fat, mediastinum, subcutaneous fat and inter- and intramuscular fat – are shrunken, and the remaining fat has an abnormal appearance, being oedematous and jelly-like in consistency and of a sickly yellowish colour. The loss of intermuscular fat gives a loose, flabby appearance to the muscles which may be pale in colour if accompanied by anaemia. There is also an increase in muscle connective tissue associated with atrophy of the actual muscles.

Chemical analysis of the meat reveals an increase in water content compared with the normal and a decrease of protein, fat and inorganic salts. In extremely emaciated animals, the water content is about 80% and protein about 19%, giving a ratio of water to protein of over 4 to 1. In lean but healthy animals, the percentage of water is rarely above 76.5% and the protein content about 22%, making the water–protein ratio less than 4 to 1. The ratio between water and protein may be of value in distinguishing between carcases that are very thin and those that are emaciated.

The lymph nodes, especially in young emaciated animals, are enlarged and oedematous. The marrow of long bones is red, watery and poor in fat content, the fat in some cases being replaced by wet, slimy material (*serous atrophy of fat*).

An emaciated carcase does not set in the normal manner and has a moist appearance on its surface and in the body cavities. Changes in the consistency of the fat are best seen around the base of the heart, in the mediastinum, in the kidney region or between the spinous processes of the vertebrae.

Judgement is based on the degree of loss of condition, efficiency of setting, presence of concurrent disease and results of laboratory examinations.

Both conditions, especially where unassociated with concurrent disease, are among the most difficult to assess on meat inspection. This is particularly the case in regions where conditional approval for manufacturing purposes and/or heat treatment is not authorised. Regard has to be given to the extent of emaciation, presence/absence of oedema and concurrent disease.

In borderline cases, it is advisable to detain the carcase for 12 hours. If after this time there is considerable drying of the body cavities with absence of serous infiltration of muscles combined with negative laboratory tests, the carcase may receive a more favourable judgement.

Emaciation and oedema frequently coexist and are suggestive of pathological emaciation.

The Codex Alimentarius Commission Alinorm 93/16A *Recommended Final Judgement* for 'General chronic conditions such as anaemia, cachexia, *emaciation*, loathsome appearance, degeneration of organs' is total condemnation.

Depending upon the *extent* of the condition the following conclusions may be drawn:

1 Approved as fit for human consumption, with distribution restricted to limited areas
2 Meat showing minor deviations from normal but fit for human consumption
3 Conditionally approved for human consumption after heat treatment, if economically justified

Total condemnation is always warranted if the condition is caused by chronic infection and laboratory examination has established presence of infection, recent use of antimicrobial substances or drug residues.

Contamination

Contamination with *faeces* is one of the greatest hazards to public health encountered in meat inspection. This is most commonly due to presentation of heavily soiled and/or wet animals to hurried or poor 'bunging' technique and full stomachs and intestines rupturing on removal. Food business operators could greatly reduce this risk by the introduction of mechanical bungers such as the Jarvis or Jupiter systems for cattle and pigs, by tying or bagging the 'bung' in cattle and sheep or by applying ligatures, clips or elastrator rings or 'rodding' the oesophagus.

Contamination of the carcase with purulent material, bile or faeces should always be removed by trimming.

Parasitic conditions

Ascaris suum

Found in pigs, *A. suum* is a large roundworm the migrating larvae of which cause typical white spots on the liver rendering in aesthetically unfit. The largest nematode of the pig is up to 40 cm long. Its life cycle is direct.

Eggs are passed in the faeces of pigs and are very resistant to temperature extremes. The egg is viable for more than 4 years in the environment. After ingestion, the egg hatches in the small intestine, and the larva penetrates the intestinal mucosa and travels to the liver and then via the circulation to the lungs and onto the small intestine via the bronchi, trachea and pharynx.

An effect of the migrating larvae on the lungs is 'milk spot' or 'white spot' which appears as cloudy whitish spots of up to 1.0 cm in diameter on the surface of the liver and results from a fibrous repair of inflammation reactions to the passage of larvae in the livers of previously sensitised pigs.

Echinococcus granulosus: *Hydatidosis and hydatid cyst*

This is a small tapeworm of the dog with intermediate hosts which include domestic and wild ruminants, man and primates, pigs and lagomorphs. Eggs are passed in the faeces of the dog. After ingestion by the intermediate host, for example, sheep, the ova hatch and the oncospheres penetrate the gut wall and travel to the liver (70%) or lungs (25%) and occasionally to other organs and tissues (5%). Transmission to humans is not via consumption of infested bovine organs but rather through the handling of infected dogs or contaminated soil, water or food (Fig. 9.21).

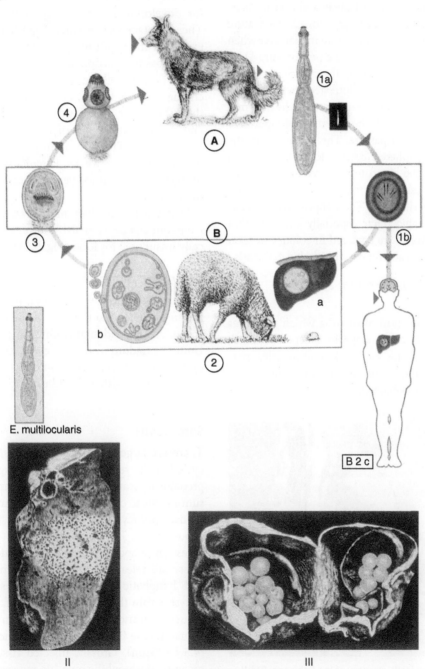

Figure 9.21 Life cycle of *Echinococcus multilocularis* (Courtesy of Pro A.T. Trees).

In the liver and lungs, the hydrated cyst is 7–20 cm in diameter but in the abdominal cavity where unrestricted growth is possible they may be much larger and may contain several litres of fluid. Brood capsules may be formed.

In animals, the majority of infections are only evident at the abattoir, in contrast to man where the hydatid, in its pulmonary or hepatic site, is often of pathogenic significance. Control is based on the regular treatment of dogs and prevention of them eating material containing hydatids.

Taenia hydatigena (known as Cysticercus tenuicollis in larval stage)

This is the largest of the intestinal dog tapeworms with the cysticerci found in the abdominal cavity and liver in intermediate hosts (sheep, cattle, deer, pig, horse), the mature *Cysticercus tenuicollis* being about 5–8 cm in diameter when they emerge as 'bladder worms' on the peritoneum. Dogs and cats are infected by consuming the cysticercus in the tissues of the intermediate host. If untreated, these may survive for several months up to a year or more. The intermediate host is infected through the ingestion of tapeworm eggs in infected faeces on pasture. The ova hatch in the intestine, and the oncospheres, infective to sheep, cattle and pigs, are carried via the blood to the liver in which they migrate for about 4 weeks before they emerge on the surface and attach onto the peritoneum. These appear in the liver as serpentine haemorrhagic tracts especially near the thin edge. At first, these tracts are dark red in colour but soon become brown or green and finally whitish due to fibrosis.

Taenia ovis (previously known as Cysticercus ovis)

Taenia ovisis is a tapeworm of the dog which measures 1–2 cm and forms its cystic stage in sheep. Cysticerci, 3–9.5 cm in size, are found in the skeletal muscles, particularly the heart, diaphragm and masseter muscles 3 months after ingestion (Fig. 9.22).

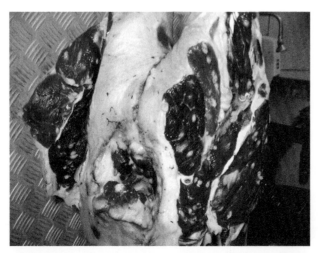

Figure 9.22 *C. ovis* in a lamb, courtesy of Ian Robinson, RMHI.

Fasciola hepatica: *Liver fluke*

Adult fluke in the bile duct lay eggs into the bile which travel to the intestine. Eggs that are passed in the faeces develop and hatch, releasing motile ciliated miracidia, and if certain conditions are correct will find their way to an intermediate host, for example a snail of the genus *Lymnaea*, most commonly *L. truncatula*. In infected snails, development proceeds through the sporocyst and radial stages to the final stage in the intermediate host, the cercaria. These are shed from the snail as a motile form and attach themselves to grass blades and encyst there to form the infective metacercariae. It takes a minimum of 6–7 weeks up to several months for development from miracidium to metacercariae. These metacercariae when ingested by the final host excyst in the small intestine, migrate through the gut wall, cross the peritoneum and penetrate the liver capsule. The young flukes tunnel through the liver parenchyma for 6–8 weeks, enter the small bile ducts and then the larger ducts and sometimes the gall bladder and reach sexual maturity. The pre-patent period is 10–12 weeks. The minimum period for completion of life cycle is 17–18 weeks. *Fasciola hepatica* can survive in untreated sheep for years. In cattle, it is usually less than 1 year.

Damage to the liver in wet seasons in the United Kingdom can be extensive and render the liver aesthetically unsuitable for food (Fig. 9.23).

Paramphistomiasis

Paramphistomiasis, rumen fluke, has become a common finding adhering to the wall of the rumen of cattle and sheep, as an incidental finding at post-mortem, in the United Kingdom in recent years (see Fig. 9.24). The life cycle is similar to *Fasciola*, in that snails act as an intermediate host with miracidium, sporocyst, rediae and cercariae stages.

Sarcocystis

There are large numbers of *Sarcocystis* species. The life cycle has the sexual reproductive stage occurring in the predator or scavenger host which come infected by consuming meat containing infected sarcocysts. These are shed as sporocysts or sporulated oocysts in the faeces after about 1 week. The intermediate host (prey) is infected by ingestion of sporocysts in contaminated food and water. These are released in the intestine, penetrate the blood and lymphatic systems and after several generations encyst within the muscle, heart, liver, lung and neuronal tissues. In muscle, the cysts lie within and between individual muscle fibres and have a characteristic cigar shape ($4.5 \times 0.35 \mu m$). Grossly, infected tissue generally has a greenish, eosinophilic myositis appearance. The final host

(a)

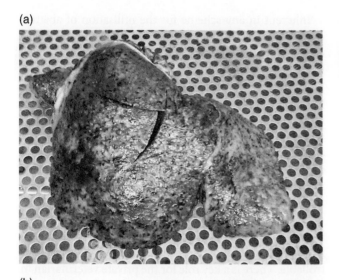

(b)

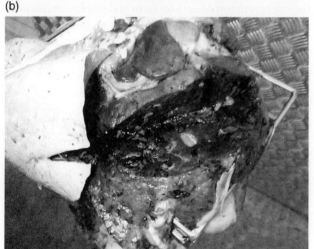

Figure 9.23 Lesions of *F. hepatica*, liver fluke.

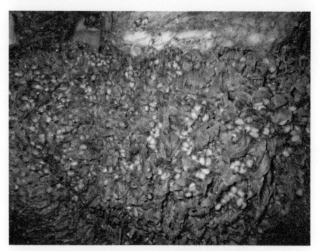

Figure 9.24 Paramphistomiasis, bovine rumen fluke.

1 Approved for human consumption
2 Totally condemned
3 Partially condemned

The category of *conditionally approved for human consumption* is utilised in some countries: carcase meat which is hygienically unsatisfactory or which in some way may be hazardous for human and animal food is treated, for example, by heating or freezing under official supervision, in such a manner that makes it safe for human consumption.

In certain regions, meat classed as *inferior meat*, namely, safe hygienically but of a lower standard, may be sold as raw meat without undergoing any treatment. Such meat must be labelled so as to indicate that it is of inferior quality and sold under close supervision by the controlling authority. It includes meat of abnormal colour, odour or taste, with slight oedema or poorly bled and, like the following category, is found in those countries where there is a scarcity of protein.

Lastly, meat may be *approved for human consumption, with distribution restricted to limited areas*. This category also occurs in those countries where meat is at a premium and includes meat from animals in an area under quarantine because of an outbreak of contagious animal disease. In this case, there must be no risk to public health, and the meat must be restricted in sale to the affected area to avoid the possible spread of disease. The category would also include meat from animals vaccinated in a restricted area.

It is the duty of the official control staff to arrange for the *health marking of the carcases* when passed and to ensure the proper disposal of unfit material. It remains important in Europe that checks to ensure the efficient and hygienic removal of the SRM associated with BSE from the carcase and viscera and their correct animal by-product categorisation, marking and disposal.

becomes infected by ingestion of mature sarcocysts, usually by eating contaminated meat of the intermediate host.

Humans may also serve as intermediate hosts and suffer myositis and vasculitis, but this tissue phase is rare, and the source of such human infection has never been determined. Human intestinal illness, with clinical signs of nausea, abdominal pain, and diarrhoea that lasts up to 48 hours, as followed ingestion of sarcocysts of *S. suihominis* in uncooked pork and *S. hominis* in uncooked beef. The extent of human illness from ingestion of infected meat has not been documented, although the meat from infected animals will be condemned on aesthetic grounds.

Courses of action

The *decisions made at post-mortem inspection* vary in different parts of the world depending mainly on local disease incidence, local economy and the presence or absence of facilities for the heat treatment of meat conditionally approved for human consumption. The main decisions in most countries, however, are as follows:

Utilisation of post-mortem data

As virtually all food animals end up in the slaughterhouse, whether prime livestock or end-of-production cull animals, for example, cull cows and sows, it is without doubt the critical and most efficient point of production at which to carry out surveillance for animal disease.

This disease data has the potential to be used for:

1 Reduction of losses due to disease and injury through feedback to livestock producers and private veterinary practitioners
2 Demonstration of trends and variations in animal disease incidence due to husbandry methods, season, geographical location, etc.
3 Tracing of affected herds as part of national disease control programmes
4 Extent, cost and reasons for condemnations due to disease and injury
5 Measurement, benchmarking and improvement of animal welfare on farm – fighting and tail biting in pigs
6 Use of information regarding animal housing and husbandry, including breeding data, to improve standards on the farm, including those of animal hygiene
7 Demonstration of certain subclinical conditions
8 Forecasting of disease outbreaks in conjunction with meteorological data
9 Enhancement of the clinical competence of the practising veterinary surgeon regarding data on client's slaughtered stock, especially casualty animals
10 Provision for research investigations
11 Quality control check on inspection standards

The slaughter establishment has therefore an important role to play in epidemiology and preventive veterinary medicine, not only in relation to post-mortem findings but also following examination of the live animal prior to slaughter. Harley *et al.* (2012) reviewed the uses that the data could be put to in improving animal welfare, highlighting the financial loss to the producer.

With the exception of a few countries, the potential of post-mortem data is regrettably not being fully exploited. Among the reasons for this deficiency are lack of coordination between those in charge of meat inspection and primary production, the practical difficulties in slaughter line recording (e.g. fast rail speeds, inadequate inspector manning levels) and traditional livestock marketing systems, through intermediaries and markets.

Many variations of systems are in existence. Those countries which possess cooperative livestock/meat systems, for example, the Netherlands and Denmark, are better placed to organise an efficient recording and feedback of information to producers.

Inherent in any scheme for the utilisation of abattoir data is the need for precise diagnoses, standard nomenclature for the diseases encountered and recognised forms of presentation of the disease data. There is no point in referring back vague or inaccurate information to livestock producers. Equally important is efficient identification of live animals as well as of their carcases and offal, which must be correlated. The system in the abattoir must include full details of the carcase and species, disease condition, part of carcase affected, weight of meat and offal condemned and, if necessary, be supplemented by the results of laboratory examinations. The disease conditions to be recorded should be of a type that is readily identified, of economic importance in the animal health and/or public health sphere and easily controllable. There is a key role for the private veterinarian in the interpretation of data on farm and implementation of controls and preventative herd health programmes.

Previous barriers to implementation of post-mortem feedback systems have largely been eliminated by web-based electronic communications. Post-mortem data recorded on the slaughter floor onto a specifically produced web site with controlled access can be instantaneously downloaded by the farmer via smartphone technology. Such as a system developed in Northern Ireland has added post-mortem data from pig slaughterhouses to information already available for the grades of pigs, delivered through an app to the producers' phone with analysis as a weekly download.

While the EFSA opinions question the efficacy of post-mortem inspection for public health purposes, they emphasise the significance of the process for animal health purposes and particularly its use on farm.

Control of hygienic production

While the responsibility to produce safe food lies with the operator, meat inspection has a critical role to play in inspection and verification of hygienic production systems and particularly the absence of visible contamination of the meat. In addition, it is important that all inspections must be carried out with due regard for hygiene. It is essential that the official inspectors set and achieve the highest standards of hygienic dress, appearance and operations if they are to have any hope of enforcing high standards within the plant. Operational hygiene has been dealt with in Chapter 8.

Before the day's slaughter commences, the inspector must verify that the premises, equipment and facilities are hygienic and in good working order and that meat operatives are properly clothed and adequate in number. Slaughter should not be allowed to commence until a satisfactory situation obtains. This *pre-slaughter check* may take the form of a visual and microbiological verification of the meat plant's own monitoring system. The preferred system is one where the operatives themselves are responsible for ensuring that the premises are hygienic, the meat inspection team merely verifying their checks.

The prevention of contamination must remain the aim, rather than post-production contamination reduction by means of water, organic acids, other bactericides or irradiation. Washing has been demonstrated (Ellerbroek *et al.*, 1993) to have no effect in reducing pathogen levels on the surface of the carcase and can, in fact, have a detrimental outcome by spreading the contamination over the surface of the carcase to less contaminated areas and increasing the available water remaining on the carcase. Suitably controlled, organic acids, irradiation, etc. may be useful tools in helping to ensure a safe product; they must not be allowed to mask poor manufacturing practice.

In the experience of the author, carcase meat which looks clean and smells clean, in general, has low microbiological counts. Meat microbiology is a tool that must be used intelligently to improve hygiene systems or standards within an establishment rather than to determine if meat is 'safe' or to compare the safety of meat between establishments or countries. There are just too many variables to permit simplistic rules for interpretation of results. These include differences between sampling and laboratory techniques, transport media and time, sample and culture; the variation in pathogenicity of different bacteriological strains; the retrospective nature of the results and the effect of storage conditions on the final bacterial count. This view was endorsed by Engel *et al.* (1997), who carried out a scrutiny of the effectiveness of the microbiological criteria imposed by the Dutch meat inspection regulations in place at that time.

Despite this, microbiological sampling is a useful tool especially if used with a food safety management system (FSMS) designed to prevent contamination of the meat with potential hazards and can be used to set HEIs leading to a final FSO at consumer level. Within meat inspection, the FSMS usually incorporates the principles of hazard analysis and critical control points (HACCP).

Hazard analysis and critical control points (HACCP)

HACCP is a system which identifies, evaluates and controls hazards which are significant for food safety. As the specific detail of HACCP as applied in different countries varies, this definition and all those quoted are those to be found in documentation issued by *Codex Alimentarius*, in particular Recommended International Code of Practice, General Principles of Food Hygiene, as revised.

It builds upon the good manufacturing practice, described in Chapter 8, and through a process of logical steps identifies the risks to food safety and identifies points in the production process where the application of controls will eliminate or reduce that risk to acceptable levels – the critical control points (CCPs).

International acceptance of the approach was first underlined during the Uruguay Round of the General Agreement on Tariffs and Trade (GATT) 1994, when the inclusion of the Codex Alimentarius Commission's recommendations on the application of HACCP was specifically identified as the baseline for consumer protection under the Agreement on the Application of Sanitary and Phytosanitary Measures.

Implementation of an HACCP system

Many books and manuals are available which describe how to implement an HACCP system within a food processing setting. The information included here is merely intended to provide a brief overview. The concept is no longer new, and over the years, understanding of its effective use has developed and practical deployment improved. It is now widely accepted that the concept works best if the principles are applied flexibly to meet the identified targets FSO but then implemented rigidly – to do what the HACCP plan says you are going to do.

The first step in preparation is to construct a process flow diagram of the process to be controlled, including step by step the introduction of all raw materials and each part of the process. This must be detailed and the accuracy validated repeatedly against what is happening on the factory floor (Fig. 9.25).

All HACCP systems comprise the following sequential steps:

1 **Hazard analysis.**
   The first step in applying the HACCP system to a food manufacturing operation is to identify and quantify the microbiological, physical and chemical hazards and risks within the operation. The following definitions are important:
   a. *Hazard* is a biological, chemical or physical agent in, or condition of, food with the potential to cause an adverse health effect.
   b. *Severity* is the seriousness (magnitude) of the hazard.
   c. *Risk* is an estimate of the likely occurrence of a hazard.
   The analysis requires the specialist knowledge of a multidisciplinary team and should include food microbiologists, engineers, veterinarians, cleaning experts and so on. A step-by-step investigation of the

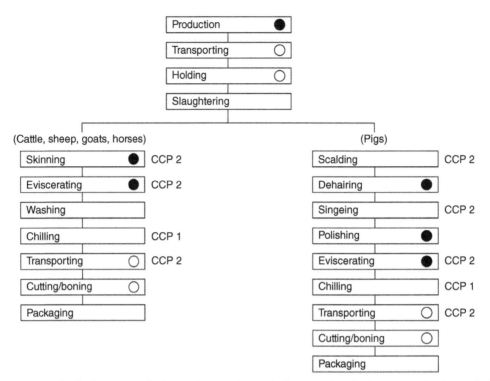

Figure 9.25 Flow diagram for fresh meat production and processing. ○ indicates a site of minor contamination. ● indicates a site of major contamination; CCP1, effective CCP; CCP2, not absolute (International Commission on Microbiological Safety of Foods (ICMSF)).

process is carried out, from the specification required for the raw material through the manufacturing process to the distribution chain.

Epidemiological investigation of historical episodes of premature spoilage or food poisoning in which the product was implicated can provide valuable information about potential hazards. All of the data emerging from this analysis should be collated into a flow chart and all of the hazards identified and evaluated with regard to their severity and likely frequency of occurrence.

2 **Determination of the CCPs.**

The classical definition of a *CCP* is a step at which control can be applied and is essential to prevent or eliminate a food safety hazard or reduce it to an acceptable level.

The proper identification of CCPs can make the difference between an effective HACCP programme and one that, by the identification of too many points in the system which must be considered as critical, becomes ineffective. A decision tree is often used as a useful tool to determine if a particular control is in effect a real CCP. However, informed professional judgement is key.

3 **Establish critical limits.**

Is a criterion which separates acceptability from unacceptability.

Increasing emphasis has been placed on quantitative, rather than qualitative, criteria which indicate whether

or not an operation is under control. Quantitative criteria, such as time, temperature, pH and the concentration of various chemicals, can be measured and indicate definitively that a system is or is not controlled. Qualitative criteria such as colour or smell are more difficult to determine objectively, and consequently, it is much more difficult to judge divergence from the accepted normal. Microbiological criteria are particularly difficult to quantify in absolute terms under practical conditions. A great deal of standardisation of sampling and laboratory techniques is required before values can be compared. Attempts to quantify in numerical terms the infective dose of a particular pathogen are fraught with difficulties owing to differences in pathogenicity of different strains and varying susceptibility between different groups of consumers. In any case, the retrospective nature of microbiological criteria usually renders them unsuitable as critical limits within an HACCP system, where real-time measurements are required so that corrective actions can be taken.

4 **Establish a system to monitor control of the CCP.**

Monitor. The act of conducting a planned sequence of observations or measurements of control parameters to assess whether a CCP is under control.

This is best carried out by the operatives themselves or by their supervisors rather than by a special team of quality assurance staff. The integration of the checks into the routine of the manufacturing process and the ownership of the quality assurance by the workers are important aspects of a successful system. The methods selected for monitoring must give immediate results so that any problems detected can be corrected immediately. Traditional microbiological checks, where the results may not be available for 36 hours or more, are therefore of little value.

A number of new approaches to microbiological monitoring are, however, becoming commercially available. Some of these techniques are suitable for determining total counts of bacteria, while others determine the presence of specific pathogens. Techniques utilising monoclonal antibodies and DNA probes in combination with automatic instruments are being developed which can give results in hours. A microbial ATP bioluminescence assay has been shown to be an accurate and rapid method for determining the levels of generic bacterial contamination on beef and pork carcases (Siragusa *et al.*, 1995). The technique can distinguish between microbial and non-microbial ATP, but sensitivity is variable at microbial levels below 10^4 (Siragusa and Cutter, 1995). The entire test, including sampling, takes only 5 minutes to complete.

5 **Corrective action:** Establish the corrective action to be taken when monitoring indicates that a particular CCP is not under control.

Procedures must be established so that immediate action can be taken upon detection of deviation from the established criteria. This may involve rectifying an out-of-control situation before an operation is allowed to commence or halting the manufacturing process. Consideration must always be given to the action that needs to be taken to rectify the food that has been produced during the period that the CCP was not fully or partially controlled. This decision may result in an adjustment to the frequency of monitoring in order to reduce the volume of potentially non-compliant product.

6 **Verification:** Establish procedures for verification to confirm that the HACCP system is working effectively.

Verification checks are carried out systematically by the quality assurance staff and the veterinary inspection team. It is important that duplication of effort by the in-house and regulatory inspectors is avoided and that all checks are complementary. Verification may involve some microbiological checks of end product, structures and equipment. All checks should be carried out at a statistically significant frequency and in a systematic, targeted manner.

7 **Documentation:** Establish documentation concerning all procedures and records appropriate to these principles and their application.

Many HACCP systems in meat plants have died under the weight of paper they generate. If, after implementation has occurred, it is discovered that too many CCPs were identified and that the monitoring process is unnecessarily complicated or cumbersome, there must be sufficient flexibility in the system to allow adjustments to be made. Another risk with cumbersome documentation is that the completion of the form can rapidly become the monitoring personnel's primary objective rather than merely a tool to meet the overall objective of safe food.

An HACCP system is not something which should, or can, be imposed by either the in-house quality assurance staff or the regulatory authority, though both bodies must be intimately involved. For the system to work properly, the entire workforce within the food factory, including all managers, supervisors, operatives, fitters and cleaning staff, must be dedicated to the success of the system and involved in its operation. This requires a considerable investment of time in training for all staff.

Worldwide food safety standards

The worldwide standards for food safety are established and described by the Codex Alimentarius Commission, established in 1963 by the FAO and WHO. The commission's science-based standards, guidelines and recommendations are used as a legal reference point by the World Trade Organisation in international trade agreements and disputes.

In addition to these standards, there are a wide range of private food standards whose requirements are demanded by retailers and customers. Some seek to provide assurance on quality including safety, while others merely seek to exploit a niche market or gain marketing advantage over competitors. However, all have a tendency to cloud and confuse the regulatory environment as to what is legal requirement versus what is voluntary and to add increased costs to the processor and consequently the final consumer.

The primary private standard is arguably ISO 22000 entitled 'Food safety management systems – Requirements for any organisation in the food chain'. Other major certification schemes include EurepGAP, the British Retail Consortium (BRC), the International Food Standard (IFS), the Safe Food Quality Standard (SQF) and the Dutch Code. All have differing requirements and apply to all or specific sectors of the food chain. All have their own systems of verification and third-party audit.

While most private and regulatory standards are now based on Codex Alimentarius standards, there are significant differences that can act as a barrier to export and market access. Increasingly, for those wishing to export or break into the major retailer sector, statutory requirements are merely a basic requirement with the private standard representing the opportunity to differentiate a position in the market. Many within this sector wonder why they have to pay for two quality systems.

References

Berends, B.R., Snijders, J.M.A. and van Logtestijn, J.G. (1993) *Veterinary Record*, 133, 411–415.

Biss, M.E., Hathaway, S.C. and Johnstone, A.C. (1994) *British Veterinary Journal*, 150, 377.

Blackmore, D.K. (1983) *Nordisk Veterinaer Medicin*, 35, 184–189.

EFSA. (2010) *Scientific Report Submitted to EFSA – Development of Harmonized Schemes for the Monitoring and Reporting of Cysticercus in Animals and Foodstuffs in the EU*, www.efsa.europe.eu/en/supporting/pub/34e.htm (accessed 30 April 2014).

Ellerbroek, L.I., Wegener, J.F. and Arndt, G. (1993) *Journal of Food Protection*, 56 (5), 432–436.

Engel, H.W.B., van den Berg, J. and Fenigsennarucka, U. (1997) *Tijdschrift voor de Diergeneeskunde*, 112, 536.

Goodhand, R.H. (1983) The Meat Hygienist (May/June), No. 38, 4.

Harley, S., More, S., Boyle, L. et al (2012) *Irish Veterinary Journal*, 65, 11.

Hathaway, S.C. and McKenzie, A.I. (1989) *Veterinary Record*, 124, 189–193.

Hathaway, S.C. and Pullen, M.M. (1990) *Journal of the American Veterinary Medical Association*, 196, 860–864.

Hathaway, S.C., McKenzie, A.I. and Royal, W.A. (1987) *Veterinary Record*, 120, 78.

Heath, D.D., Lawrence, S.B. and Twaalfhoven, H. (1985) *New Zealand Veterinary Journal*, 33, 152.

Huey, R.J. (1996) *Veterinary Record*, 138, 511–514.

Johnston, A.M. (1994) *British Veterinary Journal*, 150, 315.

McCool, C.J. (1979) *Australian Veterinary Journal*, 55, 214–216.

Mousing, T., Kyrval, J., Jensen, T. et al. (1997) *Veterinary Record*, 140, 472–477.

Siragusa, G.R. and Cutter, C.N. (1995) *Journal of Food Protection*, 58(7), 764–769.

Siragusa, G.R., Cutter, C.N., Dorsa, W.J. and Koohinaraie, M. (1995) *Journal of Food Protection*, 58(7), 770–775.

Szazados, I. (1991) *Magyar Allatorvosok Lapja*, 46(1), 27–43.

White, T.L. and Moore, D.A. (2009) *JAVMA*, 235(8), 937–941.

Further reading

Amore, G. (2012) *EFSA Journal* 2012, 10(6);2764

Andreoletti, O., Budka, H., Buncic, S. et al (2011) *EFSA Journal*, 9(10), 2351.

BCVA (2010). *Guidance for Veterinary Surgeons on the Emergency Slaughter of Cattle*, http://www.bcva.eu/bcva/news/new-guidance-veterinary-surgeons-emergency-slaughter-cattle-booklet (accessed 21 April 2014).

EFSA Panel on Biological Hazards (BIOHAZ) (2013) *EFSA Journal*, 11(6), 3266.

European Food Safety Authority (2011) *EFSA Journal* 2011, 9(10), 2371.

Hald, T. (2012) *EFSA Journal*, 10(6), 2741.

10

Poultry production, slaughter and inspection

Poultry meat production throughout the world has been increasing both in quantity and in sophistication. The annual production has increased over the past 20 years: eggs produced by broiler breeders increased between 1 and 1.5, number of chicks between 0.8 and 1.2 and percentage of breast meat by 0.25–0.3%.

In addition, the eviscerated yield has gone up by 0.2–0.25% annually, the feed conversion ratio to 2 kg has improved by between 0.04 and 0.05%, and the weight, at 42 days, has increased on average 55–60 g/year. Those trends are expected to continue, and broiler selection now involves the criteria of live weight, liveability, skeletal strength, conformation and feed conversion (See table 10.1).

Production of poultry

The broiler industry in the United Kingdom is concentrated in the hands of fewer than 10 large organisations, most of which have their own parent stock farms and hatcheries. In these companies, broilers may be grown on company farms or on specialist contract units. Other companies do not have breeding farms or hatcheries but purchase day-old broilers, usually on long-term contract, from specialist suppliers. Twelve million birds are produced each week by four companies. Chickens, turkeys, geese, ducks and end-of-lay hens are processed as well as pheasant, quail, partridge and guinea fowl.

Broiler chickens should be placed in houses which have been thoroughly cleaned and disinfected. The surrounding area and the equipment in the house must be clean and disinfected (Fig. 10.1).

Adequate floor space for each bird is essential for its growth, health, quality and general well-being. The amount of space to allow is determined by a combination of the following factors: the weight of the bird at killing age, type of housing, climatic region and time of the year. EU Directive 239/2010 sets a maximum stocking density of 33 kg/m² with the possibility of member states allowing higher stocking densities if certain requirements are met. In the United Kingdom, the government has decided that under certain conditions conventionally reared chickens may be kept to a maximum of 39 kg/m². The stocking densities may need to be reduced in summer.

Chicks should be placed in a house with a temperature of 29–31°C at 1 day old, the temperature being reduced by 2°C a week to a final temperature of 18–21°C at 35 days.

A continuous adequate supply of clean water is essential as dehydration must be avoided at all times. Water and feed intake are directly related. There is a trend towards using nipple drinkers, to replace the conventional hanging bell drinkers.

Commercial chicks are generally given a starter ration containing 23% protein between 0 and 11 days of age, grower ration of 21% protein between 12 and 22 days of age and finisher of 20% protein or less from 23 days of age onwards. Commercial broilers are killed between 32 and 40 days of age.

Though commercial broilers are produced intensively in standard poultry sheds, there is a demand for high welfare broilers.

The growing of improved welfare chicken with windowed houses, lower stocking, 30 kg/m², and environmental enrichment, with straw and/or vegetables is increasing dramatically. The birds are fed a vegetarian diet which is of a lower density than that which is fed to conventional broilers. The actual stocking density is based on retailer requirements. These birds are killed at 34–42 days of age (Fig. 10.1).

Gracey's Meat Hygiene, Eleventh Edition. Edited by David S. Collins and Robert J. Huey.
© 2015 John Wiley & Sons, Ltd. Published 2015 by John Wiley & Sons, Ltd.

The stocking rate - number of birds per square metre floor space - of free-range birds should not exceed the following criteria: for chickens 13 birds but not more than 27.5 kg live weight; for ducks, guinea fowl and turkeys 25 kg live weight; and for geese 15 kg live weight. The birds are reared in the conventional manner for the first 2 days, but the temperature of the house is decreased more quickly so that the environmental temperature is around 21°C at between 14 and 21 days.

Some birds are housed in one building from day-old to processing, while others are reared in conventional sheds and then moved. They have to live in the secondary accommodation for at least 28 days. The lower temperatures promote good feather growth (Fig. 10.2).

The birds, for at least half of their lifetime, must have continuous daytime access to open-air runs comprising an area mainly covered by vegetation of not less than 1 m² per chicken or guinea fowl, 2 m² per duck and 4 m² per turkey or goose.

Birds are fed a ration of about 24% protein for the first few days, but this is soon decreased to 17%. The feed in the fattening stage must contain at least 70% cereals. For chickens, the house must be provided with pop holes of a combined length equal to or greater than that of the longer side of the house, at the rate of 4 m/100 m² available floor area.

They must not be killed until they are at least 56 days of age, turkeys 70 days and geese 112 days.

Traditional free-range birds must have access to a larger area than free range, and there are extra requirements as detailed in Commission Regulation (EEC) No. 1538/91.

The production of these types of poultry obviously adds greatly to the cost, and for free-range birds, this would be approximately twice that for conventional broilers.

Poussin or Cornish game hens are normal conventional broilers which are killed between 21 and 33 days of age.

There are, worldwide, around three main breeding companies producing different strains of broiler. The companies which produce broiler meat are vertically integrated. That means they control the production of the eggs which produce the chick, the growing of

Table 10.1 Slaughterings of poultry meat

Year	Number slaughtered (million)		
	Broilers	Boiling fowls	Turkeys
2005	827.19	37.1	19.22
2006	813.12	35.72	17.87
2007	805.02	36.9	15.56
2008	791.6	39.16	15.89
2009	799.02	39.86	15.48
2010	862.55	41.15	15.57
2010 was a 53-week year			

Source: Courtesy of Defra.
Boiling fowls include spent commercial layer hens, spent layer breeders and spent broiler breeders.

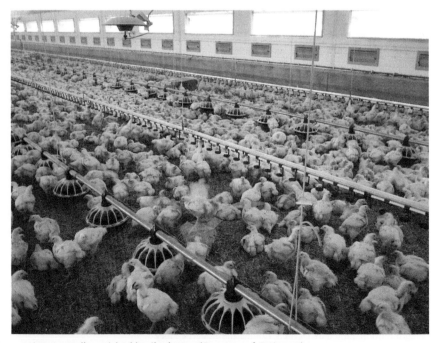

Figure 10.1 An indoor environmentally enriched broiler house (Courtesy of G Liggett).

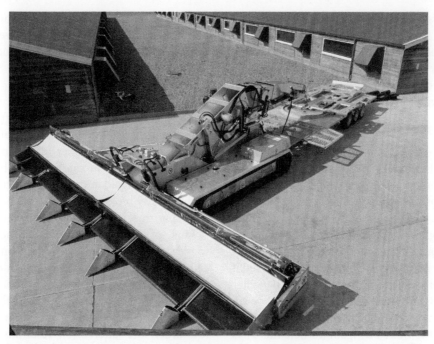

Figure 10.2 Automatic poultry harvester (Reproduced with permission from Tom Pearson, CM Agriculture Ltd).

the birds and the slaughter and further processing of the meat.

Poultry feedingstuffs

The raw materials present in the bird's food are carefully sourced and are examined for quality and chemical and microbiological purity. Animal feed is a potential source for the transmission of infection to poultry flocks.

The animal feed industry is multifaceted, comprising importers and processors of raw materials, merchants, suppliers of by-products from agricultural operations and food manufacturers and others such as feed additive and supplement manufacturers, commercial compounders, integrated producers and on-farm mixers.

The feed industry uses numerous products and by-products from other industries. Some, such as cereals, are untreated, while others like oilseeds are available as cakes or meals following processing to extract oil. Raw materials may be sourced from all over the world, although cereals in Europe are mainly of EU origin due to import tariffs discouraging imports. Poultry feed production (some 3.7 million tonnes per annum in the United Kingdom in 2010) accounts for around one-third of the annual production of all compound feeds.

Legislative controls on feed are harmonised at an EU level which is incorporated into the Animal Feed (England) Regulations 2010, with similar parallel legislation in the devolved areas of the United Kingdom.

The Feed (Hygiene and Enforcement) (England) Regulations 2005 prohibits the marketing of unsafe feed and requires traceability procedures to be in place.

European legislation was introduced in 2001 limiting the use of processed animal proteins (PAP) in animal feeds as a result of BSE. The European Commission's TSE roadmap is suggesting reintroducing feeding of PAP in poultry and pig feeds. Methods of feed analysis are contained in the Feed (Sampling and Analysis and Specified Undesirable Substances) (England) Regulations 2010.

A code of practice for the control of *Salmonella* in animal feed and feed ingredients has also been set up by the UK Government in consultation with industry bodies (revised in 2009). The code encourages the application of HACCP principles. In order to ensure that animal feed is of an acceptable quality, it is necessary to source the raw materials from suppliers complying with the relevant codes of practice in the case of other raw materials.

The raw materials should be stored in suitable buildings which prevent pests gaining access. On-farm storage bins and silos should be similarly treated. Transport of raw materials and finished feeds should be in dedicated vehicles which are thoroughly inspected before use to ensure they are clean and dry. Feed mills must be constructed of appropriate, food-grade, materials and must be regularly cleansed, disinfected and sampled for evidence of contamination. There must be segregation of raw materials from finished feeds to minimise the risk of cross-contamination.

Staff need to know the importance of good hygiene practice and should receive appropriate training.

Pelleting of feed improves the overall feed intake, and pellets are easier to handle in automated feed delivery system. The process creates temperatures high enough to reduce the numbers of pathogenic bacteria which may be present, although it does not provide a total kill. To achieve this, a separate heat treatment process involving holding the feed for a minimum time at a minimum temperature is required. This is an effective way of tackling the problem of *Salmonella* contamination of poultry feed.

Poultry flock health

All poultry farms should have a veterinarian, specialising in poultry, who will advise on the health and management of the flock. Visits should be made, at least annually, to ensure the knowledge of practices and facilities on the farm. All events which are outside the normal, for example, increased mortality, poor weights or poor feed conversion, should be thoroughly investigated. The chances of eliminating microbial contamination from poultry meat will be improved if steps are taken to ensure that birds entering the slaughter and processing chain are either free from infection or are identified as contaminated and treated accordingly.

The situation in the United Kingdom, where there has been considerable success in tackling the *Salmonella* problem, involves testing all flocks of broilers and turkeys for *Salmonella* 1 or 2 weeks prior to slaughter. This enables positive flocks to be handled with special care and attention during processing. This will entail slaughter at the end of the day or week, maximum chlorine levels of 0.5 ppm in the water and perhaps lower line speed and/or attention to prevent rupture of the intestines.

Healthier birds are produced on a single-age farm ('all-in/all-out' system). The farm is depopulated at the end of each crop or cycle and thoroughly cleaned and disinfected. Tests are carried out to ensure freedom from, for example, *Salmonella*, prior to restocking. Should *Salmonella* be isolated, cleaning and disinfection are repeated until a negative result is obtained.

The need for close liaison with the farm is even more important in the case of poultry than with other species because of their size, large numbers involved in slaughter and dressing, high rates of slaughter and the use of antibiotics, anticoccidial drugs, etc. in their rearing. Adequate withdrawal periods are essential for all drugs. This period of time should be adhered to when 'thinning' occurs, that is, when a number of birds are removed from the house in order to give extra room to allow the remaining birds grow larger.

The withdrawal of feed prior to loading for transport to slaughter, in order to reduce crop and intestinal tract contents, can also help to reduce the level of contamination. Published FAO literature recommends a minimum period of 4 hours prior to birds arriving at the poultry plant, but extending the period to 10 hours may result in faeces becoming more fluid, thus increasing the chances of cross-contamination between birds in transit. The UK Advisory Committee on the Microbiological Safety of Food recommends that a period between 6 and 10 hours should be allowed between feeding and kill.

Catching and crating

This operation should be carried out with care in order to avoid injuries and unnecessary suffering to the birds. Crates must be in good repair and of good design and must not be over- or under-filled, since both situations can lead to injury. The catchers must be well trained and supervised to avoid injury and downgrading of the birds. Only healthy birds should be crated; diseased or otherwise abnormal birds should be killed on the farm.

One of the most difficult, labour-intensive and unpleasant tasks as far as working conditions and unsociable hours are concerned is that of collecting, crating and loading birds at the point of production. Depending on the quality and commitment of the staff employed, this area can be one where bird welfare is of a high or a low order, the latter often resulting in high levels of downgrading of carcases because of the injuries inflicted.

The majority of bruises resulting in downgrading occur during catching and transportation. The incidence of bruising is also directly related to the length of the journey.

In recent years, systems have been developed to improve catching (or harvesting) and transportation. For the time being, however, broilers are still caught by hand and carried by one leg. This has to be done with great care to avoid injury. Turkeys must always be carried by two legs.

Poultry harvesting procedures can be divided into four basic systems (Loose crates, Fixed crates, Modular system, Novel mechanical methods).

Loose crates

Empty plastic crates are taken from the lorry into the shed, where a team of catchers fill the individual crates. As with all systems, fewer birds are placed in each crate in summer to reduce the risk of heat stress. The birds are passed into the crate through a flapped opening at the top. For unloading, there is a larger aperture in the side or top of the crate through which the birds may be removed. Once a crate has been filled, it is taken to the lorry. Self-stacking crates can be placed on pallets in the shed for handling by a forklift vehicle. Loose crates provide a flexible system at low capital cost but a high labour input (Fig. 10.5).

Fixed crates

The crates are fixed on to the lorry. The birds are carried out of the shed to the lorry and are placed by the handful into one of the lower crates. Numbers in each crate depend on size and weather conditions. When the correct number has been placed in the crate, the hinged flap is fastened. For loading the upper crates, a loading platform is attached to the side of the lorry, from which two men can operate. The remainder of the catching team pass the birds to these men. Once again, great care has to be taken to prevent injuries to the birds. The system has the advantage of better protection from inclement weather than provided by loose crates while in transit, but the capital cost is greater, although the labour requirements are marginally lower.

Modular system

The modular system, probably the most common in broiler processing in the United Kingdom, has been of great benefit in lowering the amount of bruising and other injuries to birds and has obvious improved welfare considerations. Basically, a module is a metal frame containing 4–16 crates or compartments. The empty modules are taken into the house by a forklift truck. The birds are caught by hand and put directly into the compartments, thus avoiding the need for multiple handling or carrying the birds for long distances before crating.

Modules tend to be bulky and heavy, weighing about 0.75 tonne when fully loaded. The floor of the poultry house needs to be firm, and 15 m of concrete is needed at the front of the shed for the lorry.

Modules allow for rapid catching and loading and a three-man team can load 6000 birds/hour. They can be loaded from either side and the large open top of each drawer ensures that minimal damage is inflicted on the birds. The modules are stacked two high on the lorry and the outside can have a curtain, which makes them suitable for all climatic conditions.

Dump modules have been used with limited success. In these, the birds are offloaded at the poultry plant by tilting the module and 'dumping' the birds on to a conveyor belt. These were developed with the intention of improving welfare, with expected lessening of fractures and bruising, but present-day thinking is to try to develop methods of stunning the birds in their crates prior to shackling.

Novel mechanical methods

These include herding systems where the birds are herded on to a conveyor and a fully automatic harvesting system which consists of a catching unit, a truck unit and a crate-loading unit. The birds are directed by long rubber fingers, on vertical rotating reels, on to a belt conveyor up to a crating area. The crating system consists of a trailer with a special rotating platform and a loading conveyor which has a hydraulic lifting device so that all drawers of the module can be filled automatically. For other mechanical methods see figures 10.2 and 10.3.

Reception and unloading

The reception area or lairage is the area where birds are held before unloading. It should be under cover and of sufficient size to hold all the transport vehicles awaiting unloading. In warm weather, additional ventilation provided by fans is necessary. In addition to good ventilation,

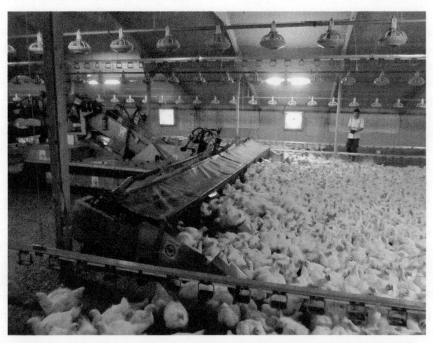

Figure 10.3 Automatic poultry harvester (Reproduced with permission from Tom Pearson, CM Agriculture Ltd).

control of relative humidity is also essential, and this should not be allowed to rise above 70%.

The method of unloading will obviously depend upon the type of crate used. Loose crates are unloaded from the vehicle and placed on a conveyor system which carries them to the hanging station. It is important that the crates are not thrown around roughly and that the birds are gently but firmly hung on the rail. The crates continue around on the conveyor, are washed and brought back to the vehicle, which should have been cleaned.

For unloading the birds from fixed crates, the vehicle is driven between two vertically moving platforms. The hangers standing on the platforms open the crates at the side, take out the birds and hang them on the killing line which is behind them. No crate conveyor system is required but the crates are extremely difficult to clean. In addition, the hangers have to turn through 180° every time a bird is removed and hung on the line.

Some of the modular systems effect unloading through hinged doors in the side in a manner similar to that for fixed crates. Another system raises the modules hydraulically to a high-level unloading platform, so that the drawers are at the required level. The birds are taken from the open drawers and hung on the shackles by a 90° rotation of the unloading operative. The 'Easyload' module is removed from the transport vehicle, either by a forklift truck or automated unloader, and fed into an automated system which presents it to a drawer push-out unit. This transfers the plastic drawers to a covered conveyor leading to the hanging station. The open drawer allows unrestricted access for the hanging operatives, greatly reducing bird damage and manpower requirements. The birds are hung directly on the killing line.

Each operator can hang 1000–1100 birds/hour. The hanging area can be enclosed to incorporate dust extraction and light density control, thus aiding health and safety for the operators and welfare of the birds, which allows them to be quiet and lessens stress during transfer onto the killing line.

The empty 'Easyload' drawers are automatically inverted to remove all loose debris and are then immersed in a pre-soak tank before being thoroughly washed and sanitised. The empty drawers continue through the drawer re-inverter to be automatically reloaded into the returning empty module frame. The module frames are also automatically washed (Fig. 10.4).

The layout of this system lends itself to separate clean and dirty areas within the arrival bay.

Pre-slaughter inspection

On arrival at the plant, every consignment should be checked to determine the condition of the birds and to ensure, for example, that during transit they have not

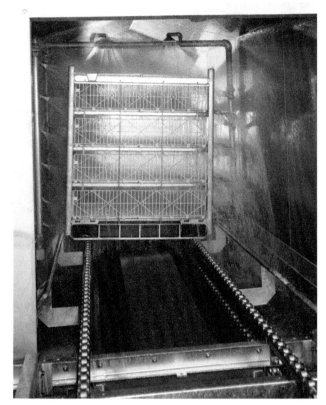

Figure 10.4 Washing crate module (Reproduced with permission from Stork Poulty Processing, Boxmeer, The Netherlands).

become trapped by the heads, legs or wings. This is a legal requirement, and all birds must be assessed by the site official veterinarian (OV).

The lighting in the hanging-on area should be sufficient to enable staff to see the birds and identify problems but not so bright as to disturb the birds. On removal from the crate or module, birds should be checked to see whether they are suffering from a condition which may cause them pain or distress. These birds should be killed immediately either by dislocation of the neck (small birds) or by stunning knife (small and large birds). This must be done by a licensed slaughterman. Runts and diseased birds, which may have been inadvertently crated, should also be killed and not shackled.

Shackling

When correctly handled, most birds remain still after a short period of wing flapping when first placed in the shackles. Broilers will generally have settled within 12 seconds and turkeys 20 seconds. A method of reducing wing flapping is for the shackler to run his or her hands down the bird's body or to briefly hold on to its legs. A strip of smooth plastic sheeting installed parallel to the conveyor line, along which the breasts of the suspended birds rub, also has a quietening effect. It is important that this sheeting extends into the stun bath.

Turkeys must not be suspended for more than 3 minutes and other birds for 2 minutes before being stunned or killed.

Stunning and slaughter

Electrical stunning

Stunning is usually carried out in an electrically charged water bath by dragging the heads of the birds through water in which an electrode is submerged. The shackles of the killing line simultaneously touch an earth electrode, causing an electric current to run through the body of the bird. Effective stunning requires careful observation of the birds and adjustment of the equipment.

The water level is critical, and it is essential to avoid water flowing down the inlet chute and causing a pre-stun shock, which may make the birds raise their heads, thus avoiding contact with the water of the actual stunner.

Research has shown that a water bath stunner using a 50 Hz AC supply and providing a current of 148 mA per bird will result in a stun/kill of 99% of birds, with only 1% of birds leaving the water bath stunned but still alive. However, 105 mA per broiler would be acceptable provided both carotid arteries are severed within 15 seconds to ensure death before birds can begin to recover.

Problems with conventional water bath stunners have been identified through observation in commercial processing plants and experiments in the laboratory. Owing to differences in the electrical resistance of the individual birds, there is little control over the stunning current and hence the effectiveness of stunning. A prototype poultry stunner has been developed which controls the current delivered to individual birds. The machine is capable of operating at typical commercial speeds of 6000 birds/hour. It can provide a constant current to each individual bird provided there is no significant current pathway between adjacent birds. A constant current stunning system will control the current flow through individual birds at an optimal level which will ensure an effective stun and at the same time minimise the carcase quality problems produced by high currents.

Less commonly used stunning instruments are the dry stunner, usually incorporating an electrically charged metal grid or plate, and hand-operated stunner.

The most reliable indicator that a bird is properly stunned by the low-current or high-frequency method is the electroplectic fit. The characteristics of this condition are the neck arched with the head directly vertical, open eyes, dilated pupils, absence of corneal reflex, wings flexed, rigidly extended legs and constant rapid body tremors after 4 seconds.

When cardiac arrest is induced, these signs are shorter lasting and less pronounced and are followed by a completely limp carcase, no breathing (absence of abdominal movements in the vent area), loss of nictitating membrane reflex and dilated pupil. The comb reflex can also determine whether sensibility has resumed after stunning or neck cutting.

Although cardiac arrest is preferable from a welfare standpoint, the use of high stunning currents on the quality of the carcase is said by some to be associated with wing haemorrhages, red skin condition, including red wing tips and pygostyles, poor plucking, broken bones (in particular furculum) and ruptured blood vessels causing blood splashing in the breast muscle.

Gas stunning

Although electrical stunning is the most common method of stunning poultry prior to slaughter under commercial conditions, methods of stunning/killing poultry using gases, while the birds are still in their transport containers, have been approved under the new EC Directive. Gas stunning/killing will enable shackling to be performed on the freshly killed birds, and this would eliminate the live bird handling at the processing plants. The two gas stunning/killing methods that are being approved in the United Kingdom are anoxia induced with 90% argon or other inert gases and a mixture of 25–30% carbon dioxide and 60% argon or other inert gases in air. In both systems, the oxygen levels must not exceed 2% (Fig. 10.5).

The birds would be stunned/killed while they are in their transport containers. This would result in the birds leaving a stunning unit in large numbers, and all the carcases would have to be uncrated and shackled rapidly to allow prompt neck cutting. It is inevitable that the time between the end of gas stunning and neck cutting would be longer than that practised under the conventional electrical stunning system. Although research has shown that the efficiency of bleeding in broiler chickens was not impaired when their necks were cut immediately after gas stunning/killing, delayed neck cutting after gas stunning of broilers could increase the prevalence of carcase downgrading conditions associated with a poor bleed out. This does not happen with turkeys, the difference being attributable to a difference in carcase cooling rate or other factors.

Gas stunning/killing methods accelerate the rate of post-mortem pH fall in poultry, and this would allow early filleting in broilers (between 2.5 and 4 hours after slaughter). Generally with anoxia, there are fewer carcase and meat quality defects. Many fewer defects are found in the breast region, including haemorrhages, but there is an increase in broken wings caused by convulsions.

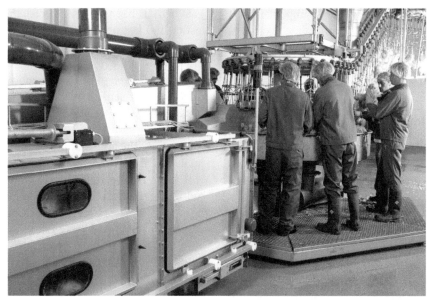

Figure 10.5 Multi-phase controlled atmosphere stunning (Reproduced with permission from Stork Poulty Processing, Boxmeer, The Netherlands).

Neck cutting

This should be carried out within 15 seconds of the bird emerging from the stunner. Mechanical neck cutting is the norm for broilers when the bird's head is guided across a single revolving circular blade or between a pair of revolving blades. Accurate positioning of the head is essential. When cardiac arrest is not produced at stunning, the most humane method of producing rapid brain death is to sever both carotid arteries. In practice, this is difficult, but not impossible, to achieve without having an effect on the further processing of the carcase.

Decapitation is also becoming popular followed by head maceration.

Where a mechanical killer is used in the United Kingdom, it is mandatory to have an operative present to manually kill any bird which has missed the automatic system. Operatives who kill the birds have to be licensed by the local authority (Fig. 10.9).

Birds are killed manually by passing a knife across the side of the neck at the base of the bird's head, which should sever a jugular vein and carotid artery. Again, it is better to sever both carotids, but care has to be taken to avoid damage to the carcase.

Whichever method is used, a sharp instrument is essential. Automatic killing of turkeys has not been introduced because of the problem of major variation in bird size within the flock.

Scalding and defeathering

The minimum time for bleeding between neck cutting and entering the scald tank in the United Kingdom is 2 minutes for turkeys and geese and 1.5 minutes for chickens

and other birds. The birds, on the conveyor, pass through a bleeding tunnel, the blood being collected and pumped into a holding tank.

The birds are scalded either by immersion in hot water or by spray scalding. Spray scalding is more hygienic but also more expensive, and therefore, scald tanks are more commonly installed. The temperature of the water is dependent on the type of final product. For the fresh, chilled market, a soft scald of 50–53°C is used as this does not damage the skin, thereby preventing discoloration and drying (barking) on air chilling (Fig. 10.6).

For the frozen market, a hard scald at a higher temperature, 56–58°C, is used as this facilitates feather removal and the birds need only remain in the tank for 2–2½ minutes instead of 3½ minutes for the soft scald. In the United States, there is a statutory requirement for an overflow from the scald tank of about 1 L/bird for hygiene reasons. Various chemicals can be added to assist feather removal and to try to prevent cross-contamination (but see the following text).

The scald tank immersion results in large numbers of organisms being released into the water; in addition, faecal material in the tank dissociates to form ammonium urate and uric acid, which form a natural buffer system, thereby maintaining scald tank pH at around 6, the point at which salmonellas are most heat resistant. The overall effect is that salmonellas, campylobacters and other organisms, including spores, can survive. Research has shown that the addition of quaternary ammonium, acetic acid, etc. to the scald tank would adjust the pH, the principal controlling factor in the survival of salmonellas and campylobacters, and therefore improve the

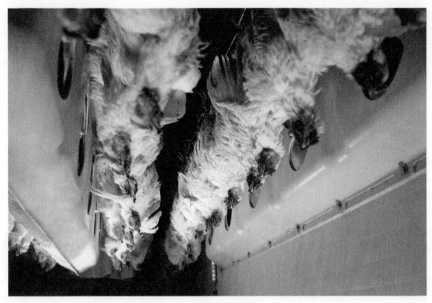

Figure 10.6 Aeroscalding – scalding without immersion into scalding (Reproduced with permission from Stork Poulty Processing, Boxmeer, The Netherlands).

hygiene. At present, this cannot be used because of the requirements to demonstrate no carcase residues and to use only potable water.

There is no doubt the operation of scalding from a hygiene standpoint is fraught with hazards; the temperature of the scald water, type (immersion, spray with hot water or steam), duration of scalding, static, agitated or countercurrent bathwater, type of tank(s), etc. all affect the degree of water bath contamination. Work by Slavik *et al.* (1995) on the numbers of *Campylobacter* and *Salmonella* on chicken carcases scalded at three different temperatures would appear to confirm that the higher the temperature, the greater the contamination (Table 10.2).

Alternative methods of scalding are being devised to improve the situation. Lower bacterial contamination has been achieved with spray scalding and plucking in a single operation (Veerkamp and Hofmans, 1973). Clouser *et al.* (1995) found that a spray scalding system for turkey carcases was superior to traditional scalding (Fig. 10.6).

Improvements in immersion scalding have been made by stirring the water in order to achieve an ideal mixing, division of the scald tank into several smaller ones and high-pressure (800 bar) treatment of scald water. All these have shown improvements in scald water quality. Lowering the pH with organic acids may affect product quality, and the addition of trisodium phosphate may cause corrosion of equipment. The ideal solution has not yet been found.

Defeathering

Feathers are removed mechanically, immediately after scalding, by a series of online plucking machines. These consist of banks of counterrotating, stainless steel domes

Table 10.2 Numbers of *Campylobacter* and *Salmonella* (log mpn/carcase) on chicken carcases scalded at three different temperatures

Bacterium	Scald	Trial Temperature (°C)		
Trial		1	2	3
Salmonella	52	3.00	3.17	3.09
	56	3.16	3.17	3.34
	60	3.50	3.48	3.36
Campylobacter	52	3.64	3.30	4.18
	56	3.39	2.94	3.39
	60	4.08	3.59	3.98

Source: From Slavik *et al.* (1995).

or discs, with attached rubber 'fingers'. Rubber flails mounted on inclined shafts are sometimes used for finishing.

The machines should be close to the scald tank and to each other to lessen the effect of cooling. Generally, birds which have been scalded at higher temperatures require 50% less defeathering capacity. The machines are adjustable to allow for differing bird sizes, and this must be carried out to prevent mechanical damage to the carcase.

Continuous water sprays are usually incorporated within the machines for flushing out feathers. Feathers are commonly taken to a centralised collection point via a fast-flowing water channel located below the machine. Dry feather systems using a conveyor belt in conjunction with a vacuum or compressed air arrangement are sometimes used. Any feathers remaining on the bird after plucking, including pin feathers, are removed by hand.

For ducks, wax stripping is used. The ducks are dipped in a bath of hot wax and then passed through cool water sprays so that the wax hardens. The hardened wax, with the feathers attached, is hand stripped. The plucked carcases are then spray washed. There is evidence to suggest that the combination of scalding at 60°C followed by immersion in molten wax at 87°C to aid final removal of the feathers has a beneficial effect on the microbiological status of the finished product.

Defeathering machines are major sites of potential cross-contamination in primary processing. Rubber fingers can score the carcase and can also harbour contamination in the 'cobweb' of tiny cracks which form when the rubber becomes brittle. In addition, the spinning action of the plucker heads form aerosols which can spread contamination. Moreover, since the atmosphere inside the machinery is both warm and moist, microbial growth is encouraged.

Following feather removal, the birds are spray washed, and at this point, the *whole-bird* post-mortem examination takes place. It is here that obviously diseased birds, badly bled and badly bruised carcases, are removed. The heads of the birds are removed by an automatic head and windpipe puller. By pulling the heads off rather than cutting them off, the oesophagus and trachea are removed with the heads. This loosens the crop and lungs, which assists in their removal by the automatic evisceration machines.

The birds then pass through an automatic foot cutter. The severed feet remain on the shackles and are removed mechanically on the return line. In the case of large turkeys, retention of the sinews is considered unacceptable. Instead of cutting off the shanks, an automatic sinew puller is used, and this draws up to nine of the main sinews.

The carcases are re-hung on the evisceration line after removal of the feet. This is now done automatically in most slaughterhouses, using a transfer system available from several equipment manufacturers. In this case, the foot cutter and transfer device are combined in one unit. This lessens the risk of cross-contamination. The empty, returning, killing line shackles pass through a shackle washer on their way back to the bird arrival area (Fig. 10.7).

Evisceration

In the EC, the evisceration area must be physically separated from the defeathering area.

Chickens are usually suspended from the shackles of the evisceration line conveyor by engaging the hock joints two-point suspension. Turkeys are commonly hung by a 'three-point' suspension which includes the head as well as the legs. This presents the bird horizontally, making cutting around the vent and evisceration easier (Fig. 10.8).

Evisceration is mainly carried out mechanically, but manual evisceration is still practised. On automatic lines, a cut is made around the vent, a spoon-shaped device is inserted into the opening, and the viscera are withdrawn. The viscera may remain attached for inspection, hanging over the back of the carcase connected by their natural tissues or hung separately (Fig. 10.9).

Contamination of the carcase surface with Enterobacteriaceae species may ensue if intestines, etc.

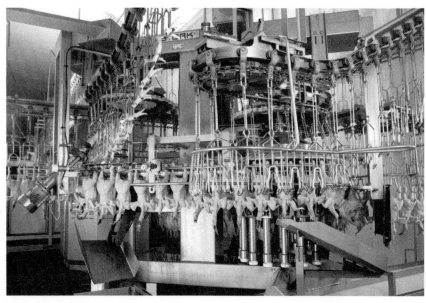

Figure 10.7 Transfer from defeathering into eviscerating line (Reproduced with permission from Stork Poulty Processing, Boxmeer, The Netherlands).

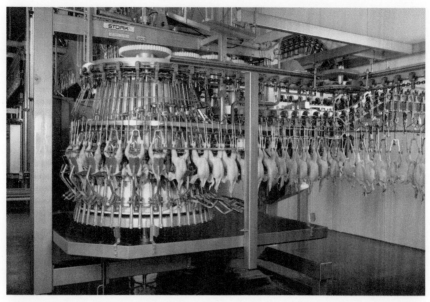

Figure 10.8 High-speed automated evisceration (Reproduced with permission from Stork Poulty Processing, Boxmeer, The Netherlands).

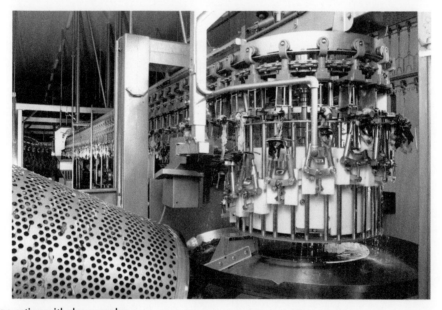

Figure 10.9 Liver harvesting with drum washer.

are damaged. This is not an uncommon occurrence because the machinery used is not able to adjust for the natural variation in the size of birds being processed. A new type of equipment, however, holds the birds horizontally by the head and hocks so that, when the viscera are removed from the body cavity, they emerge sideways. They are placed on a tray beside the bird rather than hung with it and hence do not come into contact with the carcase.

It is at this stage that a further inspection takes place which will observe changes in the internal organs. After inspection, the viscera are separated into edible and inedible offal. The edible fraction, sometimes being washed in chlorinated water (in the EU, the maximum concentration of chlorine allowed in potable water is 0.5 ppm), is sorted, chilled and packed.

The eviscerated carcase is spray washed, internally and externally (Fig. 10.10). This gives a visually clean bird and also decreases carcase contamination. The carcase should be washed not only after final inspection but between the different stages involved in evisceration, as it has been shown that by doing so the numbers of coliforms and salmonellas on carcases are reduced because there is insufficient time for attachment to occur. A suitable carcase washer comprises a small cabinet containing an appropriate arrangement of spray nozzles (Fig. 10.11 and 10.12).

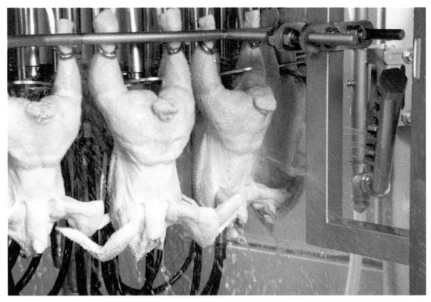

Figure 10.10 Inside and outside washing (Reproduced with permission from Stork Poulty Processing, Boxmeer, The Netherlands).

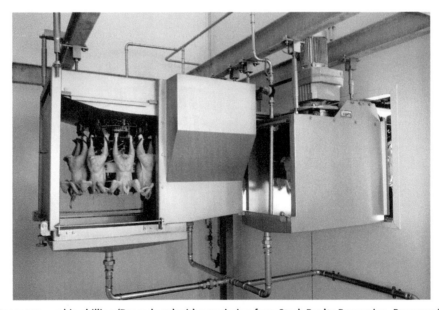

Figure 10.11 Moistener spray cabin chilling (Reproduced with permission from Stork Poulty Processing, Boxmeer, The Netherlands).

The heart, liver and gizzard (the giblets) may be pooled and inserted into the body of chickens which are to be frozen. Giblets are more frequently contaminated with *Salmonella* than other sample sites, and chickens which contain them are more often contaminated than those without giblets. The carcase and skin of these chickens are more frequently contaminated with *Salmonella enteritidis* PT4 than these sites in chickens not containing giblets, irrespective of whether the giblets themselves were contaminated.

The same study also found that frozen chickens were significantly more regularly contaminated than chilled chickens.

Partial evisceration (or effile) is carried out in Great Britain. In this process, the intestines are removed, but the remaining viscera are left inside the carcase. Delayed evisceration is also permissible, where uneviscerated birds are held for up to 15 days under refrigeration at no more than 4°C before evisceration and post-mortem inspection are carried out.

New York-dressed (NYD) birds are sold uneviscerated and with the head and feet left attached. The EEC marketing of NYD birds from licensed premises was banned from 1 May 1997. However, NYD birds may still be produced and marketed by exempt slaughterhouses (i.e. those producing fewer than 10000 birds/year). NYD birds

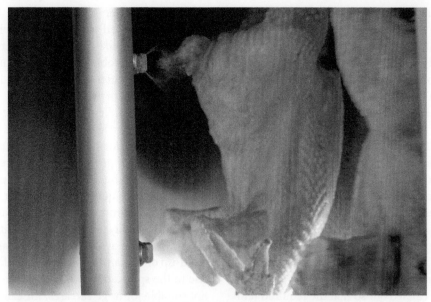

Figure 10.12 Moistener spray cabin chilling (Reproduced with permission from Stork Poulty Processing, Boxmeer, The Netherlands).

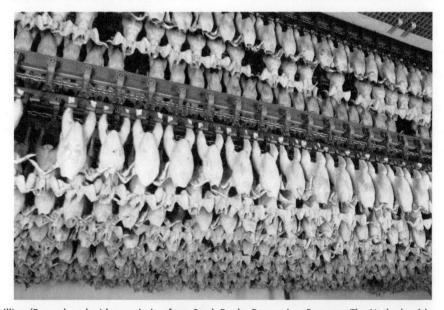

Figure 10.13 Air chilling (Reproduced with permission from Stork Poulty Processing, Boxmeer, The Netherlands).

present a particular hazard owing to the risk of leakage of faeces from the vent and, if evisceration is carried out in a kitchen, the risk of faeces or intestinal contents from ruptured intestines cross-contaminating other foods.

Chilling

In many plants, the high rate of processing (7000–1100 birds/hour) is such that there is little loss of heat from the carcase before it reaches the chilling stage, and average carcase temperatures are frequently above 30°C. Prompt and efficient chilling of the bird is essential to delay the growth of psychotropic spoilage bacteria and prevent any increase in micro-organisms of public health significance.

The type of chilling used can have an effect on the type and quantity of microbial contamination of the end product. Water chilling shows an increase in the incidence of *Salmonella* against air chilling but decreased incidence of campylobacter. Continuous, in-line, immersion chilling is still the most widely used method in many countries. Carcases move through a counterflow current of water in a state of constant agitation so that they are constantly moving into cleaner water. This washing effect also removes numerous organisms from both the inner and outer surfaces of the carcases. There may be deleterious effects if there is a significant build-up of blood and carcase material or a rise in water temperature. The addition of hypochlorite or chlorine dioxide to the water might serve to reduce the levels of contamination in the chiller, but because these compounds would quickly be deactivated on contact with skin, there would be little direct effect on carcase bacterial burdens. The main value of chlorinating chiller water is to minimise cross-contamination. Although hyperchlorination is banned in the EU, it is allowed in the United States (Fig. 10.14).

EC regulations state that the carcases must pass through one or more tanks of water or of ice and water, the contents of which are continuously renewed. Only a system whereby the carcases are constantly propelled by mechanical means through a counterflow of water is acceptable.

The temperature of the water in the tank measured at the points of entry and exit of the carcases must not be more than +16°C and +4°C, respectively.

Chilling must be carried out so that the required temperatures of fresh chilled poultry meat of not more than 4°C and for frozen poultry meat of not more than −12°C are reached in the shortest possible time.

The minimum flow of water throughout the whole chilling process must be:

2.5 L per carcase weighing 2.5 kg or less
4 L/ per carcase weighing between 2.5 and 5 kg
6 L per carcase weighing 5 kg or more

Other requirements are the length of time the carcases spend in the tanks (first tank not more than half an hour;

others, not longer than necessary), equipment to be thoroughly cleaned and disinfected when necessary and at the end of the day, calibrated control equipment and the need for microbiological monitoring.

In addition, when chlorine is used, it should be monitored to ensure correct levels.

Static water chillers involve the use of static slush ice tanks after immersion chilling and are required for larger birds, especially for turkeys which must also be 'aged' to ensure a tender product prior to freezing. The larger carcases need to be chilled for longer periods. The disadvantages of this equipment are greater than those arising from the use of immersion chillers. Water chillers are also restricted in quality products on the ground of water pickup.

Spray chillers avoid the problems associated with the build-up of contamination in the chill tanks but can give rise to the spread of bacteria through aerosols. They are not suitable for large carcases, for example, turkeys, and are costly to operate as they use high volumes of water.

Air chillers are generally used where carcases are for sale fresh. Chilling is effected either by batch in a chill room or by continuous air blast. It requires the use of low-scald temperatures to ensure a high-quality appearance (Fig. 10.13 and Fig. 10.15). The differences in microbial counts between air- and water-cooled carcases are not constant.

After initial chilling birds may be processed as whole birds or as parts (Figs. 10.17, 10.18, 10.19, 10.20, 10.21, 10.22 and 10.23).

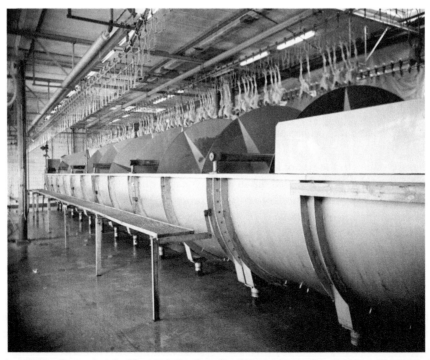

Figure 10.14 Immersion chilling (Reproduced with permission from Stork Poultry Processing, Boxmeer, The Netherlands).

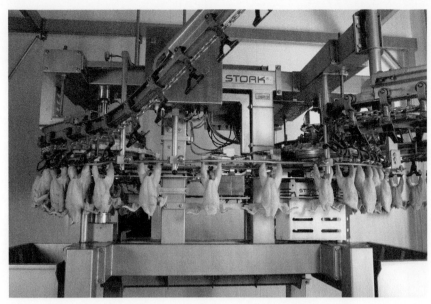

Figure 10.15 Transfer from chilling line into selection line (Reproduced with permission from Stork Poulty Processing, Boxmeer, The Netherlands).

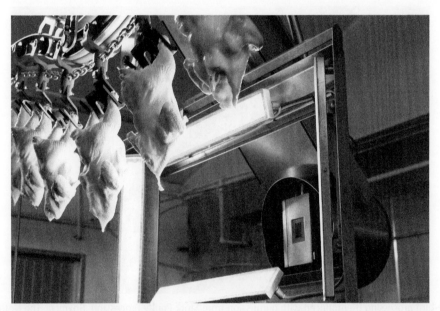

Figure 10.16 Intelligent reporting, inspection and selection system (Reproduced with permission from Stork Poulty Processing, Boxmeer, The Netherlands).

Chemical rinsing of carcases with trisodium phosphate is used in the United States.

Ante-mortem health inspection

In the EU, the traditional ante-mortem inspection, with its obvious deficiencies of not being able to inspect birds in crates or on the line adequately, has been superseded by on-farm producer declaration or a health attestation signed by a private veterinarian.

Producers with an annual production of up to 20 000 domestic fowls or 15 000 ducks or 10 000 turkeys or 10 000 geese complete a declaration which states they do not exceed the above numbers. Birds from their farm receive a pre-slaughter health inspection by the OV at the plant.

Birds from producers with an annual production in excess of the above can either have a health attestation signed by a private veterinarian which states that he or she has examined the poultry before slaughter and that in his or her opinion there are no reasons why they

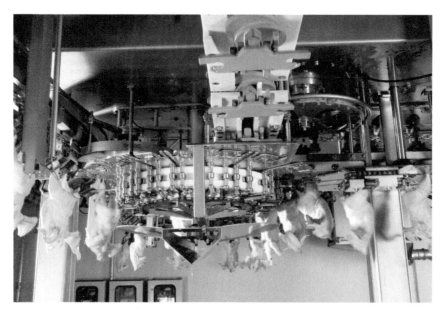

Figure 10.17 Transfer from selection line into cut-up line (Reproduced with permission from Stork Poulty Processing, Boxmeer, The Netherlands).

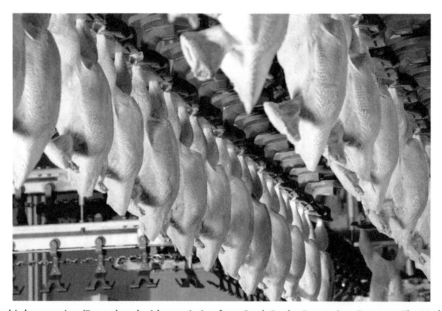

Figure 10.18 Whole-bird processing (Reproduced with permission from Stork Poulty Processing, Boxmeer, The Netherlands).

should not be slaughtered for human consumption. The veterinary pre-slaughter health inspection consists of the following:

1 Checking the producer's records, which depending on the type of bird include:
  a Date of arrival
  b Number
  c Mortality
  d Suppliers of feedingstuffs
  e Type, period of use and withdrawal periods of feed additives
  f Type of any medicinal product, with dates of administration and withdrawal (this includes vaccines)
  g Results of any previous official pre-slaughter health inspections of birds from the same specified group
  h Number sent for slaughter
  i Expected date of slaughter
2 Any additional examinations needed to establish:
  a Whether birds are suffering from a disease which can be transmitted to humans or animals
  b Whether the birds show disturbance of general behaviour or signs of sickness which may make the meat unfit for human consumption

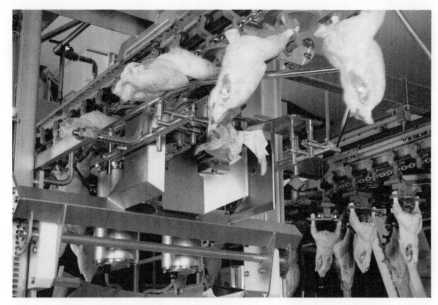

Figure 10.19 Automated cut-up line – front half cutting module (Reproduced with permission from Stork Poulty Processing, Boxmeer, The Netherlands).

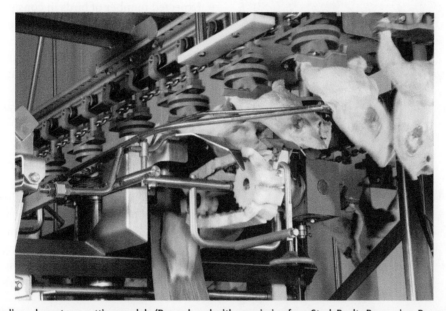

Figure 10.20 Cut-up line – breast cap cutting module (Reproduced with permission from Stork Poulty Processing, Boxmeer, The Netherlands).

3 Regular sampling of water and feed with a view to checking compliance with withdrawal periods

4 The results of tests for zoonotic agents carried out in accordance with Directive 2003/99

Alternatively, the veterinarian signs an initial declaration, given to the central competent authority, confirming that the producer's holding is under his or her supervision. The producer then submits a production report to the manager of the plant at least 72 hours before the birds are due to arrive. The information is then passed on to the OV.

If the OV is not satisfied with the information, he or she may ask for further information such as details of the hatchery, feedstuffs, growth rates, etc., and if the production report is not complete or does not provide the required information or the OV is not satisfied, he or she may order an inspection at the farm of origin to enable completion of the report. The inspection is carried out at the owner's expense. The food chain information (FCI) report consists of the following details:

- Holding of origin
- Intended date of arrival at slaughterhouse

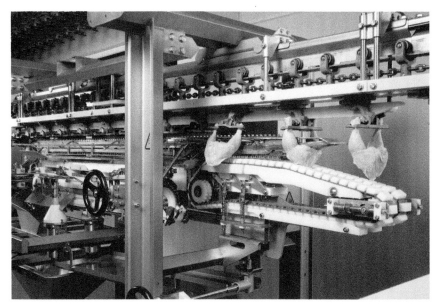

Figure 10.21 Cut-up line – leg processing module (Reproduced with permission from Stork Poulty Processing, Boxmeer, The Netherlands).

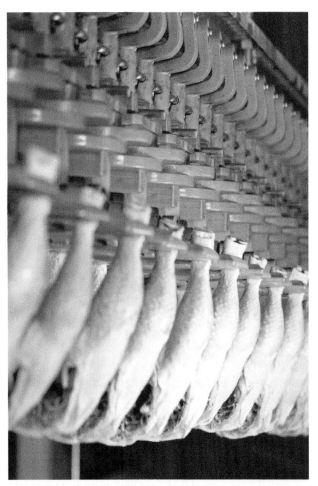

Figure 10.22 Cut-up line – leg processing module (Reproduced with permission from Stork Poulty Processing, Boxmeer, The Netherlands).

- Expected number of birds in consignment
- Mortality data (daily % in final week before slaughter and weekly mortality before that)
- Results of any on-farm veterinary inspection of flock
- Results of any laboratory tests/diagnosis carried out on birds, litter, etc.
- Dates of administration/withdrawal of all medicinal products
- Any other relevant information

The production report should be copied to the veterinary surgeon supervising the holding.

The plant OV (or a delegated poultry meat inspector (PMI)) is responsible for relaying adverse results of post-mortem inspections and dead on arrivals (DOAs) of consignments back to the holding, slaughterhouse management and veterinarian responsible for the holding as he or she or she feels necessary.

Post-mortem inspection in the plant

Plant inspection assistants (PIAs) in the United Kingdom are plant employees who have been trained to undertake post-mortem inspection on the whole bird and evisceration inspection points. They can therefore replace PMIs, who now carry out more of a supervisory role, but only with the agreement of the competent authority and after discussion with the OV. Some purchasers of poultry products insist on the independence of PMIs for inspection.

Poultry inspection assistants are taught the theory and practice of anatomy and physiology, pathology and meat inspection and also poultry welfare and legislation.

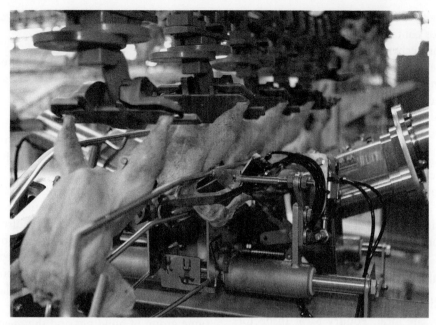

Figure 10.23 Cut-up line – wing processing (Reproduced with permission from Stork Poulty Processing, Boxmeer, The Netherlands).

Poultry must be inspected immediately after slaughter under suitable lighting (540 lux). The surface of the bird's body, excluding head and feet, except where they are intended for human consumption, the viscera and the body cavities must be subjected to visual inspection and, where necessary, palpation and incision.

Attention must also be paid to anomalies of consistency, colour and smell in the carcases, major anomalies resulting from the slaughtering operations and proper functioning of the slaughter equipment.

The OV must give a detailed inspection of a random sample of the birds rejected in the post-mortem health inspection and examine a random sample of 300 birds, taken from the entire consignment, by inspecting the viscera and body cavities.

He must carry out a special post-mortem if there are other indications that the meat from the poultry could be unfit for human consumption. In the case of partly eviscerated poultry ('effile') whose intestines were removed immediately, the viscera and the body cavities of at least 5% of the poultry from each consignment will be inspected after evisceration. If anomalies are discovered in a number of birds, then all of the consignment must be examined as previously mentioned.

In the case of NYD poultry, the birds will be examined as described earlier, no longer than 15 days after slaughter, and kept at 4°C or below.

Taking of samples for residues must be carried out by spot checks and in any event of justified suspicion. The OV also has the authority to ask for laboratory tests to be carried out to aid diagnosis or to detect pharmacological substances. Should the OV consider that hygienic processing or health inspection is not being adequately carried out, he or she can lower the line speed or stop production.

The results of the inspections should be recorded and where necessary communicated to the competent veterinary authority (of the holding from which the birds originated) and the owner of the flock of origin who will pass this information to the OV carrying out the ante-mortem inspection during the subsequent production period.

Many of the diseases listed in the following will rarely be encountered in the poultry plant.

Decision of the official veterinarian at the post-mortem inspection

Poultry meat is declared totally unfit for human consumption where the post-mortem inspection reveals any of the following conditions:

- Generalised infectious diseases and chronic localisations in organs of pathogenic micro-organisms transmissible to humans
- Systemic mycosis and local lesions in organs suspected of having been caused by pathogenic agents transmissible to humans, or their toxins
- Extensive subcutaneous or muscular parasitism and systemic parasitism
- Poisoning
- Cachexia
- Abnormal smell, colour or taste

- Malignant or multiple tumours
- General soiling or contamination
- Major lesions and ecchymoses
- Extensive mechanical lesions, including those due to extensive scalding
- Insufficient bleeding
- Residues of substances exceeding the authorised standards or residues of prohibited substances
- Ascites

Parts of the carcase which show localised lesions or contaminations not affecting the health of the rest of meat are unfit for human consumption. It is essential that condemned and suspect meat is kept separated from meat for human consumption (Fig. 10.16).

General contamination

It is the responsibility of the Food Business Organisation (FBO) to produce safe meat. Poultry Meat Inspectors confirm FBO actions and identify any specific risks.

Poultry meat, carcases and/or offal affected with general consummation by faecal material, bile, grease and disinfectants should be considered unfit for human consumption.

A hygienic trimming system must be in place if the FBO decides to trim contaminated carcases.

Any part of the carcase or offal affected with bile staining should be trimmed. Where plucking machines break the skin, the underlying musculature should be considered to be contaminated and trimmed from the carcase.

The FBO should have a system in place to deal with carcases or offal that fall on the floor. This could include trimming affected parts and consideration of the cleanliness of the floor. The OV/MHI should monitor that no contaminated meat is released for human consumption.

Guidelines on trimming poultry

Trimming must be carried out under the responsibility of the meat inspection team (supervision of trimming may be carried out by a PIA). Plant operatives should carry out most trimming. The selection of lesions or parts which require trimming must not be delegated to untrained individuals.

Minor blemishes such as bruising may be trimmed at one of the post-mortem inspection points, preferably that following evisceration, to minimise contamination of exposed meat.

Trimming of more serious conditions involving infection is usually impracticable with high line speeds, and in these cases, an adjacent trimming area should be provided.

Trimming of carcases may be delayed until after chilling, provided that:

1 There is no risk of contamination to other carcases.
2 Trimming is done under the supervision of MHI at regular times.

The OV and the FBO should agree recognised methods (i.e. marking and identification of parts to be trimmed) to ensure that trimming is properly carried out by plant staff.

The professional judgement of the OV should be used in assessing whether birds are fit for human consumption or whether rectification is required.

Poultry carcases, in licensed premises, are only allowed to be cut into parts and boned in approved cutting rooms. They must be chilled to not more than +4°C before cutting proceeds unless the slaughter room and the cutting room are near each other and located in the same group of buildings and the meat is transferred in one operation by an extension of the mechanical handling system.

Cutting must be carried out immediately, and once cutting and packaging are complete, the meat is placed in the chilling room. Packaged fresh poultry meat must not be kept in the same room as unpacked poultry meat.

Poultry disease is often multifactorial with, for example, poor ventilation along with a viral disease acting together with bacteria, for example, *Escherichia coli* (*E. coli*), to produce generalised septicaemia resulting in pericarditis, airsacculitis, perihepatitis and a congested carcase.

Yogaratnam (1995) analysed results of examinations at a poultry processing plant which received 33.65 million birds from 87 commercial broiler growing units in 1992 (Table 10.3). High carcase rejection rates of 3% or more were recorded in birds received from 13.2% of the rearing houses, distributed among 48% of the growing units. The higher rates of carcase rejection were found on the units with an average flock size of over 100 000 birds and from rearing houses with a population of more than 30 000

Table 10.3 Percentages of broiler carcases rejected because they were either DOA or diseased from farms with normal or high rates of rejection of carcases

Farm rejection rate	Percentage of carcases	
	DOA	Disease conditions
Normal	0.22	1.09
High	0.42	5.12

Source: Yogaratnam (1995).

birds. The main causes of rejection were birds DOA (0.24%), disease (1.57%) and miscellaneous conditions (0.28%). The most common cause of carcase rejection due to disease was colisepticaemia (42.8%). Septicaemia/toxaemia/fevered accounted for 29.63%, emaciation for 19.45% and ascites for 5.91%. Hydropericardium/pericarditis (1.01%), skin lesions (0.62%), joint lesions (0.31%), jaundice (0.16%) and tumours (0.01%) were also seen. The birds from units with high rejection rates had lower average slaughter weights than birds from units with normal rejection rates.

The productivity of intensively reared poultry falls as a result of disease problems as the size of the flock increases and as the number of rearing houses on one site increases.

Coliform infections

E. coli is the most commonly isolated organism from condemned carcases. *E. coli* is a normal inhabitant of the digestive tract of poultry, and large numbers are often found in the lower part of the small intestine and caeca. The serotypes most frequently causing colisepticaemia (01, 02, 08 and 078) are also likely to be found in the throat and upper trachea. These pathogenic *E. coli* probably invade the bird's body from the respiratory tract to produce the characteristic condition.

The best method of controlling colisepticaemia is to maintain the highest standards of flock management and obtain chicks only from disease-free well-managed breeding flocks and hatcheries. Pathogenic *E. coli* serotypes can be transmitted via the hatchery following faecal contamination of hatching eggs. Chicks should be the progeny of mycoplasma-free stock which have been vaccinated against IBD, infectious bronchitis and any other disease that is a local threat. The production birds, if necessary, need to be vaccinated against infectious bronchitis and IBD and provided with a coccidiostat in the feed. There is an increasing use of coccidial vaccination in speciality birds which avoids the need for a coccidiostat in the feed. The birds should be fed a well-balanced diet to avoid the consequences of mineral/vitamin deficiencies and malnutrition. Good litter management and properly ventilated houses are also vital control measures. The litter should be dry, but not dusty, and the airflow should be such that there are no pockets of stagnant air or build-up of ammonia fumes.

Lesions. The main lesions found in colisepticaemia of broilers, turkeys and ducks are congested muscles, enlarged liver and spleen with pericarditis, perihepatitis and airsacculitis.

Salmonellosis

There are two specific *Salmonella* organisms which affect only poultry. *Salmonella pullorum* causes bacillary white diarrhoea, BWD or pullorum disease, in chicks under 3 weeks of age. The disease is now eradicated from developed countries and because of the age of the bird affected would not be seen in a poultry meat plant.

Salmonella gallinarum causes fowl typhoid, an acute, subacute or chronic infectious disease of poultry, ducks, turkeys (notably in the United States), pheasants, guinea fowl, pea fowl, grouse and quail. The disease differs from other avian *Salmonella* infections in that clinical disease is usually seen in growers or adult birds, although chicks can be affected. In acute outbreaks, the first sign will be an increase in mortality, accompanied by a drop in food consumption. Depression, with affected birds standing still with ruffled feathers and their eyes closed, is seen clinically. As with most poultry diseases, the signs of ill health are mainly non-specific. In the chronic phase, there is progressive loss of condition, and an intense anaemia develops which produces shrunken, pale combs and wattles.

Lesions. Carcases of birds dying in the acute phase have a septicaemic, jaundiced appearance, with the subcutaneous blood vessels injected and prominent and the skeletal muscles congested and dark in colour. A consistent finding is a swollen friable liver that is dark red or almost black, and the surface has a distinctive copper-bronze sheen. The spleen may be enlarged and there is catarrhal enteritis.

In chronic cases (those most likely to be seen on inspection), greyish areas of necrosis may be seen in the myocardium, pancreas and intestine.

Judgement. Condemnation.

Incidence and control

In the United States, over 150 different salmonellas have been isolated from poultry. Evidence of disease in birds is most common in chicks, poultry or ducklings under 2 weeks of age. The main significance of *Salmonella* infection is as a zoonosis. The Zoonoses Directive (2003/99EC) contains provisions for community-wide controls for *Salmonella* in domestic fowl, and the Poultry Breeding Flocks and Hatcheries (England) Order 2007 reflects monitoring requirements of the directive. Defra has codes of practice for the prevention and control of *Salmonella* in breeding flocks and hatcheries and in chickens reared for meat on farms.

There are approximately 2500 different types (serotypes) of *Salmonella*. Most do not normally cause clinical disease in poultry. However, virulent strains such as *Salmonella typhimurium* DT104 have been associated with illness and mortality in chicks although cases in chickens reared for meat have been falling.

A survey carried out in the EU in 2008 showed 15.6% of broiler carcases to be contaminated with *Salmonella*, ranging from 0% in Denmark, Estonia, Finland and Luxemburg to 85.6% in Hungary (United Kingdom 3.6%).

Currently, only about 200 *Salmonella* serotypes are associated with food-borne infections in humans in any 1 year in the United Kingdom.

Salmonella virchow and *Salmonella thompson* can be invasive in humans and therefore may be as important as *S. enteritidis* and *S. typhimurium*.

Salmonellas gain access to a flock mainly through feed, but infection may also arrive through contaminated stock, wild and feral animals and personnel. There may also be a carry-over of infection from previous stock. Good biosecurity is essential including an all-in/all-out policy on farms, where all birds are of the same age and are all brought in at the same time and disposed of to allow for proper cleaning and disinfection between crops. Visitors should be discouraged and only essential staff should be allowed access. The perimeter of the farm should be identified, preferably fenced and gated securely, with parking facilities away from the buildings. Good management is dependent on a clean and tidy site. Rodent control is enhanced by the control of vegetation, including in and around ditches, with effective general management. There should be a rodent control programme. Feed spillages should be avoided, and any spills should be cleared up immediately.

Monitoring for *Salmonella* should be carried out to help reduce dissemination and ensure decontamination. There is a National Control Programme for *Salmonella* in broiler flocks (www.defra.gov.uk). Environmental samples are better than faecal, and the best sites are nest boxes, slave feed hoppers and fan outlet ducts. Other good sites on breeder farms are egg collection trays, walkways, egg sorting tables and mice. Spillage from egg trays is best in layer houses. Input sampling should include feed, residue from lorry and feed mill audit and chicks; the chick box liners should be put into an autoclave bag with peptone for transport to the laboratory. In the hatchery, trolleys and trays should be sampled as well as fluff samples.

Sampling of cleaned and disinfected houses is essential prior to restocking. Peptone water should be put in cracks on the wall half an hour before swabbing, and large fist-sized swabs should be used rather than rectal swabs. The best sites for sampling are floor sweepings, nest box floors, slave hoppers, hydrated walls and fan duct outlets.

Vaccination against *S. enteritidis* has been used. Other methods of control have included competitive exclusion (the Nurmi effect), where beneficial bacteria are given to young chicks at day old to prevent colonisation of the gut with harmful bacteria, and the use of acids in the feed to kill the *Salmonella* organisms.

Campylobacteriosis

Campylobacter is the most common cause of diarrhoea in humans in the United Kingdom although not as serious as *Salmonella* food poisoning.

The bacteria (*Campylobacter coli*, *Campylobacter jejuni*), once swallowed, multiply in the gut, and after 3–5 days (usually, range 1–10 days), the patient develops abdominal pains, diarrhoea and sometimes vomiting and fever. Although unpleasant, the illness is rarely fatal and patients usually recover within a few days. The definitive diagnosis is made by growing and identifying the bacteria in the laboratory.

The main sources for campylobacter are raw meat, especially offal, and poultry, where the bacteria may be found in a large proportion of raw broiler chickens sold in shops and supermarkets. Although present in food, they do not usually multiply; therefore, it is rarely the cause of an explosive outbreak of infection. However, the number of bacteria required to cause illness is very small – fewer than 500 can cause infection. About 3000 people are admitted to hospital annually in Britain owing to the disease. In 2003, there were 48 000 cases diagnosed. Other cases are treated by medical practitioners, but the actual figure for those affected in Britain each year may exceed 500 000.

The prevention of infection in humans involves inhibiting transmission through water, milk and food. All animals shed campylobacters into lakes, rivers, streams and reservoirs; therefore, all water destined for human consumption needs to be properly treated. In Britain, defective storage tanks have caused outbreaks affecting up to 250 people.

Milk that is not pasteurised or heat treated may contain the bacteria.

Good kitchen hygiene with the correct handling of raw meat and animal products is essential to prevent infection. Raw poultry and other types of meat should be kept separate from other food and should be properly cooked.

Incidence of campylobacteriosis

A survey carried out by the European Food Safety Authority in 2008 showed an average prevalence of campylobacter-contaminated broiler carcases in the EU of 75.8% ranging from 98.3% in the Republic of Ireland to 4.9% in Estonia (United Kingdom 86.3%).

In the United States, poultry is associated with 50–70% of human cases of campylobacter infection. *C. jejuni* is the most common isolate found in chickens. Broiler flocks are frequently campylobacter positive and 100% of birds tested can be positive. Chicken carcases are also often heavily contaminated, and numbers of campylobacter per carcase can exceed 10^6 (Fig. 10.21).

In addition, independent investigations have isolated *C. jejuni* from aseptically taken muscle samples. In epidemiological studies, there has been no effect noticed on the rate of infection in poultry units with concrete floors and surrounds as against those with earthen floors.

Farm studies carried out in Sweden showed that 16% of flocks were colonised with campylobacter. There was a seasonal variation with more positive flocks in late summer and autumn. There were differences in occurrence between farms delivering chickens to different processing companies. This might indicate different levels of farm hygiene and management. Generally, only one serotype was found in each flock, which would indicate only one source at a time, instead of infections from several different reservoirs. The most common serotypes in chickens were also the most common serotypes isolated from the surroundings, for example, ditchwater and faeces of wild birds. In general, no campylobacter, or new serotypes, were isolated in the following flocks, indicating that the infection was not permanent in the buildings and that the washing and disinfection of houses between flocks was sufficient to eliminate campylobacters.

Chickens were not colonised with campylobacter before 2 weeks of age. No connection was found between serotypes in broiler flocks and in broiler parents from which the eggs were taken. Broiler parents carried several serotypes in each flock. These epidemiological studies excluded buildings, feed, straw and day-old chicks as the source of campylobacter infection to the broiler flock. It was thought unlikely that water would be a source for the Swedish chicken flocks.

Control of campylobacteriosis

A strict and well-applied hygiene barrier seems to be the most important factor for preventing chicken flocks from campylobacter colonisation, under the assumption that the chicken house is a closed unit. It was considered that the elimination of disinfectant footbaths and the introduction of changing footwear at a well-defined hygiene barrier, 40 cm high, is essential for keeping campylobacter out of broiler farms. As campylobacter may enter from multiple sources outside the rearing units, it is important to prevent all possible ways of transmission into the house. In the United Kingdom, the main sources are the environment outside the houses, drinking water, rodents and wild birds. The organism has been found in flies, which could carry it from house to house, and people. Biosecurity of the premises is essential.

Chickens appear to become infected at around 3 weeks of age when the number of *Salmonella* in a flock peaks. However, the number of campylobacter continues to increase. When a flock becomes positive, the organism transmits to 90% of the birds in less than 1 week. After thinning of the flock, more campylobacter are found in the older birds. There can also be a significant increase in the numbers after transport to the plant. The number of organisms found in the inside of the bird is relevant to that found on the outside.

In the poultry plant, raising the pH of the scald tank with caustic soda or reducing it with acetic acid has no significant effect. Carcase washes and irradiation have yet to prove successful.

Chlamydiosis (psittacosis/ornithosis)

Chlamydiosis is sometimes referred to as psittacosis when it affects humans, mammals and birds of the parrot (psittacine) family and as ornithosis for birds other than psittacine. The cause is the intracellular parasite *Chlamydia psittaci*, which belongs to the Group B chlamydias – organisms of uncertain status occupying a position between bacteria and viruses but probably more related to the former.

The disease is worldwide in distribution, affecting all types of poultry and wild birds. It has a serious public health significance in that man may become affected, usually from close contact with birds of the parrot family. Infection occurs by inhalation of particles of infected dust (Fig. 10.22).

Lesions. The disease may be either acute or chronic, which tends to complicate the non-specific post-mortem findings. The lesions range from airsacculitis with thickened inflamed air sacs containing yellowish-white exudate to pneumonia, pericarditis, perihepatitis and enlargement of the liver and spleen.

Judgement. Affected carcases should be totally condemned. Diagnosis can be established only by laboratory examination, and cases should be reported to the regulatory authorities. Birds suspected at ante-mortem inspection of being affected with ornithosis must not be slaughtered because of the disease risk to operatives.

Miscellaneous conditions

Dead on arrival

These birds must be condemned and not processed. It is important that the catching team recognise birds which are unfit for slaughter and euthanise them on the farm.

Bruising and fractures

Causes include improper handling by the catching team and, at the poultry plant, careless shackling and defective stunning techniques and wing flapping. Any parts of a carcase with localised bruising are rejected. Severe generalised bruising indicates total condemnation.

Carcase appearance defects include red wing tips, red pygostyles, red feather tracts, engorged wing veins, haemorrhagic wing veins and haemorrhage in shoulders. Haemorrhages may occur in the muscles of the leg and breast, and broken bones include the furculum, coracoid and scapula. Unless severe, only local condemnation is required.

Fractures, without bruising, have been caused in the processing after bleeding and are due to defects in processing. It may require resetting of the machinery.

Breast blisters and hock burn

These are caused when a part of the bird comes into contact with damp litter, which causes breast blisters and hock burn. These occur more often in birds with leg weakness and may become infected, and this will require more extensive trimming. The hock burns are unsightly and in some processing plants are mechanically removed. The presence of hock burns, in some companies, affects the quality assessment of the bird and therefore the price. Attention to litter management, ensuring adequate ventilation, the avoidance of water spilling from the drinkers and good healthy birds will prevent these conditions.

Rupture of the gastrocnemius tendon. This occurs when the tendon is unable to support the bird's weight and may be followed by a greening around the area above the hock. Birds being grown to heavier than normal weights, for example, for the Christmas or Easter market, are particularly susceptible. Decreasing energy and protein levels in the earlier stages of growth helps prevent this condition. At times, infective organisms such as staphylococci and/or viruses may be responsible.

Judgement. Condemnation of the affected part; should the bird be emaciated, whole carcases condemnation.

Ascites

Ascites caused by right ventricular failure (RVF) has for many years resulted in significant mortality in broiler chicks raised at high altitude. There has been a dramatic increase in other areas which coincides with a continuing genetic and nutritional improvement in feed efficiency and rate of growth. This rapid growth requires high levels of oxygen which are not available and, combined with restricted space for blood flow through the capillaries of the lungs, leads to ascites and death. Right ventricular hypertrophy is a response to the increased workload, and this eventually leads to RVF if the volume or pressure load persists (Fig. 10.23).

Most cases of ascites occur as sudden death on the farm, but should any be found on post-mortem examination, the carcases should be condemned as the cause, other than pathophysiological, might be mycotoxins or polychlorinated biphenyl compounds containing dioxin. Liver damage may be the result of congestion of aflatoxin, coal tar products or toxins derived from plants such as cortalaria or rapeseed.

In broiler chickens in the United States and the United Kingdom, cholangiohepatitis (possibly caused by *Clostridium perfringens* or secondary to viral infection in the biliary system) is the most common cause of liver damage which results in ascites. In both meat-type ducks and breeders, amyloidosis of the liver frequently causes ascites. Feed regimes which restrict the early growth of broilers have had a significant effect in decreasing the incidence of ascites.

Slaughter liver or cholangiohepatitis

This is a condition of enlarged livers. Histologically, there is a severe, chronic hepatitis in which bile duct proliferation is a striking feature. It affects all of the liver. This may be accompanied by other changes.

Judgement. Depends on other lesions and condition of carcase.

Fatty liver haemorrhagic syndrome (FLHS)

The liver is very enlarged, pale and friable owing to the large amount of fat. There is also increased abdominal fat deposition. It may be due to nutritional imbalances, high temperatures, reduced exercise and strain of bird. It is a disease, predominantly, of older laying birds.

Vices

Vices in poultry may be considered to be undesirable behaviour, usually precipitated by some aspects of management or environment. Once started by individuals, a vice tends to be copied by other birds, and the resulting injuries can often lead to death or downgrading of carcases.

Cannibalism

Outbreaks sometimes occur without any obvious cause. Predisposing environmental conditions include excessive light in pens and cages, boredom and vent pecking, insufficient feeding and drinking space, high-density stocking and too much heat during brooding. Blood is found around the vent, through which much of the intestine may have been removed by the cannibalising birds.

Feather pecking or pulling

This is sometimes precipitated by nutritional deficiencies but may also be started by the bullying of a weak or sick bird. Overcrowding as broilers and turkeys reach slaughter age may be followed by an outbreak of feather and tail pecking, often leading to serious downgrading of the carcases of affected individuals.

Contamination

Poultry carcases may be contaminated in various ways, for example, faecal matter, paints, oils, poisons, biological residues and dirty scalding tank water. All such carcases must be condemned.

Decomposition

Carcases of poultry that have died from causes other than slaughter must be condemned, as must carcases affected with general spoilage.

Barking

This occurs when the cuticle (the outer layer of the epidermis) is damaged by too high a scald temperature and subsequent plucking. During air chilling, there is unequal drying owing to the damage and brown discoloration of the surface. This is only seen in fresh, non-frozen carcases. Dampening areas which are only slightly affected will remove the abnormal colour.

Diseases of the female reproductive system

These are relatively common non-infectious disorders in end-of-lay domestic fowl but less so in turkeys, ducks and geese.

Egg peritonitis is caused when the ova (yolk) are present in the peritoneum rather than in the oviduct. The yolk is usually viscous and gives the appearance of an 'oily peritonitis'. Impaction of the oviduct occurs when a normal egg, or more commonly a mass of inspissated yolk material, obstructs the oviduct to varying degrees.

Judgement. Condemnation.

Oregon disease

A deep pectoral myopathy of turkeys and chickens, also called green muscle disease, this myopathy is an ischaemic necrosis which develops in the deep pectoral muscle (the fillet).

The condition is only seen at necropsy or at processing, when as many as 40%, but usually less, of the spent breeding hens may be affected. It occurs less frequently in males.

The lesion may be unilateral or bilateral and in advanced cases may show a flattening of the normally convex breast muscle ('slab sided'). The actual lesions are of variable size and are clearly demarcated from the surrounding healthy tissue. Initially, there is a swollen, reddish-brown area, often associated with an excess of gelatinous fluid which later becomes green in colour,

crumbly and dry. When cooked, the green colour, due to breakdown products of haemoglobin and myoglobin, is accentuated.

Advanced lesions can be seen or detected by palpation. More recent ones can be detected by cutting into the muscle or inserting a light into the thoracic cavity after evisceration.

The lesion, although unsightly, is not harmful to the consumer and merits local condemnation only.

Over-scald

Carcases which present a cooked appearance of the flesh owing to an excessively high temperature or being held too long in the scalding tank must be condemned.

Fevered carcases

Fevered carcases are generally considered to be carcases which have congested musculature but no other signs of septicaemia/toxaemia such as pericarditis, perihepatitis or airsacculitis.

Judgement. Condemnation.

Septicaemia

Septicaemic carcases are those which have congested, darkened muscles with some or all of the following: airsacculitis, perihepatitis, pericarditis and enlarged spleen. On bacteriological examination, *E. coli* is found most often but *S. enteritidis* is sometimes isolated. The organisms present tend to be common to the whole flock.

Insufficient bleeding

In cases where no bleeding has taken place, the carcase is very red in colour. There are obvious welfare implications in this condition, and it is essential that there is a well-trained, dedicated plant operative as a manual backup to bleed any bird which may have missed the automatic neck cutter.

Emaciation

As in red meat inspection, emaciation is due to some pathological condition. It is important to distinguish emaciation from the poor condition of end-of-lay commercial egg layers, the meat of which is suitable for incorporation into soups, pies, etc., provided it passes meat inspection.

Viscera absent

Carcases presented for examination with no viscera present should be condemned.

Relevant EU legislation. Directives 2003/99, 71/118, 91/495, 92/65 and 92/116.

UK legislation. The Poultry Meat, Farmed Game Bird Meat and Rabbit Meat (Hygiene and Inspection) Regulations 2011

References

Clouser, C.S., Doores, S., Mast, M.G. and Knabel, S.J. (1995) *Poultry Science*, **74**, 723–731.

Slavik, M.F., Kim, J.-W. and Walker, J.T. (1995) *Journal of Food Protection*, **58**, 689–691.

Veerkamp, C.H. and Hofmans, G.J.P. (1973) *Poultry International*, **12**, 16–18.

Yogaratnam, V. (1995) *Veterinary Record*, **137**, 215–217.

Further reading

Bremner, A. and Johnston, M. (eds) (1996) *Poultry Meat Hygiene and Inspection*, WB Saunders, London.

Farm Animal Welfare Council. (1995) Report on the welfare of Turkeys.

Farm Animal Welfare Council. (1996) Report on the welfare of boiler chickens.

Jordan, F.T.W. and Pattison, M. (1996) *Poultry Diseases*, 4th edn, WB Saunders, London.

National Control Programme for *Salmonella* in broiler flocks, www.defra.gov.uk (accessed 15 April 2014).

11

Exotic meat production

Over recent years, there has always been a limited demand for more exotic type meats. Previously, these would have included wild-caught rabbits and hares and wild deer. More recently, rabbits, deer, ostriches, wild boar, water buffalo, bison and camelids (alpaca and llama) are being farmed with the intention of producing consistent hygienic meat and meat products. This demand is sometimes more perceived than actual, and the inability to produce a consistent product and constant market has been dominated by supply problems, lack of marketing co-ordination, cost and unfair competition with other, subsidised, meats.

Cooperatives are being formed which should help to overcome these deficiencies.

Rabbits

Rabbits are usually reared in small units, 10–200 breeding does (female rabbits) with a ratio of 1 buck to 10–20 does. The gestation period is 31 days. Stock used are New Zealand White, Californian, 'hybrids' or commercial white. The choice is based on market requirement, performance and personal preference. The does are mated at 16–20 weeks old. The bucks are used when 20–24 weeks old. The rabbits are weaned at 28–42 days old or by weight at 700 g. The average litter size is 8.68 born alive and 6.9 reared to market weight. Remating takes place, usually between 10 and 14 days after kindling. It is possible to obtain 6–8 litters per doe per year, giving over 50 rabbits reared per doe per year. Meat rabbits are marketed at 2–3 kg live weight, which can be reached from 8 weeks onwards. The food conversion ratio is approximately 3:1, but this will increase if they are fed *ad libitum* after 8 weeks of age. They are fed an 18% protein ration and 15% fibre. Rabbits cannot digest

starch easily, and the diet contains dried grass, small amounts of caustic-treated straw and cereal by-products. Supplementing the diet with hay and straw aids digestion but may slow growth.

A coccidiostat is added to the diet to prevent coccidiosis. The most commonly used one, robenidine, is not effective against *Eimeria stiedae*, the cause of hepatic coccidiosis. For treatment of this condition, the sulphonamides are effective. Ionophores which are used as coccidiostats for poultry are toxic to rabbits. It is essential that there is not a build-up of faeces in cages or beneath them which will allow ingestion of oocysts. Withdrawal periods for coccidiostats as with other medicines must be observed.

Rabbits are more easily housed in poultry-type intensive houses as these give better control over environmental conditions than the natural environment house, in which ventilation and temperature has to be controlled manually, and with the use of micro environments.

Battery cages with wire mesh flooring suitable for rabbits can be used, but it is essential that only those rabbits which do not succumb to traumatic skin diseases such as sore hocks are kept for meat production. Plastic grilles are sometimes used for adult bucks and does. These are less traumatic for the paws and acceptable from a hygiene point of view. Broiler rabbits are housed separately from the does in small groups (4–8/cage).

Slaughter

It is estimated that around 250 000 to 1 million rabbits are reared for meat in the United Kingdom. In France, 50 million are reared each year and 334 million in the EU as a whole. Commercial slaughter rabbits are usually transported in poultry-type crates, each holding about

Gracey's Meat Hygiene, Eleventh Edition. Edited by David S. Collins and Robert J. Huey.
© 2015 John Wiley & Sons, Ltd. Published 2015 by John Wiley & Sons, Ltd.

12 rabbits. The rabbits are removed one by one from the crates by a single operative, wearing rubber gloves, and each is placed with its head between the arms of the stunner and gently pushed upwards to make contact with the current. Stunning is carried out electrically with a minimum stunning current of 140 mA, which can be achieved with an application of 100 V. Following a successful stun, epileptiform activity occurs and the animal will collapse. This is characterised by cessation of breathing, salivation and increased motor activity, tonic (rigid) and clonic (kicking) phase. It is also permissible to stun rabbits by a blow to the head. Following stunning, commercial rabbits are shackled immediately, and exsanguination is carried out very quickly, within 10 seconds during the tonic phase, thereby preventing any risk of recovery.

The feet are removed and the carcase passes into the evisceration room where further dressing takes 5–6 minutes.

The main cause of death in commercial rabbits is mucoid enteropathy, a non-specific digestive upset. There is impaction of the colon and this condition is precipitated by stress, high-energy feeds and high population densities. *Escherichia coli* is the most common enteric pathogen. It causes diarrhoea in neonatal and weaned rabbits.

Inspection

In the United Kingdom, rabbit plants slaughtering in excess of 10 000 rabbits a year have to be licensed. Inspection is similar to that used in poultry, with ante-mortem and post-mortem being carried out.

Post-mortem judgements in rabbit meat inspection

Death before slaughter

Rabbits which have died before slaughter should not be presented for processing but detained at ante-mortem inspection. If, inadvertently, they are not detained at the ante-mortem point, they may be identified by the muscle, which is darker red than normal, along with the engorged vessels supplying the viscera, a more pronounced picture than with badly bled carcases (see below).

Judgement Condemn.

Badly bled carcases

In carcases which are insufficiently bled, the blood vessels appear injected, the flesh is dark, and the organs including lymph nodes are congested.

Judgement Condemn.

Injuries including bruising and broken bones

Injuries are quite common in the form of skin wounds, due to fighting or scratching, and sore hocks. Infection with *staphylococci* can follow with abscess formation.

Bruising and fractures, especially of limbs and thoracic spine, may be sustained ante-mortem, when they are normally associated with haemorrhage.

Judgement This should be based on the extent and nature of the lesion and the practicability of carrying out trimming:

1 Extensive injury or bruising, excessive blood or serum in the body tissues or multiple abscesses render the whole carcase unfit.
2 When the bruising is localised, the carcase may be passed following removal by trimming of all affected parts. When trimming, the extension of blood between muscles, bones, etc. should be considered and care must be taken to ensure that all affected tissues are removed.
3 Provided that the carcase is otherwise fit, superficial, discrete, uncomplicated bruises not exceeding 2 cm may be left untrimmed.
4 In the case of fractures, the affected tissues should be trimmed from the carcase. The cut should normally be made at a joint which ensures that all the affected tissue is removed.

Enteritis

Enteritis has many causes including *Bacillus piliformis*. The lesions vary greatly from a mild enteritis involving the whole gut to haemorrhagic enteritis with blood-stained contents. The gut contents may be either abundant and watery or sparse and mucoid, especially in the caecum.

Judgement Condemn.

Mastitis/metritis

Mastitis is usually associated with *staphylococci* or *streptococci* and metritis with *staphylococci*, *Pasteurella* or *Listeria* monocytogenes.

Judgement Judgement depends on the degree and extent of the lesions and condition of the carcase, but usually the carcase is unfit.

Tumours

It is difficult to distinguish between benign and malignant tumours in the meat plant.

Judgement Multiple or malignant tumours – reject the carcase and offal. Single benign tumour – reject the tumour and the surrounding tissue.

Pasteurellosis

Pasteurellosis is a highly contagious disease of rabbits caused by *Pasteurella multocida*. Rhinitis, bronchopneumonia, middle-ear disease, genital infection and abscesses can occur and may result in septicaemia.

Judgement This depends on the degree and extent of the lesions as well as on the condition of the carcase. Animals with mild forms of rhinitis, in good bodily condition, may be passed for food, while those with severe forms of pneumonia with fevered carcases and multiple abscesses must be condemned.

Spirochaetosis

This is caused by the spirochaete *Treponema cuniculi*. It is a local infection of vesicles, which become moist, scaly crusts on the genitalia.

Judgement In the well-nourished rabbit, removal of the affected portions is all that is necessary before releasing the carcase for food.

Tyzzer's disease

Tyzzer's disease is an acute contagious disease associated with a haemorrhagic enteritis and necrosis of the terminal ileum, large intestine and caecum (typhlitis) caused by *B. piliformis*. Focal necrotic areas may also be found in the liver and heart.

Judgement Animals which survive infection are usually in poor condition and normally merit total seizure.

Myxomatosis

Characteristic signs are conjunctivitis with a clear discharge which becomes purulent; swelling of the eyelids, base of ears and nose, giving the head a very enlarged appearance; and swelling of the anus. The oedematous ears often droop and condition is rapidly lost. The spleen is enlarged and blackish.

Judgement Condemn.

Coccidiosis

Coccidiosis is one of the most common diseases of rabbits.

Hepatic coccidiosis is recognised at post-mortem by the presence of numerous small greyish-white nodules or cysts in the liver substance which in older lesions may coalesce to form large cheesy masses. The nodules consist of hypertrophied bile ducts.

Intestinal coccidiosis may show few, if any, lesions at slaughter, especially in early cases. More advanced cases have a thickened and pale intestinal wall.

Judgement If condition is good, carcases may be passed for food, but emaciated carcases merit total condemnation.

Taenia taeniaeformis

The intermediate larva form of this cat tapeworm occurs as a whitish cyst in the rabbit liver.

Judgement Local trimming or condemnation of the affected organ is all that is normally required.

Multiceps serialis

The cystic stage of *Taenia serialis* of the dog is commonly encountered in the wild rabbit. Cysts are found in the connective tissue of the lumbar muscles and muscles of the hindlegs and occasionally at the angle of the jaw.

Judgement If only one or two cysts are present in the musculature and the rabbit is well nourished, the affected portions may be removed and the carcase passed for food.

Cysticercus pisiformis

The cystic stage of *Taenia pisiformis* of the dog is encountered in the peritoneal cavity of the rabbit, especially on the mesentery, the cysts being up to the size of a pea and filled with a clear fluid.

Judgement Their presence rarely has any deleterious effect on the carcase. Straw-coloured fluid is present in the above cysts in the early stages, but this usually progresses to pus formation and cheesy inspissated material in older lesions, warranting total seizure.

Zoonoses
Salmonellosis

Salmonellosis occurs occasionally usually due to *Salmonella typhimurium*. There may be virtually no changes to some enlargement of the liver and spleen with general carcase congestion. There is usually no diarrhoea.

Judgement Condemn.

Tuberculosis

Tuberculosis (TB) may affect rabbits due to mainly the avian and bovine types.

Judgement Condemn.

Pseudotuberculosis

Pseudotuberculosis is characterised by nodules resembling those of TB in the liver, lungs, spleen and intestines caused by *Pasteurella pseudotuberculosis*.

Judgement Condemn.

Listeriosis

Infection with *Listeria* monocytogenes may cause serious loss of condition. Some rabbits show torticollis. In addition to the emaciation, there is usually a hepatitis with the presence of numerous fine necrotic foci in the parenchyma.

Judgement Condemn.

Ringworm

The most common form of ringworm is *Trichophyton mentagrophytes* var. granulare, which can also affect man. Typical lesions appear on the head and may spread to other parts of the body.

Judgement Provided the condition is satisfactory, carcases may be passed for human consumption.

Guidelines on contamination, missing viscera and trimming

Contamination

Rabbit meat, carcases and/or offal affected with general contamination by faecal material, bile, grease, disinfectants, etc. should be considered unfit for human consumption. Where contamination of the carcase is localised, affected parts should be trimmed.

Missing viscera

Carcases presented with no viscera should not be passed as fit for human consumption.

Trimming

Trimming must be carried out under the supervision of the inspectorate. The selection of lesions or parts which require trimming must not be delegated to the management of the slaughterhouse.

Minor blemishes or bruising may be trimmed at the inspection point.

Trimming of more serious conditions involving infection, for example, septic wounds or moderate contamination by intestinal contents, is usually impractical with high line speeds, and in these cases, an adjacent trimming area should be provided.

Trimming of carcases may be delayed until after chilling provided that:

1 The carcases are segregated and remain identifiable.
2 There is no risk of contamination of other carcases.
3 Trimming is done under the constant supervision of an inspector.

Most trimming should be carried out by staff supplied by management. The mode of trimming may be adapted to suit the requirements of management, providing that all affected parts are removed. Care should be taken to ensure there is no unnecessary wastage.

Farmed deer (Fig. 11.1)

In New Zealand where one in eight farms now produce deer (there are more farmed deer than cattle), velvet antler is harvested and is worth more than the carcase. This is illegal in the United Kingdom.

Eighty per cent of New Zealand deer production is exported to Europe, with Germany taking up to 50%.

Deer are suited to a variety of management systems, and stratification of the industry is becoming apparent. Many hill farmers sell, in October and November, calves

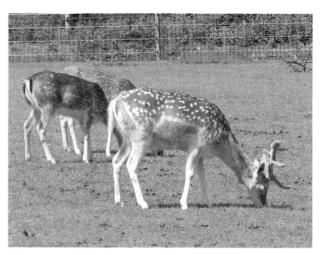

Figure 11.1 Fallow deer.

weaned in September, to be finished in lowland units. There is much interest in vertical integration, with many farmers rearing deer and slaughtering them and selling venison on the same premises. Some 60% of farmed venison is sold through farm shops after killing in the field with a rifle.

Value-added products such as roasts with a fat covering, cubed venison for stews, venison burgers, mince, haggis and sausages are being produced.

Handling and slaughter

Deer can be shot with a large rifle at very close range as they stand, unsuspecting, in a field; this has a strong welfare appeal. This should be undertaken, preferably by the regular stockmen, when deer are quiet, as will occur at a selected regular feeding site when they are being hand-fed. Under such circumstances, it may be possible to shoot 10 or more deer from a large group before the remainder become unduly disturbed. Alternatively, they can be killed in an ordinary abattoir after transport, and this appears to work well with red deer. A third slaughter option is on-farm abattoir.

Successful handling of deer depends upon understanding of their behaviour. The dominance hierarchy is very important to deer, and handlers must maintain their respect in order to avoid being the object of aggressive behaviour. It is important to be calm, confident and competent. Aggression can take the form of foreleg and hindleg kicks, and male handlers are advised to wear a cricket box or similar protection. Shields may be helpful. Stags in rut should be treated with extreme caution. Regular contact with handlers raises the fear threshold of deer and shortens their flight distance.

Red deer should be deantlered (not while in velvet) about 5 weeks prior to slaughter.

Deer in velvet should not be subjected to abattoir slaughter. Dis-budding of calves destined for slaughter rather than breeding can be carried out.

Deer must be presented for slaughter in a clean condition, and therefore, access to wallows should be stopped to reduce mud contamination of the ventral abdomen. By minimising stress, the keeping quality of the carcase is further safeguarded. As in other animals, stress causes glycogen depletion in the muscles. On death, glycogen is converted into lactic acid, creating an acidic environment. Low pH does not favour bacterial growth. An average pH of 5.6, at 24 hours post-mortem, has been recorded for red deer calves and yearlings.

During shedding out, deer must be subjected to minimum stress to ensure no bruising or other injury occurs. They should be kept in familiar groups and should not be in close confinement overnight since fighting can occur when they are left undisturbed, resulting possibly in death.

Suitable facilities are essential for loading when deer are to be transported. Transport trailers should have side-hinged solid gates to prevent the deer from jumping out. Internal partitions should be as high as possible. Some transporters cover eye-level air vents to avoid the deer being frightened by seeing vehicle lights flashing by. Deer should not be left in vehicles overnight. Hinds in late pregnancy, calves under 6 months and stags in rut should not be sent for slaughter. Bedding should be provided.

Deer are unsettled by translocation into an alien environment. On arrival at the slaughterhouse, they should not be driven off the vehicle, but allowed to come out quietly by themselves. As they move readily from dark to light, the lairage should be lit, but not to such an extent that the deer are faced with a direct light source. There should be separate facilities for bullied, ill or injured animals which allows them to still see other deer. Those that are in pain or distress must immediately be humanely slaughtered. Sticks and goads should not be used. Partitions in the lairage should be solid and at least 2.5 m high; long dark passageways should be avoided.

Strange noises, shapes and lights can push deer over the fear threshold. Yorkshire boarding, which throws a broken pattern of light, should be avoided. Deer should be kept in familiar groups in the lairage and allowed time to settle in subdued light. Some plants allow the animals to arrive so that they have a resting period overnight.

Animals may be brought out individually into the stunning crate for immediate stunning, but some slaughtering premises have found that bringing animals in pairs to the stunning crate causes less distress.

The stunning crate should admit single or pairs of animals and have solid sides, with a string mesh cover to prevent them from jumping out. The top may be draped, but the front shoulder should be left uncovered with a diffused light source to attract the deer forward. A drop-floor restrainer is an alternative to the stunning crate.

Prior to stunning, deer should not be held in the approach passages. One or two deer at a time must be placed in the stunning crate, and only when the way is clear for it to be stunned, and then bled immediately. Stunning equipment must be properly maintained and reserve equipment readily available. Deer are stunned by frontal head shot with a captive bolt pistol. Pithing is not necessary. The slaughter of a batch must be arranged such that the slaughter of the last deer is not delayed. After hoisting by a hindleg, deer are bled in the same way as cattle. Both forelegs are held to minimise the risk to the slaughter man. Carcases are usually skinned on a modified static sheep crutch. Hide pullers have been tried and a down puller for deer is commercially available. As with game venison production, because of their propensity for shedding hair, contamination with hair is a problem. A skilled skinning operative makes a huge difference to how well the carcase is presented at final inspection, and flood-washing is not required to remove the hairs. A low-pressure wash removes bone dust around the sternum and neck flap.

Meat inspection has followed existing protocols. The possible presence of TB has to be kept in mind. Blood splashing on the diaphragm and abdominal wall is sometimes seen, more in young males, but the aetiology is obscure. Bruising provides a good indicator of the adequacy of the handling of the deer, and a study of the age and site of lesions can result in the detection of the cause. Focal bruising can be caused by deer placing the forelegs on the backs of other deer or by butting with an antler stump.

Health monitoring can be carried out at the abattoir by the recording and feedback of pathological findings and the taking of liver samples for deficiency estimations.

There is considerable variability in the size of young red deer stags, which may range from 46 to 146 kg live weight and typically kill out at 55%. The carcases must be hung in a chill room so that air can circulate freely between them, drying the surface and cooling the carcase. If chilling is too rapid, cold shortening of the muscles will occur and produce tough meat. Electrical stimulation of carcases immediately after slaughter hastens rigor mortis and assists in the production of tender meat.

The field slaughter of farmed deer is usually practised on farms which operate a farm shop retail outlet. Ante-mortem inspection by a veterinarian must be carried out within a 72-hour period prior to slaughter. After shooting, the deer are bled and transported to an approved dressing facility on the farm. Alternatively, the bled whole carcase can be transported to a licensed abattoir or a farmed game processing facility to arrive and be dressed within 1 hour of slaughter, or if the transporter can be refrigerated to between 0 and 4°C, dressing can take place up to 3 hours after slaughter. In both situations, the carcases must be inspected by a meat inspector within 24 hours after slaughter.

Park deer

Wild mammals living within an enclosed territory under conditions of freedom similar to those enjoyed by wild game (i.e. deer parks) are not considered to be farmed game.

Most deer park owners operate a culling system in which the deer are shot as they graze. After shooting, the carcase is immediately bled and eviscerated and transported to the deer larder for completion of dressing. Small numbers of deer handled in this way can be sold direct to the consumer but are subject to public health checks provided in national rules.

Where a deer park culls large numbers of deer or where the carcases are sold to wholesale establishments, the construction and hygiene requirements and the timing of the operation are detailed in the Wild Game Directive 92/45/EEC, Regulations (EC) No. 852/2004 and 853/2004. In general, after shooting and bleeding, the carcase is eviscerated, and the viscera are identified with the carcase. It has to be dispatched within 12 hours to a processing house. Alternatively, the carcase and viscera can be dispatched within 12 hours to a collecting centre where they will be chilled and maintained at a temperature not exceeding 7°C until dispatched to a processing house within a further 12 hours, with certain exemptions for remote areas. All parts must be inspected within 18 hours of entering the processing house. Wild game meat declared fit for human consumption must bear a health mark.

Wild deer

Game venison is seasonal, with 50% of the red deer output occurring over a 4-week period.

Venison is low in cholesterol; the fat is not marbled through the muscle fibres although it still has a distinctive flavour.

Killing

In England and Wales, the legal firearm for culling deer is a rifle with a calibre of at least 0.240 in and a muzzle energy of at least 1700 foot-pounds, firing a soft-nosed or hollow-nosed bullet. Deer are shot either in the neck or chest. A chest shot should ensure rapid unconsciousness due to blood loss. When aiming at the neck, novice stalkers are often advised to err on the high side in order to ensure that the shot does not strike the foreleg. If the vertebral column is hit, the animal will immediately collapse.

Sticking should take place as soon as possible.

Deer may be shot two or three miles from the larder, and carcases routinely 'gralloched', that is, have the green offal removed, on the hill. Professional stalkers, as game processors, are aware of public health aspects and grade carcases according to presentation. After gralloching, carcases are dragged to the nearest track and loaded on to transport. Nowadays, the Argocat has replaced the traditional deer pony.

On arrival at the larder, the pelvis and sternum are split; the pluck is removed, including the kidneys; and the body cavities are rinsed with clean water and dried with disposable paper towels. The pluck is bagged and tagged and hung with the carcase, which is also tagged for identification. The skin is left on. Red deer like to wallow, and so splitting the pelvis, which is done to aid cooling of the haunches, is now discouraged as this can often lead to unacceptable contamination with mud and hair.

The temperature of the venison should be 7°C. Portable air conditioners are now used in many larders.

The carcase should be delivered with its pluck to the game plant within 24 hours of shooting.

After skinning, which is normally performed on a cradle, the carcase is examined by a veterinarian.

Disease is frequently less of a problem than contamination. Contamination with gut contents results from poor shooting and poor gralloching, particularly if the rectum has been imperfectly removed. In the case of poorly shot animals, large quantities of rumenal contents may be carried in the wake of the bullet under the scapula, leading to forequarter condemnation. Deer shed hair very easily and contamination with hair is another serious problem. Hair debris is best removed with the use of copious water. The professional stalker is the key person in the production of clean game venison.

The heart, liver and mediastinal lymph nodes are incised, and the kidneys and lungs are palpated. Any abscesses are treated as suspect TB, although only 0.1% of carcases have been found to be affected, predominately with the avian strain. Typically lesions range from small, chalky, white foci in the liver or lungs to miliary abscesses, throughout the carcase. TB in deer was made a notifiable disease in Great Britain in May 1989. Feeding indoors can exacerbate the incidence of mycobacterial infections.

Occasionally tumours, milk spots and flukes are seen in the liver. Fluke infection is rarely serious, not normally producing the same degree of pathology as in cattle and sheep. In the rut, stag livers are often very pale. Cardiac lesions are rare. Pneumonia is also rare, although roe deer are very susceptible to the lungworm *Protostrongylus rufescens. Cysticercus tenuicollis* is another common parasite and *Taenia hydatigena* is occasionally seen.

A major cause of death in wild deer, particularly in February, is the warble fly, *Hypoderma diana*. Young animals may have very heavy warble fly burdens, resulting in extensive meat losses.

Keds, lice and ticks are common. Ticks may transmit the spirochaete *Borrelia burgdorferi*, which could pose a zoonotic hazard to stalkers and slaughtermen from Lyme disease. Streptothrix infections from bone cuts are another hazard, causing 'slaughter finger'.

In a survey carried out by the Arun District Council/Forest Commission in 1986/1988, 2.13% of 1967 culled deer were totally condemned, in deer larders, and 1.77% partially condemned. The main causes were emaciation (10) and tumours (7).

Ostriches

The domestication of ostriches for the purpose of farming for the production of feathers began near Grahamstown, South Africa, in 1867. Since that time, a greater value has been placed on ostrich skin, which produces a top-quality leather, and a market has been developed, particularly within Europe, for ostrich meat. Although classified as 'poultry', the ostrich produces a red meat, beef-like in texture, containing lower levels of fat, calories and cholesterol than other red or white meat-producing species, which is particularly attractive to the 'health-conscious consumer'.

The ostrich (*Struthio camelus*) is the world's largest living bird, belonging to the order Ratitae or running birds. Emus (from Australia) and rhea (from South America) are also ratites. The ostrich is the only living bird with two toes.

The mature ostrich averages 2–3 m in height (to the top of its head). It can weigh up to 150 kg. The ostrich can kick forward, but not backwards or sideways. The large extended toe has a long nail and can quite easily split a person open from head to foot. No one should underestimate the danger of the captive ostrich, particularly in the breeding season. Ostriches, particularly males, will attack with the minimum of provocation, in fact with no encouragement at all. Placing a hood over the bird's eyes helps to calm it. The ostrich has exceptionally good eyesight and when alarmed stands upright with its long neck extended. Ostriches have a life span of 30–70 years.

There are different production systems. Ostriches may be left in colonies, with 8 males and 12 females in 10 acres, or in trios of 2 females and 1 male or in pairs. In Great Britain, ostrich farming has to be licensed under the Dangerous Wild Animals Act, implemented by the local authority.

The production of *eggs* by the female is very variable. They seasonally produce from 0 to 160 eggs, with an average of around 40/laying hen. The first 3 months is the most critical period in the ostrich's life.

The mortality up to 6 months is around 25% and between 6 and 14 months around 5%. Chicks may be fed rations containing 12.5 MJ/kg and 23% protein, although many are fed an 18% protein ration. They must be allowed plenty of exercise and not allowed to grow too quickly in the early stages, in order to prevent leg problems. Older birds are fed a 14.0% protein ration with 9.2 MJ/kg. Different age groups are fed different rations. The feed conversion rate will vary according to the source of the dietary supply and varies from 2:1 from hatchery to 4 months to 10:1 from 10 to 14 months, when African Black ostriches will weigh approximately 95 kg live weight.

In South Africa, a high proportion (70%) of the value of the bird is in the skin. Any damage, for example, kick mark scars, bruising or fresh wounds, results in downgrading by the tannery, and therefore, the welfare of the ostrich is of prime importance to the abattoir staff. Birds arriving at the abattoir with fresh wounds are generally returned to the farm to heal. Ostriches should always be moved in a calm and unhurried manner. They should not be separated from each other, as this is known to be stressful. Birds may be led by an operative moving ahead of the birds, calling encouragement, occasionally reinforced by the use of the arm and hand to mimic an ostrich. A further operative follows behind the group being moved.

In the United Kingdom, it is likely that, in the immediate future, slaughter will take place mainly on the farm of origin.

If ostriches are transported to a meat plant, unloading facilities must be suitable for their purpose and have non-slip flooring and the minimum possible incline. Horizontal surfaces should be provided with solid sides or barriers to a height of 2.0 m for unloading ostriches.

Lairages or holding pens should be provided without right-angled corners (e.g. octagonal pens constructed of metal tubes which are round in cross section), be constructed so as to prevent birds from slipping or falling, and be without gaps in which birds might trap their legs, toes, head or wings and without steps or other obstructions which may cause them to jump and fall or cause other injury.

If larger numbers of birds are handled, they should be moved in small groups (up to six birds) through a pre-stun race. The race should be wide enough for one bird and have solid sides up to a height of 2.0 m and be designed so that the head, neck or wings cannot become trapped.

Restraint (Fig. 11.2)

Before stunning, animals must be restrained in an appropriate manner in order to ensure avoidable pain, suffering, agitation or injury. Restraint is required to ensure that stunning is carried out accurately and effectively; it does not mean that the bird must be immobilised before stunning. To assist in hoisting and shackling after stunning, birds may be loosely hobbled at this point, although their legs must not be tied in any way that may cause them to fall.

The birds should be brought up the raceway one at a time. When the bird goes through the door, one operative, wearing rubber gloves, holds the beak or uses a crook to bring the head down into a position easily accessible to the stunning equipment.

Stunning

The electrodes should be designed and applied to ensure maximum contact area with the head and must be cleaned regularly to maintain optimum current flow. The use of saline sponges in the stunning tongs may increase contact area and current flow. The stunning tongs must span the brain, either laterally (on either side of the head and around the eyes) or vertically (to the top and bottom of the head). If the birds are hooded during stunning, allowance must be made for the possible effect of the hood directing current away from the brain, especially if the hood is wet. An application of 400 mA or greater, with 11 V for 2–6 seconds, causes insensibility for 60 seconds. There will be a short phase of initial kicking after which the bird will fall; it will be rigid with its legs flexed beneath it, and the neck may arch over the back before falling forward (the tonic phase). This is followed by kicking of varied intensity (the clonic phase). An effectively stunned

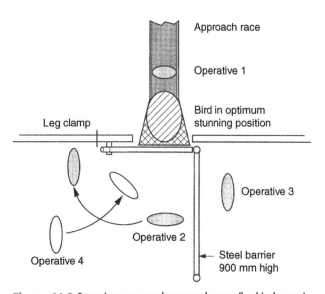

Figure 11.2 Stunning area and approach race (by kind permission of Dr Steve Wotton).

bird will not show any signs of rhythmic breathing. A return to rhythmic breathing in a stunned bird indicates that it may be recovering from the stun.

Existing knowledge of mechanical stunning of ostriches suggests that the tonic phase does not occur, and stunning produces an extended period of up to 4 minutes of severe convulsions. Mechanical stunning should only be used for emergency slaughter when electrical stunning is not available.

At Grahamstown RSA, four operatives carry out the stunning procedure: one guides the bird into the stunning area, one holds the beak, one applies the electric current, and the fourth rocks the bird backwards with legs flexed into the body during the tonic phase, assisted by the first operative from behind. This enables the application of a leg clamp at the tarsometatarsal bone, thus restraining the bird sufficiently to permit shackling. At this point, the stunning tongs are removed, and the fourth operative ring/chain shackles the bird via the big toes and attaches the shackle to a chain hoist.

Extended application of the stunning current, for up to 10 seconds, has been shown to delay the onset of kicking (clonic phase), facilitate restraint of legs and reduce the risk of injury during shackling and hoisting.

Bleeding must be carried out without delay after stunning, and the cut must sever at least one of the carotid arteries or the vessels from which they arise. The ostrich, like other birds, has an asymmetric arrangement of blood vessels in the neck, and bleeding should be achieved by a complete ventral cut of the neck immediately below the head to sever both carotid arteries and the jugular veins or by thoracic sticking to sever the major blood vessels from which the carotid arteries arise. Although bleeding from a high neck cut is initially profuse, the total bleed-out time is prolonged, and birds should be allowed to bleed for approximately 14 minutes in a bleeding area before manual plucking takes place.

Dressing

The birds are then skinned, which should be done carefully to prevent dander contamination.

A longitudinal incision is made in the neck, the skin is reflected, and the oesophagus is exposed and tied. The neck is kept for edible purposes and placed at the inspection point. Electronic identification devices must be removed from the carcase at the time of slaughter to prevent entry into the food chain.

The vent is freed from its attachments, tied and placed in a plastic bag. Evisceration is performed by a mid-abdominal incision above the breast plate. Ribs are cut on both sides of the breast plate. Thoracic viscera are exposed by pressing the breastplate down. The bagged vent is pulled into the abdominal cavity, and the intestinal tract is removed, together with the liver and spleen. Intestines are placed in a separate tray for inspection, and the liver and spleen are placed in the viscera inspection tray adjacent to the head and neck. The lungs may stay on the carcase or they may be eviscerated with the heart. They are then placed in the viscera inspection tray. Kidneys are visually inspected in the carcase and after removal. Different evisceration procedures may be carried out provided they are carried out hygienically and allow for proper inspection.

Ratites are susceptible to similar diseases as other poultry. The digestive tract is the most common site of infection by pathogenic bacteria. Necrotic enteritis caused by *Clostridium* spp. affects ostriches 2 weeks of age and over.

Ostriches should be observed at rest and in movement. This inspection procedure is similar to that for other animal species. A healthy bird is alert, has an erect neck and at times lowers and raises its head. It walks with a springy gait and appears as if walking with its heels in the air. It is inquisitive, and pecks at its environment. It may be aggressive. The urine is thick, white and clear and the faeces are firm. The feathers are clean and well separated, and the body appears well rounded. The tail is fluffed up and erect.

The main reason for condemnation is airsacculitis.

Changes after slaughter

The pH decline patterns of ostrich muscles are very rapid, with pH 5.85 in some muscles 1.5 hours after postmortem. Shortly after this, the pH rises so that in general the pH is not much below 6.0, which may be considered between normal and moderately DFD meat. It is not known whether this is due to pre-slaughter stress or an inherent ostrich muscle characteristic. The effect will be a shortened shelf life.

Since the subcutaneous fat layer is either absent or very thin when present and is concentrated in specific areas only (mainly abdominal), cold shortening of muscles may be anticipated if carcases are chilled below 10°C while the muscles are still physiologically reactive. Electrical stimulation of the carcase normally provides a solution for this problem, allowing even hot deboning without inducing shortening.

Commercial squab production

Squab, a young pigeon just before it starts flying, is a speciality poultry product which can be raised on either large or small commercial scale. Squabs are very tasty because the meat is very tender and lend themselves very well to barbecuing and other methods of cooking. About 2 million squabs are marketed each year in the United States.

Almost all squabbing pigeons are confined; 15–18 pairs can be kept in a 3×3.5 m pen. Production is labour-intensive as it requires constant attention over the flock. Squabs can be marketed as early as 25 days after birth. A good breeding pair can produce 12 squabs for market each year.

Further reading

Adams, J. (1986) *The Slaughter and Inspection of Wild Deer*, Arun District Council.

Adams, J. and Dannatt (1989) *The Culling and Processing of Wild Deer*, Arun District Council.

Alexander, T. L. (1990) Slaughter of farmed deer, Veterinary Public Health Association (VPHA) Proceedings, November 1990.

Alexander, T. and Buxton, D. (eds) (1994) *Management and Disease of Deer*, 2nd edn, Veterinary Society Publication.

Animal Welfare Act 2006.

Fletcher, T. J. (1990) Deer farming in Britain. VPHA Proceedings, November 1990.

MAFF (1996) Guidance Notes on the Slaughter of Ostriches: Welfare.

Defra: Animal Welfare Codes of Recommendation for the Welfare of Livestock. Deer: Rabbits XXX.

Rafferty, G. C. (1990) Wild venison, VPHA Proceedings, November 1990.

The Commercial Meat Rabbit Producer's Handbook, The British Commercial Rabbit Association XXX.

Webster, J. (2011) *Management and Welfare of Farm Animals. The UFAW Farm Handbook*, Wiley-Blackwell, Chichester.

The Wild Game Guide Final Revision June 2013, Food Standards Agency, London XXX.

12

Food poisoning and meat microbiology*

Part 1: Food poisoning

Types of food poisoning

Food poisoning includes bacterial and viral infections; chemical contamination of food, plant or animal toxins; and food allergies.

Food allergies, or hypersensitivity to certain foodstuffs, are not uncommon and together with other allergic diseases may be increasing. The *allergens* are generally protein in nature, for example, milk, eggs, cheese, fish, shellfish and pork, but also mushrooms, tomatoes, etc. Hypersensitivities to nuts, such as peanuts, are well documented, and food ingredients are carefully scrutinised by susceptible individuals. In some cases, the reaction can be so acute and severe as to require a few individuals to carry acute medical supplies. Nuts and cereals are also vehicles for *aflatoxin* produced during the growth of fungi, either before or after harvest. The tendency to sensitivity to certain foodstuffs may be hereditary, and a documented case in the literature describes an allergy to hens' eggs which persisted throughout four generations. As many as 30% of all people may be allergic to one or more foodstuffs.

Chemical contamination is not common and usually occurs by accidental contamination, through fraud or perhaps some unintentional chemical reaction between a foodstuff and its container. The metals encountered include copper, lead, arsenic and antimony. In England and Wales, outbreaks caused by chemical contamination have been due to the presence of zinc in acid fruits which have been stored or cooked in galvanised containers. In Germany, the storage of prepared foodstuffs in zinc containers is prohibited by law. Water is at particular risk from chemical contamination (usually accidental) such as by aluminium or phenols. Lead may, of course, be leached from lead pipes or even from soldered lead capillary joints. Not only metals are involved; a large outbreak of illness occurred in Spain following chemical adulteration of cooking oil.

Inherently poisonous substances can occur in normally edible plants and animals including certain fungi, berries, fish and shellfish. This is well recognised in the case of mushrooms, where some types are toxic. Less well known are foods that are poisonous unless properly prepared, for example, red kidney beans. Other foods in the right circumstances can acquire toxins from the environment. This is a particular problem with shellfish, which can filter out the algal toxins that cause paralytic and diarrhoetic shellfish poisoning in consumers. In some instances, breakdown products can produce illness, as in the case of scombrotoxin poisoning when bacterial action in scromboid fish, such as mackerel and tuna, converts histidine to histamine. A similar type of illness has been associated with cheese.

Surveillance of food poisoning

There are several different methods of gathering statistics on food-borne disease, and it is important to recognise the limitations posed by each of these. The three most important sources of data are:

1 Notifications of food poisoning
2 Surveillance of laboratory-confirmed infections
3 Investigation of outbreaks of food poisoning

Each of these surveillance methods provides valuable, but incomplete, information, and none on its own will measure the true extent of all food-borne disease. Specifically, most of the information gathered relates to

*Additional editing by Malcolm J Taylor, Senior Scientific Officer, Food Science Branch, Agri-Food-Biosciences Institute, Belfast BT9 5PX, UK.

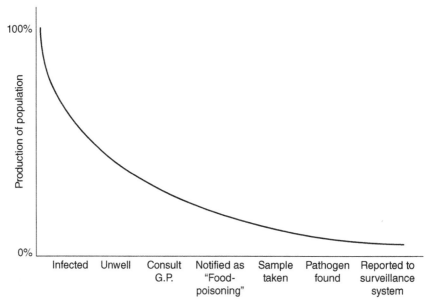

Figure 12.1 Surveillance for food-borne illness.

infectious causes of food poisoning. It is estimated that only between 1 and 10% of all food-borne illness is even counted by the various surveillance systems, and this varies from cause to cause (Fig. 12.1).

In any population, not all of those who become infected become ill. Of those who are unwell, only a proportion will seek medical help and can be counted as 'notifications'. Those who do not require medical assistance are not included in any surveillance system. If the clinician suspects 'food poisoning', then that patient *may* be formally notified, for which the GP will receive a notification fee. The number of notifications may be supplemented, for example, Health Officials and Environmental Health Officers in the United Kingdom, including cases they become aware of during their investigation. The doctor may submit appropriate samples for laboratory investigation, and this forms the basis of laboratory surveillance. The sample taken may affect the result; for example, vomitus is more appropriate for a viral agent than is a stool sample. Unless the sample is submitted within 24 hours of onset of illness, a viral cause is likely to be missed. If a pathogen is identified, then the result should be recorded by the laboratory surveillance. When no pathogen is identified, it does not, of course, mean that none were present but rather that the laboratory did not identify anything. This will depend on the organisms under scrutiny. When an outbreak occurs, it is likely that there will be greater investigation of the source of infection than might be the case when only a single patient is unwell. Causes of outbreaks may be different from the causes of sporadic infections, and it may not be possible to extrapolate.

Laboratory reports of enteric infections

Routine reporting from medical laboratories gives a useful picture of the importance of pathogens present in the population. It does, of course, only record the results from *samples* actually submitted to laboratories and can therefore be distorted by any factors which might influence sampling, for example, increased media attention. Results can also be influenced by the likely success of identifying a pathogen when present, and this success may change as laboratory methodologies improve. For example, during the 1980s, better techniques for the recovery of *Campylobacter* spp. became routinely available, and this undoubtedly contributed to the overall increase in numbers reported during the 1980s and 1990s. However, since the early 1990s, methods have been standardised and should not be the explanation for the continuing increase for *Campylobacter* spp., 200,000 reported EU cases in 2010.

Other extraneous events also play a part when identifying laboratory-confirmed cases. A change in policy occurred when the Advisory Committee on the Microbiological Safety of Food recommended in 1995 that *all* stool samples be screened for *Escherichia coli* O157. Previously, many laboratories were selective and had perhaps restricted the examination for this organism to stools from children or from patients with bloody diarrhoea.

The variation in laboratory methods and sample submissions may partly explain the geographical differences seen throughout the United Kingdom.

Outbreak surveillance

Investigation into outbreaks can give valuable information on the organisms involved, the food vehicles and the factors contributing to the cause of the outbreak. The main limitation is that the majority of cases of food poisoning occur as single cases or involve a single household only, and it is much more difficult to confirm a source of infection – even if an investigation is carried out.

Outbreaks are investigated in most parts of the world, although there is no common approach in the way this is performed. Lack of standardisation makes comparison of reports from different countries very difficult, even though the World Health Organisation and the EU have co-ordinated programmes.

Reports of food-borne disease outbreaks within the EU are included within the annual "European Union Summary Reports" on zoonoses produced by the European Food Safety Authority (EFSA) in co-operation with the European Centre for Disease Prevention and Control (ECDC) (www.efsa.europe.eu/en/zoonosesscdocs/zoonosesconsumrep.htm).

General considerations

There are many and varied sources of the organisms causing food poisoning. Most originate directly from animals, particularly *Salmonella* spp., *Campylobacter* spp. and *E. coli*. Others not only have animal sources but survive or even increase within the environment. This includes, for example, the *Clostridia* spp., *Listeria* spp. and *Bacillus* spp. Yet others have people as the source or reservoir – particularly *Staphylococcus* and viruses. Other human gastrointestinal infections such as dysentery (*Shigella* spp.) can be passed by contaminated food, although this is not the main route of spread.

Regardless of the origin of the organisms involved, they all have one factor in common. *There has been failure to adequately control the hygiene and temperature control of the whole food chain.* This chain, when it involves animals, can be divided into a number of separate stages:

Animal feed, for example, the feed mill
On farm, for example, suckled calves
During processing, for example, abattoir and cutting plant
Further processing and distribution, for example, butchers
Final preparation, for example, domestic or commercial
  kitchen

Each of these is important in the prevention of food-borne disease, and satisfactory practices must be in place. No single part of the food chain bears the total responsibility for the prevention of food poisoning.

Food-borne disease is not static and constantly changes and evolves. The traditional illnesses such as bovine tuberculosis (TB) caused by milk, which have often determined the procedures historically used in meat inspection, have largely been controlled. In the case of TB, this has been achieved by reducing the infection in animals, by identifying and removing infected animals and by treating risk foods, for example, milk, by pasteurisation.

These traditional zoonotic diseases were usually examples where the food, meat or milk, was itself carrying the pathogen when the animal was slaughtered or milked. The more current problems associated with food poisoning are usually the consequence of the food becoming contaminated either at the time of production or subsequently. This has placed an even greater emphasis on the need for *strict hygiene and temperature control.* That this is not always achieved is emphasised by the continuing and apparently increasing problem of food-borne infections.

Not all food-poisoning organisms cause illness in animals; many bacteria are part of the 'normal' intestinal flora, for example, *Yersinia* spp. and *Clostridium* spp. Even with those which can cause animal illness, this may be the exception rather than the norm. Campylobacter infection is a good example of this, the organisms being widespread in animals and birds yet rarely making them ill. But other organisms, such as *Salmonella* spp., do cause considerable animal ill health, although it is not usually the 'sick' animals that enter the food chain, rather recovered or carrier animals which are still shedding the pathogen.

Most of the organisms causing problems are spread by the faecal route, and the main problem is to prevent food becoming contaminated with animal faeces.

Food-borne pathogens

Most cases of food poisoning are caused by bacteria which arise from animal, human or environmental sources. Viral infections are unlikely to be from animals and may be due to direct human contamination or indirectly through the environment, for example, from shellfish contaminated by discharged human sewage.

Bacterial food poisoning may take one of two forms: infection with living organisms or intoxication with pre-formed toxins such as with *Staphylococcus aureus*. The feature which chiefly distinguishes the two types clinically is the incubation period, that is, the interval between eating the food and the development of symptoms. Where *pre-formed toxins* are present, the conditions are somewhat analogous to chemical poisoning, and symptoms will develop very rapidly, usually within a few hours. If *living organisms* are ingested, time will elapse before their multiplication in the body has proceeded sufficiently to provoke the usual reactions of diarrhoea and vomiting.

A summary of bacterial causes of food poisoning is given in Table 12.1.

Table 12.1 Bacterial causes of food-borne infection

Agent	Normal incubation period	Normal duration	Main clinical symptoms	Commonly associated foods
B. cereus emetic toxin	1–5 hours	<24 hours	Vomiting	Cereals, rice
B. cereus enterotoxin	8–16 hours	<24 hours	Abdominal pain, diarrhoea	Cereals, rice
Campylobacter spp.	3–5 days	2–7 days	Abdominal pain, diarrhoea (sometimes bloody), headache, fever	Poultry, cooked meats, milk
Cl. botulinum	12–36 hours	Extended	Swallowing difficulties, perhaps as respiratory failure	Preserved foods, e.g., canned, bottled
Cl. perfringens	10–12 hours	24 hours	Abdominal pain, diarrhoea	Stews, roasts
E. coli 0157	12 hours–10 days	Possibly extended	Abdominal pain, diarrhoea (may be bloody). May lead to renal failure	Beefburgers, meat, dairy products
L. monocytogenes	3–21+ days	Varies	Fever, headache, spontaneous abortion, meningitis	Soft cheeses, patés, poultry meat
Salmonella spp.	12–36 hours	2–20 days	Abdominal pain, diarrhoea, fever, nausea	Meat, poultry, eggs, dairy products
Staph. aureus	2–6 hours	12–24 hours	Vomiting, abdominal pain, diarrhoea	Cooked meat, human source
V. parahaemolyticus	12–24 hours	1–7 days	Abdominal pain, watery diarrhoea, headache, vomiting fever	Shellfish
Y. enterocolitica	3–7 days	1–3 weeks	Acute diarrhoea, abdominal pain, fever and vomiting	Pig meat products

Campylobacter spp.

Campylobacters, although long recognised by veterinarians as a cause of animal disease, were not associated with human enteric infection until 1975. Since then, the number of isolates in the United Kingdom and across the EU has steadily increased until they have become the most numerous cause of human bacterial enteric infection. Undoubtedly, improved laboratory methods have contributed to this rise, although, in addition, a true increase has occurred.

The traditional animal strains of *Campylobacter fetus fetus* and *C. fetus venerealis* rarely cause human infection and the most common types in the EU are *C. jejuni*, *C. coli* and *C. lari*. Serological sub-typing is not as well developed as that for salmonella, and most isolates are not further sub-typed. This makes epidemiological investigation very difficult as it is not easy to confirm the origin of human infection. A baseline study carried out within the EU in 2008 estimated that 70% of batches of broilers presented for slaughter were colonised.

Unlike many other food-borne organisms, *Campylobacter* spp. are fastidious in their growth requirements. They are Gram-negative and microaerophilic, requiring a low oxygen concentration (5%). They are slender, curved and highly mobile and grow best at 42–43°C and not at all below 30°C. They are most unlikely to multiply on food at room temperature. They are not heat resistant and can be killed by cooking. As though to compensate for their inability to grow on food, they have an extremely low infective dose, with as few as 500 cells being sufficient to cause human infection.

Infection in humans With a reported incidence in humans of 44 confirmed cases per 100,000 of the human population, there is an estimated 9 million cases of human illness per annum within the EU.

The normal incubation period is 3–5 days, but some evidence exists that this can be considerably extended. A characteristic of infection is acute abdominal pain, which can be so severe as to be mistaken for appendicitis, sometimes precipitating unnecessary surgery. This pain is often accompanied by bloody diarrhoea and fever, but vomiting is rare. Most infections resolve spontaneously within one week, while others can be prolonged. Complications during the acute phase are unusual and only exceptionally does death occur. There is, however, increasing evidence that there may be longer-term sequelae to campylobacter infection including both reactive arthritis and even peripheral polyneuropathy (Guillain–Barré syndrome).

Source of human infection The lack of a routine discriminatory typing scheme has often hindered investigation of the source of human infections. Unlike salmonellosis, most cases of campylobacter infection are not recognised as part of an outbreak, and detailed investigation is not carried out. The exceptions to this are outbreaks associated with milk and water, when hundreds of patients can be involved. The Advisory Committee on the Microbiological Safety of Food investigated infections with campylobacter and reported in 1993 that poultry was the most common vehicle of infection. While it is now considered that 60–80% of human infection can be linked to poultry, it should be remembered that the types of campylobacter affecting humans can also be isolated from all species of animals (including pets) and a wide range of foods including, milk, water and cooked meats. Person-to-person spread is also important.

The low infective dose for campylobacter means that cross-contamination is a particular risk since a relatively small amount of contamination may be sufficient to establish human infection. This cross-contamination must be prevented throughout the whole food chain with efforts being made to reduce the prevalence of the bacteria on farm through good biosecurity as well as through interventions during transport of the birds, in the slaughterhouse and during storage and retail.

Salmonella spp.

Within the EU, *Salmonella* are the second most common food-borne pathogen with around 100,000 confirmed cases annually. Given the constraints upon surveillance discussed earlier, this figure has been estimated by the EFSA Panel on Biological Hazards to represent a true incidence of 6 million cases.

The salmonellae constitute a large group of over 2200 different serotypes, although only 100–200 different serotypes are identified in any one year in the United Kingdom. They are members of the Enterobacteriaceae, are Gram-negative and can readily grow on a wide range of media including foods. They are temperature sensitive and readily destroyed by cooking.

The different serotypes are identified by means of the somatic (O) and flagellar (H) antigens using the "Kauffmann–White scheme". Further sub-typing can be carried out by phage typing and, increasingly, molecular methods such as plasmid profiling.

Some salmonellae usually only affect a single animal species including, for example, *S. typhi* in humans, *S. abortus ovis* in sheep and *S. pullorum* in poultry. Most salmonella species including those associated with food poisoning can infect many species of animal, although they may not cause illness in all of these. A good example of this is *S. enteritidis*, now the most common salmonella in humans, which is widespread, but usually causes no illness in poultry.

Within the EU, *S. enteritidis* and *S. typhimurium* serovars account for approximately 70% of confirmed cases of human infection.

While not as resistant as the spore-forming organisms such as the *Clostridium* spp., *Salmonella* spp. can exist for many months in the environment, especially if protected from extremes of temperature and sunlight. This means that recycling through the environment is an important route for animal (and human) infection (Fig. 12.2).

This ability of salmonella to exist within different self-contained compartments makes eradication difficult. Control is a more practical option, although specific salmonellae such as *S. pullorum* have to all intents and purposes been eradicated in commercial poultry. There is considerable ongoing effort being expended by the poultry industry to reduce salmonellae causing human illness, in particular *S. enteritidis*.

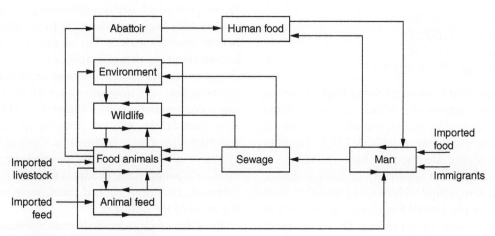

Figure 12.2 Salmonella recycling in food animals.

Infection in humans The incubation period in people is variable but is usually between 12 and 36 hours. The typical presenting symptom is diarrhoea, but this may be accompanied by nausea and abdominal pain, although vomiting is not usual. There may also be headache and fever. While the infection is normally self-limiting and does not require antibiotic treatment, occasionally, with more invasive salmonellae such as *S. virchow*, bacteraemia can occur. The infection is rarely fatal in people.

Source of human infection People can become infected following a failure of personal hygiene after contact with infected animals (or other infected people). Environmental contamination, especially *untreated water*, is also important. Most cases are thought to be the result of food-borne infection and highlight the importance of controlling hygiene in the food chain. Meat can become contaminated during the slaughter process either from intestinal contents or from faecal contamination on the hide. As with any faecally spread organism, *it is essential that clean animals are presented for slaughter to help minimise the latter and that the abattoir operates hygienically to prevent both.*

Escherichia coli O157

Verotoxigenic *E. coli* infections, particularly serogroup O157, were first reported in the United Kingdom in 1983. Since then, despite a relatively low notification rate of 0.45 cases per 100,000 population across the EU, they have become recognised as a major source of human morbidity and mortality due to the potential serious consequences of infection.

E. coli are ubiquitous inhabitants of the intestinal tracts of animals and man. A variety of serogroups cause infections, usually in a single animal species, for example, bowel oedema in pigs. In humans, a number of different disease syndromes are recognised, including:

Enteropathogenic *E. coli* (EPEC)
Enteroinvasive *E. coli* (EIEC)
Enterotoxigenic *E. coli* (ETEC)
Enterohaemorrhagic *E. coli* (EHEC)

Some of these EHEC have the ability to produce one or more toxins (verotoxins), which can be detected using tissue culture (Vero cells), and are often referred to as verotoxin-producing *E. coli* (VTEC). Together with other virulence factors, they have the ability to cause human illness but apparently no animal illness. While several serogroups such as O111 and O26 have been involved in the United Kingdom, the majority of infections are caused by serogroup O157. In other countries, other serogroups have been reported as more important than O157. As with campylobacter, a small infective dose – perhaps as few as 10 cells – is required to cause human illness, but unlike campylobacter, they can multiply on food.

Infection in humans The low infective dose plays a major part in the spread of these bacteria. Incubation is normally 1–10 days and a considerable spectrum of symptoms can be seen. These range from asymptomatic infection, abdominal pain and diarrhoea, bloody diarrhoea and haemorrhagic colitis to haemolytic uraemia resulting in renal failure. Although the total number of cases, with about 1000 reported each year in the United Kingdom, is low, the consequences are serious. In one series of cases in Scotland, 59% of cases required hospitalisation, 15% required renal dialysis, and 3% died. Serious systemic disease is a particular feature in the old and the young. Following a large milk-borne outbreak in Scotland in 1994, several children required renal transplants. Conversely, many people appear to carry and shed the bacteria yet show no signs of infection.

Source of human infection Various studies have identified three main routes of transmission: consumption of contaminated food or water, direct or indirect contact with animals and person-to-person spread. Beefburgers were recognised as a significant vehicle of infection following a large outbreak across several states in the United States in 1993 in which 732 people were affected and 195 hospitalised with four deaths. However, a wide range of foods have been implicated, including apple juice, vegetables, potatoes, bean sprouts and water. Contamination of the food with animal faeces is thought to cause most of the problem.

Cattle are considered to be the primary reservoir of VTEC with an estimated 0–17% of cattle carrying VTEC O157. As with all organisms found in animal faeces, control is based on minimising carcase contamination. This begins on the farm by reducing the number of animal carriers, but at present, not much is known about the natural transmission of *E. coli* O157 to devise a control strategy. *The most important measure is to ensure that only clean animals*, with the minimum of faecal contamination, *are slaughtered*. This was a major recommendation of the Pennington group which reported after a large outbreak in Central Scotland (at Wishaw) in 1996 in which 496 people were affected and 20 elderly people died. Products from a single butcher's premises, including cooked meat, were implicated as the cause of the outbreak.

Slaughter of clean animals must be accompanied by the hygienic operation of the whole slaughterhouse and effective control of the food chain. Ultimately, *thorough cooking* will kill the organisms. The low infective dose means that contamination unlikely to cause problems when *Salmonella* spp. or *Campylobacter* spp. are present may be enough to cause infection if *E. coli* O157 prevails.

Antimicrobial resistance

A particular concern with *Salmonella* spp. and *E. coli* is the occurrence of antimicrobial resistance genes. Of particular concern are the extended spectrum beta-lactamases (ESBL) and/or AmpC-producing bacteria. ESBL are plasmid-encoded enzymes found in Enterobacteriaceae that confer resistance to a variety of beta-lactam antimicrobials, including penicillins; second-, third- and fourth-generation cephalosporins; and monobactams. Both ESBL and AmpC-producing organisms have the potential to be transmitted from animals to humans in food.

Yersinia enterocolitica

Yersinia enterocolitica was identified as a human pathogen in the late 1930s. It is a Gram-negative non-spore-forming bacterium which grows over a wide range of temperatures (0–40°C) and optimally at 29°C. The range of growth temperatures allows multiplication at refrigeration temperatures. It is widespread in the intestinal tract of animals and is readily recovered from the environment, including water and soil. It can be divided into biotypes, serotypes and phage types. Different types are associated with different parts of the world. In Europe, serotype O3 is most commonly recorded in humans and is also associated with pigs.

Infection in humans The incubation period is about 3–7 days, and infection causes acute diarrhoea, abdominal pain, fever and vomiting. It is more common in children, although cases in adults may be followed by longer-term problems including skin rashes and arthritis. Infection is usually self-limiting, but in people with some other underlying pathology, septicaemia with a high mortality may follow. About 500 cases a year are reported in the United Kingdom.

Source of human infection This organism is often associated with pig meat products, either fresh or cured. The ability to grow at refrigeration temperature means that contaminated food, even if properly chilled, can cause infection. Such foods can also cross-contaminate other foods in the kitchen.

Listeria monocytogenes

Of the several *Listeria* species, only *L. monocytogenes* is thought to cause human infection. It is widely distributed in animals, birds, humans and the environment but has only been recognised as a food-borne pathogen since the 1980s. Like *Yersinia* spp., *L. monocytogenes* can grow at a wide range of temperatures (0–42°C) and especially well at 30–37°C. *Listeria* spp. can also grow slowly at refrigeration temperatures. A wide range of serotypes exist, but most human infection is associated with types 4 and 1/2.

Infection in humans Most human cases are sporadic, and the extended incubation period (several weeks) can make identification of the source very difficult. Unlike the case with most food-borne pathogens, the illness produced is systemic rather than intestinal. Most infected people are symptomless, and as many as 5% of the population are faecally excreting at any one time. Illness is most likely to be seen in people with reduced immunity, when the symptoms range from a 'flu-like' illness through fever and septicaemia. There is a particular risk to pregnant women (who have a naturally reduced immune capability) and the unborn child, when the mortality can be as high as 30%. Although there was a significant rise in reported cases of listeriosis in the late 1980s, this was not maintained in subsequent years. Listeriosis is now relatively uncommon, with about 100 cases reported each year in the United Kingdom.

Source of human infection This is often not identified because of the length of the incubation period. The organisms are ubiquitous and widespread in animals and the environment. Listeriosis can cause animal disease, including abortion in ewes and meningitis in younger sheep. A wide range of foods have been implicated including cheese, paté and poultry meat. Vulnerable groups, especially pregnant women and the immuno-compromised, are advised not to eat risk foods such as patés and soft cheeses.

Clostridium perfringens

The mode of action of food poisoning with *Clostridium perfringens* is through the consumption of large numbers of bacteria which rapidly form enterotoxin in the small intestine. It is a Gram-positive spore former, requiring anaerobic conditions for growth. In the United Kingdom, a better understanding of food hygiene, in particular the importance of thorough cooking and rapid cooling, has resulted in a decline in the importance of this pathogen.

Five types (A–E) of *Cl. perfringens* are known to exist, but only type A has been implicated in food poisoning. The clostridia form part of the normal intestinal flora of animals and are widespread in the environment.

Infection in humans The rapid production of enterotoxin in the intestine results in a short incubation period of 10–12 hours. The toxin causes diarrhoea and abdominal pain but not usually vomiting. Illness normally lasts 24 hours and is self-limiting. Subsequent complications and death are rare.

Source of human infection The clostridial spores survive normal cooking, and the heating process may in fact stimulate them to germinate. As food cools, very rapid multiplication can take place, since optimal growth occurs at 43–47°C. The heating process of cooking also drives off oxygen, creating the anaerobic conditions necessary for growth. These conditions are most likely to be found when large volumes of food are cooked and cooled, particularly large joints of meat or stews and casseroles. Thorough reheating (above 75°C) will kill any vegetative cells present and prevent food poisoning. Most cases occur as outbreaks, which may be large and are often associated with hospital or commercial catering. About 50 outbreaks are reported in the United Kingdom each year.

Staphylococcus aureus

Unlike most bacterial food poisoning, illness caused by *Staph. aureus* is due to the consumption of pre-formed toxin and not the bacteria, which may be absent. The toxin is heat stable and may survive for 1½ hours at boiling temperature, even though the staphylococci themselves are destroyed. Five major enterotoxins are known to be produced (A–E) of which type A is the most common. The Gram-positive cocci can grow over a wide range of temperatures (10–45°C) with the optimum at 35–40°C.

Infection in humans The presence of pre-formed toxin results in a short incubation period of 2–6 hours. The symptoms are primarily nausea and vomiting, with additionally diarrhoea. The illness may also be so acute as to cause fainting or collapse. Most patients recover within 12–48 hours.

Source of human infection *Staph. aureus* infection usually follows contamination from a human source. The organism can cause wound or skin infections and is present in the nose of up to 40% of healthy people. A failure of basic hygiene, including covering skin lesions, results in contamination of food and subsequent multiplication and toxin production. The foods usually implicated are cooked meats, poultry and dairy produce. This has been an uncommon cause of food poisoning in the United Kingdom since the 1950s, with around 10 outbreaks reported each year.

Clostridium botulinum

Botulism is one of the most feared causes of food poisoning because, although it is exceptionally rare, it is a severe disease with a high mortality. *Clostridium botulinum* is a Gram-positive spore-forming obligate anaerobe producing one or more of seven toxins (A–G). Toxins A, B and E have been associated with human disease. Types A and B are more commonly linked with meat and vegetables, while type E is associated with fish. The toxin is not thermostable and can be destroyed by cooking at 80°C for 30 minutes.

Infection in humans The clostridia produce potent neurotoxins and the symptoms reflect muscular paralysis. Symptoms can appear within 2 hours but may take as long as 5 days. There can be an initial short period of diarrhoea with vomiting and subsequent constipation. Blurring or double vision is often the first systemic sign, accompanied by dry mouth and difficulty in swallowing. The patient is usually mentally alert and there is no loss of sensation. Paralysis can extend to the limbs and eventually result in respiratory failure. The effects of the toxin may persist for several months.

Source of human infection *Cl. botulinum* is ubiquitous and can be found on a wide range of foods. Toxin production only takes place when growth occurs. This can happen during preservation processes, such as smoking or fermentation of fish and meat, which result in a suitable anaerobic environment. Improperly bottled or canned foods can also allow growth to take place.

Botulism is very rare in the United Kingdom. The first reported outbreak occurred in 1922 in Loch Maree in Scotland when eight people became ill after eating potted duck paste and all died. The largest outbreak occurred in 1989 when 27 cases (one death) were caused by hazelnut yoghurt. In total, only 10 outbreaks have been described in the United Kingdom.

Vibrio parahaemolyticus

Vibrio parahaemolyticus is a Gram-negative rod usually found in seawater where the temperature is above 10°C. It can multiply rapidly at ambient temperatures but is easily killed by cooking.

Infection in humans   The incubation period is 12–24 hours, after which profuse diarrhoea and abdominal pain develop. Less commonly, fever and vomiting may be present. The symptoms may persist for 7 days.

Source of human infection   The organism is found in seawaters, especially if the temperature is greater than 10°C. Fish and shellfish from affected waters may cause illness if inadequately cooked or if subsequently re-contaminated. It is rarely acquired in the United Kingdom, although one incident involving locally caught crab was reported on the south coast of England.

Bacillus cereus

Bacillus cereus has been recognised as an uncommon cause of food poisoning since the 1970s. It is a Gram-positive, spore-forming, motile bacillus producing two different toxins. A heat-sensitive enterotoxin causes a diarrhoeal illness, while the heat-stable 'emetic' toxin causes vomiting. The spores are heat resistant and can survive normal cooking temperatures. The bacteria are widespread in the environment, including soil and water, and consequently contaminate many foods, particularly dry foods such as cereals. Any food such as meat, dairy products and vegetables can be vehicles of infection.

Infection in humans   The two toxins produce different disease syndromes. The more common illness is vomiting caused by the 'emetic' toxin after an incubation period of 1–5 hours. This is particularly associated with rice and pasta. The diarrhoeal illness caused by the enterotoxin has an incubation period of 8–16 hours. Both forms of infection usually last no longer than 24 hours and complications are rare.

Source of human infection   Many foods are contaminated with a few spores and these can survive the initial cooking. If food is subsequently kept at ambient temperature, the spores germinate and the vegetative cells multiply rapidly, producing toxin in the food. The 'emetic' toxin is not destroyed by further heating, but the enterotoxin can be inactivated by thorough reheating. This latter toxin can, however, also be produced in the intestine of the patient following consumption of the vegetative cells. The disease is controlled by keeping cooked foods either hot or at refrigeration temperatures. About 30 outbreaks a year are described in the United Kingdom.

Part 2: Meat microbiology

Bacteriological examination of carcases

In the healthy and physiologically normal animal, those organs which have no direct contact with the exterior may be regarded as virtually sterile, though the actual operation of slaughter and dressing has a significant potential to introduce bacteria to the blood, tissues and organs. These micro-organisms are usually a mixed flora of non-specific micro-organisms of environmental as well as faecal origin but can include pathogens such as *Salmonella*, *Campylobacter*, *E. coli* and other food-poisoning organisms. In addition, specific pathogens may be present in organs or tissues such as the spleen, muscular tissue or lymph nodes, and their presence can only be attributed to a generalised septic or bacteraemic infection in the animal at the time of slaughter. Where such organisms are of intestinal origin, their entry into the systemic circulation may be explained by a breakdown in the natural resistance of the animal with migration of the organisms from the intestinal tract. Haematogenous invasion may, however, occur from other naturally infected cavities of the body for the same reason. Such systemic invasion is most likely to occur in animals that are ill or exhausted, which should be identified during the ante-mortem inspection. Subsequent bacteriological examination of the flesh and organs post-mortem would provide definitive material assistance to an inspector charged with assessing the fitness or otherwise of a carcase for human food.

Indications for examination

The examination of food of animal origin for fitness requires the three stages of ante-mortem, gross post-mortem and, where necessary, further laboratory tests.

There is no justification for conducting a bacteriological examination on a carcase or its organs when they exhibit marked pathological changes of a non-infectious nature. Such conditions or evidences of severe systemic disturbance are themselves sufficient to justify condemnation of the carcase. A bacteriological examination can never substitute for a careful organoleptic examination; its value is as a supplementary test to assist judgement when septicaemic or bacteraemic infection is suspected. The only thing to be gained from a bacteriological examination of such overtly unfit material is the identification of the infecting organism – this in itself may be sufficient reason.

A bacteriological examination may be considered obligatory in the case of animals which:

1 Have been slaughtered in emergency
2 Have been slaughtered on account of a disease associated with systemic disturbances

3 Show pathological changes on post-mortem inspection that lead to doubt as to the suitability of the meat for human consumption, even though the animal was found healthy on ante-mortem inspection
4 Have been shown by bacteriological tests to have been excreting food-poisoning organisms prior to slaughter or which emanate from a herd in which the presence of food-poisoning organisms has been officially reported
5 Have not been eviscerated within 1 hour of slaughter or where the parts of the slaughtered animal necessary for post-mortem examination are absent or have been handled in such a way as to make satisfactory judgement impossible

Material submitted

The following samples may be taken for submission to the laboratory for bacteriological examination:

1 Two *complete muscles*, with their fascia, one from a forequarter and one from a hindquarter, or cubes of muscle, each side measuring not less than 7.5 cm
2 The *prescapular or axillary lymph node* from the other forequarter of the carcase and the *internal iliac node* from the other hindquarter, including the surrounding fat and connective tissue of the nodes
3 The *spleen*, which should not be incised except in cases where the organ is considerably enlarged, in which case a piece as large as the hand should be taken.
4 A *kidney*
5 *In the case of small animals*, the whole *liver* with the gall bladder; in other animals, a portion of liver twice the size of a fist and including the portal vein, or the caudate lobe and including the portal vein, and also the portal lymph nodes and gall bladder
6 *Parts showing pathological change* and which, in view of their position, are suspected of containing pathogenic bacteria, together with the associated lymph nodes (e.g. in the case of pneumonia, a portion of the lung and associated lymph nodes)
7 A portion of the *small intestine* along with a number of *mesenteric lymph nodes* in those cases where animals have suffered from enteritis and have been reported to be excretors of *Salmonella* organisms or animals known to emanate from a herd infected with such pathogens.

Laboratory experience has shown that the *liver* frequently contains intestinal bacteria which have gained entry by way of the portal vein. As this invasion may occur after slaughter, the demonstration of organisms in the liver is of no real significance unless the organisms isolated are of a specific pathogenic type. Similarly, the *kidney* should theoretically be of value in bacteriological examinations, but in practice, bacterial invasion rarely occurs *post-mortem*.

Microbiological sampling and interpretation

Provided care is taken in the interpretation of results, microbiological examination of meat is of value in the assessment of wholesomeness, of the integrity of the hygienic processing system and methods adopted during slaughter, of dressing and processing techniques and of the efficiency of methods of preservation. It can also indicate the potential shelf life and help to identify potential health hazards.

One of the difficulties associated with microbiological examination is the lack of a standard technique accepted and applied uniformly between different countries. There are variations in sampling techniques, times of sampling, culture media, parts of carcase to be examined, number of samples, which bacteria to assess, counting methods, etc., all of which require standardisation if comparisons are to be drawn and if the results are to be uniformly interpreted. Sampling methodologies are stipulated by both legislative and customer specifications, as are the interpretations of the analyses.

The bacterial status of the meat is dependent on a number of factors, namely, the condition of the animal at slaughter, the spread of contamination during slaughter and the processing and temperature during storage and distribution. Thus, as discussed previously, meat may be contaminated with a range of bacteria which may be significant in spoilage or may be pathogenic. The quality and safety of meat is dictated by the nature and numbers of spoilage and pathogenic species which form the total flora. The microbiology of meat is therefore normally considered under two criteria:

Total bacterial counts (TBC) also known as aerobic colony count (ACC), aerobic plate count (APC) and total viable count (TVC) provide an indication of gross levels of contamination.

Specific counts of species of spoilage or pathogenic bacteria of particular significance, for example, *Salmonella* spp., Enterobacteriaceae and generic *E. coli*.

Before microbiological analysis can be carried out, it is necessary to obtain samples from the carcase under investigation. This may be achieved by taking either superficial or deep samples, or both if necessary.

Superficial samples may be taken by removing primarily destructive (surface samples) or non-destructive (swab or sponge) samples. They provide an indication of the levels of surface contamination present on the carcase. Surface contamination may originate from contact with contaminated surfaces, tools, operatives and airborne contamination. These organisms are of environmental as well as of faecal origin and generally contain the organisms which will form a spoilage flora – for example, *Pseudomonas*, lactic acid bacteria and members of the family Enterobacteriaceae, *Moraxella*, *Brochothrix and Acinetobacter*. Destructive surface sampling is used commonly in poultry where, for example, a 10 g sample of neck skin is hygienically collected for laboratory analysis.

Non-destructive surface sponge or swab method

Using a sterile technique, a sterile sponge or swab, usually 10×10 cm, is moistened with 10 ml of diluent. The swab is then applied to a given site on the carcase, over a prescribed area. This may be achieved using a template applied to the surface with the standard area of, for example, 100 cm² wiped 10 times or wiped over a standard length of carcase – for example, 50 or 100 cm. The swab is then hygienically enclosed in a plastic bag and sent for laboratory processing.

The nature of the swab or the sponge, the pressure applied during sampling and the detail of the process all affect the outcome, making comparison of results difficult.

Deep samples are used to determine the levels of systemic contamination/infection within a carcase. Such contamination is not normally of environmental origin, having resulted from pre-existing disease or infection. Bacteria isolated from deep samples tend to be pathogenic in nature. Deep samples of meat must be taken with care in order to avoid contamination by superficial organisms. Such samples can be obtained using sterile scalpels and forceps or, in the case of frozen meat, a cork borer or an electric drill fitted with a bore-extracting bit. The surface should first be prepared by flaming, followed by an aseptic dissection of about 10 g of meat.

Destructive sampling may use surface slices where a known weight (usually 10 or 25 g) is removed with sterile scalpels and forceps and then homogenised in a suitable diluent, for example, Ringer's solution, using a stomacher or other means, to provide a 1:10 dilution before plating on appropriate culture media.

Alternatively, excision of surface material a few mm thick of a fixed surface area (5 cm² from each of 4 carcass locations, rump, flank, brisket and neck) using a similar methodology may be used.

Non-destructive sampling method using rinses and washes prepared by washing or rinsing one part by weight of the meat in 10 parts by weight of the sterile diluents is now more frequently used in the EU. Samples of 1:10 dilutions may also be prepared from comminuted forms of the meat since surface washing and rinsing do not give a true picture of the degree of contamination.

The US Department of Agriculture has mandated a rinse method for sampling poultry carcases for generic *E. coli* as a tool to verify process control (http://www.fsis. usda.gov/wps/wcm/connect/3efc7f8e-e6a2-4997-91ba-9c579c2a1f14/Guideline_for_Ecoli_Testing_Slaughter_Estab.pdf?MOD=AJPERES) where microbial counts of over 1000 cfu/ml are considered to be unsatisfactory (cfu – colony-forming units).

The UK Food Standards Agency (FSA) supports a web page (www.ukmeat.org) dedicated to providing the UK meat industry with information on microbiological criteria regulations, how to comply with the regulation, how to undertake the testing, a place to record results and advice on how to undertake corrective action when the criteria are not met. Detailed sampling methodologies across several species are provided (Fig. 12.3).

Microbiological laboratory analysis

The meat sample or the rinses from swabs or sponges form the material for the microbiological analysis. The majority of such samples are commonly sent by refrigerated transport to commercial testing laboratories for microbiological analysis. In brief, the solid samples are homogenised in a suitable quantity of diluent to suspend the organisms. A dilution series is then prepared by decimally diluting this original bacterial suspension. This dilution series ensures the growth plates are not subsequently overgrown by a large inoculum of bacteria. All suspensions are then plated out on a suitable growth medium.

A general growth medium such as a total count agar (TCA) will allow the growth of almost all organisms present that are capable of growth under the selected incubation conditions (non-selective media). TCA is normally incubated aerobically at 20 and 35°C to assess the levels of psychrotrophic and mesophilic Gram-positive and Gram-negative organisms present. The plated samples can also be incubated anaerobically to assess anaerobic and facultative anaerobic populations. On completion of incubation, the number of organisms per gram of sample or per cm² may be back calculated

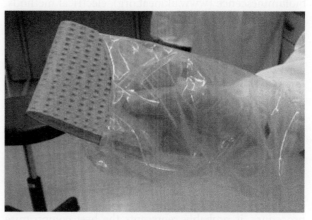

Figure 12.3 Non-destructive surface sampling swab.

depending on the original sample size and the levels of dilution employed. The colonies on these primary plates can be subcultured to purify bacterial colonies in order to help identify the organisms.

The medium used for growth may be selected specifically to provide information on one particular group/genus of pathogens or spoilage bacteria (selective media). Thus, specific agars have been developed for almost every pathogen based on the resistance of those particular pathogens to certain antimicrobial substances. For example, *Listeria monocytogenes* is resistant to nalidixic acid, cycloheximide, acriflavine and fosfomycin, and the inclusion of these in the media (Oxoid) restricts the growth of contaminating organisms, allowing a determination of the levels of these target organisms.

Despite being both simple and cheap, the *plate count* procedure is not an ideal method for measuring bacterial numbers. The most significant drawback is the time interval before a result is obtained, based on the visualisation of colonies, which may range from 2 to 7 days. In addition, the accuracy of this method, together with the representativeness of the sample tested, impacts directly on the variability of results recorded. Thus, manually completed plate counts are only accurate $\pm 2 \log_{10}$.

The automation of the plate count procedure, removing operator error as a source of inaccuracy, through the use of media preparators, automatic dilution and spiral plate makers and automatic video-based colony counters, for example, spiral plater (Whitley, Interscience, SciRobotics), Soleris (Neogene), and VIDAS (bioMerieux), are also available. These are valuable improvements and while expensive to buy are becoming easier and less expensive to operate; however, there are still delays in obtaining results associated with the analysis incubation time.

A number of *rapid methodologies* have been developed as alternatives to conventional microbiological methods. These include the use of hydrophobic grid membranes, bioluminescence (www.ukmeat.org), electrical methods, radiometry, microcalorimetry, biochemical reactions, immunological and serological reactions, nucleic acid (DNA) probes, DNA amplification (polymerase chain reaction) and flow cytometry. It is outside the scope of this chapter to consider each in detail. Such methods are now more commonly being adopted by industry, as on-site conventional microbiological culture has over recent years all but disappeared having been being replaced by low-cost off-site commercial microbiological testing. Manufacturers of such alternatives have both significantly reduced assay costs as well as reduced assay times. Despite the many problems associated with plate count procedure, it probably represents the best compromise between cost and performance and is the method which

is most widely accepted – it is in fact still the standard against which all other techniques are compared.

Bacteriological standards for meats

Various authorities, for example, the EU, the WHO Codex Alimentarius Commission and the FSA (United Kingdom), have laid down acceptance criteria for different types of meats. Although, as of yet, there are no universally accepted standard for the interpretation of bacteriological findings, the following are frequently used:

Microbiological criteria, which are mandatory criteria with legal backing

Microbiological specifications, which are generally contractual agreements between a manufacturer and a purchaser to check whether the foods are of the required quality.

Microbiological guidelines, which are non-mandatory criteria usually intended as a guide to good manufacturing practice

The International Commission on Microbiological Specifications for Foods (ICMSF of the International Association of Microbiological Societies) has stated that any microbiological criterion for food should contain the following information:

1 A statement of the micro-organisms and/or toxins of concern
2 Laboratory methods for their detection and quantification
3 The sampling plan
4 The microbiological limits
5 The number of samples required to conform to these limits

The ICMSF recommended that the *total viable count* at 35°C (or at 20°C in the case of chilled meats) should be less than 10^7/g and that *Salmonella* should be detected

---

The EU Microbiological Criteria Regulation No. 2073/2005 has defined:

Microbiological criterion is a criterion defining the acceptability of a product, a batch of foodstuff or a process, based on the absence, presence or number of micro-organisms and/or on the quantity of their toxins/metabolites, per unit(s) of mass, volume, area or batch.

Food safety criterion means a criterion defining the acceptability of a product or batch of foodstuff applicable to products placed on the market.

Process hygiene criterion is a criterion indicating the acceptable functioning of the production process. Such a criterion is not applicable to products placed on the market. It sets an indicative contamination value above which corrective actions are required in order to maintain the hygiene of the process in compliance with food law.

in not more than one of five 25 g samples. The ICMSF also recommended that *frozen poultry* when examined by rinsing should give a count at 20°C of less than 10^7/ml of the rinsing solution and that *Salmonella* should be detected in not more than one of five 25 g samples of the poultry meat.

The Commission of the European Union Code of Good Hygiene Practices gives indications on the microbiological checks on the general hygiene of conditions of production in establishments producing fresh meat, giving specifications on the nature of these controls, their frequency as well as the sampling methods and the methods for bacteriological examination (also www.ukmeat.org). These checks form part of the validation and verification of the mandatory food safety management system, which will incorporate the principle of the hazard analysis and critical control points (HACCP), which the operator must put in place and implement.

The monitoring of the safety management system may be used to assess the nature and degree of bacterial contamination on walls, floors, equipment and fittings and the hands and clothing of personnel. Tests at various operational stages, for example, at the beginning and end of work and after cleansing procedures, should provide criteria which can be reasonably maintained under everyday conditions. The results should be interpreted carefully, and allowance made for factors such as the time of year, time of day, type of stock being handled, cleanliness of animals, staff quality, etc.

While microbial counts form the basis of food microbiological criterion, they have limitations and should be interpreted with care for the following reasons:

1 Bacteria in food are not stable like heavy metals; their populations change constantly. Different strains of bacteria vary in toxin and allergen production and in invasiveness.
2 Food usually contains a variety of micro-organisms, some or all of which may enhance or inhibit each other.
3 Time of sampling, usually at plant or retail shop, gives no indication of the final microbial count in the consumer's home, long after sale.
4 The number of organisms or amount of toxin or allergen which affects man is not known.
5 Environmental conditions, for example, temperature, pH and type of sampling, markedly influence bacterial growth.

Part 3: Meat decomposition and spoilage

Decomposition is the process by which organic matter is broken down into a simpler form, primarily in meat protein but also fats and carbohydrates, by the action of bacteria, moulds and yeasts, reducing the meat into a number of simpler chemical substances, many of which are gaseous and foul smelling. All forms of foods in their natural state remain in a fresh and edible state for only a comparatively short time. Foods are rapidly colonised by bacteria, moulds or yeasts, which are the main causes of spoilage, a consequence of decomposition by factors such as enzyme action and oxidation.

Enzymes, present in all living cells, catalyse the complicated chemical reactions taking place in the cells. The process of *autolysis* – self-destruction or self-degradation – is essentially brought about by enzymes and at a rate which varies markedly in the different tissues. In general, it is highest in those tissues in which protein is synthesised in large amounts and which have high water contents, for example, gastrointestinal mucosa, testes, pancreas and adrenals. The *water contents* of some types of meat and offal are given in Table 12.2. Tissues such as the liver, kidneys and endocrine glands have slower autolytic rates, and the tissues with the lowest metabolic rates such as the skin, muscles, bone, heart and blood vessels have the lowest autolytic rates of all.

All forms of food are subject to natural deterioration, their shelf life being dependent on their structure, pH, composition, water content, presence or absence of bacteria and/or damage and conditions of storage. It is accepted that meat from fatigued animals spoils faster. The pH of the meat from these animals, on the completion of rigor mortis, is in the region of 6.5 rather than the lower normal value in a rested animal of around 5.6. Such a low pH (pH 5.6) slows the growth of bacteria, as this is outside their optimal pH range, thus slowing down the functioning of the enzyme systems and the transport of nutrients into the microbial cells.

Bacteria, moulds and yeasts are affected by factors such as temperature, moisture, availability of oxygen, nutrients and the presence or absence of growth inhibitors. Control of one or more of these factors inhibits microbial growth and lengthens the shelf life. In addition to microbial spoilage, physical damage which occurs

Table 12.2 Water content of meat and offal

	Water in grams/100 g of meat
Liver, ox, raw	73.3
Chicken breast, raw	73.7
Beef steak, raw	68.3
Chicken, boiled	61.0
Beef, corned, canned	58.5
Bacon, Danish, tank-cured	46.9
Bacon, English, dry-cured	36.3
Meat, dehydrated	7.5

during handling, transportation and processing can be regarded as a form of spoilage, as can the presence of insects, other pests and chemicals. Such physically damaged foods are more susceptible to spoilage by microbial action.

Fresh meats may be initially contaminated from many different sources – soil, dust, faeces, water and equipment – as well as from the hands and clothing of personnel. In addition, although it was originally thought that the flesh of healthy animals at slaughter was sterile, it is now known that it can harbour organisms, mostly Gram-positive mesophiles. Depending on the types of bacteria present, meatborne disease or spoilage or both may result, especially if substandard handling methods are adopted.

The main types of bacteria involved in the spoilage of meat belong to genera listed below with their characteristics.

Gram-positive organisms

1 *Brochothrix*. Grows under both aerobic and anaerobic conditions – optimum temperature 20–25°C – but can grow at temperatures as low as 0°C and optimum pH 7.0.
2 *Carnobacterium*. Grow anaerobically at high CO_2. Some can produce antimicrobial peptides and bacteriocin.
3 *Micrococcus*. Some are salt tolerant, some thermoduric and some psychrophilic. Cause spoilage of salted and chilled meats. Optimal growth temperature 25–30°C.
4 *Staphylococcus*. *Staphylococcus albus* is responsible for spoilage and *Staph. aureus* for food poisoning. Salt tolerant. Optimum temperature 37°C but can grow below this temperature.
5 *Streptococcus*, for example, *Str. faecalis*, *Str. faecium and Str. durans*. Wide temperature range for growth, 10–45°C. Some degree of salt tolerance.
6 *Lactobacillus*. Mainly mesophilic with some thermoduric and psychrophilic strains. a_w limit (water activity) value for growth −0.91. Can grow at pH of less than 4.5.
7 *Leuconostoc*. One of the lactic acid bacteria. Can produce slimes especially in high-sugar foods. Some are salt tolerant and some can elaborate flavours due to diacetyl production. Produced H_2O_2 which gives spoiled meat its green discolouration.
8 *Bacillus*, for example, *B. subtilis* (mesophilic), *B. thermophilus* and *B. coagulans* (thermoduric). Very active biochemically with strains that are saccharolytic (able to split carbohydrates), proteolytic and lipolytic. Some forms can cause flat sours in canned meats. Limit of a_w value for growth is 0.95.
9 *Clostridium*. Originate from soil and animal intestine. Proteolytic and putrefactive, for example, *Clostridium sporogenes* and *Cl. histolyticum*. Saccharolytic, for example, *Cl. perfringens* and *Cl. butyricum*.

Psychrophilic, for example, *Cl. estertheticum* and *Cl. gasigenes*. Limit of a_w value for growth is about 0.95 with no growth at a pH of less than 4.5. An important member is *Cl. botulinum*. Clostridia work with Lactobacillus and Leuconostoc (lactic acid bacteria) to produce large amounts of gas (H_2 and CO_2).
10 *Arcanobacterium (Actinomyces) – formally Corynebacterium*. Fine, non-sporing rods. Limit of a_w value for growth, 0.98–0.95. No growth below pH of 4.5. Some strains sensitive to reduced pCO_2.
11 *Microbacterium*. Limit of a_w value for growth, 0.98–0.95. No growth below pH 4.5. Psychrotrophic, insensitive to reduced a_w and able to spoil meat stored at chilling temperature with reduced relative humidity.

Many of the organisms tested earlier are able to grow under reduced and elevated pO_2 (partial pressure of oxygen). The former situation is made use of in vacuum packaging; the latter along with a reduced initial load of spoiling organisms, lowered temperature and a_w and increased pCO_2 has enabled chilled meat to achieve a shelf life of over 6 months within modified-atmosphere packaging.

Gram-negative organisms

1 *Pseudomonas*. The predominant bacteria associated with spoiled meat. Widely distributed in soil, freshwater and seawater and decomposing organic matter. Grow well in protein foods with the production of slime, pigments and odours. Preference is for a high a_w. Many are psychrophilic, but temperature range is wide.
2 *Flavobacterium*. Pigmented colonies (orange and yellow) causing discolouration of meat and other foods such as eggs, butter and milk. Some types are psychrophilic.
3 *Acinetobacter*. Able to oxidise ethanol to acetic acid.
4 *Achromobacter*. Similar in action to *Pseudomonas*. Forms slime. Includes *Alcaligenaceae* and *Burkholderiales*.
5 *Halobacterium*. Obligate halophiles spoiling meats high in salt content.
6 *Moraxella*. Sometimes classified as acinetobacter, for example, *M. liquefaciens*.
7 *Enterobacteria*. Abundant in the soil and intestines of man and animals. Commonly found in large numbers in raw foods of animal origin and also in cooked foods that have been contaminated in various ways. *E. coli is* indicative of faecal or sewage pollution. Spoilage of meat by fermentation of carbohydrates to acid and gas causing 'off' odours. The verotoxic strain *E. coli* O157:H7 is an important food-poisoning bacterium. Includes *Klebsiella*. Non-motile, non-sporing rods and the pathogenic *Salmonella*, *Shigella* and *Proteus* belong to the same group.

The main types of spoilage organisms on chilled fresh meats belong to the previous groups, which are responsible for *slime* formation during storage. These particular bacteria are found almost everywhere in nature, and it is practically impossible to avoid their contamination of carcases during dressing procedures. The time taken for slime to develop on raw meats is directly related to the initial number of organisms on the carcase surface. It is thus especially important to pay attention to efficient methods of hygiene at slaughter, during carcase dressing, refrigeration, storage and transportation. Chilling procedures do not prevent the activity of spoilage organisms, which can grow at about −7°C; critically, temperatures below 2°C will delay the onset of slime formation. Control of the relative humidity in chill rooms, that is, reducing the a_w, can reduce bacterial spoilage but results in a loss of carcase weight and liability to spoilage by psychrotrophic bacteria (*Pseudomonas, Brochothrix, Lactobacillus, Moraxella*) and some moulds (*Cladosporium, Thamnidium, Sporotrichum*). A reduced oxygen partial pressure (pO_2) in the vicinity of stored meat is of value in curtailing spoilage, as is increased pCO_2.

The spoilage process is initially fuelled by the breakdown of carbohydrate. As time passes, however, protein molecules are broken up into simpler substances by acids, alkalis, endogenous enzymes and bacteria, the degree of decomposition varying greatly with the different agencies. Of these agencies, the putrefactive bacteria carry the process further, breaking up the protein molecule into proteoses; then peptones, peptides and amino acids; and finally indole, skatole and phenol, together with various gases including hydrogen sulphide, carbon dioxide, methane and ammonia. It is the amino acids, non-toxic in nature, which furnish bacteria with abundant and available nutritive material, and their breakdown products which give the typical appearance and odour of decomposed meat. The recognised everyday signs of decomposition are marked changes of colour to a grey, yellow or green, a softening in the consistency of the tissue, a pronounced repulsive odour and an alkaline reaction caused by the formation of ammonia.

After slaughter of a healthy animal, decomposition eventually develops in the parts exposed to the air, the time taken depending particularly on the temperature and humidity of the environment. The primary surface growth is initiated by aerobic bacteria, among these being *Pseudomonas, Achromobacter* and some coliforms. These organisms extract oxygen from the meat surface and produce conditions suitable for the growth of anaerobic bacteria, for example, *Cl. sporogenes*, which can also grow within the deeper tissues where there is no oxygen. After surface putrefaction of meat has commenced, the process spreads gradually by way of the nerve and connective tissue sheaths and along the surfaces of blood or lymph vessels. The rapidity of the extension of the putrefactive process throughout a carcase is greatly influenced by the condition of the animal before slaughter. In exhausted animals or in those that have suffered from fever (especially from a septic cause) where the meat is alkaline, decomposition sets in very rapidly and quickly reaches the deeper parts.

The condition known in Britain as *heated beef* or 'heat shortening' and in North America as *sour side* is caused by inability of the freshly killed carcase to dissipate heat rapidly when carcases are hung too close to each other, thus preventing a proper current of air around the sides. This usually affects the prominent areas of the hindquarters and ribs. In mild cases where hot sides of beef have not been in close contact for too long, there is merely a blanching of the surface with no major loss of quality. A more significant consequence of slow cooling results in enzymes that enable ageing being destroyed, culminating in pre-rigour changes which impacts significantly on meat tenderness and eating quality. The condition is also observed in rabbits, hares and game which are packed in hampers or baskets while still warm and is known in the trade as *green struck*.

In animals that have died and have not been eviscerated, both external and internal decompositions occur simultaneously, owing partly to the high blood content of the meat and partly to the invasion of the abdominal veins by putrefactive bacteria from the intestines. The first bacterium to invade the carcase from the bowels after death is *E. coli*, which in warm weather may reach the joints within 24 hours; these bacteria use up the oxygen in the carcase and pave the way for penetration by anaerobic bacteria, for example, *Cl. perfringens*, from the bowel. The presence of a greenish hue, first apparent on the kidney fat and peritoneal wall, with the diaphragm soft and flaccid and lying close to the ribs, is a strong indication that evisceration of the animal has been delayed and calls for a severe judgement on the carcase. Lambs coming straight off grass and slaughtered in hot sultry weather have been known to exhibit evidence of incipient decomposition within 1 hour of dressing. Pigs in which evisceration has been delayed, particularly in the summer months, may show a greenness of the abdominal fat in 12 hours, while the kidneys, and also the liver, may exhibit a superficial black colouration; in the kidneys, this pigmentation is frequently confined to the anterior poles where blood collects due to hypostasis. This colouration, known as *sulphiding* or *pseudomelanosis*, is due to the formation of iron sulphide by chemical action between hydrogen sulphide from the digestive tract and iron from the blood haemoglobin.

In the case of *shot deer* which cannot be gutted immediately, it is customary among sportsmen to incise the abdominal wall, as a current of air cools the abdominal viscera and delays migration of putrefactive bacteria from the intestinal tract. Venison, which is particularly rich in connective tissue and therefore exceedingly tough after slaughter, requires conditioning by hanging before it is rendered palatable. It can hang for long periods without decomposition, and it is stated that the muscular tissue of deer possesses antibacterial substances which have an inhibitory action on a great number of putrefactive bacteria as well as on the bacteria responsible for food poisoning; in this way, conditioning or ripening can take place in venison un-associated with decomposition.

The smaller animals such as *game* or *hares* lose heat rapidly after death and at an atmospheric temperature of 16–18.5°C. Small carcases such as rabbits cool to air temperature in about 12 hours, whereas larger carcases such as sheep require about 24 hours. As this rapid heat dissipation inhibits the growth of putrefactive bacteria, it is practicable to consign feathered game and hares to market without removal of the abdominal viscera and packed in crates or baskets.

In British fresh *sausage*, the early stages of decomposition usually take place simultaneously throughout the meat substance, but all the accepted changes associated with decomposition may not be present. Valuable indications of unsoundness in fresh sausage, as distinct from smoked, are stickiness on the surface of the casing; in the early stages, a sour rather than a foetid odour as a result of the activity of lactic acid bacteria and *Brochothrix thermosphactum*; easy separation of the sausage meat from the casing; and a grey colour on section of the sausage. The odour of early decomposition may be detected by a boiling test, especially if a little lime water is added to the water before boiling.

It is important to remember that while the spoilage organisms indicate their presence by off colours, odours and tastes as well as changes in consistency, most food-poisoning organisms give no indication of their presence in food. Some, such as *B. cereus*, *E. coli* and *Pseudomonas*, as well as causing spoilage, can also on occasions cause food poisoning. *E. coli* is commonly found in foods of animal origin and is an indication of sewage pollution of water and unhygienic methods of preparation. The factors responsible for the onset of food poisoning (mainly lack of hygiene and careless storage of cooked and uncooked foods at temperatures suitable for bacterial growth) are virtually the same as those that lead to the spoilage of food.

Decomposition of fat

Rancidification is the chemical decomposition of fats, oils and lipids and follows oxidative, hydrolytic or microbial pathways. The problem of *fat rancidity* crops up in the storage of practically every foodstuff. An unpleasant odour or flavour in fat may be due to absorption of foreign odours, as in the tainting of meat or butter stored in a chamber previously used for fruit, atmospheric oxidation or the action of micro-organisms, which may give rise to extensive hydrolysis of fat. A small amount of free fatty acids, however, has little effect on flavour; it is more likely that the tainted flavour normally accompanying bacterial growth is mainly due to nitrogenous breakdown products of connective tissue.

Rancidity from atmospheric oxidation does not require the presence of micro-organisms and is the most common type of deleterious fatty change. The important oxidative lipids in food are the unsaturated fatty acids, particularly oleic, linoleate and linolenate, with the susceptibility and rate of oxidation increasing with their degree of unsaturation. Oxidation continues at low temperature since little energy is required for the biochemical reaction. Exposure to light is another factor which can predispose fatty tissues to oxidation. The natural resistance of some fats, for example, chicken fat, to the development of rancidity is due to the presence of antioxidants such as vitamin E. Beef and mutton fats are relatively resistant and cause little trouble except when frozen and stored at −10°C for periods longer than 18 months.

Bacon fat, particularly when exposed to light, is much more susceptible to oxidation. The type of feeding of the bacon pig also affects the rapidity of oxidation, for example, extensive swill feeding produces a soft fat with a high proportion of unsaturated fatty acids which tend to be converted to aldehydes and ketones, imparting the acid flavour associated with rancidity. The rapid onset of rancidity, together with a yellow colouration of the fat, has frequently been observed in carcases of pigs fed on cod liver oil or fish meal. A further deleterious factor in bacon manufacture is that during curing much of the natural resistance of the pig tissues to oxidation is broken down by the specific action of the pickling salts (sodium chloride is known to have a catalytic effect in fat autoxidation), and for this reason, bacon fat is more liable to develop rancidity than pork fat. Even at −10°C oxidation of bacon fat is appreciable within a few weeks, though if bacon is smoked subsequently to curing the absorption of phenolic substances confers a certain amount of protection against oxidation during storage. The time factor in the curing of bacon and ham is therefore of particular importance with bacon which undergoes a long period of manufacture more liable to become rancid.

Marked rancidity in pig fat is usually associated with a change in colour of the fat from white to yellow, and the rancid odour may be detected if a piece of fat is rubbed between the hands. Chemical methods of assessing rancidity include the measuring of peroxides produced utilising potassium iodide. The thiobarbituric acid (TBA) test and the Kreis test both rely on the intensity of a colour change to indicate the degree of rancidity which has developed.

Microbial-associated rancidification, a further factor causing taint in fat, is the activity of micro-organisms which produce hydrolysis, resulting in the liberation of free fatty acids. Experiments show that the fat of the kidney, brisket and back of the ox develops a taint when the free fatty acids reach 2.5–3.0%. The deep intramuscular fat of meat, as is seen in the marbling of prime beef, is not affected by hydrolysis or atmospheric oxidation and is therefore likely to remain sound for long periods, but the kidney and abdominal fat, being more exposed, is likely to develop rancidity early; it is for this reason that these superficial fats are removed by the retail butcher before the carcase is hung up in the shop. Fats should be regarded with suspicion if they contain over 2% of free fatty acids, although in practice the appearance, odour and flavour are the usual guidelines.

Bone taint

The rapid dissipation of body heat from a freshly killed carcase is facilitated when the surrounding air is cool, dry and in rapid circulation. The rate of cooling is slow in heavy carcases owing to their greater thickness and also in those which carry an excessive amount of fat, with the result that a high temperature may persist in the deep-seated musculature of these animals and give rise to deleterious change. This change, known as *bone taint*, is associated with the growth of putrefactive bacteria and occurs most commonly in the region of the *hip joint of the ox and pig*, but occasionally in the *shoulder region of the ox*, especially when ambient temperatures are high. The condition, which was commonly encountered in the days when there was inadequate refrigeration and during the warm summer months, is not a serious problem today.

Bone taint, or deep-seated spoilage of meat, is undoubtedly of bacterial origin. More than one organism may be involved, but the *anaerobic spore-forming bacteria* are the most important and probably emanate from the gut of the animal. It appears likely that the organisms enter the bloodstream before death, rather than during it or at the bleeding stage, and that this entrance is facilitated by pre-slaughter exhaustion, fright, shock or a sudden strain, for example, the ascent to the top floor of the factory, which predisposes the tissues around the head of the femur to bone taint. There is practical evidence that putrefaction can commence in the blood vessels of the bone marrow.

The synovial fluid of the hip joint is also a favourable medium for bacterial growth with a pH between 7.0 and 8.0, whereas that of muscle in complete rigour is usually below 6.0. The lymph stream may also be important, for bacteria resembling those in taints have been isolated more frequently from lymph nodes than from bone marrow and muscle. These bacteria may therefore be present in the lymph nodes during life and, under suitable conditions, may spread to the surrounding muscular tissue. The odour of bone taint is apparent in both the musculature around the femur and in the bone marrow; it is very typical, quite unlike that of decomposing meat and resembles the sewage-like smell associated with gut-cleaning. The condition may be associated with a change in the muscle colouration to a grey or at times a blackish purple, but frequently, the normal red colouration is entirely preserved.

Bone taint in cattle can be reduced by avoiding bacterial contamination of the carcase with rapid cooling to 1.5°C. Experimentally, tetracycline injections immediately before slaughter and antibiotic spraying of the carcase can prevent taint. The smaller butcher can aid the dissipation of heat from the freshly killed carcase of beef by removing the fat from the kidney and the pelvic cavity. Incision of the stifle joint, to promote air access and rapid cooling, will prevent the growth of anaerobic bacteria. To avoid bone taint, the temperature at the centre of the round must not exceed 4.5°C after 48 hours. Bone taint is a local condition requiring condemnation of the affected tissues, but in many cases, when the hip joint or round of beef is affected, generous trimming of the muscle around the femur is all that is necessary.

Taint in hams

Taint in hams is also known as *souring* and is attributed by American authorities to contamination by *Cl. sporogenes*, *Cl. pufrefaciens* and *Cl. putrificum*, which are proteolytic organisms and break down proteins into amino acids and ammonia. The taints in hams and beef are fundamentally similar in origin, being in each case a deep form of decomposition which is un-associated with any surface change. Though the blood, marrow, muscle and bone of normal live pigs are free from ham-souring bacteria, these micro-organisms may be present in such tissues soon after slaughter and develop rapidly along connective tissue bands between the muscle bundles. The sticking knife undoubtedly contributes bacteria to the bloodstream, which can be demonstrated experimentally by placing pure cultures of *uncommon* bacteria on the knife blade and isolating them from the tibia and other long bones. The marrow of the femur tends to harbour fewer bacteria than the tibia, and as American authorities note, *tibia sours* are much more common. Too large a sticking wound also facilitates deep-seated contamination, for the ham-souring bacteria appear to resist the high bactericidal properties of pigs' blood.

Phosphorescence

Phosphorescence is caused by a number of organisms, for example, *Pseudomonas phosphorescens*, which are widely distributed in nature, especially in seawater, and may contaminate a chilling room. These organisms are resistant to chilling room temperatures and their invasion of cold stores can be a matter of considerable inconvenience. At the commencement of phosphorescence, which occurs in 7–8 hours when the condition is artificially produced, the surface of the meat, when seen in the dark room, shows luminous areas scattered over its surface and appears as if it were studded with stars. If decomposition develops in the meat, the phosphorescence disappears. Salted or stored meat may show various changes in colour due to bacterial action. Scattered areas, reddish in colour and not unlike beetroot juice, are caused by *Serratia marcescens*, and a similar superficial change, but blue in colour, is seen as a result of surface contamination by *Pseudomonas cyanagenus*. *Pseudomonas cutirubra* appears to be the primary cause of 'red mould' on charque, the dried salted beef of South America. Meat affected with phosphorescence or abnormal surface colouration is unsightly and repugnant, but if no putrefactive changes are present, it may safely be dealt with by trimming.

Moulds

In contrast with yeasts and bacteria, moulds are readily seen with the naked eye, appearing typically as fluffy growths on old damp newspapers, walls, rotting fruits, cheese, jam, etc. They can occur in various colours, for example, white, black, green and blue. Unlike bacteria and yeasts, they are multicellular and typically consist of a mass (mycelium) of branched filaments or hyphae which bear reproductive bodies or spores. Along with yeasts, mildews, rusts, smuts and mushrooms, they belong to the class Mycota or fungi. Like bacteria, they are present everywhere and are responsible for many beneficial and harmful activities.

Moisture, temperature and organic matter are important factors in determining the presence and activity of moulds. The majority are mesophilic and have an optimum growth temperature of 20–30°C, but several types can grow at or just below 0°C, for example, the so-called *snow moulds* and those responsible for the spoilage of refrigerated foods. Some thermophilic species can grow at 50°C and higher but not below 30°C. Although most favour moist conditions, some, for example, *Candida, Rhodotorula, Cladosporium, Fusarium, Mucor, Penicillium, Rhizopus, Thamnidium* and *Sporotrichum*, are relatively tolerant to water availability (limit of a_w value for growth is 0.88–0.80) and can grow in a pH lower than 4.5.

Moulds first appear and grow most prolifically on the cut surfaces of the lean meat. Although the spores of moulds may have a ubiquitous existence, often in the air attached to dust particles, they cannot germinate without moisture. The growth of moulds can be prevented by low temperatures and attention to humidity; thus, proper ventilation in refrigerating and storage works is necessary so that circulating air may dry the surface of food and containers. The control of moulds in food products with chemicals is neither approved nor successful; the concentration of chemical required to inhibit growth increases rapidly with humidity. The chief *causes* of mould on meat are exposure to dust and variations in temperature causing condensation on the meat surface. Intermittent freezing or temperature fluctuations in a refrigerating chamber are common predisposing causes to mould growth.

Black spot

This is the most troublesome affection of imported meat and is caused by the mould *Cladosporium herbarum*. *Aureobasidium* and *Rhizopus* may also be involved. It is liable to attack quarters of chilled beef taken from ships and placed in cold store at a temperature above −8°C; some varieties grow at −7.5°C, while all grow well at around 0°C. In beef, black spot is commonly found on the neck, diaphragm and pleura, and in frozen mutton on the legs, inside the neck or in the thoracic or abdominal cavities. The spots are about 6–13 mm in diameter and occur on the surface of the meat. The dark colour is due to the fungal threads in the superficial layers of the meat, from which the mould derives the moisture necessary for growth.

Black spot cannot be removed by gentle scraping with a knife, and microscopical examination shows that the threads of the fungus, dark green or olive in colour, are interlaced between the fat cells in the connective tissue on the surface of the carcase; they do not penetrate to a greater depth than 3 mm, and the contiguous muscular and connective tissues are perfectly normal. Black spot may at times be accompanied by bacterial spoilage, when decomposition is manifested by a softening, darkening and sliminess of the carcase surface and is associated with the growth of micro-organisms of the *Achromobacter* group. Black spot which is not too extensive and which is unaccompanied by decomposition may be removed by trimming. This is invariably practicable in quarters of chilled beef, but in frozen mutton, the mould formation may be so extensive on the inner aspect of the carcase, neck and pelvic cavity that total condemnation is required. Mould formation accompanied by bacterial spoilage requires more generous paring and, at times, condemnation of the whole quarter. It has been repeatedly borne out by practical experience that meat affected with mould, and subsequently refrozen after trimming or wiping, will develop mould more rapidly and in greater abundance than meat which, though mouldy, has not been so treated. Meat which has been trimmed or wiped to remove mould therefore requires a quick sale.

White spot

White spot is caused by *Sporotrichum* and *Chrysosporium* and is the most commonly encountered defect of imported meat. It is seen as small, flat, woolly spots, frequently accompanying black spot of similar size, but it is whitish in colour and entirely superficial in nature. The spores can develop at −8°C, grow more plentifully at −2.5°C and become profuse when the temperature is above 0°C.

'Whiskers'

This fungoid growth belongs to the closely allied genera *Thamnidium and Mucor*. The hyphae grow well at 0°C and may project more than 2.5 cm beyond the surface of the meat, but they collapse in a relatively dry atmosphere. Though the growth of these moulds ceases at temperatures below −7.5°C, they retain their viability and proliferate if the temperature rises above freezing point; thus, the presence of 'whiskers' indicates the meat has been exposed during storage to a temperature at or above 0°C.

Bluish-green moulds

Bluish-green moulds belong to the genus *Penicillium* and are frequently on cheese, on unsound fruit and also on meat. They are superficial in character and grow with difficulty at 0°C, though conspicuous growths will occur at a slightly higher temperature.

The superficial nature of white spot, 'whiskers' and the bluish-green moulds renders their removal easy by trimming. In imported forequarters of beef affected with mould, particular attention should be paid to the sawn surfaces of the vertebrae, especially the cervical and first four or five dorsal vertebrae; all affected bones should be removed (an affected pleura or peritoneum may be removed by stripping). In spite of the non-pathogenic nature of most moulds, they may impart a mouldy odour and taste if extensive and of long standing. Moulds, too, may promote rancidity of fat, and in doubtful cases, a portion of the meat should be subjected to a boiling test after the meat has been wiped or trimmed.

Assessment of decomposition

The need has long been felt for a laboratory method to establish the extent of spoilage in meat. To be of practical value, such a test must be short and simple and must provide unambiguous results which can be interpreted with confidence. During the last 50–60 years, chemical, bacteriological and physical tests have been developed although none of these can substitute for organoleptic inspection by an experienced inspector.

Chemical tests

Various chemical methods have been suggested:

1 Tests based on the detection of free ammonia.
2 The determination of the total amount of volatile bases produced during spoilage. In neither of these cases does the test give a clear indication of spoilage until the meat itself smells sufficiently to be condemned sensorially.
3 The determination of free amino acid content as an indication of decomposition has been suggested, but it is likewise unsuitable except as a guide to advanced putrefaction.
4 The production of indole, sulphur and other volatile products in decomposing meat has also been investigated, but although in fish there seems to be a relationship between spoilage and the amount of total volatile reducing substances and total volatile acids present, respectively, such a relationship has not been established in meat.
5 Tests for meat spoilage based on either the oxygen requirements of the meat or on its power of reduction have been in existence for some time but have not proved of practical value.

Bacteriological test

Bacteriological methods have been devised to relate bacterial plate counts to the quality of meat, but these do not show any close relationship between the number of bacteria present and the degree of spoilage as assessed sensorially.

pH estimation

If the pH of deep muscle does not fall to 6.1 or below within 24 hours, it is likely that the carcase will decompose more rapidly than the norm.

Chemiluminescence

Chemiluminescence was used historically as a possible 'marker' for assessing the *freshness of food*. As food deteriorates, the unsaturated fats, oils and other lipids emit light. It is suggested the technique could accurately gauge the shelf life of products which might otherwise be prematurely withdrawn; develop an indicator of the life of oil, thereby improving the flavour of food fried in the oil; and assess the effectiveness of antioxidant additives.

Further reading

Jay, J.M., Loessner, M.J. and Golden, D.A. (2006) *Modern Food Microbiology.*

The European Union Summary Report on Trends and Sources of Zoonoses, Zoonotic Agents and Food-borne Outbreaks in 2011, http://www.efsa.europa.eu/en/efsajournal/pub/3129.htm

International Commission on the Microbiological Specification for Foods (Publications) http://www.icmsf.org/publications/books.html (accessed 11 April 2014).

13

Controls on veterinary drug residues in the European Union

Glenn Kennedy

Legal framework

Policy and legislation within the European Union (EU) lies within the remit of the Health and Consumer Protection Directorate General of the European Commission. These officials are responsible for the development and implementation of EU legislation on food and feed. In the specific area of veterinary medicinal products, they oversee and approve the monitoring plans submitted by EU member states and third countries and evaluate the results of those plans. They also implement the Rapid Alert System for Food and Feed (RASFF), described later. The Food and Veterinary Office (FVO), part of the Health and Consumer Protection Directorate General, is responsible for the verification of the implementation of national and community legislation on residues in the member states and for the inspection of laboratories to ensure compliance with the required standards. In addition, the FVO carries out missions in third countries to ensure that the guarantees offered by their legislation, residue monitoring plans and laboratories are at least equivalent to those in the EU. Within the EU, the primary legislation relating to veterinary drug residue analysis is Commission Decision 96/23/EC (1996). This chapter describes the implementation of this legislation in EU member states. It should be noted that the European Commission is in the process of revising this legislation, but it is likely that the principles described will remain the same.

Licensed veterinary medicines

All pharmacologically active compounds that are administered to food-producing animals must have been evaluated for their quality, safety and efficacy as part of the registration process. The number of licensed veterinary medicinal compounds is large – encompassing antibiotics, parasiticides, sedatives, tranquillisers, anti-inflammatory agents, etc. While the list of compounds included in this category is long, it is discrete. Each compound and each formulation have a unique and individual marketing authorisation. The basic principles established by the EU for the establishment of maximum residue limits (MRLs) are set out in Regulation (EC) No. 470/2009 of the European Parliament and of the Council (2009). This has introduced a number of significant changes to previous legislation. These include:

1 *Adoption of Codex MRLs without further assessment*
Before a veterinary medicine for use in a food-producing species is authorised in the EU, its active ingredient must be assessed for safety. This will usually mean an MRL is set. However, the EU is not the only body that sets MRLs. The Codex Alimentarius of the Food and Agriculture Organisation (FAO) is an international body that sets standards for food. The EU is a member as are individual member states. All are able to assess the scientific data for substances as they pass through the Codex system. The situation was that where Codex set an MRL, a further scientific assessment by the European Medicines Evaluation Agency (EMEA) had to be carried out before it could be included in EU legislation. The new regulation makes provision for **future** MRLs passed by the Codex Alimentarius Commission to be adopted by the EU without a further risk assessment, where the EU agrees the science.

2 *Extrapolation*
The majority of the first MRLs were set for 'all food-producing animals'. Subsequently, setting MRLs for specific species has become more common. Also,

Gracey's Meat Hygiene, Eleventh Edition. Edited by David S. Collins and Robert J. Huey.
© 2015 John Wiley & Sons, Ltd. Published 2015 by John Wiley & Sons, Ltd.

since the requirement for MRLs came into force, partly driven by the cost of providing the necessary data, more than 100 pharmacologically active substances are no longer authorised for food-producing species. This effect was not foreseen or intended when the previous legislation relating to the setting of MRLs was adopted. The guidelines for carrying out extrapolation have already been established. The Commission's proposal would make the potential for extrapolation to be a compulsory part of the overall scientific assessment of an application. This work would be carried out by independent assessors. It would not automatically require companies to provide additional data.

3 *Biocides*

In future, the MRL procedure for veterinary medicines will also be used to set MRLs for some biocides used in animal husbandry (such as disinfectants). The Commission is doing this because the previous EU law (article 10 of the Biocides Directive 98/8/EC) required MRLs to be set where 'relevant' for some in biocides. That directive did not establish the procedure for setting MRLs, and the Commission saw the current proposal as an opportunity to address this. Pharmaceutical companies would not be required to pay any extra fee for the work of assessing existing products for MRLs. However, if a new active ingredient comes forward for assessment, the company will have to pay the costs of the MRL assessment.

4 *Medicines for horses*

The new regulation gives extra flexibility regarding the availability of veterinary medicinal products for horses, which are categorised as food-producing animals in EU legislation. Some leeway for substances to treat horses has already been provided through Council Regulation 1950/2006. This established a list of substances for horses which are considered **essential**, but for which there is no MRL. Although MRLs were not set, the substances were reviewed by the EMEA, and a minimum 6-month withdrawal period was introduced. This is to ensure that consumers are not exposed to unacceptable residues. The European Parliament has proposed to widen the criteria by which substances can be added to the list. As well as substances which are considered 'essential for the treatment of equidae', the new regulation would add substances 'which bring added clinical benefit compared to other treatment options available for equidae'. Again, the EMEA would be involved in assessing the substances that would be subject to a minimum 6-month withdrawal period. These two measures are again to ensure consumers are not exposed to unacceptable residues.

5 *Withdrawal periods under the 'cascade'*

EU medicine legislation (Directive 2001/82) allows for the use of some medicines outside of their authorisation where there is no authorised medicine available to treat a particular disease or condition in an animal. This is known as the cascade. This process is subject to a number of restrictions. One of these is a set of blanket minima for the withdrawal periods that must be applied to such 'off-label' administrations. Another change allows the Commission to modify these withdrawal periods or establish other withdrawal periods (article 30.2 (a)). This will be done in accordance with the procedure referred to in article 89(2) of Directive 2001/82.

Hormones and ß-Agonists

Under the terms of Council Directive 96/22/EC, as amended by Directives 2003/74/EC (2005) and 2008/97/EC (2008) of the European Parliament and of the Council, the possession and use in food-producing animals of substances having a hormonal or ß-agonistic action are forbidden within the EU. This legislation:

1 Forbids the import into the EU of any food of animal origin from any country that allows the use of stilbenes and their derivatives or thyrostatic drugs in any animal food-producing species.
2 Requires the establishment of a split system for the import into the EU of food of animal origin from any country that allows the use of hormones or ß-agonists in food-producing animals. Food imported into the EU must have been produced without the use of hormones or ß-agonists at any time in their lives. There are limited exceptions to this rule. These exceptions are listed in articles 4, 5, 5a and 7 of the Directive. These exceptions relate to the use of certain products for clinical reasons and do not allow the administration of these compounds, under any circumstances, for the purposes of growth promotion.
3 Requires checks to be made on imports from third countries (i.e. non-members of the EU) to ensure compliance.

Prohibited compounds

Table 2 of Commission Regulation (EU) No. 37/2010 (2010) contains a list of compounds whose use in food-producing animals is prohibited within the EU. Their use is forbidden because no acceptable daily intake for their residues could be set and because residues of the substances concerned, at whatever limit, in foodstuffs of animal origin constitute a hazard to the health of the consumer. The compounds listed in Table 2 are *Aristolochia* spp., chloramphenicol, chloroform, chlorpromazine, colchicine, dapsone, dimetridazole, metronidazole, nitrofurans and ronidazole. Residues of these compounds must not be present in food imported into the EU from third countries. However, third countries may authorise the use of these compounds in their domestic production. They may also authorise their use in animals (farm and aquaculture) destined for the EU market – providing that residues are not present.

Unauthorised and unlicensed compounds

There are also a small number of compounds which may not be used in food-producing animals within the EU. Notably, these include malachite green (never evaluated as a veterinary medicinal product – as a consequence, no safety data are available), phenylbutazone (licensed for use only in horses, but not in horses that may be slaughtered as food), carbadox and olaquindox (formerly licensed in the EU but which lost their marketing authorisations because of concerns over the safety of these materials – particularly to farmers and feed mill employees).

Regulatory limits: MRLs, MRPLs and RPAs
Licensed veterinary medicines

Part of the approval process, referred previously, normally involves the establishment of an MRL for each drug in each species in which its use is licensed in a range of edible tissues. These MRLs are listed in table 1 of Commission Regulation (EU) No. 37/2010 (2010).

One complication exists in relation to specified feed additives (alternatively known as zootechnical feed additives). Under separate legislation dealing with animal feedingstuffs (Regulation (EC) No 1831/2003 of the European Parliament and of the Council, 2003) and for historical reasons, a range of pharmacologically active compounds – coccidiostats and histomonostats – have been approved for incorporation into animal feedingstuffs and for feeding to food-producing animals without the need for the establishment of MRLs. This anomaly is being addressed and MRLs are progressively being introduced for the coccidiostats (currently, there are no licensed histomonostats in the EU).

Illegal drugs

For illegal drugs, a different situation applies. The use of these compounds is forbidden in the production of food of animal origin. Therefore, residues are unacceptable, as their presence indicates that an illegal treatment has occurred. The consequence of this is that a "zero tolerance" approach to the presence of residues may seem to be a logical way of evaluating residues. Any amount is an offence. This was the approach that was adopted by EU

member states in 2002 and 2003 when it was discovered that a significant proportion of food (mainly poultry and aquaculture products from South and Southeast Asia and South America) contained residues of the compounds listed in table 2 of Commission Regulation (EC) No. 37/2010 (2010) – most notably the nitrofurans and chloramphenicol. Thus, consignments were declared as being 'compliant' or 'non-compliant' on the basis of the limits of detection applied in the various testing laboratories. However, the limits varied considerably between laboratories leading to pressure being brought to bear on the European Commission by third countries who wanted a minimum standard to be adopted – to allow for harmonisation between member states.

The Commission agreed that the 'minimum required performance limit' (MRPL) should be used as the reference point for action (RPA) when dealing with illegal veterinary drugs (Commission Decision 2005/34/EC, 2005). Prior to this decision, the MRPL had been intended as an internal quality control tool for laboratories in EU member states. However, with the adoption of this decision, its purpose changed radically. If the concentration of an illegal drug detected in a sample or imported consignment exceeded the MRPL, then severe enforcement action would follow. If the concentration was between the limit of detection ($CC\alpha$) and the MRPL, the sample or imported consignment would still be regarded as non-compliant – but it would be allowed into the food chain. Depending on the frequency of any such findings, more severe enforcement action might be considered necessary.

However, the number of compounds covered by MRPLs is comparatively small. To date, they have been established only for chloramphenicol (0.3 µg/kg), the nitrofuran metabolites (1.0 µg/kg), medroxyprogesterone acetate (5.0 µg/kg) and malachite (and leucomalachite) green (2.0 µg/kg, sum of both compounds). Under Regulation (EC) No. 470/2009 of the European Parliament and of the Council, a procedure for setting 'RPAs' for substances that are not authorised for use in the EU has been introduced. RPAs may be set in any matrix (irrespective of whether it is 'food' or not). If a sample is found to contain residues at or above any RPA that may be set, the food is deemed non-compliant with community legislation and should not be placed on the market. If residues below the RPA are found, the cause should be investigated to identify any illegal action and apply appropriate penalties. The legislation allows member states to refer substances to the European Food Safety Authority (EFSA) for its opinion. It is anticipated that existing MRPLs will become RPAs.

For those compounds not covered by an established RPA/MRPL, a non-compliant result remains as was the case in 2002. Any confirmed finding of a prohibited or unauthorised substance is deemed to be not in compliance with community legislation and should not be placed on the market. Thus, any sample with a confirmed concentration in excess of the detection limit (again, more properly CCα) is regarded as being non-compliant.

The National Residue Control Plan in EU member states

Compound groups

Council Directive 96/23/EC (1996) describes in detail the sampling that EU member states must carry out to satisfy their obligations. The compound groups that must currently be covered are shown in Table 13.1.

The regulation emphasises that official sampling must be unforeseen and effected at no fixed time or day of the week. For Group A substances, surveillance should be aimed at detecting the illegal administration of prohibited substances. To this effect, sampling should be targeted on the basis of criteria including sex, age, species, fattening system, background information and evidence or history of abuse. Commission Decision 98/179/EC

Table 13.1 Compounds to be included in an EU National Residue Control Plan

Group A: Substances having an anabolic effect and unauthorised substances	
Group A1	Stilbenes, stilbene derivatives and their salts and esters
Group A2	Antithyroid agents
Group A3	Steroids
Group A4	Resorcylic acid lactones (RALs), including zeranol
Group A5	ß-Agonists
Group A6	Compounds in table 2 of Regulation No. 37/2010 (2010)
Group B: Veterinary drugs and contaminants	
Group B1	Antibacterial substances
Group B2	Other veterinary drugs
	Anthelmintics
	Anticoccidials
	Carbamates and pyrethroids
	Sedatives
	Non-steroidal anti-inflammatory drugs (NSAIDs)
	Other pharmacologically active substances
Group B3	Other substances and environmental contaminants
	Organochlorine compounds (OCs) including PCBs
	Organophosphorus compounds (OPs)
	Chemical elements
	Mycotoxins
	Dyes
	Others

(1998) extends the criteria for sampling to include secondary sexual characteristics, behavioural changes, the level of development of the animals and their conformation. For Group B substances, surveillance should be aimed primarily at controlling compliance with the MRLs for veterinary drugs and pesticides and monitoring the concentration of environmental contamination.

Sampling levels for each species

Annex IV of Council Directive 96/23/EC (1996) sets out the minimum sampling frequency for each species.

In bovines, the number of animals sampled must at least equal to 0.4% of bovine animals slaughtered the previous year. Of these, 0.25% must be tested for Group A substances (with a minimum of 5% of the total being tested for each sub-group), half of the samples being collected from live animals on farm and half being collected at the slaughterhouse. The remainder of the animals sampled (0.15%) shall be tested for Group B substances, with at least the following distribution: 30% for Group B1 substances, 30% for Group B2 substances and 10% for Group B3 substances. The balance may be allocated at the discretion of the member state.

In pigs, the number of animals sampled must at least equal 0.05% of porcine animals slaughtered the previous year. For Group A substances (0.03% of animals), at least 1 farm per 100 000 pigs slaughtered the previous year must be visited. Each sub-group in Group A must be checked with at least 5% of the total number of samples. The balance may be allocated at the discretion of the member state. For Group B substances (0.03% of animals), the same breakdown as for cattle is used.

In sheep and goats, the number of animals sampled must at least equal 0.05% of sheep and goats over 3 months of age slaughtered the previous year. For Group A substances, at least 0.01% of animals slaughtered must be sampled. Each sub-group in Group A must be checked with at least 5% of the total number of samples. The balance may be allocated at the discretion of the member state. For Group B substances (0.04% of animals), the same breakdown as for cattle is used.

In horses, the number of samples taken is at the discretion of the member state and is to be in relation to the problems identified.

In broiler chickens, spent hens, turkeys and other poultry, at least one sample must be taken, for each category, per 200 tonnes (dead weight) of production, with a minimum number of 100 samples for each group if production of that category of poultry exceeds 5000 tonnes. Half of the samples must be tested for Group A substances (20% of those being collected at farm level). Each sub-group in Group A must be checked with at least 5% of the total number of samples. The balance may be allocated at the discretion of the member state. The remaining half of the samples must be tested for Group B substances, using the same breakdown as cattle.

In finfish, at least 1 sample per 100 tonnes of annual production is to be collected. One-third of the samples should be tested for Group A substances, the samples being collected at farm level on fish at all stages of production, including fish ready to be placed on the market for consumption. The remaining two-thirds of the samples should be tested for Group B substances and should preferably be collected at farm level on fish ready to be placed on the market or at a processing plant, providing that full traceability is possible. Other aquaculture products should be included in the sampling plan in proportion to their production as additional samples to those taken for finfish products.

In milk, at least 1 sample per 15 000 tonnes of production, with a minimum of 300 samples, must be taken at farm level or dairy level, providing that full traceability is possible. Seventy per cent of the samples must be analysed for at least four compounds from at least three of the following groups: A6, B1, B2a and B2e. A further 15% of the samples should be tested for residues of Group B3, and the remaining 15% may be allocated at the discretion of the member state.

In eggs, at least 1 sample per 1000 tonnes of annual production, with a minimum of 200 samples must be collected. Seventy per cent of the samples must be tested for at least one compound from each of the following groups: A6, B1 and B2b. The remaining samples may be allocated at the discretion of the member state but must include some samples for Group B3a.

In rabbits, 10 samples per 300 tonnes for the first 3000 tonnes of annual production and 1 sample for each 300 tonnes of production thereafter must be collected. Analyses for Group A compounds must be performed on 70% of samples. Of those, 70% should be allocated to Group A6 compounds and the rest to the remainder of Group A subgroups. The remaining samples (30%) should be tested for Group B substances, with at least the following distribution: 30% for Group B1 substances, 30% for Group B2 substances and 10% for Group B3 substances. The balance may be allocated at the discretion of the member state.

In farmed game, at least 100 samples must be collected. Analyses for Group A compounds must be performed on 20% of samples, the majority being analysed for Groups A5 and A6 compounds. A further 70% of samples should be tested for Group B substances, with the following distribution: 30% for Group B1 substances, 30% for Groups B2a and B2b substances, 10% for Groups B2c and B2e substances and 30% for Group B3 substances. The balance (10%) may be allocated at the discretion of the member state.

In wild game, at least 100 samples must be collected. These samples must be analysed for chemical elements only.

In honey, 10 samples per 300 tonnes for the first 3000 tonnes of annual production and 1 sample for each 300 tonnes of production thereafter must be collected. Of these, 50% should be allocated to Groups B1 and B2c and 40% to Groups B3a, B3b and B3c. The balance (10%) may be allocated at the discretion of the member state.

Relationship between species and substance to be analysed (Table 13.2)

Follow-up actions

Licensed veterinary medicinal products   When violations are found, member states are required to carry out an investigation in the farm of origin to determine why the limit was exceeded. They must take all measures necessary to safeguard public health and may restrict animal movements off the farm for a set period. If repeated infringements are found from a farm or establishment, intensified checks must be carried out for a period of at least 6 months, products or carcases being impounded pending the results of analysis of the samples. Any results showing that the MRL has been exceeded must lead to the carcases/products concerned being declared unfit for human consumption.

Prohibited and unauthorised substances   Where unauthorised substances or products or licensed products are discovered in the possession of non-authorised persons, they must be placed under official control, until investigations are complete and a representative number of samples taken for analysis. Where illegal treatment is established, the competent authority must ensure that the livestock concerned is immediately placed under official control – preventing movement of affected animals off the farm in question, except under official control. If illegal treatment is confirmed, following additional analysis, the positive animal(s) must be slaughtered and the carcases/products declared unfit for human consumption. If half or more of the samples are non-compliant, the farmer may be left a choice between a check on all the suspect animals present on the farm (at the farmer's expense), or slaughter of these animals. For at least 12 months thereafter, the farmer shall be subject to more stringent checks for the residues in question.

Sampling in third countries   Residue monitoring requirements for third countries wishing to export food of animal origin to the EU are also outlined in Council Directive 96/23/EC (1996). Article 29 (1) of the Directive states that a third country must submit a

Table 13.2 The residue or substance group measured for each commodity type

Group	Compound type	Bovine, ovine, porcine, caprine, equine	Poultry	Aquaculture and finfish	Milk	Eggs	Rabbit, wild/ farmed game[a]	Honey
A1	Stilbenes, salts and esters	X	X	X			X	
A2	Antithyroid drugs	X	X				X	
A3	Steroids	X	X	X			X	
A4	RALs and zeranol	X	X				X	
A5	ß-Agonists	X	X				X	
A6	Annex IV compounds	X	X	X	X	X	X	X
B1	Antibacterials	X	X	X	X	X	X	X
B2a	Anthelmintics	X	X	X	X		X	
B2b	Anticoccidials	X	X			X	X	
B2c	Carbamates and pyrethroids	X	X				X	X
B2d	Sedatives	X						
B2e	NSAIDs	X	X		X		X	
B2f	Others							
B3a	OCs and PCBs	X	X	X	X	X	X	X
B3b	OPs	X			X			X
B3c	Elements	X	X	X	X		X	X
B3d	Mycotoxins	X	X	X	X			
B3e	Dyes	X		X				
B3f	Others							

[a] Elements only for wild game.

plan setting out the guarantees and residue testing programme which it offers concerning the monitoring of food of animal origin destined for the European market for the groups of residues and substances set out in Annex I of that Directive. The plans submitted by third countries must offer a level of protection to the consumer that is at least equivalent to that offered by member state's monitoring plans. Third countries must establish a central competent authority that is responsible for:

- Drawing up a residue monitoring plan
- Co-ordinating the activities of the central and regional departments
- Residue monitoring and co-ordinating the prevention of the fraudulent use of substances and products on farms
- Collecting the results and sending them to the Commission, by not later than 31 March of each year

Monitoring of compliance with this Directive is accomplished by regular audits of legislation, controls and laboratory monitoring by officials of the European Commission's FVO, who may be accompanied by national technical experts to assist in the evaluation process.

Testing procedures and performance characteristics

Testing procedures

Within the EU, there are no official, prescribed methods of analysis for residues of veterinary medicinal products in food of animal origin. All member states are free to implement whatever strategies they wish to meet the EU's legislative requirements. However, all methods employed by the member states must meet the performance criteria laid down in Commission Decision 2002/657/EC (2002). The key criteria set out in this document will be described later in this chapter in section 'Analytical methods: Technical aspects'. Most EU member states operate a two-tier testing system to minimise the cost and maximise the efficiency and coverage of their testing programmes. Traditionally, broad-spectrum, high-throughput, low-cost screening tests have been used to sift samples into those which are 'negative' and those which are 'potentially positive'. Such tests now span the entire analytical spectrum from microbiological growth inhibition tests, commercial ELISA test kits, high-performance liquid chromatography (HPLC), to mass spectrometry (MS) (MS, single quadrupole, or MS^n, triple quadrupole, ion trap, etc.). All 'potentially positive' samples must then be confirmed using a second specific analytical test – increasingly, MS, coupled to either liquid chromatography (LC) or gas chromatography (GC), is used. All veterinary drug residue testing laboratories in the member states must be accredited to ISO 17025, must perform satisfactorily in proficiency testing schemes and are subject to regular audits by the European Commission's FVO to ensure the quality of their analytical work. There is no mandatory requirement for third country laboratories to be accredited to ISO 17025. However, without such accreditation, it is difficult to ensure equivalence. Similarly, there is no mandatory requirement for third countries to follow the same validation guidelines as member states. However, methods must be validated; otherwise, equivalence cannot be demonstrated.

CCα and CCβ

The performance characteristics CCα and CCβ were introduced to control the performance of analytical methods. In effect, CCα takes the measurement uncertainty associated with an analytical method into account at the level of interest. CCβ has no regulatory function.

For MRL substances, CCα is the drug residue concentration in a sample where there is 95% certainty that the true concentration is above the MRL. At concentrations below CCα, the sample is compliant. At concentrations equal to or greater than CCα, the sample is non-compliant, with a statistical certainty of at least 95%.

For banned substances, CCα is the drug residue concentration in a sample where there is 99% certainty that the sample is non-compliant (i.e. that the drug is present in the sample). At concentrations below CCα, the sample is compliant. At concentrations equal to or greater than CCα, the sample is non-compliant, with a statistical certainty of at least 99%.

Further details concerning analytical methods are to be found later in this chapter under technical aspects.

Sampling of imported food

Legal basis for sampling of imports from third countries

In addition to reviewing the residue monitoring plans and results from third countries by means of a desk evaluation and by FVO audit, compliance with the guarantees offered by third country plans submitted by third countries may be verified by means of veterinary checks at EU Border Inspection Posts (BIPs). The system of veterinary checks on animals and animal products is set out in Council Directive 91/496/EC (1991) (animals) and in Council Directive 97/78/EC (1998) (animal products). There is no statutory minimum (or maximum) level and frequency of sampling set out in these direc-

tives. Neither is a sampling level set in Commission Regulation (EC) No. 136/2004 (2004), laying down the procedures to be followed by EU BIPs.

Frequency of sampling of imports from third countries

All consignments containing food of animal origin must be subjected to a documentation check and to a physical check, which may include an examination for the presence of unacceptable residue levels (Annex IIIc of Council Directive 97/78/EC (1998)). Member states are obliged to inform the European Commission each year of the results of residue checks carried out on animals and animal products imported from third countries. There is no stipulated frequency of such import checks. A Commission recommendation on veterinary checks on animal products or products of animal origin entering the European Community from third countries (VI/2062/94) suggested that at least 1% of consignments be checked for residues (chapter VII, 4 b). However this document was never formally adopted by the Commission.

Interpretation of non-compliant results

Imported consignments that contain residues of licensed veterinary medicinal products in excess of EU MRLs may not be legally placed on the EU market and will be rejected. Imported consignments that contain residues of any of the illegal drugs at a concentration in excess of the MRPL (where set) may not legally be placed on the EU market and will be rejected or destroyed at the discretion of the member state. Where no MRPL has been set, the consignment will be rejected when the confirmed concentration exceeds CCα. It should be noted that interpretations and actions in different EU member states may vary in this case, too – as action is at the discretion of the member states.

The Rapid Alert System for Food and Feed (RASFF)

Legal basis and description of the RASFF

Regulation (EC) No. 178/2002 of the European Parliament and of the Council (2002) laid down the general principles and requirements of food law, established the EFSA and laid down procedures in matters of food safety. It also established the EU RASFF. The purpose of the RASFF is to provide the control authorities with an effective tool for exchange of information on measures taken to ensure food safety. Weekly summaries of notifications made under the RASFF are published on the Internet. These are available at http://ec.europa.eu/food/food/rapidalert/index_en.htm. It deals with issues relating to unsafe animal feedingstuffs or unsafe food products of animal origin. The nature of the hazard detected, the food/feed category affected and (usually) the concentration detected are summarised on these tables. In addition, further information on the origin, distribution and extend of the threat is listed. In the main, these are self-explanatory. However, some columns need further comment.

RASFF notification types

Alert notifications

These are sent when a food or feed (either domestic produce or imports from third countries) presenting a serious health risk is on the market and when rapid action is required. The RASFF member that identifies the problem and takes the relevant actions (e.g. withdrawal of the product) triggers the alert. The goal of the notification is to give all RASFF members the information to confirm whether the product in question is on their market, so that they can also take the necessary measures.

Border rejection notifications

These concern food and feed consignments that have been tested and rejected at the external borders of the EU (and the European Economic Area (EEA)), when a health risk has been found. The notifications are sent to all EEA border posts in order to reinforce controls and to ensure that the rejected product does not re-enter the EU through another border post.

Information notifications

These are used when a risk has been identified about food or feed placed on the market, but the other members do not have to take rapid action. This is because the product has not reached their market or is no longer present on their market or because the nature of the risk does not require rapid action.

RASFF news

This lesser category contains any information related to the safety of food and feed products which has not been communicated as an alert or an information notification, but which is judged interesting for the control authorities.

Notification basis

Some information on the status on the point in the feed and food chain at which the problem was detected is provided:

1 Border control – consignment detained
   Controls at the border posts of the outer EU/EEA borders when the consignment was detained, pending testing results.

2 Border control – consignment released
   Notification initiated through a sample taken at a border post for analysis, but the consignment was not detained, having been released to the market.
3 Official control on the market
   A result obtained as a result of a test performed on a product on the EU/EEA internal market.
4 Company's own check
   A notification initiated through a company notifying the outcome of an internal control measure to the competent authority.
5 Consumer complaint
   Notification initiated through a consumer lodging a complaint with the competent authority. Notifications initiated through reported food poisoning outbreaks are classified under this category.

Action taken

This represents the action already taken by the notifying country at the time of notification. If 'no action taken' is given for an alert notification, this normally indicates that the product is not on the market of the notifying country but that it may be on the market of other member countries.

Distribution status

This indicates knowledge existing at the time of notification about the possible distribution of the product on the market. This does not necessarily mean that the product is already on shop and supermarket shelves, available to consumers, as often it is not.

Actions taken following infringements

If a particular residue problem is identified as a result of positive results, alert notifications, adverse findings following an inspection by the FVO, etc, the European Community or individual member states may reinforce checks at the point of import (article 30 of Council Directive 96/23/EC (1996) and article 24 of Directive 97/78/EC (1998)). These give member states powers to intensify action in the event of serious or repeated infringement of community legislation.

In the case of unauthorised substances, these require that the Commission is informed of the problem (RASFF) and that the next 10 batches/consignments from the same source are impounded and inspected. If the additional checks confirm non-compliance with community legislation, the offending consignment may be returned to the country of origin, or destroyed, at the discretion of the national competent authority. The Commission must be informed of the results of the more stringent checks. All reasonable efforts are made to avoid trade disruption. However, in certain cases where there is an evident structural problem in complying with requirements, the European Commission has imposed protective measures, including import bans, pending satisfactory resolution of the problem in the affected third country. Such protective measures can include:

- Certification by the third country of absence of specific residues from each individual consignment (e.g. this was imposed on aquaculture exports from Thailand in respect of residues of the nitrofurans and chloramphenicol).
- Mandatory testing by EU member states of a proportion (up to 100%) of individual consignments from a third country for a specific residue (e.g. 100% testing was required of all poultry imports from Brazil in respect of residues of the nitrofurans).
- A complete ban on imports of food of animal origin from a third country (e.g. a complete ban on the import of food of animal origin was imposed on China).

In the case of authorised substances, a similar system applies. However, the imposition of import restrictions for repeated non-compliant results of a licensed veterinary medicine with an established MRL would, very much, be a last resort.

Analytical methods: Technical aspects

This technical section will be of interest mainly to analytical chemists but may be useful as background to official veterinarians.

Method specificity

A system of identification points (IPs) has been introduced to ensure the specificity of analytical methods. The concept of IPs is applicable to both qualitative and quantitative methods of analysis. The basic idea of IPs is that a laboratory is allowed to use any molecular spectrometric technique or combination of techniques in order to obtain the minimum number of IPs necessary for the proper identification of a component. The minimum number of IPs that must be obtained for identification of unauthorised substances is set at four. For authorised substances, the minimum number of IPs required for proper identification is set at three. However, in order to qualify for the IPs required for confirmation:

- A minimum of at least one ion ratio shall be measured.
- All relevant measured ion ratios shall meet the criteria described in the following text.
- A maximum of three separate techniques can be combined to achieve the minimum number of IPs.

Table 13.3 The relationship between mass fragments and IPs earned

MS technique	IPs earned per ion
Low-resolution mass spectrometry (LR-MS)	1.0
LR-MS^n precursor ion	1.0
LR-MS^n transition products	1.5
High-resolution MS (HR-MS)	2.0
HR-MS^n precursor ion	2.0
HR-MS^n transition products	2.5

Each ion may only be counted once.
GC-MS using electron impact ionisation is regarded as being a different technique to GC-MS using chemical ionisation.
Different chemical derivatives of an analyte can be used to increase the number of IPs only if the derivatives employ different reaction chemistries (e.g. trimethylsilyl and heptafluorobutyryl derivatives).
For substances in Group A of Annex I of Council Directive 96/23/EC, if the following techniques are used in the analytical procedure – (i) HPLC coupled with full-scan diode array spectrophotometry (DAD), (ii) HPLC coupled with fluorescence detection, (iii) HPLC coupled to an immunogram or (iv) two-dimensional TLC coupled to spectrometric detection – they may contribute a *maximum* of one IP, providing that the relevant criteria for these techniques are fulfilled.
Transition products include both daughter and granddaughter products.

For authorised substances, the use of HPLC with single wavelength ultraviolet absorbance is no longer acceptable for use as a confirmatory method. HPLC with fluorescence detection or GC-/LC-MS or MS^n detection is acceptable for the confirmation of authorised substances. For unauthorised substances, only GC- or LC-coupled MS or MS^n techniques are acceptable for use as confirmatory methods.

Table 13.3 shows the number of IPs that each of the basic mass spectrometric techniques can earn. However, in order to qualify for the IPs, a minimum of at least one ion ratio must be measured, all measured ion ratios must meet the criteria described earlier, and a maximum of three separate techniques can be combined to achieve the minimum number of IPs.

When mass spectrometric determination is performed by fragmentography, the molecular ion shall preferably be one of the selected diagnostic ions (the molecular ion, characteristic adducts of the molecular ion, characteristic fragment ions and all their isotope ions). The signal-to-noise ratio for each diagnostic ion shall be ≥3:1. The relative intensities of the detected ions, expressed as a percentage of the intensity of the most intense ion or transition, shall correspond to those of the calibration standard, either from calibration standard

Table 13.4 Maximum permitted tolerances for relative ion intensities using a range of mass spectrometric techniques

Relative intensity (% of base peak)	Electron impact – GC-MS (relative)	Chemical ionisation – GC-MS, GC-MS^n, LC-MS, LC-MS^n (relative)
>50%	±10%	±20%
>20–50%	±15%	±25%
>10–20%	±20%	±30%
≤10%	±50%	±50%

solutions or from spiked samples, at comparable concentrations, measured under the same conditions, within the tolerances specified in Table 13.4.

Performance characteristics

As stated earlier, the EU does not require the adoption of 'official methods' for the control of residues. Member states and their control laboratories are free to adopt whatever methods they wish, providing that they meet the criteria set out in Commission Decision 2002/657/EC (2002). This document has replaced the concepts of limit of detection and the limit of quantification with the performance-based concepts of CCα and CCβ, as described in ISO 11843. This can cause some confusion until it is clear that these parameters relate to performance of the method at the 'level of interest'. The level of interest depends on whether the substance is *authorised* (when the level of interest is the MRL, does this sample contain the drug at a concentration above or below the MRL?) or *unauthorised* (when the level of interest is zero, does this sample contain the drug?).

CCα, the decision limit, is defined as the concentration at and above which it can be concluded with an error probability of α that a sample is non-compliant. For most purposes, CCα is the more important parameter as it is the point at which a sample is deemed to be non-compliant.

CCβ, the detection capability, is the smallest content of the substance that may be detected, identified and/or quantified in a sample with an error probability of β. In the case of substances for which no permitted limit has been established, the detection capability is the lowest concentration at which a method is able to detect truly contaminated samples with a statistical certainty of $1 - β$. In the case of substances with an established permitted limit, this means that the detection capability is the concentration at which the method is able to detect permitted limit concentrations with a statistical certainty of $1 - β$.

For authorised substances, α and β are both set at 0.05. In the case of authorised substances, the decision that needs to be taken is, 'Does this sample contain an identified (at least 3 IPs earned) authorised substance at a concentration in excess of the MRL?' In this case, the level of interest is the MRL. Thus, if the MRL for an authorised substance is 100 µg/kg, CCα will be higher than the MRL (e.g. 115 µg/kg). The numerical difference between the MRL and CCα reflects the measurement uncertainty of the analytical method. If an analysis of a sample shows that it contains an identified drug at a concentration equal to CCα, there is a 95% certainty that the sample contains the drug at a concentration in excess of the MRL.

For unauthorised substances, α is set at 0.01 and β at 0.05. In the case of unauthorised substances, the decision that needs to be taken is, 'Does this sample contain an identified (at least 4 IPs earned) unauthorised substance?' In this case, the level of interest is zero. Thus, for an unauthorised substance, CCα will be higher than zero (e.g. 0.05 µg/kg). The numerical difference between zero and CCα reflects the measurement uncertainty of the analytical method. If an analysis of a sample shows that it contains an identified drug at a concentration equal to CCα, there is a 99% certainty[1] that the sample contains the drug. If the authorised substance has an established MRPL, CCα and CCβ should both be less than the MRPL.

Method validation

Commission Decision 2002/657/EC (2002) requires that analytical methods be validated and provides guidelines for validation. In common with other validation protocols, recovery, repeatability and within-laboratory reproducibility need to be determined. The document outlines procedures that may be adopted to measure these parameters.

For authorised substances, a set of samples of specified test material (identical or different matrices), fortified with the analyte(s) 0.5, 1.0 and 1.5 times the MRL, is prepared. For compounds with an established MRPL, at least three levels around the MRPL (e.g. 0.5, 1.0 and 1.5 times the MRPL) should be chosen. Where MRPLs have not been set for a particular unauthorised substance, the levels chosen should be as low as reasonably achievable. At each level, the analysis should be performed with at least six replicates. Repeat these steps on at least two other occasions with different operators and, where possible, different environmental conditions, for example, different batches of reagents, standards and solvents. Samples should be analysed, the identification criteria

---

[1] *The requirement that the substance must be identified (i.e. at least the minimum number of IPs has been earned) as well as the requirement that its concentration exceeds CCα means that the certainty of the decision is higher than the 99% claimed.*

applied and the concentration detected in each sample calculated. From this, the mean concentration, the standard deviation and the coefficient of variation (%) of the fortified samples should be calculated. These data may be used to calculate CCα and CCβ.

Proficiency testing

The use of proficiency tests, where different laboratories test the same materials using their own methods (providing that those methods are normally run under routine conditions), is a method of assessing laboratory reproducibility. Evaluation of laboratory performance is usually made by calculating a consensus value for the test material, based on the analytical results obtained by the participants. The calculation of a robust mean, following the elimination of outliers, is the approach most commonly adopted. This approach has some drawbacks – most notably that the consensus mean may be biased when poorly controlled methods are used by a large number of participants, leading to a wide range in analytical results. Numerical assessment of an individual laboratory's performance is usual effected with a z-score. This is essentially a measure of the deviation of the individual result from the consensus value. Underlying the use of the z-score is an assumption that individual z-scores will approximate to a normal distribution, with a mean of zero and a standard deviation of 1. Usually, z-scores are interpreted as follows: $z < 2$, satisfactory; $2 \leq z \geq 3$, questionable; and $z > 3$, unsatisfactory. The numerical values can be either positive or negative, indicating that the measurement was greater or less, respectively, than the consensus mean. The main value of a proficiency test is to highlight possible problems with an analytical method and to spur the participants with non-satisfactory outcomes to undertake some further investigation of the method and to demonstrate the implementation of corrective action.

Unfortunately, there are relatively few proficiency testing schemes available to scientists working in the field of veterinary drug residues. Some such schemes, such as those organised by the EU CRL network, are frequently available to EU member states only. Other schemes, however, are open to all participants.

References

Commission Decision 98/179/EC (1998) *Official Journal of the European Communities*, L65, 31.

Commission Decision 2002/657/EC (2002) *Official Journal of the European Communities*, L221, 8.

Commission Decision 2005/34/EC (2005) *Official Journal of the European Communities*, L16, 61.

Commission Regulation (EU) No 37/2010 (2010) *Official Journal of the European Communities*, L15, 1.

Commission Regulation (EC) No 136/2004 (2004) *Official Journal of the European Communities*, L21, 11.

Council Directive 91/496/EEC (1991) *Official Journal of the European Communities*, L268, 56.

Council Directive 96/23/EC (1996) *Official Journal of the European Communities*, L125, 10.

Council Directive 97/78/EC (1998) *Official Journal of the European Communities*, L24, 9.

Directive 2003/74/EC of the European Parliament and of the Council (2005) *Official Journal of the European Communities*, L262, 17.

Directive 2008/97/EC of the European Parliament and of the Council (2008) *Official Journal of the European Communities*, L318, 9.

Regulation (EC) No 178/2002 of the European Parliament and of the Council (2002) *Official Journal of the European Communities*, L31, 1.

Regulation (EC) No 470/2009 of the European Parliament and of the Council (2009) *Official Journal of the European Communities*, L152, 11.

Regulation (EC) No 1831/2003 of the European Parliament and of the Council (2003) *Official Journal of the European Communities*, L268, 29.

14

Health and safety in meat processing

Rosemary Lee

Accident statistics

The UK Health and Safety Executive (HSE) reported food industry injury incidence rates (i.e. injuries per 100 000 workers per year) averaged for the 3 years 2005/06–2007/08 as follows:

- Slaughtering – meat 1054
- Slaughtering – poultry 1459
- Meat and poultry products 1427
- All food and drink industry average 1470
- All manufacturing industry average 913 (HSE, 2009)

The British Meat Processors Association (BMPA) indicates that the accident rates in the meat industry put it among the worst performing sectors in the food industry (BMPA, 2009). In the United States, the injury and illness rate of meat processing is almost 3 times higher than that of the manufacturing average, while occupational ill health levels are almost 20 times higher (Horowitz, 2008). The HSE reports that the main causes of injury are as follows:

- Being struck by hand tools including knives
- Manual handling and lifting
- Slips mainly on wet or greasy floors
- Machinery such as conveyors, band saws, de-rinders, skinning machines, etc.
- Transport including forklift trucks (FLTs) at loading bays
- Falls from height – off ladders, stairs, work platforms, plant and vehicles
- Exposure to harmful substances and hot material

HSE also reports that in the food and drink industries, 5% of the workforce suffered ill health caused or made worse by work during 2001/02 (HSE, 2009). The main occupational ill health risks in meat processing are as follows:

- Musculoskeletal disorders (MSDs) from manual handling and repetitive work
- Noise-induced hearing loss
- Infections from microorganisms
- Carcinogenic risk from polycyclic aromatic hydrocarbons (PAH) from the process of smoking meat products
- Ill health from long-term working at reduced temperatures

The increased mechanisation of meat processing work which occurred in the 1980s resulted in the most dangerous aspect of the work changing to the day-to-day cumulative grind that generated crippling occupational illnesses (Horowitz, 2008). Occupational health is generally more difficult to manage than safety. The causes and consequences of poor safety at work are immediate and often relatively easy to deal with. The symptoms of occupational ill health develop over time so the connection between cause and effect is less obvious, but once the problems have been recognised and acknowledged, solutions are available.

UK legislation

The main piece of legislation relevant to all workplaces in the United Kingdom is the Health and Safety at Work Act 1974 (Health and Safety at Work Order (NI) 1978). This provides the legal framework for a comprehensive and integrated system dealing with workplace health and safety and the protection of the public from work activities. Employers must, as far as reasonably practicable, ensure the health, safety and welfare of their employees. The phrase 'so far as is reasonably practicable' allows the

Gracey's Meat Hygiene, Eleventh Edition. Edited by David S. Collins and Robert J. Huey.
© 2015 John Wiley & Sons, Ltd. Published 2015 by John Wiley & Sons, Ltd.

employer to balance the cost of taking action (in terms of time and inconvenience as well as money) against the risk being considered. An employer should keep up to date with health and safety developments affecting their industry as ignorance of reasonably practicable control measures is no defence in law. In particular, the Act covers the provision and maintenance of the following:

- Safe plant and systems of work
- Safe handling, storage, maintenance and transport of work articles and substances
- Adequate information, instruction, training and supervision
- A safe place of work with safe access and egress
- A safe working environment with adequate welfare facilities

There is an absolute duty on an employer with five or more employees to prepare and revise, as necessary, a written statement of safety policy, which details the general policy and the particular organisation and arrangements for carrying it out. The policy must be brought to the attention of all employees. The Act also imposes duties on employees to take reasonable care of their own safety and that of others who may be affected by their acts or omissions. Employees must also cooperate with the employer to ensure compliance with health and safety duties and not interfere with or misuse anything provided for health and safety. The Act gives powers to HSE inspectors to enforce the law, including in food factories, and they have the right to issue notices requiring action to be taken or to prosecute either the employer or an employee. The maximum fine that can be imposed by magistrates for health and safety offences is £20 000, and there is no limit to the level of fine that can be imposed in a Crown Court. Company directors and senior managers could also face imprisonment if they are found guilty of serious health and safety breaches.

The Corporate Manslaughter and Corporate Homicide Act (2007) sets out an offence that could lead to an organisation being convicted where gross failure in the way activities were managed or organised results in a person's death. This legislation applies to a wide range of organisations across both the public and private sectors. In England, Wales and Northern Ireland, the offence is corporate manslaughter, and in Scotland, the offence is corporate homicide. The offences do not impose additional regulatory standards but provide the courts with greater sentencing powers and a maximum sentence of 2 years imprisonment. The organisation will be guilty if the way its activities are managed or organised causes a death and amounts to a gross breach of a duty of care to the deceased. In law, a duty of care is a legal obligation imposed on an individual and requires that they adhere to a standard of reasonable care while performing any acts that could foreseeably harm others. A substantial part of this breach within the organisation must have been at a senior level. Senior level means people who make significant decisions about an organisation or substantial parts of it. This includes both centralised, headquarters functions as well as those in operational management roles.

General duties

The Health and Safety at Work Act does not provide guidance on specific aspects of health and safety. This is provided in a range of subordinate regulations and guidance. One of the roles of the HSE is to develop national standards and guidance for employers. They provide a step-by-step guide to assist businesses meet the requirements of the legislation, and the key points are detailed as follows (HSE, 2009):

1 Appoint a competent person to assist the employer meet their health and safety duties. All managers also have a level of health and safety responsibility for their staff.
2 Develop a health and safety policy. Successful health and safety management requires the effective implementation of health and safety policies. An essential requirement for management involvement at all levels is to define health and safety responsibilities in detail within the written document and to regularly check that responsibility is adequately discharged as this process leads to ownership of the policy.
3 The requirement for risk assessment is contained in the Management of Health and Safety at Work Regulations (1999), and all employers are required to carry out a suitable and sufficient assessment of the risks to employees and visitors. The findings of the assessment should be acted upon by putting sensible controls in place to prevent accidents and ill health and making sure the controls are followed. The risks in meat processing can be identified from the accident statistics and generally fall into the following categories:
   - Being struck by hand tools including knives
   - MSDs
   - Slips, trips and falls
   - Contact with machinery
   - Transport
   - Fall from height
   - Substances/microorganisms
   - Animals
   - Noise
   - Cold environment
   The hierarchy of control measures in the Management of Health and Safety at Work Regulations provides a

practical approach to resolving health and safety problems and ranks risk control measures in decreasing order of effectiveness:

- Elimination of hazard
- Substitution of hazardous processes or materials with safer ones
- Engineering controls
- Administrative controls
- Personal protective equipment (PPE)

Where possible, removing the hazard is the best option. Reliance on individual protection through PPE should normally be a last resort.

4 Provide basic welfare facilities including toilets, washing facilities and drinking water. Exact requirements are detailed in the Workplace (Health, Safety and Welfare) Regulations (1992). Showers may be required depending on the nature of the work. If these are provided, the risk from Legionella infection must be assessed and adequate controls introduced. Ventilation should be sufficient, with a warning device if an automated ventilation system fails. Temperature is to be reasonable indoors, with 16°C minimum or 13°C where physical work is involved. Lower temperatures may be required where food is handled or stored, and employers should then provide additional PPE to counteract the effects of cold. There is no maximum temperature given in the Regulations; however, if staff are working in high temperatures, management controls such as frequent breaks and access to drinking water should be introduced to control the effects. Adequate lighting should be provided; however, the safety requirements for lighting would be lower than those required for meat inspection. Emergency lighting is needed where a lighting failure may create a special risk. Facilities provided should include accommodation for clothing, changing facilities where work clothing has to be used and smoke-free facilities for rest and eating meals.

5 Provide free health and safety training and supervision. Staff should receive general health and safety training on the risks identified in their work, suitable control measures and how to report any problems or accidents. Specific risks may require more detailed training, for example, the correct use of respiratory protective equipment or the safe use of knives. The requirement for supervision is also stipulated in the Regulations to ensure the correct procedures are being followed.

6 The Safety Representatives and Safety Committees Regulations (1977) and the Health and Safety (Consultation with Employees) Regulations 1996 require employers to consult with employees. Health and safety issues should be discussed to allow staff to raise concerns and influence decisions.

7 Display the health and safety law poster or distribute the leaflet. These include basic health and safety information and let employees know who is responsible for their health and safety in the workplace.

8 Understand the Reporting of Injuries, Diseases and Dangerous Occurrences Regulations (1995) which requires employers to report work-related accidents, diseases and dangerous occurrences to the HSE.

9 Keep up to date. Managers should be aware of hazards and control measures suitable for their industry.

When two or more employers share a workplace, they must cooperate as far as is necessary to ensure compliance with all the statutory duties. The meat plant operator will take the lead in ensuring safety in the plant, but the meat inspection team manager must ensure the health and safety of their staff through communication with all parties.

Key topics requiring risk assessment

The appropriate control measures for a task are generally determined by conducting a risk assessment. The assessor must identify any foreseeable hazards, assess their risks and take action to eliminate or control them. Risk management is a problem-solving process that – when taken step-by-step – will lead to informed decisions about how best to avoid or control the impact of risks. Workers should be expected to contribute to the risk assessment process.

There are five basic steps:

Step 1: Identify the hazards
Step 2: Decide who might be harmed and how
Step 3: Evaluate the risks and decide on precautions
Step 4: Record the findings and implement them
Step 5: Review the assessment and update if necessary

Care should be taken to ensure that control measures implemented for specific hazards do not create new hazards.

Being struck by hand tools including knives

A recent study confirmed the high rate of laceration injuries in meat packing in the United States and indicated that knives were the most common contact object frequently resulting in finger injuries (Cai *et al.*, 2005). A UK HSE investigation into the nature of knife accidents in meat and fish plants reported that butchers/boners appeared to be most prone to injury, but slaughterers were involved in about one-third of the total incidents. During knife work, injuries can occur to either the non-knife hand or the knife hand. Injuries to the non-knife hand can be prevented by training staff not to make incisions towards the hand and through the wearing of

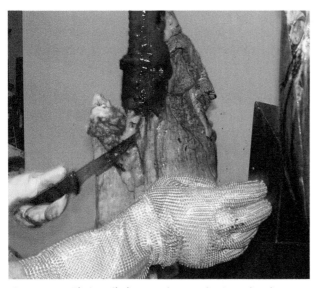

Figure 14.1 Chainmail glove on the non-dominant hand.

suitable gloves. All knife users should wear a chainmail glove on the non-knife hand (89/686/EEC and 93/68/EEC or EN 1082-1:1997) (Fig. 14.1).

These gloves can either provide wrist or whole arm protection which is recommended by the HSE. Knife slip is the most frequent cause of injury to the knife hand. Cut-resistant gloves should be worn on the knife hand. Staff training should highlight the need to keep the knife handle free from grease/fat and to grip the knife securely. Good knife design and proper handle guards will minimise this risk. Scabbards/sterilisers should be used to store knives when they are not in use, and when staff are moving around the workplace, the knife must be in a scabbard. Suitable protective aprons, such as chainmail, are recommended for deboning work or where the knife is pulled with the point towards the body. The apron should cover the body area from the mid-breast bone to mid-thigh. The weight should be borne by the wearers' shoulders and be adjusted to fit neatly against the body (DIN EN ISO 13998:2003). The lightest suitable apron should be purchased to reduce the risk of MSDs.

All employees must be trained in the use, care and maintenance of knives and other equipment such as scabbards and steels. To reduce the risk of workers accidently injuring each other with knives, there should be sufficient distance between workers. Knife workers should not be approached from their blind side, and care should be taken when sharing a steriliser. It is important to keep knives constantly clean and sharp, knife edges being sharpened 'little and often'.

The meat inspection team manager should ensure the risks from knives are assessed and suitable controls introduced. There should also ensure that all staff using knives are adequately trained.

Musculoskeletal disorders

The term MSDs refers to conditions that involve the nerves, tendons, muscles and supporting structures of the body (NIOSH, 1997). The European Agency for Safety and Health at Work (2000) defined work-related MSDs as a wide range of inflammatory and degenerative diseases of the body's musculoskeletal system. These include the following:

- Inflammation of the tendons notably in the wrists, forearms, elbows and shoulders
- Pain and functional impairment of the muscles occurring mainly in the shoulder and neck regions
- Nerve compression or entrapment syndromes mainly in the wrist and forearm
- Degenerative disease occurring in the neck, low back, hip or knee.

Woods and Buckle (2002) indicate that MSDs can result in pain, discomfort and numbness and frequently exhibit non-specific symptoms such as myalgic conditions in the upper limbs, back and lower limbs. All the definitions confirm that MSDs are characterised by pain and loss of physical function in the body, and the European Foundation of Improvement of Living and Working Conditions (EFILWC, 2007) highlight that this may limit a person's activities and restrict their participation in society.

A review of the literature (Table 14.1) indicates that MSDs are prevalent in slaughtering and meat packing operations. The main occupational risks in the food processing industry are MSDs from manual handling and repetitive work (HSE, 2007). A review of the literature indicated that in the meat industry, work-related MSDs

- affect all joints of the upper limbs;
- occur regardless of the type of animal being processed;
- occur in meat cutting, grading and wrapping operations at every stage of the production line (Toulouse and Richard, 2001).

A range of factors contribute to the development of MSDs, for example, physical, organisational, psychosocial and individual factors (NZ OSHS, 1997). High repetition rates, awkward postures and high forces are among the physical risk factors for work-related MSDs (Bernard, 1997). All these risk factors are common in the meat processing industry (Tappin et al., 2006).

In the EU, 17–30% of industrial workers report MSDs (Woolf and Akesson, 2001), and in the United Kingdom, in 2003, 14.5% of adults reported having a long-standing MSD (Office for National Statistics, 2005). The prevalence of MSDs in meat inspectors (MIs) in a period of 12 months was 82%, and as this level is much higher than that of the general population, it can be assumed that the

Table 14.1 Level of MSDs in meat processing by country

Country	Information	References
Australia	Meat processing classified as one of the highest risks for sprain and strain injuries. In 1995, the meat industry had an overall claim incidence rate five times higher than the national average and approximately one-third of these were due to work-related MSDs.	Caple (1992)
Canada	Meat and poultry processing are the highest risk industries for work-related MSDs	Yassi *et al.* (1996)
New Zealand	The meat processing sector has twice the incidence rate of the next highest industry.	Tappin *et al.* (2006)
Sweden	Survey of butchers reported that 92% had experienced pain in some part of the body in the last 3 months.	Magnusson *et al.* (1987)
United Kingdom	The main occupational health risks in meat processing are MSDs.	HSE (2008)
United States	Meat packing plants had the highest incidence rates of MSDs in 2002.	Piedrahita, Punnett and Shahnavaz (2004)
	The prevalence of upper extremity and neck symptoms was 2.4 times higher among women working in poultry processing compared to a community group.	Lipscomb *et al.* (2007)

type of work has an impact (Lee, 2008). This MIs prevalence is slightly lower than the reported rate of 92% for Swedish butchers (Magnusson *et al.*, 1987); however, this would be expected as butchery work involves more intense knife work than meat inspection.

Upper limb disorders (ULDs) are reported as being frequent in the working population with prevalence rates of 11.3% men and 15.1% women (Melchoir *et al.*, 2006). The HSE obtained spot incidence rates of ULDs in meat boning companies of 35 and 37.5% (Riley and Milnes, 2000). The prevalence of ULDs in the last 12 months among the MIs was considerably higher at 67% which would suggest that the work is increasing the prevalence of ULDs (Lee, 2008).

Low back pain (LBP) affects 60–80% of the general population in their lifetime and up to 33% of people on any given day (Anderssen, 1997; EFILWC, 2007; Walker, 2000; Woolf and Pfleger, 2003). Burton *et al.* (2006) indicate that the 12-month prevalence of LBP in industrialised countries is 15–45%. The prevalence of LBP in MIs was 52% in the last 12 months and 30% in the last 7 days which is comparable to previous surveys (Lee, 2008).

There is limited evidence available on prevalence of lower limb discomfort. However, in a recent study of MIs, 54% reported discomfort in the lower limbs in the last 12 months and 32% in the last 7 days, and this is considerably higher than reported levels in other occupations (Lee, 2008). Research on general fatigue in the lower limbs links both prolonged and static standing at work to lower extremity discomfort (Ngomo *et al.*, 2008). Discomfort causing chronic venous disorders increase with age and the number of hours spent standing, and it was recommended that standing should be combined with sitting tasks (Tomei *et al.*, 1999) (Table 14.1 and Fig. 14.2, Fig. 14.3 and Fig. 14.4).

Interventions

There are considerable constraints in developing effective interventions to reduce the occurrence of MSD's as slaughter establishments provide limited scope for work layout alterations and line speed is determined by commercial pressures. For LBP, sitting would be preferable; however, this would give a static posture and it is evident that for lower limb discomfort the person should move more. There is conflicting evidence on the benefit of mats and insoles on lower leg discomfort (Orlando and King, 2004; Hansen, Winkel and Jorgensen, 1998; Sobel *et al.*, 2007). However, both mat and shoe effects are reported as minimal compared to time-dependent effects (Hansen, Winkel and Jorgensen, 1998). A study of 12 poultry inspectors indicated that leg load was affected by the work–rest schedule and recommended not increasing the work–rest schedule above a ratio of 3:1 (van Dieen and Oude Vrielink, 1998). Dababneh, Swanson and Shell (2001) found that hourly breaks of 9 minutes from a meat processing line improved discomfort ratings for the lower limbs. Riley and Milnes (2000) recommended formal job rotation among a range of control measures in meat processing. Job rotation and regular breaks should be an integral part of the work schedule. It is apparent that any intervention would have to take a holistic approach to address the full range of MSDs present. The following points should be considered:

1 *Duration of exposure*
Look at job rotation, speed of working, breaks and provision of assistance. Take particular care when the duration of exposure is increased during overtime or peak demand working.

2 *Environment*
Make sure the temperature is reasonable and that there is adequate space and lighting. Where possible,

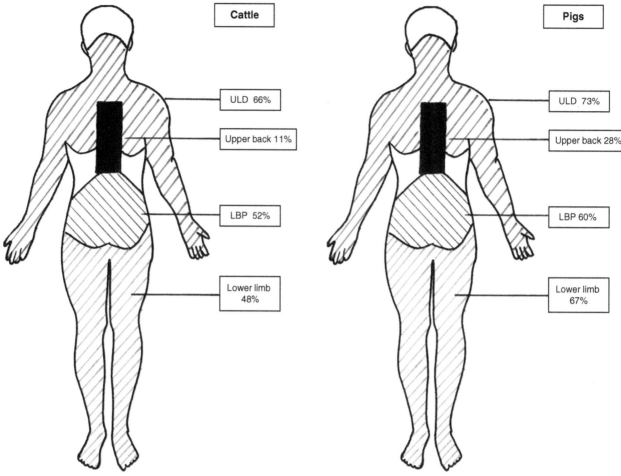

Figure 14.2 Prevalence of MSDs over the last 12 months among MIs working in cattle slaughter (Lee, 2008).

Figure 14.3 Prevalence of MSDs over the last 12 months among MIs working in pig slaughter (Lee, 2008).

seating could be introduced; however, usually on a kill line, space restricts this as well as the hygiene requirements.

3 *Risk assessment*

Reduce the injury potential in tasks where possible by tackling force, repetition and awkward posture. The use of a blunt knife causes higher force to be applied to make the cut and also increases the cutting time (Marsot, Claudon and Jacqmin, 2007; McGorry, Dowd and Dempsey, 2005). It is also important that the knife handle suits the user and is kept clean as forceful grasping due to a poor fit or slippery handle can result in ULDs. Repetition in the work is usually due to line speed and can be outside the control of the meat inspection team manager. Posture can be improved by reducing the need to work above shoulder height or below knee level due to the height of the platform, the line or the size of the carcasses. Where height adjustable platforms are used, this reduces the risk; however, in areas without height adjustable platforms, static stands may be considered to improve posture.

The position of the carcase relative to the worker is extremely important, and there should not be an excessive horizontal reach distance between the carcase and the platform. Twisting, bending and reaching due to restricted space, inadequate platform space, poor design or poor configuration and/or layout of associated equipment (such as sterilisers and tool rests) can also result in the worker adopting an awkward posture. Any improvements to the layout should be discussed with plant management.

4 *Pre-employment screening/Job placement*

This will help ensure people are not placed in jobs that will aggravate current or previous musculoskeletal conditions.

5 *Training employees*

Employees should have training and information on the nature of likely injuries and causative factors and the need to report injuries. They should also be made aware of the current medical advice regarding the importance of staying active and to continue as normally as possible.

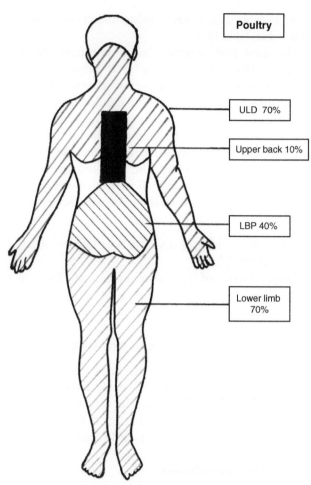

Figure 14.4 Prevalence of MSDs over the last 12 months among MIs working in poultry slaughter (Lee 2008).

6 *Monitor employees*
   Check on workers in injury-producing or aggravating tasks early in a new job, for example, after 4 weeks, to ensure no contraindications to placement.

7 *Occupational health guidance*
   Rehabilitation and monitoring of sufferers should be considered. Current research indicates that controlling the risk in the workplace has not reduced levels of disability and absence due to MSDs (Coggon, Palmer and Walker-Bone, 2007; Sprigg *et al.*, 2007). Burton *et al.* (2008) indicate that management of cases is more effective than primary intervention. Bongers *et al.* (2006) suggested that interventions which are aimed at a combination of the individual worker, the employer and organisational factors are the most effective. Work is beneficial and workers should be helped to remain at work, or in early return to work through rehabilitation programmes, to reduce future symptoms and sickness absence (Waddell and Burton, 2000). Research also advocates the need to address the

psychological factors which are present in the early stages of pain such as coping strategies, illness behaviours and fear avoidance beliefs in order to prevent the development of chronic pain (Buchbinder, 2001; Burton *et al.*, 1995; Pincus *et al.*, 2002; Waddell, 1991). There is modest evidence of the efficacy of a combined intervention of exercise and appropriate biopsychosocial education for LBP (Bongers *et al.*, 2006). 'The Back Book' has been shown to be effective in educating workers and reducing disability, and staff should be directed to the HSE website which provides the key messages on back care.

Manual handling

MSDs, usually of the lower back, can also develop as a result of **manual handling tasks** which are common in the meat processing industry, and many manual handling injuries are cumulative rather than attributable to one incident. Manual handling operations can be defined as transporting or supporting of a load including lifting, putting down, pushing, pulling, carrying or moving by hand or by bodily force. Manual handling accidents account for more than a third of all accidents reported each year to the HSE. The vast majority of manual handling accidents result in more than 3 days absence from work, most commonly as a result of a sprain or strain, often of the back. The general assessment of the risks will identify manual handling operations that require a more detailed assessment. The Manual Handling Operations Regulations establish a clear hierarchy of measures that must be followed where the general assessment indicates a possibility of risks to employees from manual handling:

a. **Avoid** the need for hazardous manual handling operations so far as is reasonably practicable.
b. **Assess** the risk of injury from any hazardous manual handling operation that cannot be avoided.
c. **Reduce** the risk of injury from hazardous manual handling operations, so far as is reasonably practicable.

Where possible, the need for the manual handling operation should be eliminated. If this is not reasonably practicable, then the meat inspection team manager should establish if the operation can be automated or mechanised. The manual handling assessment should be carried out by trained assessors who should have a thorough practical understanding of the type of manual handling tasks to be performed, the loads to be handled and the working environment in which the tasks are to be carried out. It will not be necessary to carry out the assessment each time an operation is carried out if it is repeated regularly. However, a new assessment must be carried out if there is a change to the load, the task or the handler(s). The assessment should be recorded and any required reduction of risks arranged.

All steps taken to reduce the risk of injury must be appropriate and address the problem in a practical and effective manner. If suitable mechanical assistance is available, it should be provided and used where appropriate. Staff should be trained in the use of any mechanical device or PPE supplied. Where the risk assessment identifies staff who will continue to carry out manual handling operations which may be a risk to their health, training must be provided in handling techniques. Consideration should also be given to staff with an underlying health condition that could reduce their ability to complete manual handling tasks such as previous back or knee injuries or pregnancy. The effectiveness of the measures taken should be assessed and if necessary the situation must be reappraised.

The meat inspection team manager would also be responsible for ensuring the other requirements of the Manual Handling Operations Regulations are implemented. This includes the following:

- Ensuring personnel are properly supervised and adhering to safe operating procedures
- Maintaining adequate documentation and records on all aspects of manual handling training
- Investigating any incidents relating to manual handling and initiating remedial action where necessary

Employees should be encouraged to report problems, accidents and incidents relating to MSDs that by be associated with either repetitive work or manual handling.

Slips, trips and falls

HSE figures indicate that slips and trips risks are especially important in the food industry because they occur four times more often than the average for industry and can result in serious injury. Employers should therefore assess slip and trip risks to both employees and others who could be affected and take action to control the risks. In the United Kingdom, the Workplace (Health, Safety and Welfare) Regulations 1992 states that the construction of the floor surface must be suitable, not be slippery, have effective drainage and have no holes. So far as is reasonably practical, the floor should be kept free from obstructions and accumulations of waste material. Due to the working conditions in meat processing, these requirements can be challenging. However, the HSE has provided additional guidance on how to keep floors dry (Table 14.2). If it is not possible to do this, the floor should be sufficiently rough, the environment, task and footwear suitable and individuals should walk appropriately to deal with the floor conditions. Non-slip footwear should be provided and replaced regularly.

Suitable control measures to reduce the risks of trips are detailed in Table 14.3.

The meat plant operator has responsibility for the floor condition; however, the meat inspection team manager should ensure that the risk assessment identifies any particular hazards. These should be raised with the operator. The meat inspection team manager would retain responsibility for the issuing of suitable slip-resistant footwear and ensuring renewal before the tread is worn beyond serviceability. The meat inspection team manager should also ensure all staff are aware of local deficiencies in floor surface and liaise with factory management to ensure the following:

- Adequate cleaning of floor surfaces to prevent build up of debris/blood.
- Proper ducting of waste water to maintain floors in a dry state.
- Walkways are kept clean, dry and clear of obstructions.
- All spills of oils and the like are cleaned up promptly.

Staff should be instructed in the safest way to walk on slippery surfaces (maintaining contact with the floor at all times and raising feet to a minimum extent at each step) and reminded neither to engage in nor to tolerate horseplay in the work environment (Table 14.2 and Table 14.3).

Contact with machinery

The most common machinery accidents in food/drink manufacture involve conveyors. For example, in April 2009, an employee of meat processing premises suffered a severe fracture to his arm when it became trapped in the unguarded end roller of a conveyor belt. The company and director were prosecuted by the UK HSE and fines and costs totalling £16 000 were imposed. Ninety percent of all the injuries involve well-known hazards such as in-running nips, transmission parts and trapping points between moving and fixed parts.

Under the UK Management of Health and Safety at Work Regulations and the Provision and Use of Work Equipment Regulations 1998 (PUWER), employers are required to assess the risks associated with work equipment and to either eliminate or control the risks. The term 'work equipment' covers just about every form of machine, appliance and hand tool used by people at work. If staff are responsible for operating machinery, then the risks have to be assessed and suitable control measures introduced.

Staff should

- not be permitted to operate any machinery they have not been trained to use;
- not inspect machinery while in operation;

Table 14.2 Slips risks controls

Causative factors	Practical measures for slips risks control
Environmental factors	
(a) Contamination of the floor For example, from • Spillages • wet cleaning methods • shoes • water and grease laden • vapour (poor ventilation) • natural contamination such as wet, and/or mud in outside areas • dry contamination, for example, polythene bags left on floors, product spillages or cardboard laid over spills	(1) **Eliminate contamination in the first place** If not reasonably practicable (2) **Prevent contamination becoming deposited on to walking surfaces** If not reasonably practicable (3) **Limit the effects of contamination** If there is still a risk
(b) Inherent slip resistance of the floor not maintained adequately For example, from incorrect or inadequate cleaning or maintenance or wear. **(c) The slip resistance of the floor is too low**	(4) **Maximise the surface roughness and slip resistance of the existing floor surface** If this is not enough (5) **Increase the surface roughness of the existing floor** (6) **Lay a more slip-resistant floor with higher surface roughness**
(d) Steps and slopes: do they cause sudden changes in step or not offer adequate foot hold and/or hand hold? **(e) Adverse conditions hiding the floor conditions and distracting attention** For example • low light levels • shadows • glare • excess noise • extreme temperature • bulky/awkward PPE	(7) **Ensure steps and slopes give adequate foot and hand hold and have no sudden changes** (8) **Ensure working environment allows good visibility of and concentration on floor conditions**
Organisational factors	
(f) The nature of the task • For example, the need to carry, lift, push, lower or pull loads • the need to turn, to move quickly or take long strides • distractions • having no hands free to hold on to break a fall	(9) **Analyse the tasks to see no more than careful walking is required in any slips risks area** (10) **Allocate tasks in slips risks areas only to those competent to follow slips precautions**
(g) Placing vulnerable individuals For example • poor knowledge of risks and measures • poor health and agility • poor eyesight • Fatigue **(h) Insufficient supervision** **(i) Safety culture which is not supportive**	(11) **Supervise to monitor physical controls and to see safe practices are followed** (12) **Establish a positive attitude that slips risks can be controlled**
PPE: shoe factors	
(j) Shoes offer insufficient slip resistance in combination with the floor surface, because of • type of shoe • sole material • contamination of shoes • sole pattern • wear • fit • maintenance/renewal	(13) **select suitable shoes for the floor, environment and the individual**

(continued)

Table 14.2 (Continued)

Causative factors	Practical measures for slips risks control
Individual factors	
(k) Unsafe action from staff For example, from lack of • awareness of the risk • knowledge of how slips occur • information and training or • distraction, carelessness	**(14) Train, inform and supervise employees** **(15) Set procedures for visitors**

Table 14.3 Trips risks controls

Causative factors	Practical measures for trips risks control
Environmental factors	
(a) Uneven surfaces For example, gullies, holes, steps	**(1) Eliminate holes, slopes or uneven surfaces which could cause trips risks**
(b) Obstructions For example, accumulation of articles such as work in progress or waste	**(2) Good housekeeping** **(a) Eliminate materials likely to obstruct and cause trips**
(c) Adverse environment For example, inadequate illumination to see floor properly, or glare	or if this is not reasonably practicable, **(b) Prevent material obstructing** **(3) Provide suitable lighting to permit obstructions to be seen**
Organisational factors	
(d) The nature of the task creates obstructions	**(4) Analyse the tasks**
(e) Safety culture which is not supportive	**(5) Establish a positive attitude that trips can be prevented**
Individual factors	
(f) Safe practices not followed	**(6) Train, inform and supervise employees**

• wear close fitting clothing;
• report missing machine guards;
• discard torn or fraying protective clothing which could snag on machinery parts.

Generally MIs do not operate machinery, but accidents can occur when the processing line does not operate effectively. There can be a risk at dangerous areas within the slaughter hall, that is, elevators/de-elevators, switchover points, hook return rails, etc. These locations should be highlighted in the risk assessment, and as far as possible, staff should not enter these areas. Safety helmets (BSEN 397:1995) should be worn at all times on the line and anywhere there is a risk of being struck by falling objects. Helmets should be replaced as follows:

• Normally at intervals recommended by the manufacturer or
• When the harness is damaged and cannot be replaced or
• When the shell is damaged or

• It is suspected that its shock absorption or penetration resistance has deteriorated, for example, when
  (a) the shell has received a severe impact;
  (b) deep scratches occur;
  (c) the shell has any cracks visible to the naked eye.

Accidents can also occur when staff are caught/snagged by moving offal hooks. Staff should be advised that entry to stands should never be through offal lines if hooks are sharp.

Staff should be encouraged to report near misses with machinery as well as any accidents to allow communication with the operator of the establishment. If there is a particular point of failure, this should be improved to prevent incidents. The meat inspection team manager should also liaise with factory management to ensure the following:

• All guards are fitted to machinery during operating times.
• Provision of cut-out switch in close proximity to all inspection points where inspector is within reach of fast moving lines.

- All staff are aware of position of stop buttons/cut-out switches.
- Maintenance of equipment occurs.

Transport

Workplace transport accidents in the food and drink industries are the second highest cause of fatal injury, comprising almost 30% of fatal accidents. During the 8-year period in the United Kingdom, between April 2000 and March 2008, 10 workers were fatally injured directly by workplace transport and a further 7 were fatally injured in transport-related accidents such as falls from vehicles. Each year, over 200 people in food and drink factories are struck by FLTs and other vehicles, frequently resulting in serious injuries.

The main causes of injury are as follows:

- Struck by vehicle (except FLT): 31%
- Struck by FLT: 26%
- Falls from vehicles: 22%
- Trapped between vehicle and wall: 6%
- Trapped by overturning FLT: 6%
- Trapped between two vehicles: 5%

Therefore, the priority areas which need to be addressed by the meat processing operator are as follows:

- Pedestrian safety and pedestrian/vehicle segregation
- Vehicle reversing
- Falls from vehicles

Other industry-specific hazards which can result in fatal injuries also need to be addressed, especially

- overturning of tipping lorries and trailers;
- tailgate safety on bulk delivery vehicles;
- FLTs falling from loading bays.

The risk assessment completed by the meat inspection team manager should highlight the control measures needed to provide a safe working environment. Controls that may be considered include the following:

a. Pedestrian/vehicle segregation both outside and, where possible, inside buildings.
b. Pedestrian crossing points.
c. Separate doors into buildings for vehicles and pedestrians with suitable barriers where required.
d. Designated parking areas for vehicles, including private cars.
e. Restricting access to loading yards to essential personnel wearing high-visibility clothing where necessary.
f. Reversing areas, if required, should be marked so that these are clear to drivers and pedestrians.
g. Vehicles should have reversing alarms fitted.
h. Only properly constructed cages on FLTs should be used for lifting persons.

Any site-specific hazards should be brought to the attention of the staff required to work in areas where vehicles operate.

Falls from a height

Across all industries, falls from height are the most common kind of fatal accident, and in the United Kingdom, 58 people died from a fall from height at work in 2007/08. Figures for major injuries to workers in 2007/08 show that falls from height accounted for about 12% of all major injuries. Falls from a height in the food and drink industries

- are the third highest cause of fatal injury, comprising over 20% of fatal accidents;
- are a significant cause of major injuries (broken limbs, fractured skulls, etc.) comprising over 9% of this category of accidents;
- result in about one major injury for every over-3-day absence injury;
- total more than 200 each year;
- can result in serious or even fatal injury even when the fall is less than 2 m.

The UK Work at Height Regulations 2005 apply to all work at height where there is a risk of a fall liable to cause personal injury. They place duties on employers, the self-employed and any person that controls the work of others (e.g. facilities managers or building owners who may contract others to work at height). These duty holders must ensure the following:

- All work at height is properly planned and organised
- Those involved in work at height are competent.
- The risks from work at height are assessed and appropriate work equipment is selected and used.
- The risks from fragile surfaces are properly controlled.
- Equipment for work at height is properly inspected and maintained.

There is a simple hierarchy for managing work at height:

- Avoid work at height where possible.
- Use work equipment or other measures to prevent falls where working at height cannot be avoided.
- Where the risk of a fall cannot be eliminated, use work equipment or other measures to minimise the distance and consequences of a fall should one occur.

The meat inspection team manager should liaise with factory management to ensure the following:

- Correct barriers are fitted to prevent falls.
- All inspection stands are properly serviced and maintained.
- Anti-slip strips are used, if required.

- Measures to prevent entry beneath falling platform are introduced.
- All steps provided for access to stands meet the following requirements:
- Regular rises of no more than 30 cm each.
- Handrails if overall height is greater than 45 cm.
- Steps provide good foot purchase.

The meat inspection team manager should also ensure that all staff are aware of the risks of falls from height, any control measures introduced and the requirement to never work from ordinary pallets, buckets or forks fitted to FLTs.

Substances/microorganisms

The Control of Substances Hazardous to Health Regulations 2002 (COSHH) in the United Kingdom and its amendments impose specific duties on employers to control hazardous substances at work and to protect people exposed to them. The amendments clarify good practice and introduce eight principles, which will apply to all hazardous substances. These eight principles are as follows:

a. Assess the risks.
b. Decide what precautions are needed.
c. Prevent or adequately control exposure.
d. Ensure that control measures are used and maintained.
e. Monitor the exposure.
f. Carry out appropriate health surveillance.
g. Prepare plans and procedures to deal with accidents, incidents and emergencies.
h. Ensure employees are properly informed, trained and supervised.

There is a single type of limit known as a workplace exposure limit (WEL). To achieve adequate control of exposure employers must

a. apply the eight principles of good practice;
b. ensure the WEL is not exceeded;
c. ensure that exposure to substances that can cause occupational asthma, cancer or damage to genes is reduced as low as is reasonably practicable.

The COSHH Regulations apply to a wide range of substances with the potential to cause harm if they are inhaled, ingested or come into contact with or are absorbed by the skin. These include the following:

- Substances used directly in work activities (e.g. adhesives, paints cleaning agents)
- Substances generated during work activities (e.g. fumes from soldering and welding, exhaust fumes)
- Naturally occurring substances (e.g. grain dust)
- Biological agents such as bacteria and other microorganisms

Substances are identified as hazardous if they fall into the following categories:

- Substances or mixtures of substances classified as dangerous to health under the Chemicals (Hazard Information and Packaging for Supply) Regulations 2002 (CHIP). These can be identified by their warning label as being very toxic, toxic, harmful, corrosive, irritant, sensitising, carcinogenic, mutagenic or toxic to reproduction. The supplier must provide a safety data sheet for them.
- Substances with a WEL listed in the HSE publication EH40 WELs.
- Biological agents (bacteria and other microorganisms), if they are directly connected with the work, such as with farming, or if the exposure is incidental to the work (e.g. exposure to bacteria from an air-conditioning system that is not properly maintained).
- Any kind of dust if its average concentration in the air exceeds the specified levels.
- Any other substance which creates a risk to health, but is not specifically covered by CHIP including asphyxiants, pesticides and veterinary medicines.

COSHH does not apply to the following:

- Asbestos and lead, which have their own regulations;
- Substances that are hazardous only because they are
  - radioactive;
  - at high pressure;
  - at extreme temperatures;
  - have explosive or flammable properties;
  - biological agents that are outside the employer's control, for example, catching an infection from another member of staff.

The meat inspection team manager is responsible for the following:

- Ensuring the COSHH assessments of substances hazardous to health are completed.
- Taking any action required as a result of COSHH assessments, introducing controls, arranging any health surveillance if required.
- Ensuring staff are provided with information on any risks identified, and on control measures to be followed. This may be completed through the use of a safe operating procedure/method statement, where appropriate. If a visitor or contractor could be exposed, they should also receive information on the control measures.
- Identifying health and safety training needs and ensuring that these are met.

COSHH hazards in the meat industry fall into three categories which are zoonoses, cleaning and disinfectant materials and food ingredients.

Zoonoses

Workers in the meat industry, especially in the slaughtering sector, are at risk in acquiring certain *zoonoses* (*diseases naturally transmitted between animals and man*). Analysis of surveillance figures by occupation and industry shows that the highest rates relate to poultry dressers. These can result in anything from a mild to severe disease, which in some cases may be fatal without appropriate and prompt treatment. The signs and symptoms of many of the zoonotic diseases are similar to general viral illnesses. Therefore, it is important that those who may be exposed have sufficient information to ensure they are aware of the risks and the need to receive prompt treatment. Zoonoses that may present a risk in meat processing are detailed in Table 14.4.

Generally, serious infections do not frequently occur in meat processing and for the majority standard hygiene coupled with normal safety controls are effective at controlling the risk. The use of chainmail and cut-resistant gloves reduces the risk of cuts and entry of infections into the body. Staff should also observe good personal hygiene and cover any cuts with a waterproof dressing. There should be no drinking, eating or smoking in animal holding or processing areas. Additional controls are required for some infections such as tuberculosis, brucellosis, BSE and Q fever.

General control measures for zoonoses

1 Education of workers as to the nature of zoonoses and how to minimise the risk of infection by careful handling of potentially infected stock, carcases and offal
2 Efficient veterinary ante-mortem inspection, especially with casualty animals, and the immediate alerting of staff to all disease hazards
3 High standards of personal and environmental hygiene
4 Avoidance of cuts, wounds and abrasions with prompt and efficient treatment when they occur
5 Proper meat plant construction and layout and ventilation with good staff facilities (showers, toilets, hand washing, use of bactericidal soaps, etc.)
6 Good first-aid facilities
7 Vaccination of staff where appropriate
8 Where possible, elimination of disease in domestic animals
9 Close liaison with medical expertise (Table 14.4)

Specific control measures for zoonoses

There are a number of diseases that require additional control measures. These include tuberculosis, brucellosis, BSE and Q fever. One aspect of the controls is the requirement for the respiratory protective equipment. For any respiratory protective equipment that does not operate on positive pressure, that is, disposable masks, half face masks and full face masks, the initial selection should include a face fit test to ensure it is suitable for the wearer. The test must be carried out by a competent person and the results need to be recorded. Staff should also be trained in the use of respiratory protective equipment.

Tuberculosis

The handling of tuberculosis reactor animals or their viscera has the potential to present a risk of becoming infected with tuberculosis.

Precautions

1 Tuberculosis reactors and inconclusive animals should be held or penned in a separate part of the lairage. This part must be very thoroughly cleansed and disinfected after use.
2 Staff working in the lairage should wear protective clothing, that is, brown dust coat/PVC coat, washable leggings and boots. If staff are involved in the handling of such animals, they must wear disposable gloves. These should be disposed of safely after use and hands thoroughly washed. At the end of the day, washable protective clothing must be thoroughly cleansed and disinfected and brown dust coats, if worn, despatched to the laundry as soon as possible.
3 Full protective clothing, that is, safety-type helmet, coat, apron, rubber boots, rubber gloves, hairnet and face mask (EN 149 FFP3) and safety glasses (BS2092) must be worn while post-mortem examination and sampling is being carried out on these animals. Bags containing pathological samples must be handled with the utmost care as the external surfaces may have been contaminated during collection. Disposable/ rubber gloves must be worn during packaging and this should be done in a designated area. Any surfaces which have come into contact with these bags must be thoroughly cleansed and disinfected after packaging is completed.
4 Protective clothing worn, as mentioned in point (3), while carrying out operations must be changed, or cleansed and disinfected after each session when tuberculosis reactor or in-contact animals have been slaughtered. Rubber gloves, if not disposable, should be thoroughly washed using a disinfectant soap.
5 The utmost personal hygiene should be maintained. Fingernails should be kept short and clean, and hands and exposed arms should be thoroughly washed using a disinfectant soap following removal and cleansing of protective clothing. Abrasions of the skin and even small cuts should be covered with a waterproof dressing.

Table 14.4 Meat processing zoonoses (DEFRA, 2007)

Anthrax

Causative agent	*Bacillus anthracis*
Natural hosts	Cattle, horse, pigs
Disease in humans	Cutaneous anthrax results in raised boil-like lesions with black discolouration on the skin. Pneumonic anthrax results in haemorrhagic pleural effusions, severe septicaemia, meningitis and high mortality rates.
Transmission	Cutaneous anthrax occurs through direct handling of products from infected animals. Pneumonic anthrax can be caused by inhaling spores from wool from infected carcasses.
Incidence	The risk of infection to human contacts from a confirmed animal case is very low. No cases were reported in England, Wales, Scotland or Northern Ireland since 2007.

Avian influenza

Causative agent	Type A influenza virus
Natural hosts	Birds
Disease in humans	Influenza-like illnesses
Transmission	Through breathing in the virus during exposure to infected poultry and occasionally close contact with human cases
Incidence	During 2007, there were 85 cases of AI (H5N1) infection in humans worldwide which resulted in 57 deaths in seven different countries. In 2007, the first internationally recognised outbreak of H7N2 infection affecting a number of people occurred in North West England and North Wales. Cases had a history of exposure to infected poultry premises or close contact with confirmed cases.

Bovine tuberculosis

Causative agent	*Mycobacterium bovis*
Natural hosts	Cattle
Disease in humans	Disease develops slowly, usually takes several months for symptoms to appear; symptoms include fever and night sweats, coughing, losing weight and blood in phlegm or spit.
Transmission	Breathing in infectious respiratory discharges
Incidence	There were 27 cases in GB in 2007 and none of these were linked with disease in cattle.

Brucellosis

Causative agent	*Brucella abortus*
Natural hosts	Cattle
Disease in humans	Cases of brucellosis infection in humans are associated with symptoms such as undulant fever, sweats and headache.
Transmission	Eating or drinking contaminated material, inhalation of the organism from infected animals or through skin wounds.
Incidence	In GB, where cattle herds are officially free of infection with *Brucella abortus*, brucellosis infection in humans is generally acquired abroad. There were two reports of *B. abortus* in Scotland in 2007. No cases of *B. abortus* were recorded in England and Wales in 2007. *B. abortus* is present in cattle in Northern Ireland, and in 2007, there were five cases of human *B. abortus* infection. All five cases are thought to have acquired the infection occupationally.

BSE/vCJD

Causative agent	Bovine spongiform encephalopathy agent
Natural hosts	Cattle
Disease in humans	vCJD is a rare and fatal condition of humans that affects the nervous system.
Transmission	Eating contaminated beef products. Contact with specified risk material during slaughter of infected animals.
Incidence	Five deaths from confirmed vCJD were recorded in 2007 bringing the total number of reported cases in the United Kingdom to 166 of whom 150 have died. No details of occupational links.

Camphylobacter

Causative agent	*Camphylobacter*
Natural hosts	Poultry, cattle
Disease in humans	Bacterial food poisoning
Transmission	Inhaling bacteria from infected carcasses, guts and faecal material
Incidence	*Campylobacter* infection remained the most commonly reported cause of bacterial food poisoning in humans in 2007. There are no figures for occupationally acquired infections.

(continued)

Table 14.4 (Continued)

Cryptosporidisos

Causative agent	*Cryptosporidium parvum*
Natural hosts	Infected animals
Disease in humans	The most common symptom of cryptosporidiosis is gastrointestinal illness. Other symptoms include stomach cramps or pain, dehydration, nausea, vomiting, fever and weight loss
Transmission	Through hand-to-mouth contact following contamination by handling an infected animal or through exposure to faeces.
Incidence	No details of occupationally acquired infections

Enzootic abortion

Causative agent	*Chlamydophilia abortus*
Natural hosts	Sheep, goats, cattle
Disease in humans	Symptoms in humans include gastrointestinal pain and vomiting, headache, insomnia and pneumonia.
Transmission	Human infection occurs by inhalation following exposure to infected aerosols, dust-infected bird droppings and nasal discharges and sheep foetuses and membranes.
Incidence	In 2007, there were six infections in women in GB – none of whom were pregnant. No details of occupationally acquired infections.

Leptospirosis

Causative agent	*Leptospira hardjo* *Leptospira. icterohaemorrhagiae*
Natural hosts	Cattle (*L. hardjo*) and Rodents (*L. icterohaemorrhagiae*)
Disease in humans	Cattle – flu-like illness of short duration, often with headache. Rodents – Weil's disease – fever, headache, vomiting, muscle pain, can lead to jaundice, meningitis and kidney failure – can be fatal.
Transmission	Cattle – splashing of urine Rodents – direct contact through breaks in the skin with infected urine or water contaminated with urine
Incidence	There were two cases of human leptospirosis in Northern Ireland in 2007. There were six confirmed cases in Scotland. In England and Wales, there were 74 cases in 2007 (indigenous and overseas acquired) of which 34 were indigenously acquired. Nearly half of all infections were thought to be acquired through the recreational route.

Orf

Causative agent	Orf virus
Natural hosts	Sheep and goats
Disease in humans	Causes ulcerative lesions on the face, hands and arms
Transmission	Direct skin contact with lesions on animals or by contact with virus on infected wool, hedges/fences, etc. where it can survive indefinitely
Incidence	In 2007, two human cases were reported in GB.

Q fever

Causative agent	*Coxiella burnetii*
Natural hosts	Sheep and cattle
Disease in humans	Mild illness – chills, headaches and general malaise, but rarely can progress to pneumonia, liver and heart valve damage and death
Transmission	Usually by breathing in dust contaminated by placental tissue, amniotic fluids, urine and faeces. Also direct contact with the animal and these secreta/excreta. Microorganism is resistant to drying and can survive for long periods in the environment.
Incidence	In Scotland, in 2007, there were three human cases, which is a large decrease on the 111 confirmations recorded in 2006 following a large outbreak at a slaughterhouse. In 2007, in Northern Ireland, there were five cases and 54 in England and Wales.

Ringworm

Causative agent	*Trichophyton* – various species of the fungus
Natural hosts	Humans, cattle, horses, pigs and sheep
Disease in humans	Causes inflamed, swollen, crusty skin lesions mainly on the hands, forearms, head and neck
Transmission	Direct skin contact with infected animal, spores entering through breaks in the skin
Incidence	Ringworm is likely to be one of the most common zoonotic infections; reliable data are not available on the number of cases in humans or occupational links.

(continued)

Table 14.4 (Continued)

Salmonellosis

Causative agent	Various species of the bacterium *Salmonella*
Natural hosts	Wild and domestic animals, birds (specially poultry), reptiles, amphibians and occasionally humans
Disease in humans	Diarrhoea, vomiting, fever
Transmission	Hand-to-mouth contact with faeces or contaminated objects
Incidence	A total of 13,213 cases of human *Salmonella* infections were reported in 2007 in the United Kingdom. There are no details of occupationally acquired infections.

Streptococcus

Causative agent	*Streptococcus suis*
Natural hosts	Pigs
Disease in humans	May be a severe and serious disease with meningitis and septicemia
Transmission	Breathing in infectious respiratory discharges, also direct contact (via broken skin) with contaminated meat
Incidence	The disease in humans continues to be rare with a total of 26 reports received in England and Wales between 1991 and 2007. In 2007, one case was reported in England and Wales and one case in Scotland. There were no cases in Northern Ireland.

6 When tuberculous lesions are detected at routine slaughter, the affected tissues should be handled carefully and responsibly. Suspect samples should be placed in self-seal plastic bags as soon as practicable and these should be handled as given in list point (3). Personal hygiene should include careful washing of hands/gloves with disinfectant soap. Knives should be washed and sterilised.

7 An adequate gap should be left in the line after the last reactor/inconclusive has been slaughtered in order to allow staff time to thoroughly wash themselves and their equipment.

Brucella abortus

General The risk assessment should take the following into consideration:

- The level of hazard presented by the particular animal or herd, for example, level of suspicion that brucellosis exists in the animal or herd.
- The work activity also needs to be considered, that is, how close to the animal will the officer need to be to carry out the task.
- The environment in which the work will be carried out, for example, outside or inside, in a large well ventilated building, in a small poorly ventilated building, etc. also needs to be assessed.

The level of hazard presented by individual animals, groups of animals or herds can be determined by epidemiological assessment. Animals/herds that represent the highest risk are classified as 'High-Risk' and other animals/herds where there is also an increased level of risk are classified as 'At-Risk'. Where there is any suspicion about the status of an animal, it should be assumed to be infected for the purposes of assessing any risk associated with its processing. Staff are considered to be at risk when working with brucellosis risk animals and their carcases. 'Working with' may be defined as follows:

- With regard to live animals, this includes sampling, examining, inspecting and valuing.
- With regard to carcasses, this includes sampling, examining and inspecting or any other activity which exposes an officer to an equivalent level of risk. In other words, instances where an officer is obliged to handle or inspect animal tissues.

Where an officer is within a building in which animals are accommodated but is not 'working with' them, the risk should be determined accordingly. This applies where brucellosis risk animals are penned away from the work area (i.e. crush) pending further handling. The control measures will not necessarily have to include the use of PPE (splash or respiratory protection) where other measures (separation, ventilation, etc.) are determined to be sufficient. As there is a potential for aerosol spread of the organism, precautions should be applied to all parts of any air space where staff are likely to encounter a contaminated aerosol. Where it can be demonstrated that factors such as distance and air movement provide an effective barrier to the spread of contamination, some areas may be deemed to be uncontaminated and an appropriate adjustment of the control measures may be employed. However, unless there are effective and demonstrable measures in place to limit the extent to which airborne contamination may spread, an airspace should be assumed to be contaminated throughout (Fig. 14.5).

Exposure to brucellosis presents an additional hazard to staff which may be controlled by the use of respiratory

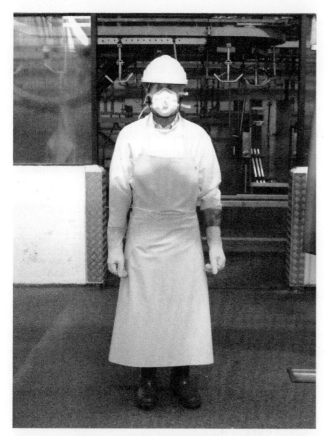

Figure 14.5 PPE for inspection of brucellosis reactors.

and/or splash protection as appropriate. Respiratory protection must be worn where there is a risk of brucella organisms being inhaled in water-based mists and aerosols. Respiratory protection[1] will be provided by the following:

- Disposable face mask to EN 149, FFP3 filter standard, OR
- Half mask reusable respirator fitted with a P3 filter OR
- Full face powered helmet respirator to EN146 THP2 standard with a P3 standard filter

Splash protection must be worn where there is a risk of body fluids or tissue etc., being splashed on the face, lips or eyes. Splash protection will be provided by the following:

- Full face visor, OR
- Goggles (indirect/non-vented) AND a face mask (disposable or half mask) OR
- Full face powered helmet respirator

The use of a face mask or respirator of the appropriate specification will also provide respiratory protection.

---

[1] Bearded staff must wear a full face powered helmet respirator to EN 146 THP2 standard with a P3 standard filter as a good seal will not be achieved by the other two protection methods noted.

Staff may choose to wear a face mask in combination with goggles to provide splash protection even though a risk assessment has determined that no respiratory protection is required.

- It is recognised that wearing a face mask may hinder communication. However, staff should manage the situation so that there is no need to remove the mask while work is being carried out, for example, the official veterinarian identifies/assesses reactor animal and leaves holding pen. Only then does he/she remove the mask and speak to others.
- Aprons, boots, etc. must be thoroughly washed and protective clothing changed once all potentially infected animals have been processed, and as necessary during their processing.
- Waterproof clothing, boots and eye protection must be suitably disinfected and thoroughly washed following work.
- Disposable PPE must be suitably disinfected prior to safe disposal.
- Any cuts/abrasions on those parts of the face not covered by goggles or any face mask/respirator worn must be covered with waterproof dressings.
- Double gloving should be used to reduce the likelihood of contamination of skin due to breakages in glove material. Gloves should be long enough to protect skin in the wrist and forearm region should the coat sleeve move up the arm.
- Where cotton coats are used, disposable plastic sleeves or disposable gloves reaching to the elbow must be worn to reduce the likelihood of seepage of material through the coat material onto skin or personal clothing.
- Contaminated cotton coats must be handled, transported and stored in an hygienic manner using appropriate bins, lockers or bags. They must be laundered using laundering services. Under no circumstances should coats used on high-risk premises be taken home for laundering.

Brucellosis H&S control measures in the lairage

- Staff taking blood samples should, if possible, sample animals from the jugular vein in the neck. Animals should be worked on singly, that is, do not work at the neck of an animal standing behind another infected/potentially infected animal. Where jugular sampling cannot be carried out safely, samples should be taken from the tail – ensuring that PPE used is adequate.
- An aborted foetus or foetal membranes should be removed from the lairage only after they have been soaked in disinfectant. They can then be disposed of to a rendering plant as high-risk material.

- Staff with beards must not test/carry out valuations on high-risk Brucellosis animals in indoor restraint facilities unless wearing suitable respiratory equipment.
- Brucellosis risk animals should, where possible, be held or penned in a separate part of the lairage at the earliest opportunity after their identification. This part must be thoroughly cleansed and disinfected as soon as possible after the animals have been slaughtered.

Brucellosis H&S control measures in the slaughter hall The following control measures should be considered as alternative methods of reducing the risk to staff, and they should be employed as an alternative to, or if necessary in addition to, the use of PPE:

- Use of off-line slaughter facilities where these exist, thereby minimising exposure of staff to carcase fluids normally released during processing.
- Slaughter brucellosis high-risk animals at the end of a kill, or at least at the end of a production section at a main work break, for example, just before lunch. Formal arrangements must be reached with the management of the establishment to facilitate this. This control measure is most likely to be effective in controlling an inhalation risk where the processing line is cleared at the work break and there is a low-pressure wash-down of the premises and equipment. The purpose of these procedures is to allow staff to discontinue the use of PPE (e.g. mask) worn during the previous work shift, on the assumption that any inhalation risk has been sufficiently reduced. Logically therefore, any control measure employed to control an inhalation risk during the affected work shift should continue until the break, even if this involves the processing of 'normal' animals until that time.
- Ideally the maximum number of brucellosis seropositive cattle slaughtered daily should be 20–25. It appears that below this number, the concentration of brucella organisms is low enough so that worker infection is less likely to occur.
- One carcase space should be left between each potentially infected animal at all points on the line where this is possible, since this appears to be effective in reducing aerosol concentration.
- To facilitate proper personal hygiene, an adequate gap should be left on the line after the last high-risk or at-risk animal in a batch is handled to allow operatives and inspectors time to wash themselves and their equipment.
- The udders of all reactor or in-contact cows should be removed intact with the teats uncut to avoid any leakage of udder contents. Staff should be aware of the danger of jets of milk from intact teats when cows are suspended for bleeding.
- The uterus must not, on any account, be opened. Unnecessary handling of, and contact with, the uterus or its contents, even for the purposes of inspection, should be avoided as the uterus is the predilection site for the organism.
- Where there is any suspicion about the status of an animal, it should be assumed to be infected for the purposes of assessing any risk associated with its processing.
- Note that retro-pharyngeal lymph nodes are a common site for infectivity.
- This information must be made available to meat plant personnel responsible for the implementation of control measures

Bovine spongiform encephalopathy (BSE)

Specified Risk Material (SRM) consists of the tissues and organs that are most likely to contain the BSE agent if animals are infected. Although there have been no confirmed cases of transmission of BSE to humans as a result of occupational exposure, there is a theoretical risk of this occurring. If BSE can be transmitted in the occupational setting, this would be most likely to occur via infected SRM in the following ways:

- Contaminating wounds and open lesions on the skin
- Contaminating an inoculation injury of intact skin (i.e. via new cuts from knives, sharp instruments or bone fragments)
- Contaminating pre-existing wounds
- Splashing into mucous membranes (eyes and mouth) or
- Being swallowed

BSE is unlikely to be transmitted by the inhalation of infectious airborne particles; however, it is recommended that appropriate precautions be taken as a safeguard where there is the likelihood of generating droplets and aerosols from infected tissue. Staff should adhere to safe working practices and avoid or minimise the use of tools and equipment or procedures likely to cause cuts, abrasions or puncture wounds and personal contamination. Where use of such equipment is unavoidable, suitable PPE should be worn to prevent cuts, puncture wounds and personal contamination. All new and existing cuts, abrasions and skin lesions should be covered with waterproof dressings and/or gloves before starting work. If cuts or puncture wounds occur while working, they should be washed thoroughly with soap and running water only. The wound should be encouraged to bleed and covered with a waterproof dressing when clean and dry. If contaminated material is splashed into the eyes or face, they should be washed with running water immediately. Hands and exposed skin (and arms and face if necessary) should be washed before eating, drinking, smoking, taking any medication, using the telephone, applying make-up, inserting contact lenses, going to the toilet, etc. Rest breaks and meals should be taken away from the main work area after removing any PPE in a separate area. Protective clothing should be disposable or, if this is not practical, must be washable and stored separately from personal clothing. This protective clothing must be cleaned before storage. The following PPE should be worn during all abattoir work:

- Overalls, protected by a waterproof apron or waterproof leggings.
- Chainmail aprons and/or leggings should be worn where a risk assessment shows that there is a risk of stabbing or cutting injuries.
- Impervious and washable boots.
- Impervious gloves that cover hands and arms if exposed.
- Protective clothing should be disposable or, if this is not practicable, must be washable and stored separately from personal clothing. This protective clothing must be cleaned before storage.
- Provision should be made for visors/face protection equipment (EN149 FPP3/BS EN 166:2002) (when a risk assessment shows the need for face protection to avoid risks from splashing).

Q Fever

Suitable PPE should always be worn when handling afterbirths or birth products. This will include a coverall, footwear such as wellington boots, gloves and respiratory protective equipment (EN 149–FFP3). Use face protection, such as a visor to specification BS EN 166:2002, for the eyes and mouth if there is a risk of splashing from urine or placental fluids. The meat inspection team manager should make sure the PPE is properly maintained, cleaned and decontaminated after use and stored in a clean area. There may be a requirement for screening of staff for pre-existing health conditions such as compromised immune system, valvular or vascular disease or for individuals who have had their spleen removed or are pregnant.

Zoonoses and pregnant women

Although the risk of developing an infection from zoonoses is no greater for a pregnant woman than for other workers, the outcome for the foetus can be severe. For example, enzootic abortion in sheep may result in abortion or stillbirth of the foetus in humans. If the pregnancy survives the infection, there appears to be no risk of long-term harm or birth defects. Listeria infection during pregnancy can cause abortion of the foetus, or premature birth. If the child is infected in the womb or during delivery, this may lead to septicaemia and meningitis, which has a high fatality rate. There can also be long-term effects in many organs, including the airways, eyes and nervous system. Q fever may lead to acute or chronic infection in the mother and rarely to an adverse effect on the foetus. Therefore, pregnant women should be excluded from work that exposes them to risk.

Enzootic abortion – pregnant women should be excluded from contact with sheep at lambing time and removed from sheep slaughter lines.
Brucella – pregnant women should be excluded from high-risk Brucella animal slaughter.
Salmonella – pregnant women should not visit poultry production establishments if salmonella is present/ suspected.
Listeria – pregnant women should avoid aborted foetuses, sick animals and untreated manure.
Q fever – pregnant women should be excluded from contact with sheep at lambing time and removed from sheep slaughter lines. They should also avoid birth products from cattle.

Non-zoonotic infections

While abattoir workers are no more at risk of developing tetanus than other occupations, nevertheless in an industry where livestock are handled and where wounds can occur, the possibility of tetanus exists.

Tetanus

Causative agent	*Clostridium tetani*
Natural hosts	Humans and animals but spores occur widely in the environment, for example, soil
Disease in humans	Exaggerated reflexes, muscle rigidity and uncontrolled muscle spasms – lockjaw
Transmission	Organism enters through a break in the skin
Incidence	In England, between 1989/90–1995/6, a total of 175 cases of tetanus were reported. The disease is becoming rarer.

Cleaning and disinfecting materials

Cleaning materials used in meat processing can be irritant or toxic. Occupational dermatitis can be caused by contact with some soaps/cleaners as well as flour and handling meat, fish, poultry and wet work. Dermatitis usually affects the hands and forearms resulting in redness, scaling and blistering of the skin. It affects an estimated 8500 people in the food and catering industries each year – about 10% of the total in all industries.

There should be a safety data sheet available for each substance which the meat processing operator should have used to complete a COSHH assessment. The meat inspection team manager should ensure that they have seen this assessment and instruct staff on any control measures to be followed.

Food

Spices and seasonings can be irritant or can cause allergies or be potential sensitisers resulting in occupational asthma. Rhinitis (runny or stuffy nose) is an inflammation of the nasal mucous membrane and can be caused by irritant dusts including spices and seasonings.

Meat tenderisers containing proteolytic enzymes are sensitisers. A sensitiser is defined as a substance that causes a substantial proportion of exposed people or animals to develop an allergic reaction in normal tissue after repeated exposure to the substance. These substances have no immediate health effects; however, if you are exposed to them frequently, they can make you allergic or sensitive to other substances, often quite suddenly. Typical reactions to sensitisers can include skin disorders such as eczema and respiratory disorders such as asthma.

Animals

All cattle are unpredictable and capable of injuring people. Extensive research shows that changes in cattle rearing methods, reduced human contact and the introduction of continental breeds have contributed to an increase in risk to personal safety when handling cattle at abattoirs (Turner, Lawrence and Lowman, 2008). These upstream factors are largely beyond the control of the operators of commercial abattoirs. The evidence clearly shows that when animals are handled in a way which suits their normal behavioural characteristics, their behaviours are more predictable and the handling process is made safer and more efficient. However, there always remains a risk when handling live cattle given that the animals can weigh several hundred kilos, move very quickly when startled, are essentially unpredictable, jump approximately 2 m almost from standing and may also have horns. Even cattle which do not deliberately intend to cause injury to a handler should be viewed as a potential threat. Around half of the fatalities that occur on farms result from either the handler slipping and accidentally being trodden by an animal or an animal accidentally slipping and crushing a handler. Ultimately, the risk of injury can only be prevented by separating cattle from people. The law requires that risks are assessed and reduced to a reasonable level where this is not achievable.

The official veterinarian should have a safe location from which to conduct the ante-mortem inspection. If the ante-mortem inspection requires that an animal be isolated or separated for further inspection or examination, there should be adequate segregation procedures which should be followed. The official veterinarian should also liaise with factory management to ensure that all reasonable steps have been taken to eliminate/minimise the risk of a live animal escaping into the slaughter hall. Staff must be aware of escape routes from slaughter hall and liaise with factory management to ensure that protocol for dealing with an escaped animal is adequate.

Noise

Hearing damage caused by exposure to noise at work is permanent and incurable. Exposure to noise can also cause tinnitus which may also occur in combination with hearing loss. Three percent of compensation cases under the government Industrial Injury Scheme were for hearing loss, which also results in about 75% of occupational health insurance claims. However, the risk of damage to hearing will be minimised if suitable controls are introduced.

In the United Kingdom, the Control of Noise at Work Regulations 2005, which build on the old regulations dating from 1990, are designed to reduce the risk of noise-induced hearing loss by lowering the current exposure thresholds and to encourage employers to reduce workers' noise exposure through risk management.

- There are two action levels for daily noise exposure: 85 and 80 dB, known as the upper exposure action value and the lower exposure action value, respectively.
- There are two action values for peak noise at 135 and 137 dB.
- There are exposure limit values (ELV) of 87 dB (daily exposure) and 140 dB (peak noise) which take into account the effect of wearing hearing protection and must not be exceeded.
- There is a specific requirement to provide health surveillance where there is a risk to health.

Generally, meat processing establishments are noisy environments. As a simple guide to identify if there is a likely problem, staff need to raise their voices to carry out a normal conversation when about 2 m apart. If it is noisy, a risk assessment is needed to determine the extent of the problem. It is important that the risk assessment is carried out by competent people. The risk assessment should be reviewed if there are changes in the workplace that affect noise. Even if it appears nothing has changed, the assessment should be repeated every couple of years.

For meat processing establishments, the control of noise is the responsibility of its management and they should identify hearing protection zones, that is, areas where the use of hearing protection is compulsory, and mark them with signs if possible. The meat inspection team manager should

- provide staff with hearing protectors if they ask for it when their noise exposure is between the lower and upper exposure action values;
- provide staff with hearing protectors and make sure they are used when their noise exposure exceeds the upper exposure action values;
- provide staff with training and information on how to use and care for the hearing protectors;
- ensure that the hearing protectors are properly used and maintained;
- arrange for health surveillance for those staff who are likely to be regularly exposed above the upper

exposure action values, or are at risk for any reason, for example, already suffer from hearing loss or are particularly sensitive to damage (Table 14.5).

Cold environment

Working in a cold environment can involve several adverse effects on human performance and health including thermal discomfort, increased strain, decreased performance and cold-related diseases and injuries. Cold can also interfere with several other factors in the workplace, modifying or aggravating the risk of common hazards and increasing the risk of cold associated injuries. In cold conditions, the body must both conserve and produce heat to maintain its core temperature near 37°C. The body regulates temperature through redistribution of blood flow or increase in metabolic rate. Redistribution of the blood flow from the skin to the central circulation is an effective means of keeping

Table 14.5 Assessing the risk from noise (Reproduced with permission from Tolley).

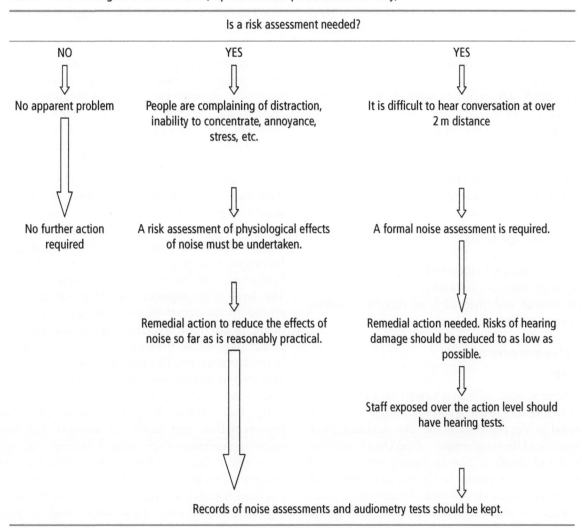

the body core warm and the skin surfaces cold. The danger associated with these actions is that the temperature in the extremities, such as the fingers and toes, may approach that of the environment with possible tissue damage. The head will stay warm even in cold temperatures, resulting in up to 25% of the total heat loss from the body which should be prevented with an insulating layer such as a hat. If the control of blood flow is insufficient to prevent heat loss, involuntary shivering will occur. Shivering usually starts in the neck, apparently to warm the critical blood flow to the brain. Voluntary activity will also increase the metabolic rate. If the blood flow and the metabolic rate cannot prevent serious heat loss, the body will suffer some effects of cold stress. The skin will be damaged first, while the body core is protected for as long as possible. As the skin temperature is lowered to 15–20°C, manual dexterity decreases. Tactile sensitivity is severely reduced as the skin temperature falls below 8°C. If the temperature approaches freezing, frostbite can occur. In the hands, joint temperature below 24°C and nerve temperature below 20°C severely reduce the ability to carry out motor tasks. Reduction of core temperature is more serious, and concentration is impaired at temperatures below 36°C and even simple activities become affected. At a core temperature around 32°C, the body can lose consciousness and heart failure may occur at about 26°C.

People suffering from certain medical conditions may be unsuited to work in cold stores. These include chronic respiratory disease, asthma, arthritis, cardiovascular disease and Raynaud's syndrome. Any staff with these medical problems should be excluded from cold store work.

According to the Cold Storage Association, the recommended protective clothing for temperatures below −5°C includes the following:

1 Thermal undergarments
2 Jacket and salopettes or all in one coverall
3 Cold store gloves with thermal liners
4 Safety boots with thermal socks
5 Safety helmet with thermal liner, thermal balaclava and thermal hood

General requirements

Accidents

All accidents at work, no matter how trivial and irrespective of whether they result in absence from work, should be entered in the Accident Book. The Accident Book takes account of the requirements of the Data Protection Act 1998 and details of how to comply are contained within the book. As entries in the Accident Book and accident forms can be 'discoverable documents' in court proceedings, for example, where an injured employee

brings a claim, it is therefore most important that they are completed fully and accurately.

Employers generally require that any accident resulting in absence from work should be reported by the line manager. In addition, in the United Kingdom, the Reporting of Injuries, Diseases and Dangerous Occurrences Regulations 1995 (RIDDOR) requires certain injuries, diseases and reportable dangerous occurrences to be reported to the HSE using the appropriate forms. The RIDDOR Regulations require that the HSE is notified without delay by telephone if a there is a death or major injury as a result of a work accident. The official forms must follow this up within 10 days. In the case of all other reportable accidents, the official forms should be sent to the HSE within 10 days.

It is also the responsibility of line management to scrutinise medical reports and certificates from general practitioners (GPs) and take the necessary action to notify the HSE when a reportable disease is diagnosed. GPs will use the common description of each reportable disease in the medical certificates that they provide to employees to submit.

Accidents, cases of ill health, dangerous occurrences, near misses and property damage within the workplace can have a high human and financial cost. It is vital therefore that appropriate arrangements are put in place to investigate all incidents. The main aim of investigation is to pinpoint the causes of incidents and take prompt and effective action to prevent recurrence. Incidents need to be examined in sufficient depth so that immediate causes and the underlying failures of systems for managing health and safety are identified.

The significance of the incident will determine the type and depth of the investigation. Consideration should be given not only to the actual consequences of the incident under investigation but also to the potential for more serious outcomes. Normally, line managers will investigate with help as required from the appropriate health and safety adviser and other specialist personnel. The level of management involved will generally be related to the actual or potential significance of the injury, ill health or loss. The more serious the event or greater its potential, the greater is the effort to be applied to the investigation. The risk assessment should also be amended to include any changes in procedures identified through the accident investigation.

In the United Kingdom, under the 'Safety Representatives and Safety Committees Regulations', safety representatives are entitled to carry out inspections where there has been a reportable accident or dangerous occurrence or where a reportable disease has been contracted. Management may be present during these inspections. Management needs to provide reasonable facilities for independent investigation by safety representatives and private discussions with the staff they represent.

First aid

The Health and Safety (First-Aid) Regulations 1981 apply to all workplaces and require employers to provide adequate and appropriate equipment, facilities and personnel to enable first aid to be given to employees if they are injured or become ill at work. What is adequate will depend on the circumstances in the workplace. This includes whether trained first-aiders are needed, what should be included in a first-aid box and if a first-aid room is needed. Employers should carry out an assessment of first aid needs to determine this (Table 14.6).

First-aid container contents

There is no mandatory list of items that should be included in a first-aid container. As a guide, where no special risk arises in the workplace, a minimum stock of first-aid items would normally be the following:

- A leaflet giving general guidance on first aid (e.g. the HSE leaflet 'Basic Advice on First-aid at Work')
- 20 individually wrapped sterile adhesive dressings (assorted sizes), appropriate to the type of work (dressings may be of a detectable type for food handlers)
- Two sterile eye pads
- Four individually wrapped triangular bandages (preferably sterile)
- Six safety pins
- Six medium-sized individually wrapped sterile unmedicated wound dressings – approximately 12 × 12 cm
- Two large sterile individually wrapped unmedicated wound dressings – approximately 18 × 18 cm
- One pair of disposable gloves

Personal first-aid kits for travelling workers would typically contain the following:

- A leaflet giving general guidance on first aid (e.g. the HSE leaflet 'Basic Advice on First-aid at Work')
- Six individually wrapped sterile adhesive dressings
- One large sterile unmedicated dressing – approximately 18 × 18 cm
- Two triangular bandages
- Two safety pins
- Individually wrapped moist cleansing wipes
- One pair of disposable gloves

These are suggested contents lists only; equivalent but different items will be considered acceptable. The contents of first-aid containers should be examined frequently and should be restocked as soon as possible after use. Sufficient supplies should be held in a backup stock on-site. Care should be taken to discard items safely after the expiry date has passed.

The meat inspection team manager should

- appoint, train and maintain training of first-aider(s) at major sites;
- ensure all staff are aware of who first-aiders are and where to find them;
- instruct all staff to seek first aid for all injuries no matter how minor.

Emergency procedures

In the United Kingdom, the Fire & Rescue Services attend more than 30 000 fires in the workplace each year. Lives are lost, thousands are injured and the economic costs mean many businesses never re-open. The Regulatory Reform (Fire Safety) Order 2005 replaces previous fire safety such as the Fire Precautions Act and requires any person who exercises some level of control in premises to take reasonable steps to reduce the risk from fire and ensure occupants can safely escape if a fire does occur. The responsible person is required to

- carry out or nominate someone to carry out a fire risk assessment identifying the risks and hazards;
- consider who may be especially at risk;
- eliminate or reduce the risk from fire as far as is reasonably practical and provide general fire precautions to deal with any residual risk;
- take additional measures to ensure fire safety where flammable or explosive materials are used or stored;
- create a plan to deal with any emergency and, in most cases, document your findings;
- review the findings as necessary.

The meat inspection team manager should ensure staff cooperate with any fire requirements and are aware of the evacuation procedures for the premises.

Other emergencies that could occur include the release of ammonia or the escape of an animal prior to slaughter.

Ammonia is a colourless gas with a strong, irritating smell and may severely burn the skin and eyes upon contact. It is widely used as a refrigerant in meatpacking, poultry and other food processing plants. Ammonia leaks in the refrigeration pipes can endanger all workers in the plant; therefore, it is important that control procedures are in place. Workers exposed to very serious leaks may develop pulmonary edema, a build-up of fluid in the lungs caused by the damaging effect of the gas. Workers may suffer permanent lung and eye problems as a result of exposure to high levels of ammonia.

As previously stated, there should also be a procedure in place to ensure the safety of staff in the premises if an animal escapes from the lairage or the stun box. These procedures should be included in the risk assessment and communicated to staff.

Training

The UK Health and Safety at Work Act requires the provision of information, instruction, training and supervision as is necessary to ensure, so far as is reasonably practicable, the health and safety at work of employees. This is expanded by the Management of Health and Safety at Work Regulations, which identify situations where health and safety training is particularly important, for example, when people start work, on exposure to new or increased risks and where existing skills may have become rusty or need updating. Training must be provided during working hours and free to your employees. Special arrangements may be needed for part-timers or shift workers. The risk assessments will identify training needs and if information needs to be provided. Training can be provided through a combination of internal and external courses. The Health and Safety (Training for Employment) Regulations 1990 ensure that learners doing work experience are covered by health and safety law. There are a number of other regulations which include specific health and safety training requirements, for example, first aid.

Table 14.6 Assessment of first-aid needs checklist

The minimum first-aid provision for each workplace is as follows
- A suitably stocked first-aid container
- A person appointed to take charge of first-aid arrangements
- Information for employees on first-aid arrangements
This checklist will help you assess whether you need to make any additional provision.

Aspects to consider	Impact on first-aid provision
1. What are the risks of injury and ill health arising from the work as identified in your risk assessment?	If the risks are significant, you may need first-aiders.
2. Are there any specific risks, for example, working with • hazardous substances • dangerous tools • dangerous machinery • dangerous loads or animals?	You will need to consider • specific training for first-aiders • extra first-aid equipment • precise siting of first-aid equipment • informing emergency services • first-aid room
3. Are there parts of your premises where different levels of risk can be identified?	You will probably need to make different levels of provision in different parts of the premises.
4. Are large numbers of people employed on-site?	You may need first-aiders to deal with the higher probability of an accident.
5. What is your record of accidents and cases of ill health? What type are they and how did they happen?	You may need to • locate your provision in certain area • review the contents of the first-aid box
6. Are there inexperienced workers on-site, or employees with disabilities or special health problems?	You will need to consider • special equipment • local siting of equipment
7. Are the premises spread out, for example, are there several buildings on the site or multi-floor buildings?	You will need to consider provision in each building or on several floors.
8. Is there shift work or out-of- hours working?	Remember that there needs to be first-aid provision at all times people are at work.
9. Is your workplace remote from emergency medical services?	You will need to • inform local medical services of your location • consider special arrangements with the emergency services
10. Do you have employers who travel a lot or work alone?	You will need to consider issuing personal first-aid kits and training staff in their use.
11. Do any of your employees work at sites occupied by other employers?	You will need to make arrangements with the other site occupiers.
12. Do you have any work experience trainees?	Remember that your first-aid provision must cover them.
13. Do members of the public visit your premises?	You have no legal responsibilities for non-employees, but HSENI strongly recommends you include them in your first-aid provision.

Do not forget that first-aiders and appointed persons take leave and are often absent from the premises for other reasons. There must be sufficient people appointed to cover these absences to enable first-aid personnel to be available at all times people are at work.

(continued)

Table 14.6 (Continued)

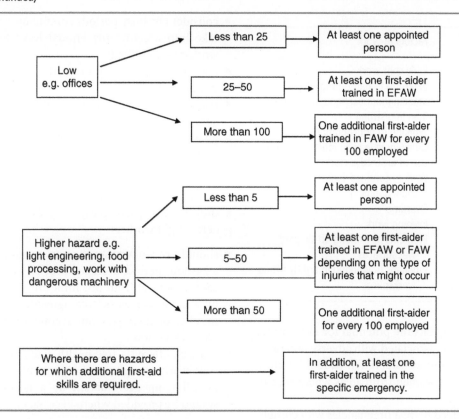

New and expectant mothers at work

Under the Management of Health and Safety at Work Regulations, employers are required to assess risks to all their employees. An amendment specifically highlighted assessment of risks at work to new and expectant mothers and the unborn child or the child of a woman who is breastfeeding. The term 'new or expectant mother' means a worker who is pregnant, who has given birth in the previous 6 months or who is breastfeeding.

The hazards that line management need to consider are physical, biological and chemical agents and working conditions. Examples are as follows:

Physical agents	Manual handling where there is a risk of injury
	Noise
	Ionising radiation
	Non-ionising electromagnetic radiation
	Extremes of heat or cold
	Movements or postures, travelling, mental and physical fatigue and other physical burdens
Biological agents	Zoonoses
Chemical agents	Carbon monoxide
	Lead

Working conditions – There are other aspects of pregnancy that may affect ability to undertake work, and management should take these matters into account in allocating duties. The impact of these will vary during the course of the pregnancy (Table 14.7).

Dexterity, agility, coordination, speed of movement and/or reach may all be impaired because of increasing size. If a risk assessment of work reveals a risk to new and expectant mothers, all the female employees who could be exposed to the risk should be informed and also given details of the control measures that are available. Many of these hazards are already covered by the specific Health and Safety Regulations, for example, COSHH. A significant risk from a chemical, which is covered by COSHH, will normally be controlled adequately if the employer is complying with the requirements of COSHH. If a significant risk cannot be avoided by normal control measures, an employer must temporarily adjust her working conditions and/or hours of work. If it is not reasonably practicable to do so, or would not avoid the risk, suitable alternative work should be sought.

Amniotic fluid is designed to cushion the foetus; however, if trauma is excessive, there is potential for damage to the foetus and for foetal death. Clearly, good advice to pregnant women would be to avoid situations where there is the potential for direct abdominal trauma. The controls necessary are for pregnant women to avoid situations where they may be in direct contact with cattle or

Table 14.7 Aspects of pregnancy to be considered by management

Aspects of pregnancy	Factors at work
Morning sickness	Early shift work
	Exposure to nauseating smells
Backache	Standing/manual handling/posture
Varicose veins	Standing/sitting
Haemorrhoids	Working in hot conditions
Frequent visits to toilet	Difficulty in leaving job/site of work
Increasing size	Use of protective clothing
	Work in confined spaces
	Manual handling
Tiredness	Overtime
	Evening work
Balance	Problems of working on slippery, wet surfaces
Comfort	Problems of working in tightly fitting workspaces

horses. Literature suggests the potential for even minor maternal trauma to be associated with adverse outcomes to the foetus. Therefore, consideration should be given to removing pregnant women from areas where slips or falls occur regularly.

There may be a need to treat pregnancies with complications differently.

Working time regulations

The basic rights and protections that the Regulations provide are as follows:

- A limit of an average of 48 hours a week which a worker can be required to work (though workers can choose to work more if they want to)
- A limit of an average of 8 hours work in 24 which night workers can be required to work
- A right for night workers to receive free health assessments
- A right to 11 hours rest a day
- A right to a day off each week
- A right to an in-work rest break if the working day is longer than 6 hours
- A right to 4 weeks paid leave per year

The meat inspection team manager should ensure compliance with working time regulations and manage working hours as required. Managing workers' hours means planning to ensure the following:

- No worker aged 18 or over works more than 48 hours in an average working week, and no young worker works more than 40 hours a week.
- All workers receive rest periods between working days to which they are entitled.

It is also good practice to

- consider any busy periods coming up;
- take into account any annual leave to which your workers are entitled;
- take into account any maternity, paternity, adoption or parental leave;
- consult with workers about what hours they find most suitable;
- give reasonable notice of any changes to working hours;
- consider flexible working.

It is especially important you plan ahead if operating a shift system, particularly in a 24-hour business. In general, night workers:

- should not work more than an average of 8 hours in a 24-hour period, averaged over 17 weeks;
- cannot opt out from this limit unless it is allowed for by a collective workforce agreement, although in a number of cases you can average night work over a 26-week period;
- must be offered a free health assessment before they start working nights and on a regular basis after that (a follow-up examination by a health professional should be provided where necessary).

In general, workers under 18 are not permitted to work at night. The meat inspection team manager should keep records to ensure workers do not exceed their night working limit, retain records of night workers' health assessments for 2 years or, if they did not accept the offer of a free health assessment, record when the offer was made.

References

Anderssen, G.B.J. (1997) in *The Adult Spine: Principles and Practice* (ed J.W. Frymoyer), Lippincott-Raven, Philadelphia, pp. 93–141.

Bernard, B.P. (eds) (1997) *Musculoskeletal disorders and workplace factors. A critical review of epidemiological evidence for work-related musculoskeletal disorders of the neck, upper extremity and low back*. National Institute for Occupational Safety and Health (NIOSH) Cincinnati. www.cdc.gov/niosh/docs/97-141/pdfs/97-141.pdf (accessed 17 April 2014).

Bongers, P.M., Ljmker, S., van den Heuvel, S. and Blatter, B.M. (2006) Journal of Occupational Rehabilitation, 16, 279–302.

British Meat Processors Association (2009) Health and Safety Guidance Notes for the Meat Industry, http://www.bmpa.uk.com/_Attachments/Resources/971_S4.pdf (accessed 17 April 2014).

Buchbinder, R. (2001) British Medical Journal, 322(7301), 1516–1520.

Burton, A.K., Balagué, F., Eriksen, H.R. *et al.* (2006) European Spine Journal, 15 (Suppl 1), S136–S168.

Burton, A.K., Kendall, N.A.S., Pearce, B.G., *et al.* (2008) Management of Upper Limb Disorders and the Biopsychosocial Model. Health and Safety Executive Research Report 596, HSE Books, London.

Burton, A.K., Tillotson, K.M., Main, C.J. and Hollis, S. (1995) Spine, 20, 722–728.

Cai, C., Perry, M.J., Sorock, G.S. *et al.* (2005) American Journal of Industrial Medicine, 47(5), 403–410.

Caple, D.C. (1992) Musculoskeletal injury prevention – meat industry prevention study. Unlocking the Potential for Future Productivity and Quality of Life: Proceedings of the Ergonomics Society of Australia (ESA) Conference, Melbourne.

Coggon, D., Palmer, K.T. and Walker-Bone, K. (2007) Rheumatology, 39, 1057–1059.

Dababneh, A.J., Swanson, N. and Shell, R.L. (2001) Ergonomics, 44(2), 164–174.

Department of Food, Farming and Rural Affairs (DEFRA) (2007) Zoonoses Report UK, http://www.defra.gov.uk/foodfarm/farmanimal/diseases/atoz/zoonoses/documents/reports/zoonoses2007.pdf

European Agency for Safety and Health at Work (2000) Work-Related Musculoskeletal Disorders in Europe. Factsheet Issue 3, Bilbao, http://osha.europa.eu/publications/factsheets/3/facts3_en.pdf/at_download/file (accessed 17 April 2014).

European Foundation for the Improvement of Living and Working Conditions (2007) Managing Musculoskeletal Disorders, http://www.eurofound.europa.eu/ewco/studies/tn0611018s/ (accessed 17 April 2014).

Hansen, l., Winkel, J. and Jorgensen, K. (1998) Applied Ergonomics, 29(3), 217–224.

Hawkins, L. (2002) *Tolley's Guide to Managing Employee Health*, Reed Elsevier (UK) Ltd, London.

Horowitz, R. (2008) Labor Studies in Working Class History of the Americas, 5(2), 13–25.

HSE (2007) Food Manufacture – Slaughtering Meat, Poultry and Fish Processing, http://www.hse.gov.uk/food/slaughter.htm (accessed 17 April 2014).

HSE (2008) Musculoskeletal Disorders (MSDs) in Great Britain, http://www.hse.gov.uk/statistics/causdis/musculoskeletal/index.htm (accessed 17 April 2014).

HSE (2009) Health and Safety Made Simple, http://www.hse.gov.uk/business/must-do.htm (accessed 17 April 2014).

Lee, R. (2008) Understanding musculoskeletal disorders in staff employed in meat inspection in Northern Ireland. MSc Thesis. University of Derby.

Lipscomb, H.J., Epling, C.A., Pompeii, L.A. and Dement, J.M. (2007) American Journal of Industrial Medicine, 50(5), 327–338.

Magnusson, M., Ortengen, R., Anderson, G.B.J. *et al.* (1987) Applied Ergonomics, 18(1), 43–50.

Marsot, J., Claudon, L. and Jacqmin, M. (2007) Applied Ergonomics, 38(1), 83–89.

McGorry, R.W., Dowd, P.C. and Dempsey, P.G. (2005) Applied Ergonomics, 36, 71–77.

Melchoir, M., Roquelaure, Y., Evanoff, B. *et al.* (2006) Occupational Medicine, 63, 754–761.

National Institute for Occupational Health and Safety (NIOSH) (1997) *Musculoskeletal Disorders and Workplace Factors: A Critical Review of Epidemiological Evidence for Work-related Musculoskeletal Disorders of the Neck, Upper Extremity and Low Back*, US, Department of Health and Human Sciences/NIOSH, Cincinnati.

Ngomo, S., Messing, K., Perrault, H. and Comtois, A. (2008) Applied Ergonomics, 39, 729–736.

NZ OSHS (1997) *Muscle Minding: A Guide for the Prevention of OOS in the Meat, Poultry and Fish Processing Industries*, Occupational Safety and Health Service, Department of Labour, Wellington.

Office for National Statistics (2005) Chronic sickness rate per 1000 reporting longstanding condition by group, by sex. General Household Survey 2003, www.statistics.gov.uk/statbase/Expodata/spreadsheets/D8791.xls (accessed 17 April 2014).

Orlando, A.R. and King, P.M. (2004) Journal of Occupational Rehabilitation, 14(1), 63–75.

Piedrahita, H., Punnett, L. and Shahnavaz, H. (2004) International Journal of Industrial Ergonomics, 34, 271–278.

Pincus, T., Burton, A.K., Vogel, S. and Field, A.P. (2002) Spine, 27(5), 109–120.

Riley, D. and Milnes, E. (2000) Reducing the risk of musculoskeletal disorders in meat boning work. ERG/00/22 Health and Safety Laboratory.

Sobel, E., Levitz, S.J., Caselli, M.A., Christos, P.J. and Rosenblum, J. (2007) Journal of American Podiatric Medical Association, 91(10), 515–520.

Sprigg, C.A., Stride, C.B., Wall, T.D. *et al.* (2007) Journal of Applied Psychology, 92, 1456–1466.

Tappin, D., Moore, D., Ashby, L. *et al.* (2006) Centre for Human Factors and Ergonomics Report, 7(1).

Tomei, F., Baccolo, T.P., Palmi, S. and Rosti, M.V. (1999) American Journal of Industrial Medicine, 36, 653–665.

Toulouse, G. and Richard, J.-G. (2001) in *International Encyclopaedia of Ergonomics and Human Factors, Volume III* (ed W. Karwowski), Taylor & Francis, London, pp. 1578–1590.

Turner, S., Lawrence, A.B. and Lowman, B. (2008) Handling beef cattle: Identifying research needs and knowledge transfer opportunities to improve human safety and animal welfare. Scottish Agricultural College, http://www.sruc.ac.uk/mainrep/pdfs/cattlehandlingreport.pdf

van Dieen, J.H. and Oude Vrielink, H.H.E. (1998) Ergonomics, 41(12), 1832–1844.

Waddell, G. (1991) *A New Health Care Delivery System for Low Back Pain and Disability*, Medical Research Council.

Waddell, G. and Burton, A.K. (2000) *Occupational Health Guidelines for the Management of Low Back Pain at Work – Evidence Review*, Faculty of Occupational Medicine, London.

Walker, B.F. (2000) Journal of Spinal Disorders, 20(13), 205–217.

Woods, V. and Buckle, P. (2002) Work, Inequality and Musculoskeletal Health. Contract Research Report 421, HSE, London.

Woolf, A.D. and Akesson, K. (2001) British Medical Journal, 322, 1079–1080.

Woolf, A.D. and Pfleger, B. (2003) Bulletin of the World Health Organisation, 81(9), 646–656.

Yassi, A., Sprout, J. and Tate, A. (1996) American Journal of Industrial Medicine, 30, 461–472.

Index

abattoirs
  in UK 4
  small units 51
abomasum 22
abscesses 117, 204
Accident Books 312
accidents 312–13
Achromobacter 272
acidity 167
  see also acids
acids 95
  see also acidity
Acinetobacter 70, 72, 272
Actinomyces pyogenes 204
activated sludge process 64–5
adenosine triphosphate (ATP) 73, 78, 109, 130–1
adhesives 91
adrenal bodies 36–7
adrenal cortex 212
adrenal glands 36–7
adrenaline 130
adrenocorticotrophic hormone (ACTH) 130, 153
aerobic digestion 64
aerosols 105
aflatoxin 259
age
  determination of 20–1, 37–9
  of cattle 37
ageing
  and cancer 212
  of meat 86
air 105–6
  circulation rates 74
alarm reaction 130
alert notifications 286
algae 91
alkalis 95
alkylphenol ethoxylates (APEOs) 111
Alternaria 72
alternating current (AC) 144
aluminium 91
ammonia 63, 72, 73, 313
anaerobic digestion 64
anaerobic glycolysis 130
anatomy 19–43
Angus 4
animal by-products 178–83

category 1 178–9
category 2 179–80
category 3 180–1
  hygiene requirements 183
animal diets 2
Animal Feed (England) Regulations 2010 225
animal health 189
animal housing 119
animal medicines 117
Animal Transport Certificate 124
animal waste 117–18
animal welfare 118–19
animal welfare officers (AWO) 136
animal-based proteins 42
ante-mortem inspection 188–92, 199
anterior mediastinal nodes 31
anterior nodes 33
anterior vena cava 152
anthelmintics 117
anthrax bacilli 78
antimicrobials 173
antioxidants 86
aphagia 213, 214
appropriate level of protection (ALOP) 192
apron washes 161, 167
Arcanobacterium 272
Arcanobacterium pyogenes 207
argon 142, 149
arsenic 187
arthritis 186, 205
arthrology 19–21
Ascaris suum 57, 215
ascites 245–6
ASPCA pens 154, 155
Aspergillus 57, 72
automatic lairage system 53
automatic pelt removal 57
avian epidemic tremor 15
axillary nodes 31

Bacillus 72, 272
Bacillus cereus 267
Bacillus circulans 84
Bacillus coagulans 84
Bacillus piliformis 251
Bacillus stearothermophilus 84
backup stunner 144

bacon
  dry-cured 71
  production 69–71
bacon fat 274
bacteria
  and canned food 81–3
  and modified atmosphere packaging 76
  and refrigeration 72
  effect of freezing 78
  non-sporing 82–3
  pathogenic 63, 78
  sticking 160
bactericidal soap 164
bacteriological standards 270–1
bacteriological tests 277–8
bacteriophages 174
balancing tanks 64
Balantidium coli 57
barking 247
barley beef system 6
bedding 115
Beef Bung Bagging Machine 171
beef
  freezing 75
  global production 3
  production systems 6–7
Beta-agonists 280
beta-endorphin 129
bilateral severance 152
bile acids 210
bile pigments 209
bilirubin 131, 209, 210
biliverdin 209
biochemical oxygen demand (BOD) 63, 64, 110, 111
biocidal active components 95–7
biocides 280
biofilms 95
biological oxygen demand (BOD) 107, 182
biological treatment systems 64
bioluminescence 109, 221
biosecurity 15, 242
birds
  pest control 51
bison 2, 5
black pith 209
black spot 276–7

Gracey's Meat Hygiene, Eleventh Edition. Edited by David S. Collins and Robert J. Huey.
© 2015 John Wiley & Sons, Ltd. Published 2015 by John Wiley & Sons, Ltd.